Integrated Evaluation of Disability

Integrated Evaluation of Disability

Ramar Sabapathi Vinayagam

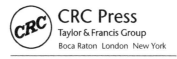

CRC Press
Taylor & Francis Group
Boca Raton London New York

CRC Press is an imprint of the
Taylor & Francis Group, an **informa** business

CRC Press
Taylor & Francis Group
6000 Broken Sound Parkway NW, Suite 300
Boca Raton, FL 33487-2742

First issued in paperback 2020

© 2019 by Taylor & Francis Group, LLC
CRC Press is an imprint of Taylor & Francis Group, an Informa business

No claim to original U.S. Government works

ISBN-13: 978-1-138-50190-4 (hbk)
ISBN-13: 978-0-367-65685-0 (pbk)

Library of Congress Cataloging-in-Publication Data

Names: Vinayagam, Ramar Sabapathi, author.
Title: Integrated evaluation of disability / Ramar Sabapathi Vinayagam.
Description: Boca Raton, FL : CRC Press, [2019] | Includes bibliographical
references and index.
Identifiers: LCCN 2018023696 | ISBN 9781138501904 (hbk. : alk. paper) | ISBN
9781351165440 (ebook)
Subjects: | MESH: Disability Evaluation | Rehabilitation--methods | Patient
Care Planning | Holistic Health
Classification: LCC RC71.3 | NLM WB 320 | DDC 616.07/5--dc23
LC record available at https://lccn.loc.gov/2018023696

Visit the Taylor & Francis Web site at
http://www.taylorandfrancis.com

and the CRC Press Web site at
http://www.crcpress.com

Dedication

My wife
Sulochana Ramar

My children
Pazhani Hariram Jothi and Maheswari Ramar
Nagarajan Ganapathy and Nalini Ramar
Mahendran Natchadalingam and Balaabhirami Ramar

Grandchildren
Kishore Nagarajan
Anjana Jothi
Manojavan Nagarajan
Sriram Jothi
Vinay Navaneethan Mahendran

Contents

Forewords

Abdulla Ahmed Eyadeh
Department of Physical Medicine and Rehabilitation
Physical Medicine and Rehabilitation Hospital
Ministry of Health
Kuwait
ISPRM (Africa and Middle East)

It is with an immense sense of appreciation and great pleasure that I write a foreword to the book on *Integrated Evaluation of Disability* by S. Ramar. To compile a book on any subject needs a lot of dedication, effort, and perseverance in addition to an in-depth knowledge of the subject. To write a book on such a difficult and diverse problem as disability takes this effort to a very high and different dimension altogether.

I consider myself very fortunate to closely witness the shaping of this book from its conception. In 2001, I had a chance to visit the Government Institute of Rehabilitation Medicine at Madras Medical College in Chennai, India to learn about their facilities and the nature of their ongoing work. During that visit, I felt elated to meet S. Ramar and understand his profound knowledge and experience in pain management including interventional pain management (IPM) for peripheral joints, electromyography (EMG) studies, and disability evaluation. It did not take too long for me to realize that Physical Medicine and Rehabilitation (PMR) Hospital, Ministry of Health, Kuwait could utilize his services. I persuaded the Ministry of Health to invite him as a consultant and to work for us, and, to this day, I am more than delighted that I made the right decision.

In 2002, he started his services in the PMR Hospital, Ministry of Health, State of Kuwait. He established an interventional pain management clinic and elevated the EMG services. He was instrumental in setting up the protocols and procedures for accreditation and constituting the operational policies. These value-added establishments and procedures paved the way for the Higher Council for Accreditation of Ministry of Health to recognize and place the PMR Hospital with full credit.

During this time, I observed his keen interest in the concept of *Integrated Evaluation of Disability*. My effort to uplift this project by negotiating with the Ministry of Health in collaboration with the World Health Organization (WHO) Project on the International Classification of Functioning, Disability and Health (ICF) was not fruitful due to some constraints. So, I continued encouraging him to pursue his ideas on *Integrated Evaluation of Disability* on his own.

In the meantime, when he became the chairman of the PMR department, the day-to-day operations demanded most of his time, sidelining his focus on this project. However, I am glad that he kept the fire alive to return with a bang with this book.

Having retired from his services from the PMR Hospital, Kuwait, he continued to work on this project with unparalleled dedication and resilience. He was relentless during this work and came out victorious.

Disability is a very complex subject, and formulating a comprehensive method to quantify disability has been a challenge. Physicians have been eagerly seeking a unified method of disability evaluation for many years. This is because disability can affect multiple systems. The same amount of functional loss assumes different dimensions of activity restrictions depending on the individual, the country, social situation, economic situation, and the context and purpose of assessment. Global deliberations on this subject are ongoing in this field.

Over the years, world bodies and governments have been striving to formulate regulations aimed at according equal opportunities to the less-abled persons in society by providing ease of access, certain rights, and privileges. This requires a valid method and a common language in quantifying and qualifying disability, understood by all health providers and officials worldwide. The definition of impairment, disability, and handicap put forth by WHO (1980) and later revised as impairment, limitation of activity, and restriction of participation (WHO—ICF 2001) demonstrates thinking in this direction.

As a person with a keen interest in the field of disability evaluation and quantification, S. Ramar has ventured into this difficult subject, putting forth this unique method of addressing the ICF—impairment of structures/functions, activity limitation, participation restriction, and environmental factors. He has also addressed areas like assistive devices, technology, and the availability of social, familial, and governmental support; thereby covering many ICF factors, which can affect the life of a person with altered ability positively or negatively. This book has adopted a novel approach to assigning an impairment score based on the homunculus representation of motor and sensory in the brain. Besides infusing the principles of the homunculus, he has taken on a great task of performing a "Modified Delphi Process" by obtaining opinions from senior experts in order to assign an optimum value of the percentage of disability. He has described the formula for combining multiple impairments and a method for combining with that of activity limitation and participation restriction to arrive at whole person disability limiting to 100%. The uniqueness of this book is its objective evaluation without any element of intuitive value.

I am sure this concept put forth by S. Ramar deserves the attention and deliberations by experts in the field of disability evaluation. His exhaustive work can serve as a reference for physicians practicing disability evaluation. Further, it will enlighten the novice about the concept of disability evaluation. The software integrated with this book on the Companion Website can solve complex computational tasks.

I wish S. Ramar all the very best.

Mayilvahanan Natarajan

Institute of Orthopaedics and Traumatology
Government General Hospital, and Madras Medical College
The Tamil Nadu Dr. MGR Medical University
Chennai, India

"My disability has opened my eyes to see my true abilities."

Robert M. Hensel, *born with Spina bifida; Guinness World Records holder*

Disability affects millions of people and their families in our country. Around 10% of the world's population live with a disability. True to the word of Mr. Robert M. Hensel identifying true ability in disability is essential in Rehabilitation. Assessment of the disability is a challenge to the medical fraternity and particularly to Physical Medicine and Rehabilitation specialists who primarily identify the inner abilities of the differently abled persons to enable them to reach their potential.

It gives me immense pleasure that Prof. S. Ramar has faced this challenge and dealt with it effectively in this book about disability evaluation. He is one of those who has strong conviction and depth of knowledge in executing any of his endeavors. I am privileged to write this foreword to this perfect manuscript. This book once again reveals his strong character and is an accomplishment of his commitment to work.

This book consists of 23 chapters, and each one of them reveals the author's hard work in compiling the data and analysis. This book includes extensive inputs from WHO ICF 2001 and the National Institute of Disability and Rehabilitation Research, which states *disability does not mean that a person is ill*—valid information even too many medical professionals.

The gradual evolution of disability evaluation to a biopsychosocial model—International Classification of Functioning, Disability, and Health of WHO-ICF—deserves special mention here. The author proposes a new novel method of *Integrated Evaluation of Disability* combining impairments, limitations, and environmental factors. As the author proposes, I believe this will only reveal the true status of disability. The author analyzes the requirement of an "Activity Participation Skill Assessment Scale," "Environmental Factors Measurement Scale," and "Personal Factors Measuring Scale," and grades the severity of the disability to quantify the limitation of activity, participation restriction, and environmental factors, and hence developed the said-scales.

He has used a unique modification of the Delphi Process to fine-tune the clinical evaluation. The integrated approach conceptualized by the author meets the long-pending need for sewing together the biological deficit and socio-environmental context. Thoughtful and non-intrusive care by the social system can mitigate much of the agony of the disabled.

The concept of assigning the percentage of impairment based on the representation of various parts of the body in the motor and somatosensory homunculus is a novel, scientific, evidence-based idea that needs special mention.

The author's *Whole Person Impairment (WPI)* is an innovative approach to calculating the impairment. In practice, the concept of impairment confines itself mostly into quantifying locomotor disabilities. The author takes a departure in planning to measure disability experienced because of dysfunctions in other systems too. In patients with multi-system disturbances, the disabilities may be overlapping, summating, or even more than summating. Dr. Ramar has consulted experts in the respective domains and carefully studied impairment due to cardiovascular, respiratory, hematological, immunological, gastrointestinal, metabolic, genitourinary, special sensory, and dermatological disturbances, in addition to those due to neurological, musculoskeletal, and congenital problems. Thus, the idea of also calculating WPI for the systemic organ disorders such as liver, kidney, hematological disorder, so on, and their sequel, will widen the scope of disability to newer disease conditions.

As the disability frequently spans more than one dimension, Dr. Ramar has taken care to furnish a method to combine them and provide an algorithm to formulate the combined disability. The exhaustive and integrative approach might frighten a busy practitioner concerned about the constraints of time. Being a busy practitioner himself for more than four decades, the author answers with a "Ready Reckoner Impairment Table" in Chapter 23 after working out 300 common situations. The software integrated on the Companion Website will make it even more comprehensive and less time demanding.

The innate talent as the teacher emerges in many places when the author uses examples of various disease conditions and their practical situations to explain his views, which will be very useful for postgraduate students to easily understand the concept of disability assessment. I am sure this book will also give way to the evolution of a universal method of assessing disability that will soon be accepted internationally.

I hope this book will become a reference guide for all people who embroil in the welfare of differently abled people.

S. Sabhesan
Institute of Psychiatry
Madurai Medical College
Madurai, India

Dr. Ramar happens to be a very close friend. We both belong to a small group of "oldies" who wear introversion next to our souls. We have graduated, specialized in our specific fields of interest, researched, worked as teachers, and continued to mature in the profession together. It has always been a pleasure to meet him inside and outside the professional domains.

I have witnessed him as a practitioner. His long and dedicated clinical evaluations, setting up of an individually tailored therapeutic paradigm, and his empathetic communication to the patient and to the caregiver have always been a treat to watch. For him, clinical evaluation has not become a conditioned reflex and continues until the last minute to be cerebral. Years have not fatigued his methodical approach even by a whimper.

I have seen him carrying on with his research. Like any other researcher, he ploughs the lonely furrow of data collection, statistical abstraction, and inferences. He has an uncanny way of reading his huge data and works intuitively to know the essential core. To my knowledge, his research is always based on his clinical observations, and that is what makes it interesting and definitive.

Psychiatry has taught that an attitudinal prejudice makes for a myopic vision and erroneous detailing. Cleansing by an enormous de-biasing had been a prerequisite at a personal level before I could venture into writing these few words. And yet, the present work has bowled me over enormously. This is an extension and elaboration of his earlier work on disability evaluation in India, two decades ago. There has been an exponential shift in the conceptualization of disability evaluation.

Quoting the case of a pianist, the author brings home the limitations of considering only the impairment as an index of disability. However, assessing impairment makes a good and workable beginning. As a physiatrist with consummate expertise in quantifying impairment, he has brought out an extensive scoring system. This medical evaluation underscores a meticulous working knowledge in not only physiatry and orthopedics, but also in neurology, cognitive aspects of behavioral sciences, cardiovascular system, respiratory system, hematology, immunology, endocrinology, urology, sexual medicine, and others and the quantifying systems in each one of the branches. Collating ideas, comments, and critiques from his colleagues from other branches of medicine, the author has made the calculation of impairment a simple task; so authentic and, yet, so simple for even a novice to gain expertise with minimal training.

Simultaneously, Dr. Ramar makes his assertion that the medical model has its limitations. The humanist inside the medico advocates a biopsychosocial model. Disability assessment undergoes a paradigm shift because disability evaluation should also assess the individual's ability/disability in domains fundamental to acquiring the skills to live, learn, and work successfully in the community. Factoring in impairment, limitation of activity, participation restriction, and environmental support in the integrated evaluation brings about a qualitative conceptual change and integrates the biological with the psychosocial. Instead of looking at the individual's structural and functional impairment only, one begins to learn how the individual is maimed in his day-to-day personal and social life and the pursuit of his goals and ambitions. The evaluation is truly objective because it measures the disability in the individual's unique socio-cultural context.

Disability is not just impairment. It is a dysfunctional state embedded in the individual's contextual background. The state's responsibility and contribution can work significantly to lessen the individual's malaise. The present work demands due consideration for such contextual support. Necessarily, it also points to where the State must focus on distributing its scant resources to address the collective felt-needs of its unfortunate citizens. Contributions from the individual support groups and the state would mitigate the sufferings of impairment at the individual level. The present work succinctly underlines various areas where minimal environmental changes can contribute significantly to the well-being of the disabled. The purpose of disability evaluation is not indulgence by doling out the largesse, but a scientific apportionment where the needy, the professionals, and the executive are on equal footing in collective planning and execution.

In the present era of multi-specialties, a working expertise culled over years of experience, but limited to a narrow domain is inescapable. It is to the author's credit that so many experts from diverse fields have shared their ideas in shaping the concept. The author's assimilation of their inputs and acknowledgement of their contributions symbolizes the openness, inclusiveness, and scientific temperament of the work.

Innovativeness in thinking, such as bringing in the homunculus model, is bound to create its own positive and negative repercussions. The author seems to be aware that as the ripples settle down, placid waters would reveal the transparency and depth of thinking. Provoking rigorous scientific debate is the hallmark of any work in science, and the little hesitant steps would pave the way for further refinement and a final leap.

The author has thanked the grace of Almighty for His Blessings in executing this work. Any reader would concur that this work is a Blessing.

Perumal Thiagarajan

Department of Medicine
Pathology, and Immunology
Baylor College of Medicine
and
Hematology Laboratory and Transfusion Medicine
Michael E. DeBakey VA Medical Center
Houston, Texas

It is my pleasure and a great honor to write a foreword for this monograph by Dr. S. Ramar. Dr. Ramar has a long and distinguished career in physiatry for the past 40 years. As the Director of the Institute for Rehabilitation Medicine in Chennai, and later as the Head of the Department of Physical Medicine and Rehabilitation, PMR Hospital, Ministry of Health in Kuwait, he has vast expertise in all aspects of disability evaluation. His passions for scholarly excellence and devotion to the practice of academic physiatry resulted in this monograph. It is evident that the author has diligently researched, critically reviewed, and meticulously appended the existing methodologies on disability evaluation. With these thorough and deliberate reviews of the current literature, Dr. Ramar has presented an *Integrated Evaluation of Disability* in various disciplines.

Chronic anemia and thrombocytopenia are responsible for most disabilities in hematological disorders. Bleeding into the joints is the major cause of morbidity in patients with disorders of coagulation. Dr. Ramar has provided simple, readily available, easy to use tools. I am certain both experts and novices will find this book extremely useful.

S. Harikrishnan

Department of Cardiology
Sree Chitra Tirunal Institute for Medical Sciences and Technology
Trivandrum, India

I was introduced to Dr. S. Ramar by my classmate and close friend, who was one of his junior colleagues in Kuwait. I realized the stature of Dr. Ramar among his colleagues from the words of my classmate.

Being a cardiologist with almost zero exposure in physiatry (except as a patient) I was a little apprehensive when Dr. Ramar asked me to review the section on cardiology and write a foreword to his book. Those who have interacted with him will realize that refusing a request from such a nice person like Dr. Ramar is too difficult.

But while reviewing the chapters in his book—*Integrated Evaluation of Disability*, I realized the enormous details he has included in his book. Chapter 9 on the impairment of cardiovascular functions has compiled all the available "functional classifications" about various cardiology disease entities, such as coronary artery disease and valvular heart disease. The compilation is so extensive that cardiology postgraduates can use it as a reference.

The concept of cardiac rehabilitation was unknown in India until recently. We now realize the importance of physiatry and rehabilitation in cardiology. The improvement in outcomes—in morbidity, quality of life, and even mortality—following structured rehab sessions in coronary artery disease, valvular heart disease, and heart failure are worth mentioning. There are only a few centers in India that are doing significant work in cardiac rehabilitation. The improvement in quality of life (QOL) after participating in a structured rehab session is gratifying as vouched by most patients.

In this context, the release of a book on functional assessment by Dr. Ramar is timely. Those who venture into the area of cardiac rehabilitation can use this well-written book for their daily practice as well as a reference document.

I congratulate Dr. Ramar for bringing out such an excellent book and wish him all the very best in life.

V. Velayutham
Department of Ophthalmology
Madras Medical College
and
Regional Institute of Ophthalmology
Chennai, India

It gives me immense pride to write the foreword of this wonderful book. It has been one of my wishes to contribute to a cause as integral as this; and here is my chance.

The world's population comprises a significant number of those who are physically disabled, and several countries make the requisite efforts to help people with special needs. While developed countries address all the concerns toward ensuring normalcy in all surroundings and situations, it is not entirely the case with developing and underdeveloped countries.

In our country, it is very difficult even to ascertain the exact prevalence of differently abled persons, and their rehabilitation can occur only after such enumeration and assessment.

The author, Dr. S. Ramar, has laboriously described even the minute details in assessing a disability and its percentage. He has also suggested how available environments have contributed positively or negatively to a person's disability.

This has a long way to go in countries like ours, though I am very certain that this book will give ample guidance and confidence in the assessment and management of situations for the disabled.

I hope that readers use the information provided here to its maximum extent and go on to yield positive results.

S. Ammamuthu
Institute of Otolaryngology
Madras Medical College
Chennai, India

Dr. S. Ramar, a good friend of mine, is an exemplary physician and teacher. He has always adopted a methodical approach toward, both his patients and research. In this book, the meticulous preparation and painstaking pursuits of the author to simplify and present a broad complex topic are evident.

This book is an essential tool for everyone interested in the objective evaluation of disability and will be of immense benefit to physicians and postgraduate students.

The author has brought out the salient features in an excellent way and has succeeded in keeping this book informative and thought-provoking.

I appreciate the diligent hard work in crafting this book. This unique book will find its niché in the evolving concepts of disability evaluation.

M.G. Rajamanickam
Department of Urology
Kilpauk Medical College and Government Royapettah Hospital
and
Department of Urology
Sri Ramachandra Medical College and Research Institute
Chennai, India

I am delighted to review Dr. S. Ramar's book, *Integrated Evaluation of Disability*. Dr. S. Ramar is one of the earliest to specialize in physical medicine and rehabilitation. He has occupied very high posts in Physical Medicine and Rehabilitation in both India and in Kuwait.

While going through his preface, I was very impressed how he developed his interest and involvement in disability evaluation. From early 1981 until 2014, he has had many opportunities to work in this area of disability assessment and evaluation and has published guidelines in this field. With such vast experiences in this field, he has incorporated all possible references to compile this book, which will serve as a great tool for the medical fraternity.

While reviewing Chapter 8 "Impairment of Urogenital Functions," I am of the opinion that Dr. S. Ramar has used ideal techniques for the assessment of the above functions.

He has compared various international guidelines from the American Medical Association Guidelines, Korean Academy of Medical Sciences, and so on, and has compiled his guidelines for evaluation of permanent impairment in urogenital functions. India only has a few references available covering this specialty; one such is the Urological Society of India's *Guidelines on Disability Assessment in Urological Diseases*.

To my knowledge, nobody in India, except Dr. Ramar, has integrated disability evaluation of persons with medical conditions related to all medical specialties. I am sure both postgraduate students and practicing doctors can utilize this well-written book for their daily day practice and as a reference document.

I highly appreciate the excellent work of Dr. Ramar and prevalent use of his ideas in day-to-day practice would be the fitting response to the innovative approach.

Preface

Long back in December 1989, the author's abiding interest in disability evaluation was triggered by an invitation to participate as a resource person in a WHO follow-up seminar to review the guidelines advocated by an expert group meeting of Disability Evaluation (1981) and in a WHO Seminar on Evaluation of Physical Impairment of Disease of Spine (1991) in New Delhi, India. His commitment and subsequent explorations culminated in his publishing a textbook in 1993 called *Objective Evaluation of Impairment and Ability in Locomotor Handicapped*, which also incorporated the Government of India's *Guideline for Uniform Definitions of Physically Handicapped* with illustrations. In 2001, as an invitee from India, he participated in a Delphi Process for a WHO collaborative project with Munich University, Germany on ICF—International Classification of Functioning, Disability and Health. With redoubled interest, he ventured, in 2006, to further the process and develop an integrated method of disability evaluation based on WHO-ICF functions, structures, activities, participation, environmental factors, and personal factors.

The optimum method of disability evaluation assesses impairment of function and/or structure, limitation of activities, participation restriction, environmental factors, and behavior of the person toward his/her disability.

The existing literature on disability evaluation has only focused on impairment and/or limitation of activities and/or earning capacity. The methods have not considered evaluation of participation, namely, the skills fundamental to live, learn, and work successfully in the community. As it has not attempted evaluation of environmental and personal factors, the rationale for assigning the percentage of disability was incomplete.

Different countries assign different percentages of impairment for similar impairment of structure or function. Global efforts were undertaken to assign a percentage of disability, for example, Disability Weight Projects, Institute of Medicine's (IOM) Enabling–Disabling Process Model, and Mathematical Model of Disability (Enabling America—Models of Disability and Rehabilitation: Evolution of Models of Disability), WHODAS 2.0 (WHO II Disability Assessment Schedule), and so on. No uniform definition has been developed yet to assign a percentage of disability. The medical field is seeking an ideal objective method of evaluation because of the inadequacy of the existing tools/scales for disability evaluation.

A simple evaluation of impairment undermines the importance of limitation of activity and participation restriction as illustrated by a professional pianist who after amputation of his fingers in the right hand would not be able to return to his profession. The author's conception of evaluation of disability to integrate impairment of function and/or structure, limitation of activity and restriction of participation, environmental barriers and behavior of the person toward his/her disability assesses the true status of disability.

As ICF has not described any methodology for disability evaluation, the author has worked on his own to develop a method based on *Integrated Evaluation of Disability*. The resultant book comprises 23 chapters, which include neurological, neuromusculoskeletal, genitourinary, cardiovascular, hematological, immunological, respiratory, digestive, visual, otorhinolaryngology systems, burns, and intellectual disability or mental retardation.

It was a Herculean task to assign an appropriate percentage of disability. The principles of the motor and sensory homunculus, a weighted score based on the severity of impairment of function/structure, opinions from physicians practicing disability evaluation including a "Modified Delphi Process," and the outcome of the pilot study on "Clinical Model" all formed the base for assigning a percentage of disability.

The author has also obtained opinions from global experts in the medical fields of physical medicine and rehabilitation, ophthalmology, orthopedic surgery, neurology, cardiology, pulmonology, hematology, urology, psychiatry, plastic surgery, phoniatry, and psychology from Belgium, India, Kuwait, the Netherlands, Oman, Romania, the United Kingdom, and the United States. Additionally, senior physicians in physical medicine and rehabilitation, cardiology, gastroenterology, hematology, ophthalmology, orthopedics, otorhinolaryngology, neurology, plastic surgery, psychiatry, pulmonology, and urology reviewed the final work. Their critiques and opinions enabled the author to improve the content.

Further, the author instituted a pilot study to apply the concepts of *Integrated Evaluation of Disability* in clinical models for about 300 clinical conditions. The pilot study offered valuable hints to further refine the intricacy of clinical methods and tools, the grading of the severity of impairment or disability, as well as assigning impairment.

The "Clinical Model" facilitated the author's efforts to develop the "Ready Reckoner Impairment Table" for about 300 clinical conditions with multiple clinical presentations.

Furthermore, *Integrated Evaluation of Disability* includes user-friendly software on the Companion Website for the book at: www.crcpress.com/cw/Vinayagam. The software integrated on the Companion Website also provides flexibility to select their method of evaluation, that is, impairment evaluation and/or limitation of activity and participation restriction or global evaluation of disability (function, activity, participation, and environmental and personal factors) depending on the laws and acts prevalent in their respective countries. It also provides a "Ready Reckoner Impairment Table." The clinician can select to feed the data into a Microsoft Excel spreadsheet for obtaining an impairment score, or simply retrieve the impairment score from the "Ready Reckoner Impairment Table." The clinician can also save the worksheet for future reference.

It is my sincere hope that this book would serve as a textbook about disability medicine for postgraduate students and physicians in physical medicine and rehabilitation, neurology, occupational medicine, ophthalmology, orthopedics, otorhinolaryngology, and rheumatology. It would also serve as a reference book on disability for postgraduate students and physicians in cardiology, pulmonology, nephrology, urology, gastroenterology, hematology, plastic surgery, psychiatry, and pain medication.

By using an integrated evaluation, this approach can be a better and preferred one in health surveys to identify the prevalence of severity of disability for future health planning: predicting health service requirements, developing policy decisions, and providing budgetary allocations. It will guide the physicians in measuring the "Rehabilitation Outcome" at the time of discharge after the rehabilitation program. It will enable the authorities in deciding the eligibility for disability benefits and insurance companies in determining the compensation for disability. It may serve as a reference book in the judiciary for their decisions in matters related to disability.

The author believes that in as much as this approach provides an easy and, yet, a scientifically sound tool in the hands of the expert for evaluation of disability, it equally provides succor to the unfortunate fellow-beings in their march toward a life of dignity and redefined ability.

Ramar Sabapathi Vinayagam
Department of Physical Medicine and Rehabilitation
Ministry of Health
Kuwait

Government Institute of Rehabilitation Medicine
Madras Medical College
Chennai, India

Department of Physical Medicine and Rehabilitation
Tirunelveli Medical College Hospital
Tirunelveli, Tamilnadu, India

Author

Ramar Sabapathi Vinayagam, MD, in 1973, obtained a medical degree from Madurai University, India, and he also trained in physical medicine and rehabilitation at the University of Madras. After working as a tutor, assistant professor, and additional professor, he became the professor and head of the Institution of Government Institute of Rehabilitation Medicine, Madras Medical College, Chennai in 2001. He assumed the position of General Secretary from 1994–1999, and was vice president of the Indian Association of Physical Medicine and Rehabilitation 2000–2002. Subsequently, he worked as a consultant 2002–2011, and was the chairman of the Department of Physical Medicine and Rehabilitation 2011–2012 in the Ministry of Health of Kuwait.

Dr. Ramar has more than 40 years of clinical experience with skills in electrodiagnostic studies, which includes electromyography and nerve conduction studies, and pain management including interventional pain management for peripheral joints, rehabilitation of stroke, rehabilitation of persons with spinal cord injury and amputation, and disability evaluation.

Dr. Ramar has served as a postgraduate teacher in physical medicine and rehabilitation; chairman, Board of Studies School of Physiotherapy, The Tamil Nadu Dr. M.G.R. Medical University, Chennai; postgraduate examiner in physical medicine and rehabilitation for universities in India and the National Board of Examinations, New Delhi. He has served as coordinator on the accreditation committee for the Physical Medicine and Rehabilitation Hospital, Ministry of Health, Kuwait; and as chairman of the Committee on Disability Evaluation, Physical Medicine and Rehabilitation Hospital, Ministry of Health, Kuwait. He has served as a resource person in WHO expert group committees and participated in the Delphi Process from India for the WHO Collaborative Project with Munich University, Germany on ICF—International Classification of Functioning in Disability and Health 2000.

He has received numerous awards and honors, including the DHADHIJI Award in 1997 from the Indian Association of Physical Medicine and Rehabilitation. In 1993, he wrote the book *Objective Evaluation of Impairment and Ability in Locomotor Handicapped*; and in 2001, he authored a chapter in the book *Neurorehabilitation Principles and Practice* (Second Edition).

Acknowledgments

I sincerely thank Abdulla Ahmed Eyadeh, former head of the Department of Physical Medicine and Rehabilitation, Physical Medicine and Rehabilitation Hospital, Ministry of Health, State of Kuwait. He triggered me to boost my interest in developing *Integrated Evaluation of Disability* based on the International Classification of Functioning, Disability and Health. He has given me books on disability as a gift to double my interest in this task. He has arranged for an opinion about our concept on *Integrated Evaluation of Disability* with our colleagues involved in disability evaluation in various specialties in Kuwait. He has also motivated me whenever I was slack in this task. It would not have been possible for me to begin this work without his great moral help.

I also should thank John L. Melvin, professor and chairman of the Department of Physical Medicine and Rehabilitation, Jefferson Medical Center, Thomas Jefferson University, Philadelphia, Pennsylvania, for his support as well as reviewing my initial work on *Integrated Evaluation of Disability*. He has also provided me with valuable scientific opinion.

I should also thank Gerold Stucki, professor and chair, Department of Health Sciences and Health Policy, University of Lucerne, director, Swiss Paraplegic Research (SPF), director, ICF Research Branch, WHO FIC CC Germany (DIMDI), Switzerland. Professor Stucki had reviewed my presentation on Disability Evaluation during the 4th World Congress of International Society of Physical Rehabilitation Medicine, Seoul. While his opinion had strengthened my performance during the congress, it had also helped me to proceed in the right direction in my work on *Integrated Evaluation of Disability*.

It is a gift from God that I have two supporting hands—one my beloved friend Perumal Thiagarajan and another my dear friend Sabhesan Sivam.

I sincerely thank Perumal Thiagarajan, professor of medicine, pathology, and immunology at Baylor College of Medicine and director, Hematology Laboratory, and Transfusion Medicine, Michael E. DeBakey VA Medical Center, Houston, Texas. He has guided me throughout my career offering valid suggestions for refining the presentation of this book as well as critiques and opinions on the Chapter 11 "Impairment of Functions in Hematological and Immunological Systems." It was an immense help from him

that he spared a lot of his time in designing most of the diagrams using Adobe Illustrator.

My sincere thanks to Sabhesan Sivam, former professor of psychiatry, Institute of Psychiatry, Madurai Medical College, Madurai, India, who has reviewed the entire book and provided valid suggestions that enabled me to improve the content. His positive, encouraging moral support in every step of my work boosted my confidence to complete this book.

I sincerely thank Papanicolaou A. C., director of the Center for Clinical Neurosciences, University of Texas Medical School, Houston, Texas, for sparing his valuable time to discuss the role of homunculus in assigning impairment in 2003 as well as for his opinion on updated information in 2007.

I wholeheartedly thank the following experts who have reviewed the preliminary work on Integrated Evaluation of Disability and provided their valid opinion in 2007 to pursue the project further.

1. Adel Al-Zayed, psychiatrist, Psychiatric Medicine Hospital, Ministry of Health, Kuwait
2. Amal Salaheldeen, phoniatrist, Physical Medicine and Rehabilitation Hospital, Ministry of Health, Kuwait
3. Andrew J. Haig, associate professor, Physical Medicine and Rehabilitation and Orthopedic Surgery, University of Michigan, Ann Arbor, Michigan, US
4. Ryad Khan, consultant, Department of Neurology, Ibn Sina Hospital, Ministry of Health, Kuwait
5. Arun Narayanaswamy, urologist, Al-Amiri Hospital, Ministry of Health, Kuwait
6. Daniël Wever, consultant and physician, Physical Medicine and Rehabilitation, the Netherlands
7. Guy Vanderstraeten, professor and head of the Department of Physical Medicine and Rehabilitation, University Hospital, Belgium
8. Hasan Ibrahim Yacoub, clinical psychologist, Psychological Medicine Hospital, Ministry of Health, Kuwait
9. Haim Ring, professor and chairman, Neurological Rehabilitation Department, Loewenstein Rehabilitation Center; past chair, Physical Medicine and Rehabilitation Department, Sackler Faculty of Medicine, Tel Aviv University; chairman, National Rehabilitation Council, Ministry of Health, Israel

10. B. Jayakrishnan, pulmonologist, Al-Rashid Allergy Hospital, Ministry of Health, Kuwait
11. John Alexander, consultant neurologist, Ibn Sina Hospital, Ministry of Health, Kuwait
12. John L. Melvin, professor and chairman, Department of Physical Medicine and Rehabilitation, Jefferson Medical Center, Thomas Jefferson University, Philadelphia, Pennsylvania, US
13. Leon, urologist, International Hospital, Salmiya, Kuwait
14. Liviu Pop, head of the Department Physical Medicine and Rehabilitation, Rehabilitation Hospital Cluj-Napoca, Romania
15. Mohamed Budir, orthopedic surgeon, Al-Razi Hospital, Ministry of Health, Kuwait
16. V. Nagarajan, consultant neurologist, Ibn Sina Hospital, Ministry of Health, Kuwait
17. Nandakumar, professor of Physical Medicine and Rehabilitation, Annamalai University, Chidambaram, India
18. Perumal Thiagarajan, Department of Hematopathology, Bayer College of Medicine, Houston, Texas, US
19. Radhakrishna Panicker, pulmonologist, Al-Rashid Allergy Hospital, Ministry of Health, Kuwait
20. Sabhesan, professor of psychiatry, Institute of Psychiatry, Madurai Medical College, Madurai, India
21. Said Al Saadany, psychologist, Psychiatric Medicine Hospital, Ministry of Health, Kuwait
22. C.A. Thiyagarajan, staff grade medical practitioner, lead clinician in Domiciliary Ventilation and Botulinum Toxin Therapy, National Spinal Injuries Centre, Stoke Mandeville Hospital, Aylesbury, United Kingdom
23. Vesna Zeljic, head of the Unit of Pediatric Rehabilitation, Department of Physical Medicine and Rehabilitation, Physical Medicine and Rehabilitation Hospital, Ministry of Health, Kuwait

I sincerely thank the following experts who have reviewed the work on Integrated Evaluation of Disability, in a group meeting held in 2010. Their critiques and comments triggered me to refine my thinking on this task.

1. Abdulla Eyadeh, former head of the Department of Physical Medicine and Rehabilitation, Physical Medicine and Rehabilitation Hospital, Ministry of Health, Kuwait
2. Ali Abdullah, consultant rheumatologist, Military Hospital, Ministry of Health, Kuwait
3. Abdulla Abu Najma, consultant orthopedic surgeon, Farwania Hospital, Ministry of Health, Kuwait
4. Abdul Razak, consultant spinal surgeon, Al-Razi Orthopedics Hospital, Ministry of Health, Kuwait
5. Ali Al Kandari, consultant neurosurgeon, Ibn Sina Hospital, Ministry of Health, Kuwait
6. Fawzia Al Kandari, consultant cardiologist, Chest Hospital, Ministry of Health, Kuwait
7. Jassem Al Hashel, consultant neurologist, Mubarak Al-Kabeer Hospital, Ministry of Health, Kuwait
8. Moodi Al Mutairi, consultant rheumatologist, Mubarak Al-Kabeer Hospital, Ministry of Health, Kuwait

I wholeheartedly thank the following panelists who participated in the Modified Delphi Process in 2012 to process the validation of clinical methods for disability evaluation.

1. Abdulla Eyadeh, former head of the Department of Physical Medicine and Rehabilitation, Physical Medicine Rehabilitation Hospital, Ministry of Health, Kuwait
2. Amal Salaheldeen, phoniatrist, Physical Medicine Rehabilitation Hospital, Ministry of Health, Kuwait
3. Biju Gopinath, physician, Department of Physical Medicine and Rehabilitation, Physical Medicine Rehabilitation Hospital, Ministry of Health, Kuwait
4. Chidambaram Ambalavanan, physician, Department of Physical Medicine and Rehabilitation, Physical Medicine Rehabilitation Hospital, Ministry of Health, Kuwait
5. Fadi Kobal, physician, Department of Physical Medicine and Rehabilitation, Physical Medicine Rehabilitation Hospital, Ministry of Health, Kuwait
6. Ghada el Sayed el Gohary, physician, Department of Physical Medicine and Rehabilitation, Physical Medicine Rehabilitation Hospital, Ministry of Health, Kuwait
7. Hamada Sayed Ahmed, physician, Department of Physical Medicine and Rehabilitation, Physical Medicine Rehabilitation Hospital, Ministry of Health, Kuwait
8. John Alexander, consultant neurologist, Ibn Sina Hospital, Ministry of Health, Kuwait
9. Lata Prasad, physician, Department of Physical Medicine and Rehabilitation, Physical Medicine Rehabilitation Hospital, Ministry of Health, Kuwait
10. Mohamed Hossam, phoniatrist, Physical Medicine Rehabilitation Hospital, Ministry of Health, Kuwait
11. Mohamed Ibrahim Dughbaj, physician, Department of Physical Medicine and Rehabilitation, Physical Medicine Rehabilitation Hospital, Ministry of Health, Kuwait
12. Nagarajan, consultant neurologist, Ibn Sina Hospital, Ministry of Health, Kuwait
13. Nishabhavan Narayanapillai Prasanth, physician, Physical Medicine and Rehabilitation, Cochin, India
14. Padmakumar, physician, Physical Medicine and Rehabilitation, Trivandrum, India
15. Periasamy, consultant neurologist, Ibn Sina Hospital, Ministry of Health, Kuwait

16. Rachel Samuel, physician, Physical Medicine and Rehabilitation, Trivandrum, India

17. Rajendra Prasad, physician, Department of Physical Medicine and Rehabilitation, Physical Medicine Rehabilitation Hospital, Ministry of Health, Kuwait

18. Ramaswamy Pillai, former professor and head of the Department of Physical Medicine and Rehabilitation, Medical College, Trivandrum, India

19. Sabhesan Sivam, former professor of Psychiatry, Madurai Medical College, Madurai, India

20. Shajan Purusothaman, physician, Department of Physical Medicine and Rehabilitation, Physical Medicine Rehabilitation Hospital, Ministry of Health, Kuwait

21. Srdjan, physician, Department of Physical Medicine and Rehabilitation, Physical Medicine Rehabilitation Hospital, Ministry of Health, Kuwait

22. Suresh Ramakrishna, physician, Department of Physical Medicine and Rehabilitation, Physical Medicine Rehabilitation Hospital, Ministry of Health, Kuwait

23. Thabath Ismail, physician, Department of Physical Medicine and Rehabilitation, Physical Medicine Rehabilitation Hospital, Ministry of Health, Kuwait

24. Uma Pandian, head of the Department of Physical Medicine and Rehabilitation, Vijaya Health Centre, Chennai, India

25. Unnikrishnan Ramachandran, physician, Department of Physical Medicine and Rehabilitation, Physical Medicine Rehabilitation Hospital, Ministry of Health, Kuwait

26. Vesna Zeljic, consultant and physician, Physical Medicine and Rehabilitation Physician, Physical Medicine Rehabilitation Hospital, Ministry of Health, Kuwait

27. Vlasta Tosnerova, associate professor, Department of Rehabilitation, Medical Faculty, Charles University, Hradec Kralove, Prague, Czech Republic

28. Wael Abdelgawad, physician, Department of Physical Medicine and Rehabilitation, Physical Medicine Rehabilitation Hospital, Ministry of Health, Kuwait

I must acknowledge the help of senior experts for their eloquent reviews of the final work in their respective fields during 2012–2017. It enabled the author to fine-tune the output of this work. Hence,

1. I sincerely thank, Dr. Mayilvahanan Natarajan, 7th vice chancellor, Tamil Nadu Dr. M.G.R. Medical University, Chennai, India, for having spared his precious time and provided his suggestions

2. I profoundly thank Harikrishnan, professor of cardiology, Sree Chithrai Thirunal Institute of Medical Sciences and Technology, Thiruvananthapuram, India, for reviewing Chapter 9 "Impairment of Cardiovascular Functions" with valid suggestions

3. I also express my sincere thanks to V. Nagarajan, consultant neurologist, Ibn Sina Hospital, Ministry of Health, the State of Kuwait, for his valid opinion and comments on Chapter 6 "Impairment of Functions of the Nervous System"

4. I immensely thank Radhakrishna Panicker, pulmonologist, Ministry of Health, the State of Kuwait, for reviewing and furnishing a valuable opinion on Chapter 10 "Impairment of Pulmonary Functions"

5. I extend my sincere thanks to Jayakrishnan, senior consultant (pulmonology), Department of Medicine, Sultan Qaboos University for his critiques and comments on my initial work on Chapter 10 "Impairment of Pulmonary Functions"

6. I thank Prabha Chandran Nair, senior consultant in Pulmonology, G.G Hospital, Thiruvananthapuram, India, for reviewing Chapter 10 "Impairment of Pulmonary Functions"

7. I also thank K. Bharathi Babu, pulmonologist, Apollo Specialty Hospitals, Madurai, India, for reviewing Chapter 10 "Impairment of Pulmonary Functions" and providing valuable suggestions

8. I profusely thank P. Jones Ronald, consultant nephrologist, Vinayaka Mission Hospital, Salem, India, for his review and valuable comments on Chapter 8 "Impairment of Urogenital Functions"

9. I sincerely thank Rajamanickam, former professor and head of the Department of Urology, Kilpauk Medical College, Chennai, India, for his review and valuable comments on Chapter 8 "Impairment of Urogenital Functions"

10. I immensely thank Ammamuthu, former director, Institute of Otorhinolaryngology, Madras Medical College, Chennai, India, for his review and critiques on Chapter 14 "Impairment of Hearing Functions"

11. V. Velayudham, former director, Institute of Ophthalmology, Madras Medical College and Research Institute, Chennai, India, had contributed to his review and opinion on Chapter 13 "Impairment of Visual Functions." Though he prematurely left us for his heavenly abode, his participation in reviewing this work will always be held in esteem and revered

12. I sincerely thank Meenakshisundaram, former professor of ophthalmology, Tirunelveli Medical College for providing his critiques and opinion on Chapter 13 "Impairment of Visual Functions"

13. I wholeheartedly thank Harshad Devarbhvai, gastroenterologist, St. John's Medical College Hospital, Bengaluru, India, for reviewing Chapter 12 "Impairment of Swallowing, Liver, and Defecation Functions" and providing his opinion and comments

14. I sincerely thank both Sunderraj Ellur, additional professor, and Dr. D. Rajeswari, junior consultant and assistant professor, Department of Burns and Plastic Surgery, St. John's Hospital, Bengaluru, India, for their critiques and opinion on Chapter 18 on "Burns: Impairment"

15. I should also thank Unnikrishnan, physiatrist, Physical Medicine and Rehabilitation Hospital, Ministry of Health, Kuwait, for reviewing the whole book and providing valid input to improve the content

16. I extend my sincere thanks to John Alexander, consultant neurologist, Ibn Sina Hospital, Ministry of Health, State of Kuwait, for his review and opinion

17. I profusely thank Peter Pauly, head of the Physical Medicine and Rehabilitation Department; Salzkammergutklinikum (Vöcklabruck, Gmunden Bad Ischl) and medical director of Villa Seilern Merkur Recration Bad Ischl; Stiefern Hauptstraasse 31, 3562 Schoenberg, Austria for his review and opinion

I sincerely thank Dr. Kn. K.S.K. Chockalingam, director, and Dr. S. Shanmugavel, principal, National Engineering College, Kovilpatti, Tamil Nadu, India, for providing me basic training in Adobe Illustrator. I also sincerely thank Mr. S. Solaisamy. senior system administrator, and Mr. R. Krishnamurthy, technical assistant, National Engineering College, Kovilpatti, India, for guiding me in drawing illustrations and figures with Adobe Illustrator.

I should thank my better half, Mrs. Ramar Sulochana, for the patient devotion of her time that helped me to pursue this work since 2006. I should also thank my son-in-law, Mr. Pazhani Hariram Jothi, for developing a macro in the Excel sheet that enabled me to continue the pilot study on the "Clinical Model," locked the worksheet excepting the data entry column as well as in incorporating hand-drawn diagram, photos harvested from nature and purchased pictures in designing the cover page. My eldest daughter, Ramar Maheswari, a software engineer, despite her pressing engagements at home and work, has taken continued interest by furnishing me with the essential software for pursuing this work. Further, she is actively engaged in preparing the necessary software for computation of the disability. My second daughter, Ramar Nalini, and my son-in-law, Mr. Nagarajan Ganapathy, extended their constant prayers for successful completion of this challenging task as well as providing much-needed equipment to pursue my work with ease. My youngest daughter, Ramar Balaabhirami, and my son-in-law, Mr. Mahendran Natchadalingam, have helped me in computing the data and assisted me in the "Modified Delphi Process."

Finally, I submit this work to Almighty for having graced me with His Blessings to take up and complete this task.

Ramar Sabapathi Vinayagam
Courtallam, India

Disclaimer

The author declares that he has written this book without any commercial or financial assistance and that he does not have any potential conflict of interest. The author has made considerable efforts to present accurate and reliable information in this book and the supporting software, Ready Reckoners and worksheets on the Companion Website. Nevertheless, the author does not take any legal responsibility for the topicality, accuracy, correctness, completeness, or usefulness of the content provided. Liability claims regarding damage caused by the use of any information contained in the book and the supporting software, Ready Reckoners and worksheets including any information which is incomplete or incorrect, will, therefore, be rejected.

Introduction to disability

1.1 MAJOR LIFE ACTIVITIES

Depending on their age, gender, and cultural background, a person with normal function can perform day-to-day activities in a way that falls within the measured range designated as normal for a human being. Major daily activities in one's life comprise meaningful communications, self-care, chores, and ability to move from one place to another. Other activities include educational/vocational pursuits, parental/family responsibilities, social and community activities, citizenship roles, and so on. The World Health Organization's Disability Assessment Schedule (WHODAS) remarks that it is easy to define disease and death, but it's hard to define disability (1).

1.2 WHO IS DISABLED?

Disability manifests when physical or intellectual impairment substantially limits or restricts a person from performing his/her major life activities. The National Institute of Disability and Rehabilitation Research states that disability does not represent illness but a person with disability utilizes health care more often than the general population (2).

1.3 DEFINITIONS OF IMPAIRMENT, LIMITATION OF ACTIVITY, PARTICIPATION RESTRICTION, DISABILITY

Impairment refers to loss or an abnormality of a structure or function. For example, disease or injury, such as in the case of diabetic gangrene or a traffic accident, causing an amputation. Also, there can be a loss or abnormality of function in terms of motor control, loss of sensation, and loss of bladder/bowel control, for example, following a spinal cord injury due to a road accident or following stroke due to a cerebrovascular accident. The World Health Organization's International Classification of Impairments, Disabilities, and Handicaps (WHO-ICIDH) 1980 describes, "Impairments (*I code*), concerned with abnormalities of body structure and appearance and with organ or system function, resulting from any cause; in principle, impairments represent disturbances at the organ level" (3). The World Health Organization's International Classification of Functioning, Disability and Health 2001 (WHO-ICF 2001) describes "Impairment as

loss or abnormality in body structure or physiological function (including mental functions)" (4).

Because of impairment, the person may not be able to sit, stand, walk, climb stairs, eat, write, attend to personal hygiene, and dress. This inability, or difficulty, is referred to as a disability as per WHO-ICIDH 1980, whereas WHO-ICF 2001 described it as a "Limitation of Activity." WHO—ICIDH 1980 describes "Disabilities (*D code*), reflecting the consequences of impairment in terms of functional performance and activity by the individual; disabilities thus represent disturbances at the level of the person" (3). WHO—ICF 2001 defined "Limitation of Activity" as "difficulties an individual may have in executing activities" (4).

Because of a limitation of activity, the person is unable to pursue educational, vocational, recreational, religious, societal or parental roles. Restriction of this performance is referred to as a "Handicap" as per WHO—ICIDH 1980 and "Restriction of Participation" as per WHO—ICF 2001. WHO—ICIDH 1980 describes "Handicaps (*H code*), concerned with the disadvantages experienced by the individual as a result of impairments and disabilities; handicaps thus reflect interaction with and adaptation to the individual's surroundings" (3) and WHO—ICF—2001 describes it as "Participation Restriction." "Participation Restriction' are problems an individual may experience in involvement in life situations" (4). As per the WHO—ICF—2001, the term "Disability" is an umbrella term covering the whole disability process, which includes impairments, activity limitations and participation restrictions (4).

1.4 CAUSES AND CLASSIFICATION OF DISABILITIES

There is increasing prevalence of disability because of increasing growth in population, aging, rising incidence of chronic diseases, and increasing longevity of life due to advancements in medical technology. The common causes of impairment are congenital disorders, injury during birth, road traffic accidents, falls, injury following land mines, injury during war, malnutrition, communicable diseases (such as HIV/AIDS), diabetes, cardiovascular diseases, cancer, and mental disorders. The resultant disability demands an increase in the need for health care and rehabilitation services (5). Box 1.1 describes the classification of disability.

> **BOX 1.1: Classification of disabilities**
>
> 1. Mobility or motor disability: Affects movement from gross motor skills, like walking, to fine motor movements involving manipulation of objects by hand
> 2. Visual disability: Complete or partial loss of vision in one or both eyes
> 3. Hearing disability: Complete or partial hearing loss in one or both ears
> 4. Mental disability: Includes learning disability, cognitive or intellectual disability, and psychological and psychiatric disability
> 5. Multiple disabilities: Combination of mobility, hearing, vision, cognition, for example, Cerebral Palsy
> 6. Disability related to medical conditions such as cardiomyopathy, chronic renal failure, epilepsy and other seizure disorders, cancer, obstructive and restrictive lung diseases, HIV/AIDS, and so on

1.4.1 Mobility disability

Mobility disability affects movement from gross motor skills, like walking, to fine motor movements involving manipulation of objects by hand.

1.4.1.1 MOTOR DISABILITY DUE TO CONGENITAL OR INHERITED DISORDERS

Motor disabilities, due to congenital or inherited disorders, include congenital skeletal limb deficiencies—namely amelia, hemimelia, or phocomelia of the lower and upper extremities with the total or partial absence of a leg or arm, arthrogryposis multiplex congenita, congenital dislocation of the knee with quadriceps fibrosis, and congenital dislocation of the hip. It also includes Klippel-Feil syndrome and myelodysplasia due to an incomplete closure of neural tube—myelomeningocele at lumbar level with flaccid paralysis of both lower limbs. It further includes sensory loss of both lower extremities, bladder and/or bowel incontinence, congenital talipes equinovarus, congenital muscular dystrophies, and inherited diseases such as osteogenesis imperfecta, facioscapulohumeral muscular dystrophy, Friedreich's ataxia, Duchenne muscular dystrophy, childhood muscular dystrophies, and others.

1.4.1.2 MOTOR DISABILITY DUE TO TRAUMA

As per the *World Report on Road Traffic Injury Prevention—2004*, WHO estimates that between 20 million and 50 million people worldwide suffer from road traffic injuries each year (6). Additionally, the WHO report documented that road traffic crash injuries cost 1% of the gross national product in low-income countries, 1.5% in middle-income countries, and 2% in high-income countries (6).

Besides traffic accidents, other causes that contribute to disabilities are birth injuries, weapon injuries, falls, industrial injuries, frostbite, and others. Birth injuries include Erb's palsy or Klumpke's palsy with complete paralysis of the arm or paralysis of the proximal or the distal arm. Disorders, which result from traumatic brain injuries, include tetraplegia, hemiplegia, monoplegia, and cerebellar ataxia. Motor disabilities due to trauma also include spinal cord injuries (with tetraplegia, hemiplegia, paraplegia, monoplegia with sensory impairment, bladder/bowel incontinence), traumatic peripheral nerve injuries, traumatic amputation of the limbs, and others.

1.4.1.3 MOTOR DISABILITY DUE TO INFECTIONS

Motor disabilities, which result from infections, comprise post-encephalitic sequelae, post-meningitis sequelae, post-polio residual paralysis, leprosy with peripheral nerve lesions and amputations, tuberculous spondylitis with spinal cord injury, transverse myelitis, mycetoma foot, and so on.

1.4.1.4 MOTOR DISABILITY DUE TO RHEUMATIC DISEASES

Motor disabilities due to rheumatic diseases include rheumatoid arthritis, ankylosing spondylitis, systemic lupus erythematosus, scleroderma, and so on.

1.4.1.5 MOTOR DISABILITY DUE TO VASCULAR DISEASES

Motor disabilities caused by vascular diseases include cerebrovascular disease with stroke, peripheral vascular disease with amputation of a leg or arm, and so on.

1.4.1.6 MOTOR DISABILITY DUE TO MALIGNANCY

Motor disabilities due to malignancy include osteogenic sarcoma, Ewing's sarcoma, chondrosarcoma, fibrosarcoma resulting in limb amputation, ependymoma, neurofibroma, meningioma, and so on.

1.4.1.7 MOTOR DISABILITY DUE TO OTHER CAUSES

Vitamin deficiency disorders (e.g., subacute combined degeneration) may cause motor disability. Motor disability may result from endocrine disorders (e.g., diabetes mellitus causing gangrene and amputation). Motor disability also might result from degenerative disorders, such as motor neuron disease, spinocerebellar degeneration, spondylotic myelopathy, and so on. Motor disability can be due to peripheral nerve lesions.

1.4.2 Visual disability

Visual disability comprises of complete or partial loss of vision in one or both eyes due to enucleation of eye, retinopathy, retinoblastoma, maculopathy, optic neuritis, cataract, corneal scar, and so on.

1.4.3 Hearing disability

Hearing disability includes complete or partial hearing loss in one or both ears, for example, sensory neural hearing loss, conductive hearing loss, and so on.

1.4.4 Mental disability

1.4.4.1 LEARNING DISABILITY

A learning disbility in perceiving or processing auditory and visual-spatial information results in difficulties in acquiring knowledge, remembering things, and learning from experiences. Persons with an isolated learning disability do not have an intellectual disability.

1.4.4.2 COGNITIVE (OR) INTELLECTUAL DISABILITY

Cognitive disability comprises of difficulties with the thought process, learning, memory, retrieval of information, communication, appropriate usage, making judgments, and problem-solving due to conditions such as Down syndrome, Alzheimer's disease, dementia, traumatic brain injury.

1.4.4.3 PSYCHOLOGICAL AND PSYCHIATRIC DISABILITIES

A psychological and psychiatric disability is usually hidden due to conditions such as schizophrenia, depression, and others.

1.4.5 Multiple disabilities

Multiple disabilities are a combination of mobility, hearing, vision, cognition. Cerebral palsy is an example of these combinations of multiple disabilities.

1.4.6 Disability related to medical conditions

Clinical conditions, such as cardiomyopathy, obstructive and restrictive lung diseases, chronic renal failure, chronic liver failure, epilepsy and other seizure disorders, HIV/AIDS, cancer, and so others, can produce disability.

1.5 TEMPORARY AND PERMANENT DISABILITIES

Disabilities may be temporary or permanent, progressive, or regressive, intermittent.

1.5.1 Temporary disability

During a period of temporary disability, the person is unable to ambulate, perform activities of daily living, to participate in vocational, avocational, and social activities partially or wholly. However, with treatment, the person regains normal activities.

1.5.2 Permanent disability

With maximum medical and rehabilitation management, the condition remains stationary, and the person remains disabled due to the limitation of activities and participation restriction in vocational, avocational, social, and civic life.

1.5.3 Progressive disability

The impairment/disability of persons with diseases such as muscular dystrophy and motor neuron disease are usually progressive.

1.5.4 Regressive disability

The impairment/disability of persons with infective polyneuritis may regress.

1.5.5 Intermittent disability

Persons with rheumatoid arthritis or multiple sclerosis may develop impairment/disability or accentuation of residual impairment/disability during periods of relapse.

1.6 SEVERITY OF DISABILITY

The WHO International Classification of Functioning, Disability and Health (ICF) uses a generic scale to quantify the impairment of bodily functions and/or structures, limitation for activities, performance restrictions, and environmental barriers/facilitators (7).

1.7 PREVALENCE OF DISABILITY

1.7.1 Global prevalence

The Department of Public Information, United Nations Development Program (UNDP) documents that 80% of persons with disabilities live in the developing countries. The World Bank estimates that 20% of the world's poorest people are disabled (Box 1.2) (8).

BOX 1.2: World Bank estimates

20% of the world's poorest people are disabled

Persons with severe and moderate disability constitute 2.9% and 12.4% respectively in a global population of 6.5 billion in 2004. There is a linear increase in the prevalence of moderate and severe disability as the age advances, that is, 5% between 0 and 14 years, 15% between 15 and 59 years, and 46% 60 years and above. The prevalence of moderate and severe disability is higher in low and middle-income countries in all ages than in high-income countries (9). World Report on Disability 2011 stated that World Health Survey covered 64% of world population in 59 countries in 2002–2004. Box 1.3 depicts the average prevalence rate of disability in persons aged 18 years and above was 15.6% as per survey (11.8% in higher income countries to 18.0% in lower income countries) (10).

BOX 1.3: World Report on Disability 2011 World Health Survey

Average prevalence rate in adult population aged 18 years and over was 15.6%.

World Report on Disability 2011 also stated that about 785–975 million persons aged 15 years and above were living with a disability based on 2004 disability estimates of World Health Survey and Global Burden of Disease. Among them, 110–190 million have considerable problems in functioning. It has estimated that more than one billion people including children, that is, about 15% of the world population suffering from a disability (Box 1.4) (11).

BOX 1.4: World Report on Disability 2011

- About 785–975 million persons 15 years and older were living with disability
- Among them, 110–190 million have substantial problems in functioning
- Estimation of more than 1 billion people including children—about 15% of the world population suffer from disability

---

1.7.2 Australia

The 2015 survey estimated that 4.3 million Australians, or 18.3% of the population, had a disability. Among them, 78.5% suffered from a physical disability and 21.5% from a behavioral and mental disability (Box 1.5) (12).

BOX 1.5: Australia—2015 survey

Disabled persons: 18.3% of the population

1.7.3 Britain

As per "Disability Prevalence Estimates 2011/12," there were 11.6 million persons with disability in Great Britain. Among them, 5.7 million were adults in the working age, 5.1 million were in "Over State Pension" age, and 0.8 million were children (Box 1.6). The estimate included persons with chronic illness, disability, with the considerable problem in activities of daily living (13). In the UK, the prevalence of disability was 17.6% using ICF components "Impairment, Activity Limitation and Participation restriction" as per census 2001 (14). The prevalence of disability was 27.2% using ICF components "Impairment, Activity Limitation and Participation Restriction" based on 2002 disability survey (14).

BOX 1.6: Great Britain 2010/11 disability prevalence estimate disabled people: 11.6 million

- Adult working age: 5.7 million
- Over state age pension: 5.1 million
- Children: 0.8 million

1.7.4 China

Institute of Population Research/WHO Collaborating Centre for Reproductive Health and Population Science, Peking University, Beijing calculated age-adjusted disability prevalence rates from nationally representative surveys conducted in 1987 and 2006. An estimated prevalence of disability increased from 52.7 million to 84.6 million in 2006. Representative survey 2006 documented the prevalence of visual disability of 15.6% (12,980) in male persons, and 25% (19,541) in female persons. The prevalence of hearing and speech disability was 39.6% (32,987) in male persons and 36.2% (28,305) in female persons. The prevalence of physical disability was 38.7% (32,279) in male persons and 34.4% (26,894) in female persons. The prevalence of intellectual disability was 12.7% (10,604) in male persons, and 11% (8,614) in female persons; and mental disabilities of 8.9% (7,405) in male persons and 10.9% (8,523) in female persons. The 2006 survey also documented 72.4% (60,316) of male persons with disability, and 72.2% (56,380) female persons with disability in the rural population. It also documented 27.6% (23,026) male persons with disability, and 27.8% (21,757) female persons with disability in urban population (Box 1.7) (15).

BOX 1.7: China 2006 Survey

Estimated prevalence of disabled persons:
84.6 million
Visual disability: 15.6% (Male), 25% (Female)
Hearing and speech disability: 39.6% (Male),
36.2% (Female)
Physical disability: 38.7% (Male), 34.4% (Female)
Intellectual disability: 12.7% (Male), 11% (Female)
Mental disabilities: 8.9% (Male), 10.9% (Female)

1.7.5 India

As per 2011 census, the provisional population of India was 1,210,193,422 (16) and 26,810,557 persons were disabled of whom males were 14,986,202, and females 11,824,355. Among the total persons with disability, 18,631,921 were from a rural area and 8,178,636 were from the urban area. Among the total persons with disability, 5,032,463 were persons with seeing disability, 5,071,007 were with hearing disability, 1,998,535 with a speech disability, 5,436,604 with movement disability, 1,505,624 with mental retardation, 722,826 with mental illness, 4,927,011 with other disabilities and 2,116,487 with multiple disabilities (Box 1.8) (17).

BOX 1.8: India—2011 Census

Provisional population: 1,210,193,422
Total Persons with disability: 26,810,557

- Male: 14,986,202
- Female: 11,824,355
- Rural: 18,631,921
- Urban: 8,178,636
- Visual disability: 5,032,463
- Hearing disability: 5,071,007
- Speech disability: 1,998,535
- Movement disability: 5,436,604
- Mental retardation: 1,505,624
- Mental illness: 722,826
- Other disability: 4,927,011
- Multiple disabilities: 2,116,487

As per 2001 census, 21.9 million (2.1% of the total population) were disabled in India. Persons with seeing disability constitute 1%, speech disability 0.2%, hearing disability 0.1%, movement disability 0.6%, and mental disability 0.2% (18). The prevalence of disability was 1.7% during the survey 2002 with the ICF component of "Impairment" (14). World Health Survey 2002–2004 documented the disability prevalence as 24.9% (WHS results are weighted and age-standardized) (14).

1.7.6 Japan

As per the "World Report on Disability," the disability prevalence was 5% during a survey in 2005 (14). Based on self-reported disability in the Japanese population 2001, there were about 6.5 million disabled persons in Japan, with a total population of about 127 million. It documents 3.5 million persons with physical disabilities, 2.6 million with mental disabilities, and 459,000 persons with low IQs—intellectual disabilities (Box 1.9) (19).

BOX 1.9: Japan—Self-reported disability 2001

Population: 127 million
Persons with disability: 6.5 million

- Physical disability: 3.5 million
- Mental disability: 2.6 million
- Intellectual disability: 0.459 million

1.7.7 United States

As per the "World Report on Disability," the disability prevalence was 14.9% in a 2007 survey Restriction" (Box 1.10) (14).

BOX 1.10: United States Disability Survey 2007 (World Report on Disability)

Prevalence of disability: 14.9%

Whereas the community survey in New York City in 2006 was different. It documents 13.7% ± 0.2 of persons with any disability within the civilian population 5 years old and above (7,560,751 ± 1,799). It further documents 5.4% ± 0.5 of persons with any disability within the civilian population 5–15 years old (1,148,352 ± 4,007), 10.3% ± 0.2 persons with any disability within the civilian population 16–64 years old (5,455,470 ± 4,248), and 43.4% ± 0.8 persons with any disability within the civilian population 65 years old and above (956,929 ± 2,239) (20).

The US Centers for Disease Control and Prevention in its morbidity and mortality weekly report documented that the prevalence of disability in 2005 was 21.8% like that of 1999, that is, 22%. There was a rise in the reported number of persons with disability from 44.1 million to 47.5 million. An estimated 8.6 million persons disabled by arthritis, 7.6 million persons, disabled by back and spine disorders, and 3.0 million persons disabled by cardiac problems contributed to leading causes of disability. The prevalence of disability in women (24.4%) was higher compared to men (19.1%) in all age groups. There was a linear increase in prevalence of disability among both sexes as the age advanced, that is, 11% between 18 and 44 years, 23.9% between 45 and 64 years, and 51.8% above 64 years (21).

The "World Report on Disability" documented that the disability prevalence was 19.3% using ICF components "Impairment, Activity Limitation and Participation restriction" as per census 2000 (14).

1.8 DISABILITY ADJUSTED LIFE YEARS—DALY

In an ideal situation, standard life expectancy at birth is set at 80 years for men and 82.5 for women when a person lives up to the age of standard life with perfect good health. A combined loss of years of life (YLL) due to premature death and years lost because of a disability (YLD) represent Disability Adjusted Life Years (DALY) (22). The Global Burden of Disease (GBD) 2010 compared DALY, YLDs, YLLs, and the percentage of death for various diseases and injuries (23).

1.9 REHABILITATION

Early identification, the intervention of diseases/injuries and prevention of disability, and rehabilitation of persons with residual disability are necessary to reintegrate them into the society as a useful, productive member. "United Nations Standard Rule on Equalization of Opportunities for Persons with Disability 1993" describes rehabilitation as a measure to enable persons with disabilities to regain their functions to an optimum level in physical, sensory, intellectual, and psychosocial status and reintegrate them into the society with a higher level of independence. It recommends awareness raising, medical care, rehabilitation, supportive services, and training of personnel providing health and rehabilitation services as preconditions to attain this goal (24).

1.10 IMPORTANCE OF DISABILITY EVALUATION

Disability evaluation serves to estimate the prevalence of severity of disability during health survey for future health planning: foreseeing and planning service needs, identifying priorities, allocating resources, and developing policy decisions.

It guides physicians to assess "Rehabilitation Outcome" at the time of discharge after the rehabilitation program.

It enables the authorities to decide the eligibility for disability benefits such as disability pension, premature retirement with salary (or) pension, compensation for work-related or accident related disability, financial assistance to remove architectural barriers in the house—adding lift, ramp, and so on. Further, it enables the authorities to extend free (or) concessional mobility/hearing aids, the exemption in car parking, concession in air tickets/train tickets. It also covers priority in housing loan, admission in special schools/regular teaching institutions, relaxation in college admission to persons with disability and preference in suitable employment in government and non-governmental organizations.

Disability evaluation is essential in deciding the compensation for disability by Insurance companies, and in Judiciary for their decision in matters related to disability.

REFERENCES

1. Üstün TB, Kostanjsek N, Chatterji S, Rehm J. *Measuring Health and Disability: Manual for WHO Disability Assessment Schedule (WHODAS 2.0)*. Geneva, Switzerland: World Health Organization; 2010. p. 3.
2. National Institute on Disability and Rehabilitation Research's long range plan in Section two: NIDDR research agenda Chapter 4: Health and function. 2000. p. 43.
3. World Health Organization. *International Classification of Impairments, Disabilities and Handicaps: A Manual of Classification Relating to the Consequences of Disease*. Geneva, Switzerland: WHO; 1980. p. 14.
4. *International Classification of Functioning, Disability and Health*. Geneva, Switzerland: World Health Organization; 2001. p. 213.
5. *Disability and Rehabilitation: WHO Action Plan 2006–2011*. Geneva, Switzerland: World Health Organization; 2014.
6. Peden M, Scurfield R, Sleet D, Mohan D, Hyder AA, Jarawan E, Mathers C. *World Report on Road Traffic Injury Prevention*. Geneva, Switzerland: World Health Organization; 2004. p. 15.
7. *International Classification of Functioning, Disability and Health*. Geneva, Switzerland: World Health Organization; 2001. p. 222.

8. *CONVENTION on the RIGHTS of PERSONS with DISABILITIES: Some Facts about Persons with Disabilities*. In: Department of Public Information UN, editor. 2006.

9. *Global Burden of Disease 2004 Update: Part 3 Disease Incidence, Prevalence and Disability*. Geneva, Switzerland: World Health Organization; 2008. p. 34.

10. World Health Organization TWB. *World Report on Disability*. Geneva, Switzerland: World Health Organization; 2011. p. 27.

11. World Health Organization TWB. *World Report on Disability*. Geneva, Switzerland: World Health Organization; 2011. p. 29.

12. *4430.0 - Disability, Ageing and Carers, Australia: Summary of Findings, 2015*. Canberra, Australia: Australian Bureau of Statistics; 2015.

13. Disability prevalence estimate 2011/2012 (England Scotland and Wales). Office from Disability Issues, and Department for Work and Pensions, Gov.UK; 2014.

14. World Health Organization TWB. *World Report on Disability*. Geneva, Switzerland: World Health Organization; 2011. pp. 271–276.

15. Zheng X, Chen G, Song X, Liu J, Yan L, Du W et al. Twenty-year trends in the prevalence of disability in China. *Bull World Health Organ*. 2011;89(11):788–797.

16. *Census of India*. New Delhi, India: Office of the Registrar General and Census Commissioner, Ministry of Home Affairs, Government of India; 2011. p. 41.

17. *Census of India*. New Delhi, India: Office of the Registrar General and Census Commissioner, Ministry of Home Affairs, Government of India; 2011.

18. Government of India, Ministry of Home Affairs. *Census of India*. New Delhi, India: Office of the Registrar General & Census Commissioner, India; 2001.

19. *Social Security programs throughout the world: Asia and the Pacific, 2008*. Washington, DC: Office of Retirement and Disability Policy; March 2009.

20. *2006 American Community Survey S0201. Selected Population Profile in the United States*. In: Bureau UC, editor. New York: U.S. Census Bureau; 2006.

21. *Morbidity and Mortality Weekly Report—United States, 2005*. In: Department of Health and Human Services USoA, editor. Atlanta, GA: Centers for Disease Control and Prevention; 2009.

22. *Health Statistics and Information Systems - Metrics: Disability-Adjusted Life Year (DALY)*. Geneva, Switzerland: World Health Organization; 2014.

23. GBD 2010 - GBD Compare [Internet]. Institute for Health Metrics and Evaluation, University of Washington; 2013. Available from: healthmetricsandevaluation.org/gbd-compare/.

24. Enable UN. *Standard Rules on the Equalization of Opportunities for Persons with Disabilities*. Geneva, Switzerland: United Nations; 2006. pp. 1–6.

Basis for *Integrated Evaluation of Disability*

2.1 METHODOLOGY FOR DEVELOPING AN *INTEGRATED EVALUATION OF DISABILITY*

There is no unified method for evaluation of disability, and different countries adopt various methods to evaluate disability. The World Health Organization (WHO) has brought out a unified definition of disability and advanced a biopsychosocial approach to interpret disability. However, it needs clinical tools for the evaluation of disability. A comprehensive study extending from 2006 to 2017 has emerged with a comprehensive method for an *Integrated Evaluation of Disability*.

Phase I (2006)—Developing a Preliminary Model of *Integrated Evaluation of Disability*: The project initiated a literature review and developed an initial model of *Integrated Evaluation of Disability* incorporating disability dimensions, such as impairment, limitation of activity and participation restriction, and environmental and personal factors.

Phase II (2007)—Review of the Preliminary Model by Experts: Experts in physical medicine and rehabilitation practicing disability evaluation from Belgium, India, Israel, Kuwait, the Netherlands, Romania, and US reviewed the preliminary model of *Integrated Evaluation of Disability* and provided their opinions.

Phase III (2008–2011)—Analysis of the Reviews and Views of the Experts: The project analyzed the expert opinions on *Integrated Evaluation of Disability*. Their reviews and views enabled the incorporation of relevant changes. Further, it developed clinical tools, "Activity Participation Skill Assessment Scale," "Environmental Factors Measurement Scale," and "Personal Factors Measuring Scale" for evaluation of disability.

The project introduced the "Modified Delphi Process" for further refinement. The panelists from Austria, Czech Republic, India, Kuwait, and the United States consented to participate in the "Modified Delphi Process."

Phase IV (2011–2013)—Modified Delphi Process: The "Modified Delphi Process" evaluated the appropriateness of non-standardized clinical methods/tools, and grading of the severity of impairment/disability. It also evaluated the method of assigning impairment, "Activity Participation Skill Assessment Scale," "Environmental Factors Measurement Scale," and "Personal Factors Measurement Scale."

Phase V (2012–2017)—Review by Senior Physicians: Senior physicians in physical medicine and rehabilitation, orthopedics, cardiology, pulmonology, plastic surgery, hematology, urology, nephrology, and psychiatry reviewed the final work and provided their suggestion. The project incorporated relevant suggestions pertinent to the *Integrated Evaluation of Disability*.

Phase VI (2014–2017)—Pilot Study with the Clinical Model: The project instituted a pilot study to apply *Integrated Evaluation of Disability* in clinical models and developed a "Ready Reckoner Impairment Table" for about 300 clinical conditions with multiple clinical presentations. The project envisioned valuable hints to improve further the intricacy of clinical methods/tools, grading of severity of impairment/disability as well as assigning impairment. Thus, it has assisted to develop an optimum method of evaluation of impairment/disability and assigning impairment.

Phase VII (2017)—Software: The project initiated the development of software to help physicians practicing disability evaluation save time when computing the whole person disability.

2.2 EVOLUTION OF METHODS OF DISABILITY EVALUATION

2.2.1 WHO—ICIDH 1980

In 1980, WHO introduced the International Classification of Impairment, Disabilities and Handicap (IDICH). Section 1.3.1 of Chapter 1 describes in detail the disability process of ICIDH 1980.

2.2.2 Medical and social models

The medical model represents disability as a problem directly caused by disease, trauma, or other health conditions (1).

It focuses mainly on the diagnosis and treatment of diseases and injuries. Thus, the disability is a discussion of the personal aspect for health-care intervention in the medical model. The medical model is limited to a narrow band of evaluation of impairment in the broader spectrum of the disability. The real disability model must also incorporated social factors. Hence, the social model concerns with reintegration of the person with a disability into the society (1,2).

Initially, physicians and authorities have used impairment evaluation only to discharge persons with disability from service, to claim compensation for work-related injuries, and to extend disability benefits. Subsequently, there is a shift in evaluation based on impairment with functional limitations and/or earning capacity. Illustration 2.1 summarizes the rationale of the medical model and social model.

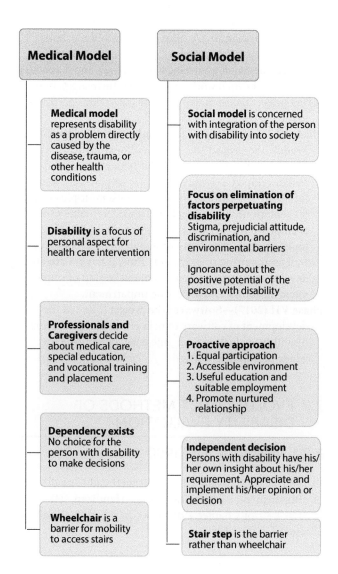

Illustration 2.1 Medical model and social model.

2.2.3 National Center for Medical Rehabilitation Research (1993)

The research plan for the National Center for Medical Rehabilitation Research (NCMRR) considers restrictions related to social policy, structural barriers, or attitudinal barriers may prevent the person to perform his/her role, and avail services and opportunities for complete participation in the society (3). The NCMRR model emphasizes the social limitations restricting the participation of a person with a disability to perform his/her major life activities. For example, these restrictions include a lack of cooperation from employers to build ramps to gain access to the public buildings by the person with a disability (4). NCMRR stresses that a broad spectrum of disability with its impact on the main life activities indicates the necessity for a continuing determination to evolve and interpret disability based on scientific and social understanding (5).

2.2.4 New Institute of Medicine (IOM) Model (1997): Enabling–Disabling Process Model

The Institute of Medicine (IOM) Enabling–Disabling Process Model (1997) states that disability dislocates the person from their prior integration into the social structures of family, community, society, and physical space. A person without a disability is integrated into society with complete access to education and employment, has the ability to perform the role of parenthood and leadership, and so on, as well as has access to physical space.

This model highlights that an occult disability becomes an overt disability when the stigma of disability displaces the person from the environment. It emphasizes providing access to the environment namely physical space (e.g., provision of ramps) (4), and to a social structure for performing parental/family roles, educational and vocational pursuits, social and community activities, and his/her role as a citizen to alleviate his/her disability. This model correctly identifies the environment as a pathway for rehabilitation-intervention.

It defines disability as an outcome due to an interaction between the person and their environment. It describes the physical, and social environment and interaction of the individual with the environment as a three-dimensional mat. The interaction of the disabled person with the environment produces deflection in the mat. The amount of displacement denotes the severity of the disability. The enabling and disabling factors control the displacement. The environmental support represents a enabling factor, and lack of environmental support represents a disabling factor (4).

2.2.5 Institute of Medicine Mathematical Model of Disability

The IOM developed a Mathematical Model of Disability for computing the real status of disability. In this model, the sum of pathology (P), impairment (I) and functional limitation (FL) denotes the potential disability (PD) (4). Disability is a function of potential disability and the environment

$$\text{Disability} = \frac{\text{potential disability}}{\text{environment}} \qquad (2.1)$$

2.2.6 World Health Organization's Disability Assessment Schedule (2000)

World Health Organization's Disability Assessment Schedule (WHODAS) describes the scope of disability evaluation in a broader perspective and the importance of diagnosis and assessment of disability (6). WHODAS focuses mainly on six domains of the main life activities namely understanding and communicating, mobility, self-care, interacting with people, life activities, and participation in society. It has not included evaluation of impairment of function and structure, environmental, and personal factors.

2.2.7 International Classification of Functioning, Disability, and Health 2001

WHO reviewed ICIDH 1980 and identified inadequate consideration to the environmental factors; no clear demarcation between impairment and disability dimensions, and disability and handicap dimension; and lack of explanation about the precise association and temporal relationship between these dimensions (7) (Illustration 2.2). Hence, International Classification of Functioning, Disability, and Health (ICF) emerged in 2001. It retained the former term "Impairment," and replaced the previous terms "Disability" and "Handicap" with "Activity limitation" and "Participation restriction." In ICF, the disability represents an umbrella term for the whole disability process, that is, impairments, activity limitations, and participation-restrictions. Illustration 2.2 depicts the primary difference in the disability process in WHO–ICIDH 1980 and WHO–ICF 2001.

2.2.7.1 IMPAIRMENTS, ACTIVITY LIMITATIONS, AND PARTICIPATION RESTRICTIONS

ICF describes *"Impairment is a loss or abnormality in body structure or physiological function including mental functions," "Activity limitations are difficulties an individual may have in executing activities,"* and *"Participation-restrictions are problems an individual may experience in involvement in life situations"* (8).

2.2.7.2 ENVIRONMENTAL FACTORS AND PERSONAL FACTORS

The intricate relationship between a person's health condition and environmental and personal factors tends to modify the severity of the disability.

Access to physical and rehabilitation medical management measures, such as physiotherapy, occupational therapy, speech therapy, artificial limbs, appliances, and mobility aids; and provision of a barrier-free environment in public buildings, bus stations, airport and park helps foster a supportive environment. A supportive environment decreases or eliminates impairment, limitation of activity, and participation restriction.

An architect sustained a fracture D8 vertebra following road traffic accident and developed spastic paraplegia. His mobility, activities, and participation in daily activities were limited or restricted. His limitation of activities also included washing his body, toileting, dressing, eating, writing, commuting on public transport, or driving his car. His restriction of participation included resuming his work as an architect, using public utility services and health care, going to the bank, gardening, and visiting his friends and relatives. He underwent physical and rehabilitation medicine management and started ambulating with a wheelchair. The environmental barriers were perpetuating his limitations due to thresholds, doorways, stairs, inaccessible toilet/bath for a wheelchair, electrical fixtures, inappropriate work table and computer desk for a wheelchair, lack of

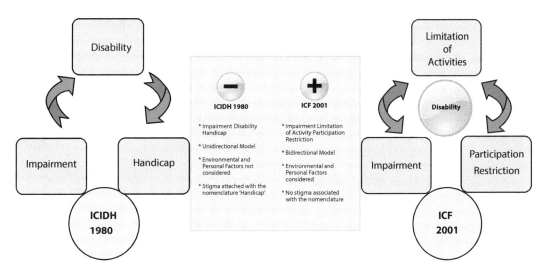

Illustration 2.2 Comparison of ICIDH and ICF 2001.

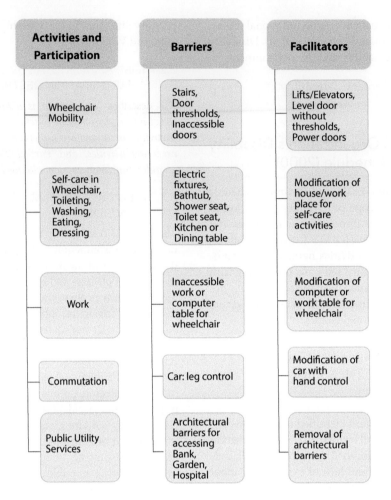

Illustration 2.3 Activities and participation, barriers, and facilitators.

leg controls for driving a car, and inaccessible roads for a wheelchair to inspect outdoor construction work. Removal of architectural barriers in his home/workplace, a hand control in the car along with training for transfer himself to the car and stowing a wheelchair, workplace modification, and psychological adaptation enabled him to resume his work as an architect. Removing the barriers and creating facilitators decreased the gap between his capacity and performance. Illustration 2.3 illustrates strongly the concept of ICF to eliminate obstacles and create facilitators for reviving his/her activity as well as participation in his/her vocational and avocational tasks.

Personal factors include age, gender, race, education, character, health status, lifestyle, personal habits, behavioral and psychological strategies, earning capacity, and social status.

2.2.7.3 BIOPSYCHOSOCIAL APPROACH

ICF emphasizes that disability is not only related to the impairment of function and/structure, but also to multiple factors emerging from the social environment. Hence the society must develop social action and provide environmental modifications for the full and efficient participation of the persons with disability in every activity of social life (1). Both environmental and personal factors have either facilitatory

or inhibitory influence on the alleviation of disability (9). Hence, ICF advanced the Biopsychosocial Approach. It integrates medical and social models of disability to encompass all dimensions of functioning including insights and perceptions about biological, personal, and social factors (1). Illustration 2.4 depicts the biopsychosocial approach of ICF.

2.2.8 World Bank (2007)

The World Bank remarks that disability is an outcome of an interaction between the person and his/her environment, and, hence, disability is not precisely specific to a person or environment (10). The social model anticipates that if the environment incorporates suitable accommodation and extends the necessary support, a person with impairment could participate fully in society by regularly performing their function and role and, thus, is not disabled (11).

2.2.9 Americans with Disabilities Act of 1990 (2009)

The Americans with Disabilities Act (ADA) refers to a physical or mental impairment as a disability. The impairment significantly limits one or more of the main life activities and

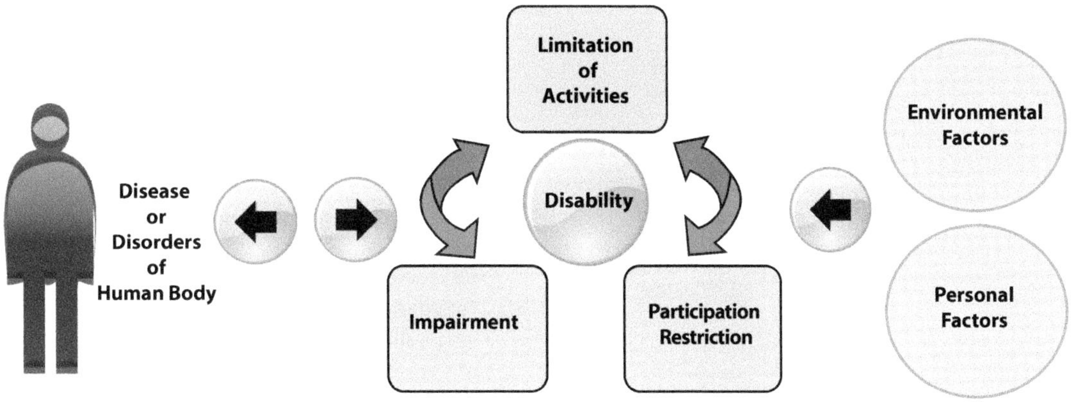

Illustration 2.4 Biopsychosocial Approach.

primary bodily functions of a person. The main life activities include self-care, manual tasks, vision, hearing, eating, sleeping, mobility, speech, breathing, learning, reading, concentrating, thinking, communicating, and working. The primary bodily functions comprise the immune functions, tissue growth, digestive, bowel, bladder functions, neurological, brain, respiratory, circulatory, endocrine, and reproductive functions (12).

2.2.10 World Disability Report (2011)

The World Disability Report remarks that there is a change in thinking from medical perspective to a social perspective, that is, from a medical model to social model. Hence, there is a tendency to relate disability due to social limitations rather than due to impairment of function because of a medical condition. It is essential not to predict or interpret disability wholly due to a medical condition or entirely due to social limitations. Hence it is necessary to assign proper weight to every aspect of disability considering the impact of both medical conditions, and social limitations imposed on the person with a disability (13). The Preamble to the United Nations Convention on the Rights of Persons with Disabilities (CRPD) accepts that disability is an evolving concept, and further emphasizes that disability is an outcome of an interaction between the person with an impairment and environmental and attitudinal barriers. It prevents the person with a disability to participate fully in the society on an equal basis with fellow citizens (13).

2.2.11 Prevailing methods of disability evaluation in other countries

Chapter 4 describes in detail about methods of disability evaluation in Belgium, France, Italy, the United Kingdom, Germany, the United States (AMA method), Japan, India, Korea, Australia, Canada, Switzerland, Kenya, South Africa, the Netherlands, and China.

2.2.12 Prevailing methods of disability evaluation based on ICF

Chapter 4 describes in detail about how the Cyprus Republic, Germany, Switzerland, Italy, and Taiwan applies the method of disability evaluation based on ICF.

2.3 INTEGRATED EVALUATION OF DISABILITY

2.3.1 Concept of the *Integrated Evaluation of Disability*

Integrated Evaluation of Disability is a holistic method. It assesses and integrates the impairment of function and/or structure, limitation of activities, participation restriction, environmental barriers/supports, and personal factors to derive whole person disability. For example, impairment of structure refers to amputation of the leg. Impairment of functions denotes loss of muscle power, loss of sensation of hand, and loss of control over urination. Limitation of activities represents a limitation in accomplishing personal demands such as self-care: washing whole body/parts of the body, toileting, grooming, dressing, eating and drinking; ability to move from one place to another; and daily chores. Restriction of participation refers to constraints in educational and vocational pursuits, relationship demands (parental/family roles), social and community activities, and citizenship roles of a country, and so on.

Environmental factors refer to access to medical management, rehabilitation facilities, elimination of architectural barriers (such as the provision of an elevator), and attitudinal barriers, such as social stigma.

Personal factors include the behavior of the person toward their disability and working and earning capacity to compute the whole person disability (Illustration 2.5).

2.3.2 Need for an integrated evaluation

The illustration *vide infra* emphasizes the need for an integrated evaluation of impairment, limitation of

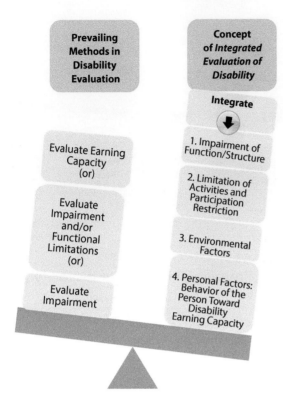

Illustration 2.5 Concept of *Integrated Evaluation of Disability*.

activity, restriction of participation, environmental support or barriers, and the behavior of the person toward his/her disability and earning capacity.

1. An agricultural worker, who had no formal education, underwent an amputation of his/her leg and can walk after being fitted with an artificial limb. The fitting of an artificial limb decreased his/her limitation of activity. However, he/she would remain unemployed, as he/she could not return to his/her agricultural work. Furthermore, alternate employment may not be possible because of his/her illiteracy and limitation of participation would persist. On the other hand, a bank employee sustained a similar amputation and received a similar artificial limb. Indeed, he/she resumes his/her job, decreased his/her limitation of activity, and eliminated participation restriction. Thus, two persons with the same level of amputation may not have the same disability. They cannot have the same percentage of disability.

2. A person with a finger amputation would derive only a small percentage of disability. However, in the case of a pianist, where loss of a finger or part of it has much higher disability because of his occupation/recreation, the percentage of disability would be higher.

3. A person with achromatopsia cannot recognize any color signal (14). He/she perceives only greyscale between black and white and lacks the full experience of color perception in their environment. This may affect his/her activities of daily living. He/she also finds difficulty in identifying the color signal in a traffic light and can drive only by locating the illumination of upper, middle, or lower lights. Thus, he/she has a greater risk of being involved in an accident. Further, color discrimination is significantly important in certain occupations requiring critical safety tasks, such as in air, marine, road and train transport systems as well as in certain trades. Hence, he/she may not be eligible for occupations, such as a pilot, trainman engineer, railroad worker, firefighter, and signalman on railways. Thus, the disability depends not only on acuity or field of vision but also on other functions of vision such as color vision.

4. A person with an IQ of 35 has a moderate impairment. His/her overall performance in major life activities would be at a low ebb. If the environment in which he/she lives has no resources for special education or vocational training for people with special needs, he/she will remain dependent on help to perform major life activities and have limited independent living. It emphasizes the need to also evaluate limitation of activity, participation restriction, and environmental support, since impairment evaluation alone may misjudge the gravity of disability.

5. The availability of and access to rehabilitation services for a person with a disability influences the severity of the disability. An individual with stroke was not able to walk, climb stairs, commute, and pursue employment. Rehabilitation programs such as physiotherapy, occupational therapy, and an appliance fitted to his/her lower extremity would enable him/her to walk with the help of elbow crutches/cane. Provision of a hand control in the car would help a person to drive and commute to work. Provision of a lift in the workplace would give a person access to the higher floors. The receipt of appropriate rehabilitation services and environmental support decreases mostly limitation of activity and restriction of participation, thus grossly reducing the severity of the disability. It underlines the need for assessing rehabilitation services (environmental support) given to the person with a disability for computing percentage of disability.

6. A person with a traumatic amputation of a leg or hand may not be able to avail artificial limb in centers far from their residence even after availing government concession for commutation. It may be due to the difficulty in meeting the daily expenses toward food and caretakers during commuting and rehabilitation management. Ithighlights the need for assessing the economic status of the person (personal factors) to compute the percentage of disability.

7. The landscape in which the person with a disability is living has an impact on the severity of disability. To illustrate, a person with stroke was fitted with an appliance, such as an Ankle Foot Orthosis (AFO), residing in a mountainous terrain has difficulty in climbing up and down the slopes with or without elbow crutches or

a cane. This reiterates the need to include the landscape of the living surroundings for evaluation of disability.

8. Similarly, there are situations where medical management could help to reduce the disability. A person with end-stage renal disease would have had a severe impairment, limitation of activity, and restriction of participation. After renal transplantation, there was no impairment of function and only negligible amount of limitation of activity and restriction of participation. This scenario underlines the need for assessing available medical or rehabilitation measures rendered to the person for quantifying their disability.

9. The behavior of the person toward his/her disability could significantly modify the severity of disability. After experiencing a stroke, a person was unable to use his left arm and leg. He would not accept his inability to use his arm and leg. He was very adamant in refusing to undergo rehabilitation management and resisted counseling to cooperate with rehabilitation management. He became bedridden and dependent for help with all his activities, including self-care, and could not resume his business. His impairment of function, limitation of activity, and restriction of participation remained permanent regardless of environmental supports, such as accessibility to medical and rehabilitation management. Whereas, an engineering graduate sustained total inability to use both his arms and legs due to a spinal cord injury during his evaluation for employment. Following medical management, he was ambulant with a wheelchair but dependent for help in his daily living activities, including self-care. He accepted his disability and decided to lead a useful, productive life with his normal mental ability. He started teaching children with disability and opened a rehabilitation program for them in his house. His endeavor in instituting teaching programs and rehabilitation management has progressed from his small house through to middle schools, to high schools, and on to a medical and vocational rehabilitation center catering to a large population. Though his impairment of function persisted and his activity was limited to wheelchair mobility; there is no participation restriction in his yeoman service to humanity. These two examples assert the significance of the behavior of the person toward his/her disability for a complete evaluation of disability. Hence, *Integrated Evaluation of Disability* incorporates all these variables.

2.3.3 Scope of an *Integrated Evaluation of Disability*

Disability evaluation serves to estimate the prevalence of disabled persons and the magnitude of the severity of disability through health surveys; to develop policy, identify service needs, establish priorities, forecast plan, and distribute resources; to plan levels of health care and lengths

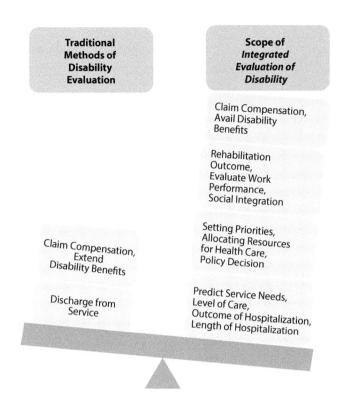

Illustration 2.6 Scope of *Integrated Evaluation of Disability*.

of hospitalization; and to measure the outcome of hospitalization and rehabilitation. Further, it enables the authorities to evaluate social integration; to decide insurance and/or accident related claims and extend benefits to persons with disabilities. Illustration 2.6 illustrates the scope of *Integrated Evaluation of Disability* and *Traditional Methods of Disability Evaluation*. Illustration 2.7 explains the basis of *Integrated Evaluation of Disability*.

2.3.4 *Integrated Evaluation of Disability*—Illustrations

2.3.4.1 FLACCID PARALYSIS—RIGHT LOWER EXTREMITY

A person with flaccid paralysis involving right lower extremity without environmental support obtains a disability of 35% (theoretical value) based on the integrated evaluation of impairment, limitation of activity and participation restriction, and personal and environmental factors. If this person receives environmental support namely an appliance—KAFO, lift/elevator in the house/workplace and modification of his/her car with hand control, his/her disability would decrease from 35% to 25% (Illustration 2.8).

2.3.4.2 END-STAGE RENAL DISEASE

A person with the end-stage renal disease would be having a severe disability—50%. However, after renal transplantation, there is the only negligible amount of disability—5%

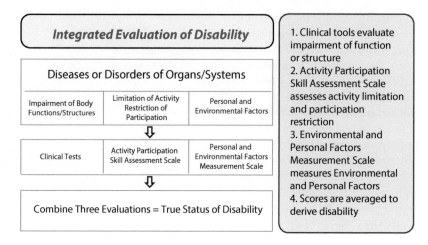

Illustration 2.7 Basis of *Integrated Evaluation of Disability*.

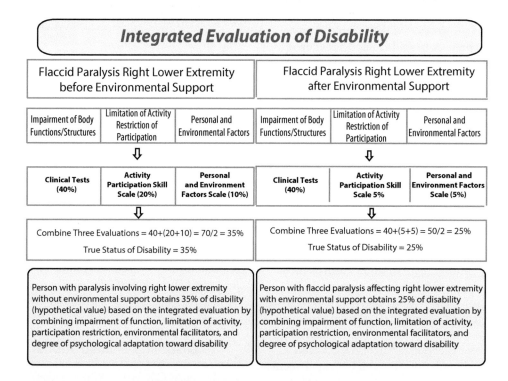

Illustration 2.8 Flaccid paralysis of lower extremity before and after environmental support.

(Illustration 2.9). It also stresses the need for assessing available medical or rehabilitation measures rendered to the person with a disability for quantifying disability.

2.3.4.3 DEAFNESS

An individual with deafness would be having a severe impairment, limitation of activity, and restriction of participation. A cochlear implant provides the perception of sounds by activation of the auditory nerve through an electronic device comprising of the microphone, speech processor, transmitter, receiver/stimulator, and an array of electrodes. A cochlear implant does not restore normal hearing but provides the perception of sounds for useful hearing in the environment (15).

This illustration again highlights the importance of assessing medical management rendered to the person for assigning a percentage of disability. The person with deafness is assigned whole person disability of 50%. The disability decreased after cochlear implant depending on the functional gain after cochlear implant (Illustration 2.10).

2.3.5 Clinical methods/tools/scales

Integrated Evaluation of Disability developed a methodology to evaluate disability by integrating impairment, limitation of activity and restriction of participation, environmental factors, the behavior of the person toward his/her disability and working and earning capacity. Clinical methods/tools

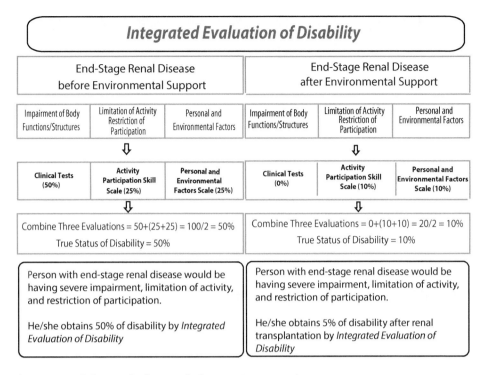

Illustration 2.9 End-stage renal disease before and after environmental support.

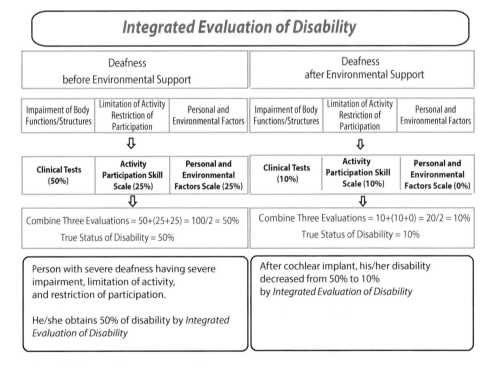

Illustration 2.10 Deafness before and environmental support.

including laboratory investigations and imaging studies, and "Activity Participation Skill Assessment Scale" (APSAS), "Environmental Factors Measurement Scale" (EFMS), and "Personal Factor Measurement Scale" (PFMS), and "Working and Earning Capacity Scale" provide a true assessment. Hence, *Integrated Evaluation of Disability* avoids subjective assumptions (Illustration 2.11) and assigns an optimum

percentage of disability to the whole person without any element of biased opinion or arbitrary judgment.

2.3.5.1 IMPAIRMENT

Integrated Evaluation of Disability has selected both standardized and non-standardized clinical methods/tools to evaluate impairment of function/structure. Non-standardized

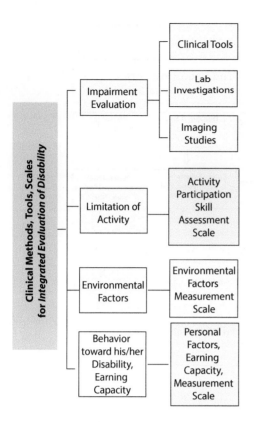

Illustration 2.11 Clinical methods, tools, scales for *Integrated Evaluation of Disability*.

clinical methods/tools underwent validation by "Modified Delphi Process" as well as a trial with "Clinical Model."

2.3.5.2 LIMITATION OF ACTIVITY AND PARTICIPATION RESTRICTION

Integrated Evaluation of Disability has developed "Activity Participation Skill Assessment Scale" (APSAS) for assessing limitation of activity and participation restriction. The "Activity Participation Skill Assessment Scale" evaluates nine domains of activity and participation namely learning-applying knowledge-acquiring skills, task management skills, communication, mobility, self-care, household activities, interpersonal skills, participation in educational-vocational pursuits, economic transaction and management, and participation in community, social, and civic life.

2.3.5.3 PERSONAL AND ENVIRONMENTAL FACTORS

"Environmental Factors Measurement Scale" (EFMS) evaluates environmental support/barriers. It evaluates mainly four types of environmental factors comprising of technological services, architectural design, social security including health services and policies, and attitudinal environment. "Personal Factors Measurement Scale" (PFMS) evaluates the behavior of the person toward his/her disability and working and earning capacity.

2.3.6 Severity scale for disability

Integrated Evaluation of Disability developed a severity scale. "No disability" refers to a score of "0" or

0%–4%. "Mild disability" denotes a score of "1" or 5%–24%. "Moderate disability" represents a score of "2" or 25%–49%. "Severe disability" describes a score of "3" or 50%–74%. "Profound disability" indicates a score of "4" or 75%–94%. "Complete disability" assigns a score of "5" or 95%–100%. The severity scale quantifies the severity of impairment, limitation of activity and participation restriction, environmental support and barriers, and behavior of the person toward his/her disability and earning capacity (Table 2.1).

2.3.7 Basis for assigning impairment or disability

Integrated Evaluation of Disability allocates impairment based on motor and sensory representation in the homunculus, a weighted score (based on the severity of impairment, limitation of activity, participation restriction, and environmental barriers), the consensus opinion of experts through the "Modified Delphi Process", and outcome of the pilot study with the "Clinical Model."

2.3.8 Combining impairment by formula

The following formula (Equation 2.2) combines impairment of different functions, namely, consciousness, sleep, intelligence, cognition, language functions; cranial nerve functions; spinal motor, spinal sensory functions of right upper extremity, left upper extremity, right lower extremity, left lower extremity, and spine; renal, bladder, bowel, genital functions; cardiac and pulmonary functions; and structural impairments, such as amputation, congenital skeletal limb deficiencies, dwarfism, and burns, to limit the impairment to maximum of 100%.

$$A + \frac{B(100-A)}{100} \qquad (2.2)$$

Example: In the formula $A + [B(100-A)/100]$, where "100" represents normal capacity of the person, "A" denotes higher impairment, for example, motor impairment of right upper extremity—60% "B" denotes lower impairment, for example, motor impairment of right lower extremity—40%. The percentage of impairment after combining with the formula $A + [B(100-A)/100]$ is 76%. After impairment his/her residual capacity is 24%.

2.3.9 Combining impairment, limitation of activity, and participation restriction

Integrated Evaluation of Disability combines the percentage of impairment, the Activity Participation Skill Assessment score, personal factors measurement score, and environmental factors measurement score. It combines percentage of biological impairment (76%), and psychosocial limitation and restriction, which is the percentage of limitation of activity and participation restriction, and personal and environmental score (74%) to obtain an average. The average is 75% (76 + 74 = 150/2). The average refers to the whole person disability, that is, 75%.

Table 2.1 Severity scale of *Integrated Evaluation of Disability*

Impairment scale	Activity Participation Skill Assessment Scale	Personal Factors Measurement Scale	Environmental Factors Measurement Scale
Impairment: 0%–4%	Performs normally all activities and participate normally in educational and vocational pursuits, social, community, and civic life	Normal behavior for activities and participation in educational and vocational pursuits, social, community, and civic life. Loss of earning capacity 1%–4%	95%–100% of environmental facilitators such as assistive technology services, architectural design, social security including health services, systems and policies, and attitudinal environment exist
Mild Impairment: 5%–24%	Performs all activities and normally participate in educational and vocational pursuits, social, community, and civic life, but taking more time than normal	Extends full cooperation for all activities and participation in educational and vocational pursuits, social, community, and public life after counseling. Post-morbid earning capacity with loss of income: 5%–24%	75%–94% of environmental facilitators exist
Moderate Impairment: 25%–49%	Performs all activities and regularly participate in educational and vocational pursuits, social, community, and civic life with difficulty and maximum effort	Provides partial cooperation for all activities and participation in educational and vocational pursuits, social, community, and public life after counseling. Post morbid earning capacity with loss of income: 25%–49%	50%–74% of environmental facilitators exist
Severe Impairment: 50%–74%	Performs all activities and participate in educational and vocational pursuits, social, community, and civic life using orthosis/ prosthesis or mobility aids or assistive devices or supportive and safety devices or visual aids or hearing aids	Extends poor cooperation for all activities and participation in educational and vocational pursuits, social, community, and civic life with depression. Post morbid earning capacity with loss of income: 50%–74%	25%–49% of environmental facilitators exist
Profound Impairment: 75%–94%	Performs all activities and participate in educational and vocational pursuits, social, community, and civic life only with personal assistance	Lack of cooperation for all activities and participation in educational and vocational pursuits, social, community, and public life with aggressive behavior. Post morbid earning capacity with loss of income: 75%–94%	5%–24% of environmental facilitators exist
Complete Impairment: 95%–100%	Inability to perform all activities and participate in educational and vocational pursuits, social, community, and civic life	Exhibits noncooperation for all activities and participation in educational and vocational pursuits, social, community, and public life with suicidal tendency. Post morbid earning capacity with loss of income: 95%–100%	1%–4% of environmental facilitators exist

2.3.10 Criteria for permanent impairment

Integrated Evaluation of Disability assesses the impairment of function and structure once the impairment is permanent. The impairment becomes permanent within about 1–2 years after maximum medical improvement stops without any further scope for advancement with the utmost medical care. It stresses that further medical treatment is unlikely to yield significant functional improvement to a level that enables the person to perform major life activities and to participate in the community, and social and civic life (Box 2.1).

BOX 2.1: Criteria for permanent impairment

1. The medical condition is stable without any further scope of improvement within about one to two years with maximum medical management
2. The clinical condition is progressively worsening with maximum medical management and without any further scope of recovery (or) improvement, for instance, motor neuron disease or Duchene muscular dystrophy
3. The clinical condition is relapsing and remitting, such as in multiple sclerosis, and the residual neurological deficit remained stationary for about 1–2 years
4. The condition deemed to have reached a status of maximum medical improvement when the surgery is contraindicated due to medical reasons

Impairment: Clinical tools evaluate impairment of function and structure

Limitation of Activity and Participation Restriction: "Activity Participation Skill Assessment Scale" assesses a person's limitation of activity, participation restriction, and adaptive behavior

Personal and Environmental Factors: "Personal Factors Measurement Scale" and "Environmental Factors Measurement Scale" measure adaptive behavior of the person toward disability and environmental support

---

2.3.11 Qualification of personnel to perform disability evaluation

ICF describes impairment as a loss or an abnormal body structure, affecting physiological and mental functions (8). Furthermore, the impairment refers to a variation or disparity in the biomedical status of the human body from population-based norms. Those who are qualified are primarily responsible for evaluating and deciding on the biomedical condition of the human body and its physical and mental functions based on these norms (16).

2.3.12 Ready Reckoner Impairment Table

Integrated Evaluation of Disability has developed a "Ready Reckoner Impairment Table" based on the outcome of a pilot study on the "Clinical Model" to assign impairment for 34 system/organ/major clinical modules with about 300 multiple clinical presentations. The clinician can retrieve the impairment score directly from the "Ready Reckoner Impairment Table" for the corresponding clinical presentation.

2.3.13 Software

The software integrated with the book on the Companion Website can help physicians to compute with ease and save time when evaluating disability.

It allows the user to choose their method of assessment either impairment evaluation or limitation of activity and participation restriction or impairment, limitation of activity, and participation restriction.

It will also allow choosing integrated assessment of disability to encompass function, activity and participation, and environmental and personal factors.

It will further permit the evaluator to select the required system, organ, extremities, or whole person for disability evaluation.

2.3.14 Roadmap to adopt *Integrated Evaluation of Disability*

Each country has different methods to arrive at the percentage of disability. The criteria may be either impairment and/or impact on daily activities and/or earning capacity. **Roadmap may provide guidance for adopting *Integrated Evaluation of Disability* based on the prevailing laws and acts in the respective countries.** Keeping pace with the need for evaluating the whole person disability, they can strive to apply integrated evaluation of impairment, limitation of activity and participation restriction, and environmental and personal factors. Illustration 2.12 represents the roadmap for using *Integrated Evaluation of Disability*.

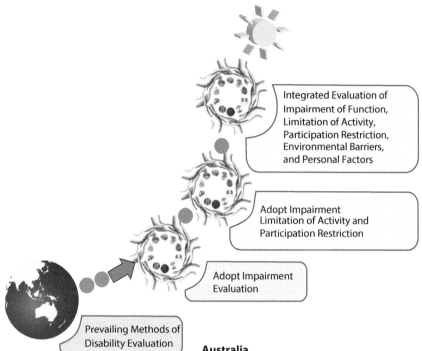

Australia
Eligible Age: Persons between 15 years and pension age
Permanent Impairment: Physical, visual, intellectual, or psychiatric conditions
Inability to work or be retrained for minimum of 15 hours per week
within 2 years following impairment
Canada
Functional limitations imposed by the medical condition
resulting in severe and prolonged physical or mental disability
preventing one to pursue gainful regular employment
Europe
Methods of evaluation of disability differ between
countries. Impairment and/or impact on daily activities and/or
occupational status
India
Impairment of function/structure and limitation of
activities
Japan
Impairment resulting in inability or limitation to
perform daily activities or impairment in their ability to work
Korea
Medically measurable permanent impairment indicating the degree of
difficulty in usual activities of daily living except job or work
US AMA
Diagnosis-based impairment evaluation using key and non-key
factors such as physical findings, clinical studies, functional impact of
the clinical condition, and burden of treatment compliance

Illustration 2.12 Roadmap to adopt *Integrated Evaluation of Disability*.

REFERENCES

1. World Health Organization. *ICF - International Classification of Functioning, Disability and Health.* Geneva, Switzerland: WHO; 2001. p. 20.
2. Kate S. Trends in rehabilitation and disability: Transition from a medical model to an integrative model (part 1). *Disability World,* 2004. Available from: www.disabilityworld.org.
3. National Institutes of Health. *Research Plan for the National Center for Medical Rehabilitation Research.* Washington, DC: US Department of Health and Human Services; 1993. pp. 23–25.
4. Brandt EN, Pope AM. *Models of Disability and Rehabilitation: Evolution of Models of Disability.* Washington, DC: National Academy Press; 1997 [cited Institute of Medicine].
5. National Center for Medical Rehabilitation Research (NCMRR) 20th Anniversary Scientific Symposium: Advancing Research to improve the lives of persons with disability National center for Medical Rehabilitation Research; 2011, December 12–13. p. 33.
6. WHO DAS II. *Disability Assessment Schedule Training Manual: A Guide to Administration, World Health Organization, Classification, Assessment, and Survey Team (CAS), Global Programme on Evidence for Health Policy (GPE).* Geneva, Switzerland: WHO; 2000. p. 9.
7. Gray DB, Hendershot GE. The ICIDH-2: Developments for a new era of outcomes research. *Arch Phys Med Rehabil.* 2000;81(12 Suppl 2):S10–S14.
8. *International Classification of Functioning, Disability and Health.* Geneva, Switzerland: World Health Organization; 2001. p. 213.
9. *International Classification of Functioning, Disability and Health.* Geneva, Switzerland: World Health Organization; 2001. p. 17.
10. Team DMaDD. *Measuring Disability Prevalence.* Washington, D.C: The Social Protection Advisory Service, The World Bank; 2007.
11. Mont D. Measuring health and disability. *Lancet.* 2007;369(9573):1658–1663.
12. *Americans with disabilities Act of 1990, and ADA Amendments Act of 2008 by the (P.L. 110-325).* In: Justice USDo, editor. United States Code; 1990 and 2008. p. 7.
13. World Health Organization TWB. *World Report on Disability.* Geneva, Switzerland: World Health Organization; 2011. p. 4.
14. Rehabilitation ISfLvRa, editor. GUIDE for the evaluation of VISUAL impairment. *International Low Vision Conference VISION-99.* San Francisco, CA: Pacific Vision Foundation; 1999.
15. *Cochlear Implants.* In: (NIDCD) N-NIoDaOCD, editor. Washington, DC: U.S. Department of Health & Human Services; 2014.
16. *International Classification of Functioning, Disability and Health.* Geneva, Switzerland: World Health Organization; 2001. p. 12.

3

Literature review and selection of clinical tools and scales

National Institute of Disability and Rehabilitation Research states that disability does not represent illness (1). It is hard to define and measure disability as it involves life activities with environmental interaction (2). Evaluation of impairment of function/structure, limitation of activity, participation restriction, environmental support or barriers, and adaptive behavior of the person toward their disability need specific clinical methods to assign an optimum percentage of disability.

3.1 SELECTION OF FUNCTIONS AND STRUCTURES FOR EVALUATION OF IMPAIRMENT

Body functions refer to physiological and psychological functions of the body. Body structures relate to anatomical systems or regions of the body—organs, limbs, and their segments. *Integrated Evaluation of Disability* has selected groups of functions and structures. It comprises neurological functions, namely consciousness functions, intellectual functions, cognitive functions, calculation functions, functions of motor planning to perform movements, sleep functions, language functions, voice functions, speech functions, swallowing function, and olfactory function. It also includes muscle power functions, muscle tone functions, muscle endurance functions, movement functions, and sensory functions. It includes musculoskeletal functions, namely mobility and stability of a joint. It further includes renal functions, micturition functions, bowel movement and defecation functions, genital functions, pulmonary functions, cardiac functions, and hematological and immunological functions.

3.2 REVIEW OF LITERATURE AND IDENTIFICATION OF CLINICAL TOOLS AND SCALES

The literature review explored clinical tests, methods, scales, practice guidelines, criteria, definitions, and parameters to choose the appropriate clinical tools for evaluating impairment of function and structure (Illustration 3.1, Tables 3.1 through 3.5).

3.3 SELECTION OF ACTIVITIES, PARTICIPATION, AND ENVIRONMENTAL FACTORS

"Activity" is an action accomplished by the person to sustain their daily life and concurs the individual's view toward his/her functioning. "Participation" is taking part in life events and refers to the social approach of functioning. "Environmental factors" refer to the factors existing in a person's immediate surroundings. It comprises of the physical, social, and attitudinal environment. Architectural barriers hinder the mobility of people with artificial limbs, appliances, crutches, wheelchairs, and walking canes at home and in the community. Structural modifications in the environment; assistive technology facilitators for communication, mobility, and transportation; and social support enable the participation of the individual with a disability in rehabilitation programs. Social support enhances the reintegration of the person into their home and society (35). Environmental factors, namely natural environment, transportation, access to health care, assistance at home, and governmental policy, have a strong association with life satisfaction of persons with disabilities resulting from spinal cord injury (36).

Integrated Evaluation of Disability has chosen specific activities to evaluate disability. It comprises of learning-applying knowledge-acquiring skills, task management skills, communication, mobility, self-care, household activities, interpersonal skills, participation in educational and vocational pursuits, economic transaction and management, and participation in community, social and civic life. *Integrated Evaluation of Disability* has also selected specific environmental and personal factors relevant to disability evaluation.

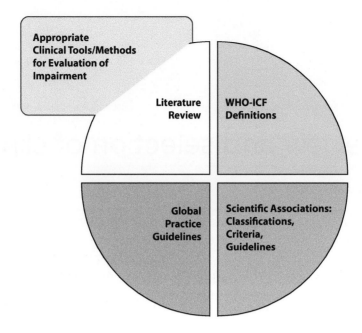

Illustration 3.1 Literature review.

Table 3.1 Exploring/searching of clinical methods/tools/definition/criteria/classification/scales: Neurological functions—Consciousness, sleep, IQ, and speech

No	Clinical methods/tools	Source
1	Impairment of function, limitation of activity, restriction of participation, and environmental and personal factors	International Classification of Functioning, Disability and Health: ICF, World Health Organization (3)
2	Definition of vegetative state	Practice parameters: Assessment and management of patients in the persistent vegetative state 1994, American Academy of Neurology (4)
3	Evaluation of sleep function	The International Classification of Sleep Disorders, Revised: Diagnostic and Coding Manual, American Academy of Sleep Medicine (5), Rules for scoring respiratory events in sleep: update of the 2007 AASM Manual for the Scoring of Sleep and Associated Events. Deliberations of the Sleep Apnea Definitions Task Force of the American Academy of Sleep Medicine (6)
4	Description of insomnia and fatal coma	Final Panel Statement (7)
5	Classification of IQ	IQ classification in Psychiatric use, *Diagnostic and Statistical Manual of Mental Disorders* (DSM-IV), American Psychiatric Association (8)
6	Evaluation of IQ	Wechsler Adult Intelligence Scale III (9). Raven's matrices (10)
7	Evaluation of stuttering	Bloodstein method (11)

Table 3.2 Exploring/searching clinical methods/tools/definition/criteria/classification/scales: Neurological functions—Cranial nerves, sensory, and motor functions

No	Clinical methods/tools	Source
8	Evaluation of smell—Olfactory Perception Function	Standard clinical test—Sniff the substance one after the other namely peppermint, almond oil, coffee, clove, soap
9	Evaluation of sensory function—Trigeminal Nerve	Standard clinical tests—Touch sensation and dissociated sensory loss
10	Evaluation of motor function—Trigeminal Nerve	Standard clinical test—Wasting and weakness of temporal masseters and pterygoid
11	Evaluation of motor function, taste sensation—Facial Nerve	Standard clinical tests
12	Evaluation of swallowing functions—Dysphagia	Swallowing Performance Status Scale (SPSS) (12–14)
13	Evaluation of muscle power—Manual Muscle Test	Medical Research Council (MRC) scale (15)
14	Evaluation of muscle tone	Modified Ashworth Scale (16)
15	Evaluation of range of motion (ROM) of joint	Standard clinical test—Goniometric or inclinometer measurement of passive range of motion of a joint
16	Evaluation of stability of joint in spine and extremities	Standard clinical tests—Abnormal mobility, drawer sign, telescopic test, etc., plain radiograph, open-mouth odontoid radiograph, Harris rule of 12's (17), plain CT, dynamic CT
17	Evaluation of sensory function	Standard clinical tests
18	Evaluation of chronic pain	Standard clinical—Visual analogue scale (18)

Table 3.3 Exploring/searching clinical methods/tools/definition/criteria/classification/scales: Cardiovascular functions

No	Clinical methods/tools	Source
19	Evaluation of functional capacity of heart	The Criteria Committee of the New York Heart Association Nomenclature and Criteria for Diagnosis of Diseases of the Heart and Great Vessels: Functional Capacity and Obj. Assessment of Patients with Diseases of the Heart 1994 (19)
20	Evaluation of heart failure	2009 Focused update incorporated into the ACC/AHA 2005 Guidelines for the Diagnosis and Management of Heart Failure in Adults, a report of the American College of Cardiology Foundation/American Heart Association Task Force on Practice Guidelines Developed in Collaboration with the International Society for Heart and Lung Transplantation (20)
21	Evaluation of functional limitations associated with cardiovascular diseases	Functional Classification of Goldman (21)
22	Evaluation of systolic (ejection fraction) and diastolic function	Evaluation of diastolic filling of left ventricle in health and disease: Doppler echocardiography is the clinician's Rosetta Stone (22)
23	Evaluation of cardiac rhythm abnormalities	2012 ACCF/AHA/HRS focused update incorporated into the ACCF/AHA/HRS 2008 guidelines for device-based therapy of cardiac rhythm abnormalities: a report of the American College of Cardiology Foundation/American Heart Association Task Force on Practice Guidelines and the Heart Rhythm Society (23)
24	Evaluation of valvular heart disease	2014 AHA/ACC Guideline for the Management of Patients with Valvular Heart Disease (24)

Table 3.4 Exploring/searching clinical methods/tools/definition/criteria/classification/scales: Functions of hematological and immunological systems

No	Clinical methods/tools	Source
25	Diagnosis of anemia	Hemoglobin concentrations for the diagnosis of anemia and assessment of severity 2011, Vitamin and Mineral Nutrition Information System (VMNIS), World Health Organization (25)
26	Evaluation of leukemia	Standard Clinical Tests—Parameters namely lymphocytosis in the blood and bone marrow, lymphadenopathy, hepatomegaly, splenomegaly, anemia, and thrombocytopenia
27	Severity classification of thrombocytopenia	Thrombocytopenia by Finnish Medical Society Duodecim, Evidence-Based Medicine (26)
28	Definitions in hemophilia	Definitions in hemophilia, Recommendation of the scientific subcommittee on factor VIII and factor IX of the scientific and standardization committee of the International Society on Thrombosis and Haemostasis 2001 (27)
29	Classification System for HIV Infection	1993 Revised Classification System for HIV Infection and Expanded Surveillance Case Definition for AIDS Among Adolescents and Adults (28)

Table 3.5 Searching clinical methods/tools/definition/criteria/classification/scales: Functions of respiratory system, digestive, and excretory systems and congenital disorders

No	Clinical methods/tools	Source
30	Asthma	Guidelines for the evaluation of impairment/disability in patients with asthma (29)
31	Evaluation of COPD	Global Initiative for Chronic Obstructive Lung Disease: Global strategy for the diagnosis, management, and prevention of chronic obstructive pulmonary disease (Updated 2013) (30)
32	Evaluation of respiratory failure	Standard clinical tests—PaO_2 and $PaCO_2$
33	Evaluation of vital capacity, FEV_1, FVC	Standard Clinical Test—Spirometry
34	Evaluation of chronic liver disease	AASLD practice guidelines: Evaluation of the patient for liver transplantation 2005 (31)
35	Evaluation of renal function	Clinical Practice Guidelines for Chronic Kidney Disease: Evaluation, Classification and Stratification—National Kidney Foundation Kidney Disease Outcomes Quality Initiative 2002 (32)
36	Classification of congenital limb deficiency	The ISO/ISPO classification of congenital limb deficiency 1991 (33)
37	Evaluation of short stature	Consensus statement on the diagnosis and treatment of children with idiopathic short stature: a summary of the Growth Hormone Research Society, the Lawson Wilkins Pediatric Endocrine Society, and the European Society for Pediatric Endocrinology Workshop 2008 (34)

3.4 REVIEW OF LITERATURE AND IDENTIFICATION OF SCALES FOR EVALUATION OF LIMITATION OF ACTIVITY, PARTICIPATION RESTRICTION, AND ENVIRONMENTAL AND PERSONAL FACTORS

Disability evaluation entails an assessment of impairment of functions and structure. It also includes measuring limitation of activity, participation restriction, and environmental support relating to the individual's personal, occupational, and social demands fundamental to acquiring the skills to live, learn, and work successfully in the community. However, it is not about the health aspect of the person with a disability. Retrieval and review of the literature revealed that the following scales, instruments, and tools exist for evaluation of functional status, functional status and quality of life measures, health-related quality of life outcome measures, and functional and social status outcome measures.

3.4.1 Functional Status Measures

3.4.1.1 PULSES

The PULHEMS (1943) profile served as a physical standard of instruction for the medical examination of army recruits and soldiers in the Canadian army (37). The US Army adopted the PULHEMS profile with some modification by incorporating mental and emotional components with the acronym PULHES. Moskowitz and McCann further modified with the acronym PULSES. In the acronym, PULSES "P" represents the physical condition, "U" represents upper limb functions, "L" lower limb functions, "S" sensory functions (speech, hearing, vision), "E" excretory functions, "S" mental and emotional status. It grades the impairment of functions as "Normal," "Mild," "Moderately Severe," and "Severe." The reliability and validity of the PULSES have been far less tested (38).

3.4.1.2 BARTHEL INDEX

The Barthel Index (1955) evaluates functional changes following a rehabilitation program of people with musculoskeletal and neurological disorders. It comprises of 10 measures of daily activities. Two measures related to mobility by walking and/or using a wheelchair on a level surface of 50 yards with or without devices or prostheses, and ascending and descending stairs. It includes eight measures related to self-care, namely nutrition, transfer activities, grooming, toileting, bathing, dressing, and bowel and bladder continence.

All of these activities are scored using a "Three-Point Scale," namely total dependence, assistance required to perform an activity, and total independence. The score 0 represents total dependence and 100 total independence (37,39,40).

3.4.1.3 KATZ ADL

Katz Activities of Daily Living (ADL) (1959) is a quantitative measure to evaluate functional changes in chronically ill persons under treatment. It comprises six measures of activities of daily living; that is, bathing, dressing, toileting (defecating, cleaning after defecation, arranging clothes), transfers (from bed to chair or chair to bed), continence (bowel, bladder), and feeding. It applies a "Three-Point Scale" from independence to dependence. It assigns an ordinal scale ranging from A to G where "A" represents total independence on all six activities and "G" total dependence on all six activities (37,39,41).

3.4.1.4 LEVEL OF REHABILITATION SCALE

The Level of Rehabilitation (LOR) scale published in 1978 evaluates In-Patient Rehabilitation Program (42). The last version of LOR III comprises of 18 items under four domains namely five in ADLs, two in mobility, five in communication, and six in cognitive functions. A "Two-Point Scale" evaluates memory, and a "Six-Point Scale" assesses remaining activities where 0 represents total dependence and 5 normal. Respective rehabilitation professionals, such as rehabilitation nurses, physiotherapists, occupational therapists, speech pathologists, and clinical psychologist complete the questionnaire (39). Velozo et al. remarked that there is a limitation of the LOR scales in patients with higher independence (43).

3.4.1.5 PATIENT EVALUATION AND CONFERENCE SYSTEM

This system was intended for functional assessment in adult rehabilitation programs to define the rehabilitation goal as well as to generate a follow-up outcome measure. The final revised version consists of 44 items under four domains—severity of impairment, self-care, motor functions, and cognitive functions. Members of the rehabilitation team evaluate these items using a seven-point ordinal scale where 1 represents total dependence, and 7 normal, scores 1–4 indicates dependent functions and scores 5 and above independent functions. Harvey and others also used this scale to develop a document after outpatient evaluation to referring physician (37,39,44).

3.4.1.6 FIM—FUNCTIONAL INDEPENDENCE MEASURE INSTRUMENT

American Congress of Rehabilitation Medicine and the American Academy of Physical Medicine and Rehabilitation supported a development of a uniform data system for the measurement of disability and outcome of rehabilitation management. It resulted in the Functional Independence Measure (FIM) Instrument in 1983 (39). The FIM instrument is widely used in rehabilitation settings. It comprises of six domains namely self-care, sphincter control, mobility, locomotion, communication, and social cognition. Each item derives a score from one to seven. Score 1 represents total assistance (performs less than 25% of a task or is unable to do the task). A score of 2 indicates maximum assistance and performs 25%–49% of the task, and a score of 3 indicates moderate assistance and performs 50%–75% of the task. A score of 4 represents minimal assistance, performs more than 75% of the task, and requires incidental hands-on help only. A score of 5 represents requiring supervision and only standby assistance, verbal prompting, or help with setup. Score 6 defines modified independence requiring the use of a device but no physical help, and 7 total independence (39,45). Ian McDowell remarked that FIM could serve as a brief assessment tool for evaluating disability (37). Stineman et al. described Activities of Daily Living, sphincter management, mobility, and executive function (ASME) staging for "Functional Independence Measure" as a common language. They developed a shorthand expression for functional consequences of disease and injury, and illustrated with a shorthand abbreviation for domains and functional independence. In ASME 5,1,6,7, the 5 represents supervision for ADL (A-5), 1 represents total dependence for sphincter management (S-1), 6 represents modified independence in mobility

(M-6), and 7 represents complete independence in executive function (E-7) (46). Granger et al. emphasized that FIM is useful in designing precise treatment programs and predicting outcomes of medical rehabilitation (47).

Cohen and Marino compared five generic Functional Status Measures—Barthel Index, Katz Index, FIM Instrument scale, Patient Evaluation Conference System, and LOR Scale. They have remarked that Barthel Index, LOR scale, Patient evaluation and conference system, and FIM instrument evaluate the disability, and FIM instrument serves as the best measure of disability (39).

3.4.2 Disability: Functional status and quality of life measures

3.4.2.1 WHOQOL—100

This instrument measures the quality of life under six domains—physical factors, psychological factors, status of independence, social rapport, environmental factors, and spiritual, religious or personal beliefs.

The World Health Organization Quality of Life (WHOQOL) scale can help serve in medical practice to select the best choices in patient care and improve a physician's understanding of how the disease affects a person's quality of life. It also assesses the effectiveness and relative merits of different treatment modalities, to evaluate health care, to assist research, and to help in policy making (37,48,49).

3.4.2.2 DISABILITY INTERVIEW SCHEDULE

The disability interview schedule comprises four domains, that is, mobility (walking, stairs, transfer, and travel), self-care, domestic duties (shopping, cooking, cleaning, washing clothes) and occupation. This schedule measures the prevalence and severity of disability in the epidemiological survey (50,51).

3.4.2.3 LAMBETH DISABILITY SCREENING QUESTIONNAIRE (VERSION 3)

This questionnaire serves to detect disability with a health survey. It comprises of questions relating to ambulation, mobility, self-care, sensory functions (seeing, hearing, speech), and social activity (cooking, household work, visiting family/friends, hobbies/spare time activities, paid work) (52,53).

3.4.2.4 OECD LONG-TERM DISABILITY QUESTIONNAIRE

Long-Term Disability Questionnaire (1981) of the Organization for Economic Cooperation and Development (OECD) compares disabilities and evaluate changes in disability over a specified period in the participating countries—Canada, Finland, France, West Germany, the Netherlands, Switzerland, the UK, and the United States.

The questionnaire measures disability relating to vision, hearing, mobility, feeding, self-care, and communication (53,54).

3.4.2.5 THE FUNCTIONAL STATUS RATING SYSTEM 1981

This system evaluates functional status in self-care, mobility, communication, psychosocial adjustment, and cognition (53,55,56).

3.4.2.6 FUNCTIONAL AUTONOMY MEASUREMENT SYSTEM—SMAF

This *système de mesure de l'autonomie fonctionnelle* (SMAF) measures the functional autonomy of the elderly persons. It evaluates mental functions, communication, mobility, ADL, and Instrumental Activities of Daily Living (IADL). The "Five-Point Scale" assesses each item where 0 is total independence, 0.5 with difficulty, 1 needs supervision, 2 needs help, and 3 total dependence. Physicians, nurses, or social workers use this measure to evaluate functional autonomy (57,58).

3.4.3 Health-related quality of life outcome measures

Health-related quality of life instruments evaluate outcome measures among people with disabilities and the general population regarding their health, level of independence, social relationships, environment, and spiritual activities.

3.4.3.1 NOTTINGHAM HEALTH PROFILE

The Nottingham Health Profile (NHP) evaluates emotional status, social isolation, sleep, energy, pain, physical mobility, vocation, social life, family life, sex life, housework, hobbies, and holidays (59–62).

3.4.3.2 SICKNESS IMPACT PROFILE

The Sickness Impact Profile (SIP) measures the perception of illness by the person. It includes sleep and rest, nutrition, ambulation, mobility, and restricted movement. Furthermore, it includes behavior during work, integration with family members, household activity, communication, leisure and recreation, intellectual functioning, emotional reactions, thoughts and inner feelings, hygiene, and participation in social activities. SIP assesses the outcome of health care (63).

3.4.3.3 SHORT-FORM 36

Short-Form 36, developed from the RAND Medical Outcome Study (MOS), measures health status as well as medical care outcome. It evaluates limitations or restrictions of physical activities, social participation, performing his/her role as a parent, citizen, member of the society, and so on, pain, stress and anxiety, energy and strength, and general health under eight domains of health status (64). Freeman et al. remarked that there is limitation of applying SF 36 as an outcome measure in multiple sclerosis due to lack of comparative supportive evidence from other relevant measures (65).

3.4.3.4 QUALITY OF WELL-BEING SCALE

It assesses the quality of life as it relates to the functional performance of mobility, physical activity, and social participation. It is a preference-weighted scale. Patient groups and the general population allocate weights by average ratings for different health states. Weight 0.0 represents death and 1.0 represents normal (62,66,67).

3.4.3.5 EUROQOL (EQ-5D)

The EQ-5D includes a questionnaire relating to mobility; self-care; education, work, household activities, family interaction, recreation; pain or discomfort; and anxiety/depression. It applies a "Three-Point Scale" to grade the severity of the problem (68).

3.4.3.6 HEALTH UTILITY INDEX

Health Utility Index (HUI) consists of a questionnaire relating to vision, hearing, speech, ambulation, dexterity, emotion, cognition, and pain (69–71).

Andresen and Meyers remarked that EQ-5D and HUI require additional work to assure their applicability for disability outcome research (62).

3.4.4 Functional and social status outcome measure

3.4.4.1 CRAIG HANDICAP ASSESSMENT AND REPORTING TECHNIQUE

The Craig Handicap Assessment and Reporting Technique (CHART) (1992) assesses physical activity, mobility, employment, participation in social activities, and economic self-reliance. The revised CHART also evaluates cognition. Each domain derives a maximum score of 100. The maximum score represents normal performance. Administration of CHART requires an interview either in-person or by telephone (72–74).

3.4.4.2 COMMUNITY INTEGRATION QUESTIONNAIRE

Community integration questionnaire provides a measurement of community integration after traumatic brain injury. It consists of a questionnaire relating to reintegration into home and society, as well as pursuing education, gainful employment, and so on. It needs an in-person or telephone interview to complete the questionnaire (72,75).

3.4.4.3 LONDON HANDICAP SCALE

It evaluates mobility, physical ability to take care of himself/herself, occupation, participation in social life, orientation and awareness about the surroundings, and economic self-reliance and independence. It involves a personal discussion or telephone interview for answering the questionnaire. The categories on each dimension have a weight based on several levels of disadvantage. Total weights of all categories range from 0 to 100 where 0 denotes maximal handicap and 100 denotes no handicap (72,76).

3.4.4.4 ASSESSMENT OF LIFE HABITS SCALE

It assesses nutrition, physical fitness, self-care, communication, household activities, mobility, responsibility, interpersonal relationships, community participation, education, occupation, and recreation. It obtains a response from the person about their ability to perform an activity, namely "no difficulty," "some difficulty," "accomplished by substitution," and "not accomplished." It also assesses the nature of assistance required, that is, "no assistance" or "technical aid" or "adaptation" or "human assistance." It assigns the score according to the nature of responses using a scale 0–9. Further, it applies a "Five-Point Scale" to rate the level of satisfaction from "very dissatisfied" to "very satisfied" (72,77,78).

3.4.4.5 FRENCHAY ACTIVITIES INDEX

Frenchay Activities Index measures an outcome after stroke rehabilitation. It comprises of 15 questions. It includes cooking, cleaning cookware and cooking area, washing clothes, household work and house maintenance, shopping, and social visits. It also includes outdoor walking more than 15 minutes, pursuing a hobby, reading books, driving a car or traveling in the bus, long distance driving, maintenance of a car, gardening, and gainful employment. The score ranges from 15 to 60. Persons with stroke or their relatives answer questionnaire either by personal interview or by mail (72,79,80).

Dijkers et al., in their review, remarked that a person with a disability would agree about "positive social outcome" only if he/she attains "reintegration into the society as a useful, productive member including participation in family and community life" (72).

Functional Status Measures, functional status and quality of life measures, health-related quality of life outcome measure, and functional and social status outcome measures have limitations in evaluation of all facets of disability namely impairment of function and structure (Illustration 3.2).

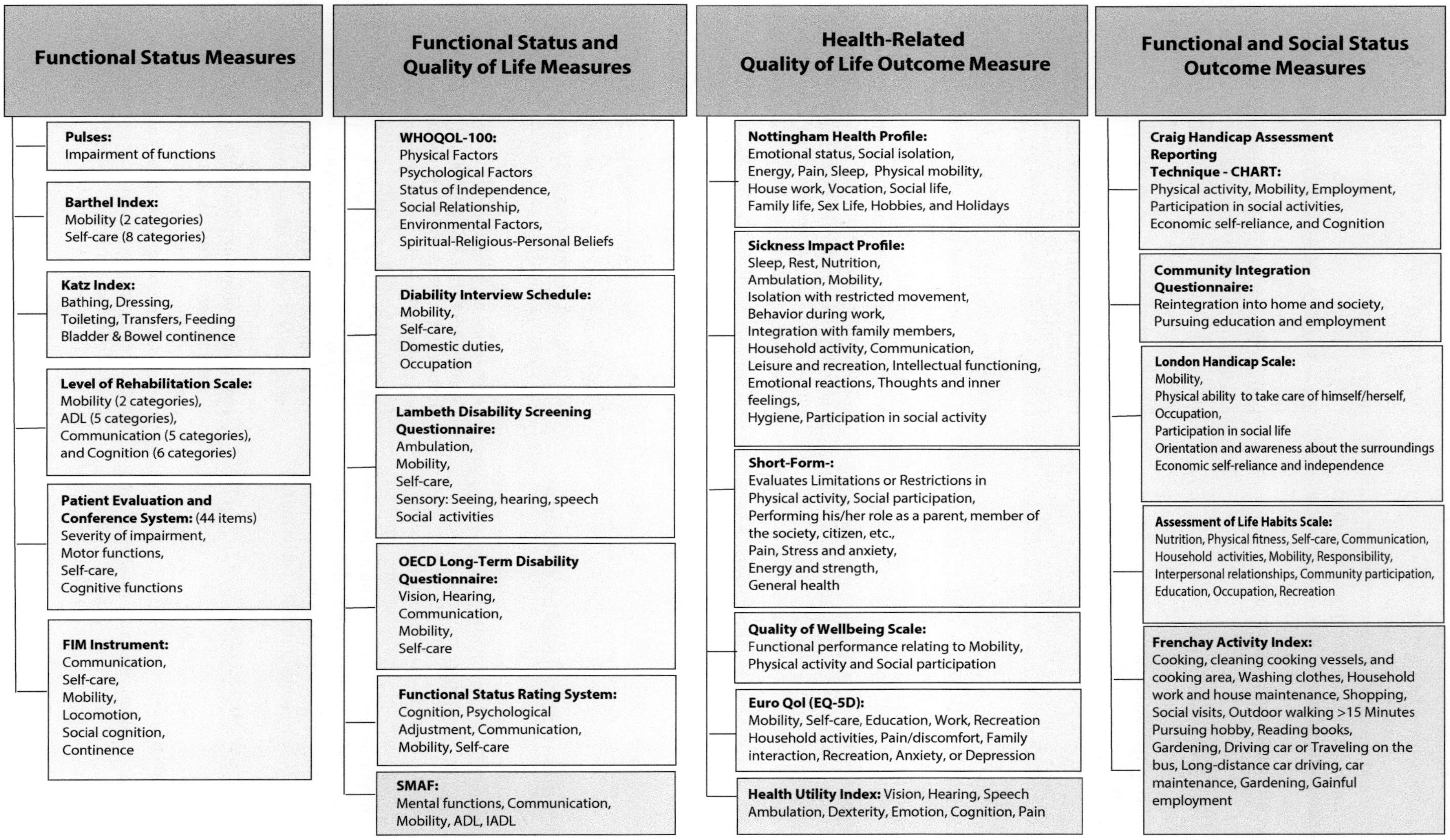

Functional Status Measures

Pulses:
Impairment of functions

Barthel Index:
Mobility (2 categories)
Self-care (8 categories)

Katz Index:
Bathing, Dressing,
Toileting, Transfers, Feeding
Bladder & Bowel continence

Level of Rehabilitation Scale:
Mobility (2 categories),
ADL (5 categories),
Communication (5 categories),
and Cognition (6 categories)

**Patient Evaluation and
Conference System:** (44 items)
Severity of impairment,
Motor functions,
Self-care,
Cognitive functions

FIM Instrument:
Communication,
Self-care,
Mobility,
Locomotion,
Social cognition,
Continence

Functional Status and Quality of Life Measures

WHOQOL-100:
Physical Factors
Psychological Factors
Status of Independence,
Social Relationship,
Environmental Factors,
Spiritual-Religious-Personal Beliefs

Diability Interview Schedule:
Mobility,
Self-care,
Domestic duties,
Occupation

**Lambeth Disability Screening
Questionnaire:**
Ambulation,
Mobility,
Self-care,
Sensory: Seeing, hearing, speech
Social activities

**OECD Long-Term Disability
Questionnaire:**
Vision, Hearing,
Communication,
Mobility,
Self-care

Functional Status Rating System:
Cognition, Psychological
Adjustment, Communication,
Mobility, Self-care

SMAF:
Mental functions, Communication,
Mobility, ADL, IADL

Health-Related Quality of Life Outcome Measure

Nottingham Health Profile:
Emotional status, Social isolation,
Energy, Pain, Sleep, Physical mobility,
House work, Vocation, Social life,
Family life, Sex Life, Hobbies, and Holidays

Sickness Impact Profile:
Sleep, Rest, Nutrition,
Ambulation, Mobility,
Isolation with restricted movement,
Behavior during work,
Integration with family members,
Household activity, Communication,
Leisure and recreation, Intellectual functioning,
Emotional reactions, Thoughts and inner feelings,
Hygiene, Participation in social activity

Short-Form-:
Evaluates Limitations or Restrictions in
Physical activity, Social participation,
Performing his/her role as a parent, member of
the society, citizen, etc.,
Pain, Stress and anxiety,
Energy and strength,
General health

Quality of Wellbeing Scale:
Functional performance relating to Mobility,
Physical activity and Social participation

Euro Qol (EQ-5D):
Mobility, Self-care, Education, Work, Recreation
Household activities, Pain/discomfort, Family
interaction, Recreation, Anxiety, or Depression

Health Utility Index: Vision, Hearing, Speech
Ambulation, Dexterity, Emotion, Cognition, Pain

Functional and Social Status Outcome Measures

**Craig Handicap Assessment
Reporting
Technique - CHART:**
Physical activity, Mobility, Employment,
Participation in social activities,
Economic self-reliance, and Cognition

**Community Integration
Questionnaire:**
Reintegration into home and society,
Pursuing education and employment

London Handicap Scale:
Mobility,
Physical ability to take care of himself/herself,
Occupation,
Participation in social life
Orientation and awareness about the surroundings
Economic self-reliance and independence

Assessment of Life Habits Scale:
Nutrition, Physical fitness, Self-care, Communication,
Household activities, Mobility, Responsibility,
Interpersonal relationships, Community participation,
Education, Occupation, Recreation

Frenchay Activity Index:
Cooking, cleaning cooking vessels, and
cooking area, Washing clothes, Household
work and house maintenance, Shopping,
Social visits, Outdoor walking >15 Minutes
Pursuing hobby, Reading books,
Gardening, Driving car or Traveling on the
bus, Long-distance car driving, car
maintenance, Gardening, Gainful
employment

Illustration 3.2 Functional scales/outcome measures.

3.5 WORLD HEALTH ORGANIZATION'S DISABILITY ASSESSMENT SCHEDULE—WHODAS 2.0

The World Health Organization Disability Assessment Schedule (WHODAS) 2.0 is a generic assessment instrument to measure health and disability at the population level or in clinical practice. It evaluates cognition, communication, self-care, interpersonal interaction, life activities, and participation in social activities. It has a full version of 36 items, a short-version of 12 items, and 12 + 24 item version. The person, interviewer, or the proxy can administer the scale (81).

Integrated Evaluation of Disability was tending to apply WHODAS 2.0 for evaluation of disability because WHODAS 2.0 has undergone extensive field tests across the world and it has good reliability, item response characteristics, and strong factor structure. Health and health-related interventions apply WHODAS 2.0 to design and to monitor their impact. There is no provision to evaluate impairment and environmental factors in WHODAS 2.0. WHO is developing a module for bodily impairment for the forthcoming WHODAS (82). At present, it limits the use of WHODAS 2.0 in *Integrated Evaluation of Disability*. Furthermore, WHODAS 2.0 rates the difficulty as mild, moderate, severe, and extreme. The rating performed by the disabled person, the interviewer, or the proxy has an element of subjectivity. Exaggeration or even malingering might prompt to gain a higher percentage of disability when the person with a disability or the proxy fills up the questionnaire. WHODAS 2.0 says that if a respondent with a spinal cord injury has a personal assistant, who helps him/her in daily bathing, the item derives a score of 1 for "None." Though personal assistance removes the difficulty, the person with disability develops dependency. Without the personal assistance he or she cannot function. Hence, higher grading is necessary for personal assistance.

3.6 "ACTIVITY PARTICIPATION SKILL ASSESSMENT SCALE," "ENVIRONMENTAL FACTORS MEASUREMENT SCALE," AND "PERSONAL FACTORS MEASUREMENT SCALE"

Integrated Evaluation of Disability developed "Activity Participation Skill Assessment Scale," "Environmental Factors Measurement Scale," and "Personal Factors Measurement Scale" and "Personal Factors Measurement Scale" to evaluate limitation of activity, participation restriction, and environmental and personal factors including working and earning capacity (Illustrations 3.3 through 3.5).

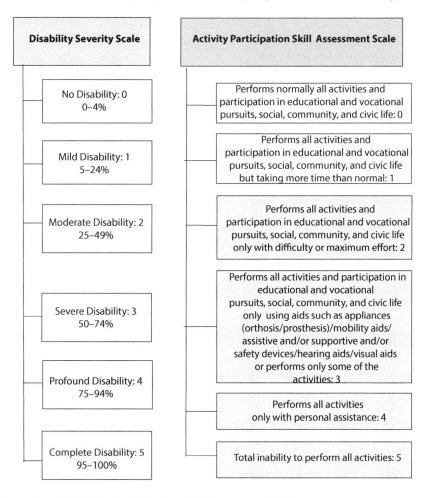

Illustration 3.3 Severity scale and Activity Participation Skill Assessment Scale.

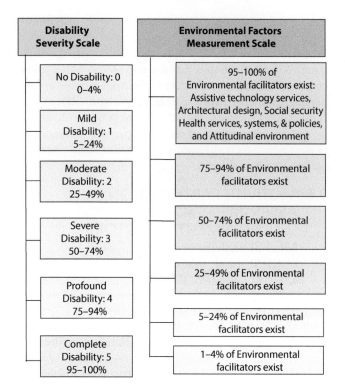

Illustration 3.4 Severity scale and Environmental Factor Measurement Scale.

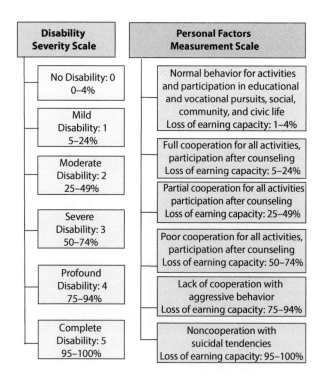

Illustration 3.5 Severity scale and Personal Factors Measurement Scale.

WHO-International Classification of Functioning, Disability and Health (ICF) quantifies bodily functions and structures, activities and participation, and environmental factors using a generic scale (83). *Integrated Evaluation of Disability* developed the disability severity scale to quantify limitation of activity, participation restriction, environmental and personal factors.

Integrated Evaluation of Disability has chosen nine domains of activity and participation namely learning-applying knowledge-acquiring skills, task management skill, communication, mobility, self-care, household activities, interpersonal skills, participation in educational-vocational pursuits, economic transaction and management, and participation in community, social and civic life.

Integrated Evaluation of Disability developed "Environmental Factors Measurement Scale" to assess a hundred variables under four domains of environmental factors namely technological services, architectural design, social security including health services and policies, and attitudinal environment.

If there is any tendency for the person to malinger and not corroborate with the clinical findings, it is necessary to refer the person to occupational therapy services for activity evaluation and medical social work service for participation evaluation.

This scale assigns a score of 100% for maximum limitations of activity/restriction of participation/environmental barriers and 0% for absence of limitation of activity/restriction of participation/environmental barriers.

"Personal Factors Measurement Scale" measures eight variables relating to the behavior of the person toward his/her disability and three variables relating to working and earning capacity. Chapter 22 describes in detail about the personal factors and working and earning capacity.

3.6.1 Modified Delphi Process

"Activity Participation Skill Assessment Scale" underwent validation by the "Modified Delphi Process." "Activity Participation Skill Assessment Scale," "Environmental Factors Measurement Scale," and "Personal Factors Measurement Scale" underwent a trial with a "Clinical Model" in a pilot study. Chapter 5 elaborates in detail about "Modified Delphi Process."

3.6.2 WHODAS 2.0 and Activity Participation Skill Assessment, Environmental Factors Measurement Scales

Both "Activity Participation Skill Assessment Scale," and WHODAS 2.0 are ordinal scales. "Activity Participation Skill Assessment Scale" applies a hand scoring approach using a weighted score 0, 1, 2, 3, 4 for evaluation of limitation of activity, participation restriction by the physician. WHODAS 2.0 uses simple hand scoring approach for busy clinical settings and a complex scoring approach (item response theory) for comparative analysis across populations or subpopulations (82,84). WHODAS 2.0 applies a scale of "None," "Mild," "Moderate," "Severe," and "Extreme or Cannot Do" (Illustration 3.6).

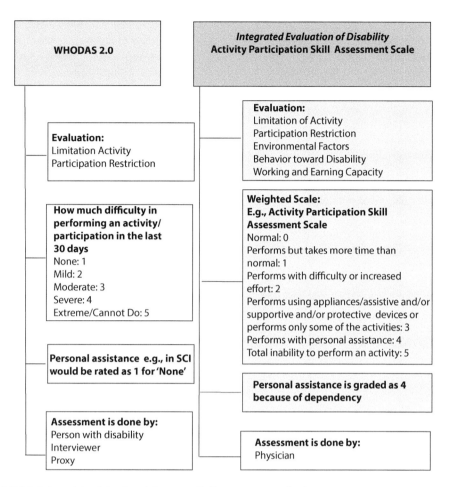

Illustration 3.6 WHODAS 2.0 and Activity Participation Skill Assessment Scale.

REFERENCES

1. National Institute on Disability and Rehabilitation Research's long-range plan in Section two: NIDDR research agenda Chapter 4: Health and function. 2000. p. 43.

2. Üstün TB, Kostanjsek N, Chatterji S, Rehm J. *Measuring Health and Disability: Manual for WHO Disability Assessment Schedule (WHODAS 2.0)*. Geneva, Switzerland: World Health Organization; 2010. p. 3.

3. *International Classification of Functioning, Disability and Health: ICF*. Geneva, Switzerland: World Health Organization; 2001.

4. American Academy of Neurology. Practice parameters: Assessment and management of patients in the persistent vegetative state (summary statement). American Academy of Neurology Quality Standards Subcommittee. *Neurology*. 1994;45:1015–1018.

5. *The International Classification of Sleep Disorders, Revised: Diagnostic and Coding Manual* [Internet]. Chicago, IL: American Academy of Sleep Medicine; 2001.

6. Berry RB, Budhiraja R, Gottlieb DJ, Gozal D, Iber C, Kapur VK et al. Rules for scoring respiratory events in sleep: Update of the 2007 AASM Manual for the Scoring of Sleep and Associated Events. Deliberations of the Sleep Apnea Definitions Task Force of the American Academy of Sleep Medicine. *J Clin Sleep Med*. 2012;8(5):597–619.

7. Chronic Insomnia: Final Panel Statement. *NIH State-of-the-Science Conference on Manifestations and Management of Chronic Insomnia in Adults*. NIH Consensus Development Program, Office of Disease Prevention, U.S. Department of Health & Human Services; 2005.

8. *IQ Classification in Psychiatric Use Diagnostic and Statistical Manual of Mental Disorders (DSM-IV)* [Internet]. Washington, DC: American Psychiatric Association; 1994.

9. Wechsler DW. *Wechsler Adult Intelligence Scale-III (WAIS - III)*. San Antonio, TX: The Psychological Corporation; 1997.

10. Raven JC. *Standard Progressive Matrices*. London, UK: H. K. Levis; 1958.

11. Bloodstien O. *A Handbook on Stuttering*. Chicago, IL: National Easter Seal Society; 1987.

12. Nguyen NP, Frank C, Moltz CC, Vos P, Smith HJ, Nguyen PD et al. Analysis of factors influencing aspiration risk following chemoradiation for oropharyngeal cancer. *Br J Radiol*. 2009;82(980):675–680.

13. Karnell MP, MacCracken E. A database information storage and reporting system for videofluorographic oropharyngeal motility (OPM) swallowing evaluations. *Am J Speech Lang Pathol*. 1994;3:54–60.

14. Salama JK, Stenson KM, List MA, Mell LK, MacCracken E, Cohen EE et al. Characteristics associated with swallowing changes after concurrent chemotherapy and radiotherapy in patients with head and neck cancer. *Arch Otolaryngol Head Neck Surg*. 2008;134(10):1060–1065.

15. Compston A. Aids to the investigation of peripheral nerve injuries. Medical Research Council: Nerve Injuries Research Committee. His Majesty's Stationery Office: 1942; pp. 48 (iii) and 74 figures and 7 diagrams; with aids to the examination of the peripheral nervous system. By Michael O'Brien for the Guarantors of Brain. Saunders Elsevier: 2010; pp. [8] 64 and 94 Figures. *Brain*. 2010;133(10):2838–2844.

16. Bohannon RW, Smith MB. Interrater reliability of a modified Ashworth scale of muscle spasticity. *Phys Ther*. 1987;67(2):206–207.

17. Torretti JA, Sengupta DK. Cervical spine trauma. *Indian J Orthop*. 2007;41(4):255–267.

18. Wewers ME, Lowe NK. A critical review of visual analogue scales in the measurement of clinical phenomena. *Res Nurs Health*. 1990;13(4):227–236.

19. The Criteria Committee of the New York Heart Association. *Nomenclature and Criteria for Diagnosis of Diseases of the Heart and Great Vessels: Functional Capacity and Objective Assessment of Patients with Diseases of the Heart*. Boston, MA: Little, Brown; 1994. pp. 253–256.

20. Hunt SA, Abraham WT, Chin MH, Feldman AM, Francis GS, Ganiats TG et al. 2009 Focused update incorporated into the ACC/AHA 2005 Guidelines for the Diagnosis and Management of Heart Failure in Adults A Report of the American College of Cardiology Foundation/American Heart Association Task Force on Practice Guidelines Developed in Collaboration with the International Society for Heart and Lung Transplantation. *J Am Coll Cardiol*. 2009;53(15):e1–e90.

21. Goldman L, Hashimoto B, Cook EF, Loscalzo A. Comparative reproducibility and validity of systems for assessing cardiovascular functional class: Advantages of a new specific activity scale. *Circulation*. 1981;64(6):1227–1234.

22. Nishimura RA, Tajik AJ. Evaluation of diastolic filling of left ventricle in health and disease: Doppler echocardiography is the clinician's Rosetta Stone. *J Am Coll Cardiol*. 1997;30(1):8–18.

23. Epstein AE, DiMarco JP, Ellenbogen KA, Estes NA 3rd, Freedman RA, Gettes LS et al. 2012 ACCF/AHA/HRS focused update incorporated into the ACCF/AHA/HRS 2008 guidelines for device-based therapy of cardiac rhythm abnormalities: A report of the American College of Cardiology Foundation/American Heart Association Task Force on Practice Guidelines and the Heart Rhythm Society. *J Am Coll Cardiol*. 2013;61(3):e6–e75.

24. Nishimura RA, Otto CM, Bonow RO, Carabello BA, Erwin JP III, Guyton RA et al. 2014 AHA/ACC guideline for the management of patients with valvular heart disease. *J Am Coll Cardiol*. 2014:63:2438–2488.

25. *Haemoglobin Concentrations for the Diagnosis of Anaemia and Assessment of Severity*. Vitamin and Mineral Nutrition Information System (VMNIS). Geneva, Switzerland: World Health Organization; 2011.

26. Duodecim FMS. Thrombocytopenia. In: *EBM Guidelines. Evidence-Based Medicine* [Internet]. Helsinki, Finland: Wiley Interscience; 2007.

27. White GC 2nd, Rosendaal F, Aledort LM, Lusher JM, Rothschild C, Ingerslev J et al. Definitions in hemophilia. Recommendation of the scientific subcommittee on factor VIII and factor IX of the scientific and standardization committee of the International Society on Thrombosis and Haemostasis. *Thromb Haemost*. 2001;85:560.

28. *1993 Revised Classification System for HIV Infection and Expanded Surveillance Case Definition for AIDS Among Adolescents and Adults*. Atlanta, GA: Morbidity and Mortality Weekly Report, Centers for Disease Control and Prevention; 1992.

29. Association ATSMSotAL. Guidelines for the evaluation of impairment/disability in patients with asthma. *Am Rev Respir Dis*. 1993;147:1056–1061.

30. Global Initiative for Chronic Obstructive Lung Disease. Global strategy for the diagnosis, management, and prevention of chronic obstructive pulmonary disease (Updated 2013) [Internet]. Global Initiative for Chronic Obstructive Lung Disease, Inc. 2013.

31. Murray KF, Carithers RL Jr. AASLD practice guidelines: Evaluation of the patient for liver transplantation. *Hepatology*. 2005;41(6):1407–1432.

32. *Clinical Practice Guidelines for Chronic Kidney Disease: Evaluation, Classification and Stratification* [Internet]. National Kidney Foundation Kidney Disease Outcomes Quality Initiative; 2002.

33. Day HJB. The ISO/ISPO classification of congenital limb deficiency. *Prosthet Orthot Int*. 1991;15(2):67–69.

34. Cohen P, Rogol AD, Deal CL, Saenger P, Reiter EO, Ross JL et al. Consensus statement on the diagnosis and treatment of children with idiopathic short stature: A summary of the Growth Hormone Research Society, the Lawson Wilkins Pediatric Endocrine Society, and the European Society for Paediatric Endocrinology Workshop. *J Clin Endocrinol Metab*. 2008;93(11):4210–4217.

35. *Impact Assessment Guidelines*. In: European Commission, editor. European Commission; 2009. p. 35.

36. Whiteneck G, Meade MA, Dijkers M, Tate DG, Bushnik T, Forchheimer MB. Environmental factors and their role in participation and life satisfaction after spinal cord injury. *Arch Phys Med Rehabil*. 2004;85(11):1793–1803.

37. McDowell I. *Measuring Health: A Guide to Rating Scales and Questionnaires*, 3rd ed. New York: Oxford University Press; 2006. p. 62.

38. Moskowitz E. PULSES profile in retrospect. *Arch Phys Med Rehabil*. 1985;66(9):647–648.

39. Cohen ME, Marino RJ. The tools of disability outcomes research Functional Status Measures. *Arch Phys Med Rehabil*. 2000;81(12 Suppl 2):S21–S29.

40. Mahoney FI, Barthel DW. Functional evaluation: The Barthel Index. *Md State Med J*. 1965;14:61–65.

41. Katz S, Downs TD, Cash HR, Grotz RC. Progress in development of the index of ADL. *Gerontologist*. 1970;10(1):20–30.

42. Carey RG, Posavac EJ. Program evaluation of a physical medicine and rehabilitation unit: A new approach. *Arch Phys Med Rehabil*. 1978;59(7):330–337.

43. Velozo CA, Magalhaes LC, Pan AW, Leiter P. Functional scale discrimination at admission and discharge: Rasch analysis of the Level of Rehabilitation Scale-III. *Arch Phys Med Rehabil*. 1995;76(8):705–712.

44. Harvey RF, Jellinek HM. Functional performance assessment: A program approach. *Arch Phys Med Rehabil*. 1981;62(9):456–460.

45. Keith RA, Granger CV, Hamilton BB, Sherwin FS. The functional independence measure: A new tool for rehabilitation. *Adv Clin Rehabil*. 1987;1:6–18.

46. Stineman MG, Ross RN, Fiedler R, Granger CV, Maislin G. Functional independence staging: Conceptual foundation, face validity, and empirical derivation. *Arch Phys Med Rehabil*. 2003;84(1):29–37.

47. Granger CV, Hamilton BB, Linacre JM, Heinemann AW, Wright BD. Performance profiles of the functional independence measure. *Am J Phys Med Rehabil*. 1993;72(2):84–89.

48. WHO. *WHOQOL: Measuring Quality of Life – The World Health Organization Quality of Life Instrument*. Geneva, Switzerland: World Health Organization; 1997.

49. Division of Mental Health WHO. *Field Trial WHOQOL -100: The 100 Questions with Response Scales*. Geneva, Switzerland: WHO; 1995.

50. Bennett AE, Garrad J, Halil T. Chronic disease and disability in the community: A prevalence study. *Br Med J*. 1970;3:762–764.

51. McDowell I. *Measuring Health: A Guide to Rating Scales and Questionnaires*, 3rd ed. New York: Oxford University Press; 2006. pp. 88–90.

52. Charlton JRH, Patrick DL, Peach H. Use of multivariate measures of disability in health surveys. *J Epidemiol Community Health*. 1983;37:304.

53. McDowell I. *Measuring Health: A Guide to Rating Scales and Questionnaires*, 3rd ed. New York: Oxford University Press; 2006. pp. 89–93.

54. McWhinnie JR. Disability assessment in population surveys: Results of the OECD common development effort. *Rev Epidemiol Sante Publique*. 1981;29:417.

55. Forer SK, Miller LS. Rehabilitation outcome: Comparative analysis of different patient types. *Arch Phys Med Rehabil*. 1980;61(8):359–365.

56. Forer SK. *Revised Functional Status Rating Instrument*. Glendale, CA: Rehabilitation Institute, Glendale Adventist Medical Center; 1981.

57. Hebert R, Guilbault J, Desrosiers J, Dubuc N. The functional autonomy measurement system (SMAF): A clinical-based instrument for measuring disabilities and handicap in older people. *Geriatrics Today: J Can Geriatrics Soc*. 2001;4:141–147.

58. McDowell I. *Measuring Health: A Guide to Rating Scales and Questionnaires*, 3rd ed. New York: Oxford University Press; 2006. pp. 122–140.

59. Hunt SM, McEwen J. The development of a subjective health indicator. *Sociol Health Illn*. 1980;2(3):231–246.

60. Hunt SM, McEwen J, McKenna SP. Measuring health status: A new tool for clinicians and epidemiologists. *J R Coll Gen Pract*. 1985;35(273):185–188.

61. McEwan J. *The Nottingham Health Profile*. New York: Springer; 1990.

62. Andresen EM, Meyers AR. Health-related quality of life outcomes measures. *Arch Phys Med Rehabil*. 2000;81(12 Suppl 2):S30–S45.

63. Gilson BS, Gilson JS, Bergner M, Bobbit RA, Kressel S, Pollard WE et al. The sickness impact profile. Development of an outcome measure of health care. *Am J Public Health*. 1975;65(12):1304–1310.

64. Ware JE Jr, Sherbourne CD. The MOS 36-item short-form health survey (SF-36): 1. Conceptual framework and item selection. *Med Care*. 1992;36(6):473–483.

65. Freeman JA, Hobart JC, Langdon DW, Thompson AJ. Clinical appropriateness: A key factor in outcome measure selection: The 36 item short form health survey in multiple sclerosis. *J Neurol Neurosurg Psychiatry*. 2000;68(2):150–156.

66. Kaplan RM, Ganiats TG, Sieber WJ, Anderson JP. The quality of well-being scale: Critical similarities and differences with SF-36. *Int J Qual Health Care*. 1998;10(6):509–520.

67. Andresen EM, Rothenberg BM, Kaplan RM. Performance of a self-administered mailed version of the quality of well-being (QWB-SA) questionnaire among older adults. *Med Care*. 1998;36(9):1349–1360.

68. Cheung K, Oemar M, Oppe M, Rabin R. *EQ-5D: User Guide - Basic Information on How to Use EQ-5D*. EuroQol Group; 2009.

69. McDowell I. *Measuring Health: A Guide to Rating Scales and Questionnaires*, 3rd ed. New York: Oxford University Press; 2006. pp. 683–694.

70. Furlong WJ, Feeny DH, Torrance GW, Barr RD. The Health Utilities Index (HUI) system for assessing health-related quality of life in clinical studies. *Ann Med.* 2001;33(5):375–384.

71. Horsman J, Furlong W, Feeny D, Torrance G. The Health Utilities Index (HUI): Concepts, measurement properties and applications. *Health Qual Life Outcomes.* 2003;1:54.

72. Dijkers MP, Whiteneck G, El-Jaroudi R. Tools of disability outcomes research: Measures of social outcomes in disability research. *Arch Phys Med Rehabil.* 2000;81(Suppl 2):S63–S80.

73. Mellick D. *The Craig Handicap Assessment and Reporting Technique.* The Center for Outcome Measurement in Brain Injury; 2000. Available from: http://www.tbims.org/combi/chart.

74. Whiteneck GG, Charlifue SW, Gerhart KA, Overhoiser JD, Richardson GN. Quantifying handicap: A new measure long-term rehabilitation outcomes. *Arch Phys Med Rehabil.* 1992;73(6):519–526.

75. Willer B, Ottenbacher KJ, Coad ML. The community integration questionnaire. A comparative examination. *Am J Phys Med Rehabil.* 1994;73(2):103–111.

76. Harwood RH, Rogers A, Dickinson E, Ebrahim S. Measuring handicap: The London Handicap Scale, a new outcome measure for chronic disease. *Qual Health Care.* 1994;3(1):11–16.

77. Noreau L, Fougeyrollas P. Long-term consequences of spinal cord injury on social participation: The occurrence of handicap situations. *Disabil Rehabil.* 2000;22(4):170–180.

78. Fougeyrollas P, Noreau L, Bergeron H, Cloutier R, Dion SA, St-Michel G. Social consequences of long term impairments and disabilities: Conceptual approach and assessment of handicap. *Int J Rehabil Res.* 1998;21(2):127–141.

79. Holbrook M, Skilbeck CE. An activities index for use with stroke patients. *Age Ageing.* 1983;12(2):166–170.

80. Schuling J, de Haan R, Limburg M, Groenier KH. The Frenchay Activities Index. Assessment of functional status in stroke patients. *Stroke.* 1993;24(8):1173–1177.

81. Üstün TB, Kostanjsek N, Chatterji S, Rehm J. *Measuring Health and Disability: Manual for WHO Disability Assessment Schedule (WHODAS 2.0).* Geneva, Switzerland: World Health Organization; 2010. p. 3.

82. Ustun TB, Chatterji S, Kostanjsek N, Rehm J, Kennedy C, Epping-Jordan J et al. Developing the World Health Organization disability assessment schedule 2.0. *Bull World Health Organ.* 88(11):815–823.

83. *International Classification of Functioning, Disability and Health.* Geneva, Switzerland: World Health Organization; 2001. p. 222.

84. WHO DAS II. *Disability Assessment Schedule Training Manual: A Guide to Administration World Health Organization Classification, Assessment, and Survey Team (CAS), Global Programme on Evidence for Health Policy (GPE).* Geneva, Switzerland: WHO; 2000. p. 9.

Methods for assigning impairment

4.1 PREVAILING METHODS OF ASSIGNING PERCENTAGE OF DISABILITY

There is no uniform definition for assigning impairment, as countries assign different disability scores for a similar impairment of structure or function.

4.1.1 Earl D. McBride—Disability Evaluation: Principles of Treatment of Compensable Injuries 1955, 1964

McBride measures disability based on physical impairment and functional factors. Physical impairments include anatomical and physiological tissue damage, pain, limitation on work restoration, and limitation on working condition, reactionary influences like poor rehabilitation services; and functional factors including quickness of action, coordination of movements, strength, endurance, safety, security, and adverse employability (1–3).

4.1.2 Henry H. Kessler's *Disability: Determination and Evaluation* (1970)

Kessler in his book *Disability: Determination and Evaluation* documents that evaluation of function alone indicates the basis for measuring ability or disability (4).

4.1.3 Veterans Administration—United States 1976

Physician's Guide: Disability Evaluation Examinations 1976 documents loss of earning capacity following diseases, injuries, or residual deficits serves to grade disability from 0 to 100% (5).

4.1.4 Disability weights: 1999–2002–2008

Disability weight refers to a single numerical value representing multiple aspects of disability (6). In disability weights, 0 accounts for no disability and 1 extreme disability. In the Dutch Disability Weights Study, panel members value the disease by applying the Person Trade-Off (PTO) Method (7). Essink-Bot and Bonsel describe disability weights as reflecting the relative severity of the consequences of the diseases and stages of the disease. There are many methods available to value the disability weights, namely—Visual Analogue Scale (VAS) and Trade-Off Methods (Standard Gamble, Time Trade-Off, Willingness to Pay, and Person Trade-Off). The disease label adds vital information for valuation. The General Health Classification, namely Health Utilities Index or EQ-5D, provides the status of the disability associated with the disease. They also value disease stages as mild, moderate, and severe to interpret the severity of disability (8). Box 4.1 summarizes the salient features of disability weight. The health state and duration of health state are valued, for example, if the length of health status and disability weight are independent (8).

The 2004 Global Burden of Disease (GBD) Study developed disability weights for about 500 clinical conditions resulting in disability. It classified disability based on disability weights as Mild Severity: Class—I and Class—II; Moderate Severity: Class—III, IV, and V; and Severe Disability: Class—VI and VII. Class I has a disability weight of 0.00–0.02, and Class VII has a disability weight of 0.70–1.00 (9).

Disability weight of common neuromuscular diseases namely mental retardation, dementia, amputation, incontinence, infertility, and erectile dysfunction reported in different projects were compared (7,9–12).

Disability weight uses society's preferences for measuring different health states to derive the Disability Adjusted

---

BOX 4.1: Disability weight

Disability weight is a single numerical value representing multiple aspects of disability where 0 represents no disability and 1 represents extreme disability.

Disease label adds vital information for valuation.

Panel members value the disease by applying, for example, Person Trade-Off method.

Disability weight does not indicate the personal life experience of the disability or the ground reality about the disability or society's value for the person with disability.

Clinically and conceptually, it is not usual practice to infer disability from diagnoses.

- Weight: Class I: 0–0.02; Class VII: 0.7 and 1.

BOX 4.2: New Institute of Medicine (IOM) Model: Enabling–Disabling Process Model

Occult disability becomes overt disability when a person is displaced from the environment.

Rehabilitative methods serve as enabling processes to restore function and improve the access to the environment, for example, building ramps.

Environment acts as a pathway for rehabilitation-intervention.

Institute of Medicine (IOM) Mathematical Model of Disability:

Potential disability (PD) = pathology (P)

+ impairment (I) + functional limitation (FL)

$$\text{Disability} = \frac{\text{potential disability}}{\text{environment}}$$

Life Years (DALY). It measures only society's idea about good health. Disability weight does not indicate the personal life experience of the disability or the ground reality about disability or society's value for the person with a disability (13).

Disability is usually not inferred from disease (14). Ideally, disability is evaluated based on impairment of function and structure, limitations of activities, participation restriction, environmental supports and barriers, and behavior of the person toward his/her disability *but not inferred from diagnosis or on the subjective assumptions for various diseases based on the respondent opinion.* The severity of disability may also vary based on the environmental support availed and the behavior of the person with a disability. Thus, there is a limitation with applying the Disability Weight for *Integrated Evaluation of Disability.*

4.1.5 New Institute of Medicine (IOM) Model (1997): Enabling–Disabling Process Model

The disability displaces a person from their prior integration into social structure; that is, family, community, society, and physical space. On the contrary, a person with normal ability integrates into the community with complete access to education and employment. This allows him/her to perform the role of parenthood and leadership, and so on, as well as promotes access to physical space. The Institute of Medicine's (IOM) model stresses that when the disability displaces a person from the environment, occult disability manifests as an overt disability. The rehabilitative methods serve as an enabling-process to restore function and improving access to the environment, for example, building ramps (15). This model correctly identifies the environment

as a pathway for rehabilitation intervention. The "Three-dimensional mat" illustrates disability by applying physical, social factors, and interaction of the person with the environment. The amount of displacement in the mat denotes the severity of the disability. The environmental support specifies the enabling factor, and lack of environmental support determines the disabling factor. The enabling and disabling factors determine the amount of deflection in the mat (15). Box 4.2 describes "New Institute of Medicine (IOM) Model: Enabling–Disabling Process" including mathematical model.

4.1.6 Mathematical Model of Disability

The Mathematical model describes a method for computing disability percentages. In this model, the sum of pathology (P), impairment (I), and functional limitation (FL) denotes potential disability (PD) vide formula Equation 4.1 (15).

$$\text{Potential disability}\left(\text{PD}\right) = \text{pathology}\left(\text{P}\right)$$

$$+ \text{impairment}\left(\text{I}\right) + \text{functional limitation}\left(\text{FL}\right)$$

$$\text{Disability} = \frac{\text{potential disability}}{\text{environment}} \quad (4.1)$$

The mathematical model logical for computing disability percentages. Though it is possible to assign an objective numerical value for impairment and functional limitation, it may not be possible to assign an actual numerical value for pathology. Hence, it may not be feasible to apply the mathematical formula to compute the percentage of disability.

4.1.7 Assessing disability in Europe: Similarities and differences—2002

In Europe, methods of evaluating disability differ between countries. Each country follows its own methods. The methods may be "Barema," or assessing residual functional capacity of the person and their loss of earnings or work capacity. It also includes methods based on the American Medical Association's *Guide to the Evaluation of Permanent Impairment*, or "*Socio-Vocational Method*," or methods based on clinical history and medical examination (Social Limitation and Works Incapacity). The Barema method defines disability by an arbitrary ordinal scale providing progressive disability values or assessing care needs to look after the person with a disability (16). Box 4.3 describes a summary of disability evaluation in Europe.

4.1.7.1 BELGIUM

In Belgium, the BOBI applies medical diagnosis and identifies impairments for the evaluation of disability (16).

4.1.7.2 FRANCE

The French Barema uses the concepts of WHO-ICIDH for the assessment of the impairments and incapacities of persons with disabilities. Evaluation of disability includes clinical diagnosis, medical management, resultant disability, and its impact on daily life. It applies Balthazar's rule to combine multiple disabilities. It classifies disability as mild (0%–50%), moderate (50%–80%), and severe (≥80%). It labels permanent disability after the medical condition becomes stable within the time limit of one year (16).

4.1.7.3 ITALY

The Italian Barema bases evaluation of disability on anagraphic data, present and past vocational history, present and past family history, the clinical evaluation including laboratory and other investigations, final diagnosis, prognosis, functional limitations, and nature of the permanent disability. It applies reduction formula

$$IT = IP1 + IP2 - (IP1 \times IP2) \qquad (4.2)$$

where IT refers to "Total Invalidity," IP1 refers to "Partial Individual Disability Factor 1," and IP2 refers to "Partial Individual Disability Factor 2" in multiple disabilities (16).

4.1.7.4 GERMANY

The German Barema is based on recent developments in medical science in all areas of assessment to elicit permanent effects of health injury (16).

4.1.7.5 SPAIN

Spain's Disability Evaluation applies the method based on the limitations of day-to-day activities of life to computing degree of disability. Zero percent disability refers to the absence of impairment in day-to-day activities of life. Slight disability (1%–24%) refers to clinical signs, symptoms, and complications resulting in minimal difficulty in day-to-day activities of life but can perform the activities. *Moderate disability* (25%–49%) refers to clinical signs, symptoms, and complications producing significant difficulty in day-to-day activities of life but independent in self-care. Severe disability (50%–70%) refers to clinical signs, symptoms, and complications producing significant inability in day-to-day activities of life and may affect some self-care activities. Very severe disability (>70%) refers to clinical signs, symptoms, and complications producing an inability to perform all day-to-day activities of life (16).

4.1.7.6 UNITED KINGDOM

In the United Kingdom, capacity for work is the basis for Workmen's compensation scheme, and pensions for war veterans. Hence disability allowances are based on functional evaluation by eliciting the ability to perform all types of work (16).

BOX 4.3: Assessing disability in Europe

Belgian Official Disability Rating Scale (BOBI): Disability rating scale applies medical diagnosis and identification of impairments for the evaluation of disability.

French Barema: Evaluation of disability is based on clinical diagnosis, medical management, and resultant impairment and its impact on daily life.

Italian Barema: Evaluation of disability is based on anagraphic data, vocational history, family history, clinical evaluation, final diagnosis, prognosis, functional limitations, and nature of permanent disability.

German Barema: Evaluation of disability relies on recent developments in medical science to measure permanent effects of injury to health.

Spain Disability Evaluation: Degree of disability is based on the limitations of day-to-day activities of life.

United Kingdom—Workman's Compensation Scheme, Pension for War Veterans: Disability allowances are based on a functional evaluation that measures the ability to perform all types of work.

4.1.8 United States—American Medical Association—*Guides to the Evaluation of Permanent Impairment*: 2007

American Medical Association (AMA) *Guides to the Evaluation of Permanent Impairment* assign whole person impairment based on consensus opinion from multiple medical specialties and cumulative experience. It combines the consequences of anatomical impairment with the functional impairment. It bases impairment evaluation on key factors namely history, physical examination, clinical investigations/studies; non-key factor namely functional history grade modifier, and burden of treatment compliance. It follows "Hierarchy" (Step-Up Method) in assigning whole person impairment, for example, amputation of the index finger, that is, converts digital impairment into hand impairment, then into upper extremity impairment and finally into whole person impairment. It defines impairment class from 0 to 4 with modification by a non-key factor. It assigns whole person impairment only when the person with the disability reached the status of maximum medical improvement. In this guide, the whole-person impairment 0% refers to normal state and 100% refers to a state approaching death (17). Box 4.4 summarizes salient features of the AMA Guides for the evaluation of permanent impairment.

BOX 4.4: United States: American Medical Association's *Guides to the Evaluation of Permanent Impairment*

Whole person impairment is based on a consensus from multiple medical specialties as well as from cumulative experience.

Combines the consequences of anatomical impairment with the functional impairment.

Impairment evaluation is based on key factors namely history, physical examination, clinical investigations/studies; non-key factor that is, functional history grade modifier, and burden of treatment compliance.

It follows "Hierarchy" in assigning whole person impairment.

It defines impairment classes from 0 to 4.

It assigns whole person impairment only when the person with the disability reaches the status of maximum medical improvement.

4.1.9 Japan—Permanent Disability Social Insurance Programs

National Pension and Employees' Pension Insurance programs provide a pension for persons with permanent disability. It defines disability as long-term impairment and limitations in daily living, not a limitation in their ability to work. It classifies eligible individuals into three groups. Group—I denotes

---

BOX 4.5: Pensions for the Permanently Disabled Population—Japan

Group I: Long-term impairment with inability to perform his/her daily activities without constant attendance

Group II: Long-term impairment with significant limitations to perform his/her daily activities resulting in inability to live independently

Group III: Some restrictions in daily activities with impairment in performing their work

---

long-term impairment with the inability to perform his/her daily activities without constant attendance. Group II indicates long-term impairment with significant limitations to perform his/her daily activities resulting in an inability to live independently. Group III means some restrictions on everyday activities with impairment in performing their work (18). Box 4.5 describes eligibility categories for availing disability pension.

4.1.10 India—Guidelines for the Evaluation of Various Disabilities and Procedure for Certification: 2001 and 2009

Guidelines for the Evaluation of Disability, the Government of India, define impairment as total, partial loss, or deviation in anatomical structure and physiological and psychological function of a human being. Disability evaluation includes impairment of function or structure, resultant functional limitations, and restriction or lack of ability to perform an activity optimum for a person. The person is deemed to have a disability if his/her disability is ≥40% as certified by a medical authority (19). Box 4.6 summarizes the "*Guidelines for Evaluation of Various Disabilities and Procedure for Certification.*"

BOX 4.6: India—Guidelines for Evaluation of Disability

Disability evaluation includes impairment of function or structure, resultant functional limitations, and restriction or lack of ability to perform an activity optimum for human being.

The person is deemed to have disability if the disability is ≥40% as certified by a medical authority.

4.1.11 Korea—Development of the Korean Academy of Medical Sciences Guideline for Rating Physical Impairment: 2009

The *Guideline for Rating Physical Impairment* in Korea considers permanent physical impairment only after sufficient medical treatment is given and after the patient becomes stable. There should be evidence of structural and functional

Doctors perform an objective evaluation of physical or medical impairment with scientific basis.

Considers permanent physical impairment only after sufficient medical treatment is given and after the patient becomes stable.

There should be evidence for structural and functional impairment confirmed by existing medical diagnostic methods.

Assigns maximum whole person impairment of 100%.

Impairment refers to the loss of functional capacity due to his/her clinical condition affecting his/her ability to work. It emphasizes to decide the impact of impairment rather than assessing his/her clinical condition.

It evaluates functional capacity based on what the person can do or could do and not based on what the person wishes to do.

Impairment becomes permanent if the clinical condition is diagnosed based on clinical evidence by the appropriately qualified medical practitioner, completely treated, stabilized, and persisting for more than 2 years

It assigns impairment only if the impairment is permanent.

It classifies functional impairment as mild (5 points), moderate (10 points), severe (20 points), and extreme (30 points).

Persons are eligible for disability support pension if their points are 20 and above.

impairment confirmed by existing medical diagnostic methods. Korean Academy of Medical Sciences (KAMS) assigns maximum whole person impairment of 100%. The doctors perform an objective evaluation of physical or medical impairment on a scientific basis (20). Box 4.7 provides a brief outline of the *Guideline for Rating Permanent Physical Impairment* in Korea.

4.1.12 Australia: Social Security Determination: 2011

As per Part 1 under Section 3 (Interpretation) of the Social Security Determination 2001, impairment refers to the loss of functional capacity due to a clinical condition affecting the person's ability to work. It includes evaluation of functions such as cognition which mainly covers the limitation of activities and work capacity. It emphasizes determining the impact of impairment rather than assessing the person's clinical condition. It evaluates functional capacity based on what the person can do, or could do, and not based on what the person wishes to do. It assigns impairment only if the impairment is permanent. It assesses functions requiring physical exertion and stamina, upper limb functions, lower limb functions, spinal functions, mental health functions. It also assesses functioning related to alcohol, drug and other substance use, brain function, communication function, intellectual function, digestive and reproductive function, hearing and other functions of the ear, visual function, continence function, functions of the skin, and functions of consciousness for work-related impairment. Impairment becomes permanent if the clinical condition is diagnosed based on clinical evidence by the appropriately qualified medical practitioner, and thoroughly treated, stabilized, and persisting for more than two years. It classifies functional impairment as mild, moderate, severe, and extreme, and assigns 5, 10, 20, and 30 points respectively. Persons are eligible for a disability support pension if their points are 20 and above (21). Box 4.8 summarizes about Australia Social Security Determination 2011 relating to impairment.

4.1.13 Canada Pension Plan Disability: 2014

Disability evaluation includes assessment of the medical condition, its progression, functional limitations imposed by the medical condition, coexisting medical conditions, the impact of the treatment on the medical condition, and opinions provided by the physician and/or other health professionals and clients. The medical condition must result in severe and prolonged physical or mental disability preventing him from pursuing gainful regular employment for availing Canada pension plan disability benefits (22). Box 4.9 depicts the summary of the method of disability evaluation and eligibility for a disability pension in Canada.

Disability Evaluation: Assessment of the medical condition and its progression

Functional limitations imposed by the medical condition

Coexisting medical conditions

Eligibility for Disability Pension: Functional limitations imposed by the medical conditions resulting in severe and prolonged physical or mental disability preventing to pursue gainful regular employment

- Impact of the treatment on the medical condition
- Opinion provided by the medical practitioners and/or other health professionals and clients

4.1.14 Switzerland

In Switzerland, disability refers to a permanent total or partial earning incapacity based on the evaluation of biomedical status and impairment (23). Disability evaluation also needs to assess work incapacity for planning to return to work program (24).

4.1.15 Kenya

Kenya evaluates disability based on impairment.

4.1.16 South Africa

It defines disability as physical, sensory, psychological, developmental, learning, and neurological impairments resulting in limitation of activity and restriction of participation in community and social life due to economic, physical, social, attitudinal barriers, and/or cultural factors (25). In South Africa, a person is eligible for disability benefits if they cannot support themselves financially due to the limitation of their daily functioning and are unfit to obtain an employment to fulfill daily needs because of their health condition.

4.1.17 Netherlands

In the Netherlands, the Social Insurance Institute assigns a doctor to evaluate a person seeking a disability pension. The doctor assesses the impact of physical and mental impairments on the patient's work capacities, daily routines, and hobbies. The person is declared fully disabled as per labor qualifications if their loss of theoretical income is more than 80%. If the loss of income is less than 35%, he/she is not eligible for disability pension. If the loss of income is between 35% and 85%, he/she receives a partial pension. The person with a permanent and total disability receives 75% replacement rate, a person with a non-permanent disability receives 70% replacement rate, and the person with a partial disability receives 70% of the difference between previous and current wages (26).

4.1.18 China

In China, permanent or temporary impairment refers to physical, mental, or sensory impairment resulting in limitation of the capacity to perform essential activities in the normal way for a person within their social context. The 1987 disability survey applied the World Health Organization's (WHO's) International Classification of Impairments, Disabilities, and Handicaps (ICIDH), and the 2006 survey administered WHO's International Classification of Functioning, Disability and Health (ICF) (27).

4.2 PREVAILING METHODS OF DISABILITY EVALUATION BASED ON ICF

4.2.1 World Bank

The World Bank states that the impact of disability during life situations or experience should guide assessing disability instead of diagnosis, impairment, and functional limitations. ICF aids to coordinate information related to disability based on self-report functional questionnaires, functional capacity evaluations (FCEs), standardized rehabilitation assessment tools, (28) and administrative records. Provision of assistive devices, vocational rehabilitation, and social assistance determines the ability to work and take care of oneself. It emphasizes transparency in disability determination.

4.2.2 Cyprus Republic

The Cyprus Republic developed a project to implement a new system of assessing the functions and disability based on ICF. It includes a study, preparing a manual, providing training for professions, and creating awareness. The evaluation procedures involve preparation of the assessment file, evaluation of the medical and functional assessment, and completion of the evaluation process in three stages by a team comprising social worker, medical doctors, and rehabilitation professionals. It assesses every person and assigns a score based on the impairment of bodily functions and structures and limitation in daily activities at school, work, and in life. The document does not provide details about the clinical measuring tools for the evaluation of impairment, activities, and participation, and environment. It classifies disability into mild with minimal impairment, minimal limitation of activity with social participation; and moderate with reduced impairment with/without low intellectual capacity, limitation of activity with significant restriction of social participation. The classification also includes a high degree of disability with the inability to function in social roles with the substantial limitation of social participation; and severe disability with physical and psychological dependence for self-care, and severe limitation of activity and maximum limitation in social participation. It grades work-related disability into the first degree of total loss of working capacity and self-care capacity, second degree with complete loss of working capacity and preserved self-care capacity, and third-degree disability with half of the working capacity of more than 50% of the working hours. It applies the ICF generic scale to grade the severity of impairment and limitation of activity. It classifies disability into physical, psychiatric, mental, visual, and hearing disability.

4.2.3 Germany

Twenty-Three German and Swiss experts identified 105 categories of ICF activities and participation to assess the impact of joint contractures on activity limitations and participation restrictions in elderly persons (29).

4.2.4 Italy

Italy bases its disability evaluation on ICF. It is linked with outcome measures comprising 42 categories for myasthenia gravis. It requires additional research to verify its psychometric properties (30).

4.3 *INTEGRATED EVALUATION OF DISABILITY*—GUIDELINES FOR ASSIGNING IMPAIRMENT

4.3.1 Basis for assigning impairment/ structure

Integrated Evaluation of Disability aims to assign appropriate and optimum percentage of disability to the whole person without any element of biased opinion or arbitrary judgment. It applies the principles of the motor and sensory homunculus (31), weighted score for impairment of functions/structure, "Modified Delphi Process," and conclusion from a pilot study in the "Clinical Model" formed the base to define the percentage of impairment. Illustration 4.1 highlights the basis of assigning impairment in *Integrated Evaluation of Disability*.

4.3.1.1 HOMUNCULUS

Motor and sensory homunculus represent the various parts of the body in a distorted profile in the brain. There was a wider area of representation in the homunculus for the body parts performing dexterity skills, language and speech, and complex sensory function. The study of brain mapping with cortical stimulation by Penfield and Rasmussen does not indicate the exact percentage of representation of each part in the homunculus (31).

The topographical profile of the motor cortex in the human being, as illustrated by Penfield and Rasmussen, shows a high degree of representation of the hand, mouth, and face in contrast to lower animals. In the sensory homunculus (Figure 4.1), the face, wrist and hand, and ankle and foot occupy a larger area of sensory processing than other parts of the body.

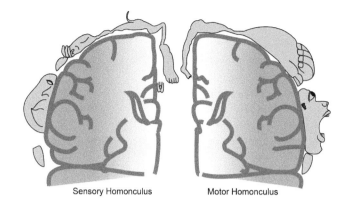

Sensory Homonculus   Motor Homonculus

Figure 4.1 Motor and sensory homunculus.

The size of these areas is directly proportional to the number of specific sensory receptors in the corresponding peripheral area of the body (31).

Review of literature revealed usefulness of newer technology, such as magnetoencephalography (MEG) (32), functional MRI (fMRI), and positron emission tomography (PET) in redefining the diagnosis of clinical conditions by mapping of the brain.

As voluntary effort cannot activate complete motor/sensory area, MEG/fMRI/PET can only reveal the epicenter of activity. Hence, there is a limitation of these methods in defining the boundary of individual parts of the body in the homunculus by brain mapping to assign appropriate impairment. Cortical stimulation still serves as the gold standard for brain mapping, as it can map the eloquent motor and sensory area on the surface of the brain to define the boundaries of the homunculus (33,34).

Integrated Evaluation of Disability is so well thought out that in the absence of other evidence-based methods, motor and sensory homunculus can still serve as a basis to relate and to distribute motor and sensory impairment for various segments of upper extremity and lower extremity. A person with a normal hand with nonfunctional proximal segments can perform functions using their upper extremity with minimal limitations, whereas a person with normal proximal segments with a nonfunctional hand cannot perform any function. It proclaims that the concept of homunculus can be one of the determinants to assign impairment for both motor and sensory loss to various segments of upper and lower extremity in the *Integrated Evaluation of Disability*.

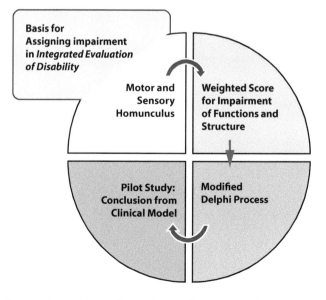

Illustration 4.1 Basis for assigning impairment in *Integrated Evaluation of Disability*.

4.3.2 Defining severity of impairment

Integrated Evaluation of Disability defines the severity of impairment based on the magnitude of the loss of function or structure, the burden of disease (e.g., AIDS), and the burden of treatment (e.g., chemotherapy in malignancy). It also includes the need for the replacement of

---

BOX 4.10: **Defining severity of impairment**

1. Magnitude of impairment of function/structure
2. Burden of disease
3. Burden of treatment
4. Need for replacement of implanted device
5. Failure of implanted device
6. Failure of treatment with risk of mortality
7. Disfigurement
8. Stigma

implanted devices, such as a pacemaker or prosthesis, and failure of the implanted device (e.g., cardiac pacemaker or implantable cardioverter defibrillator—ICD). It further includes failure of treatment, such as in malignancy, end-stage heart/renal/hepatic failure, the stigma associated with certain conditions like AIDS, Hansen's disease, and disfigurement to define the severity of impairment. Box 4.10 summarizes the factors determining the severity of impairment.

4.3.3 Severity scale—Impairment

Integrated Evaluation of Disability has developed a severity scale to classify the severity of impairment. The scale levels are mild, moderate, severe, profound, and complete impairment (Illustration 4.2).

4.3.4 Sub-grades of severity scale

Integrated Evaluation of Disability selects an intermediate score between zero and mild impairment, median score between mild and moderate impairment, median score between moderate and severe impairment, and median score between severe and complete impairment to sub-grade the severity scale (Table 4.1).

4.3.5 Weighted score

Integrated Evaluation of Disability applies the principle of "weighted score" for grading functional or structural impairment. Weighted score assigns an impairment of, for example, 1% for "attention," 2% for "memory," 3% for "orientation/perception," 4% for "visuospatial perception," and 5% for "abstraction or organization and planning or judgment."

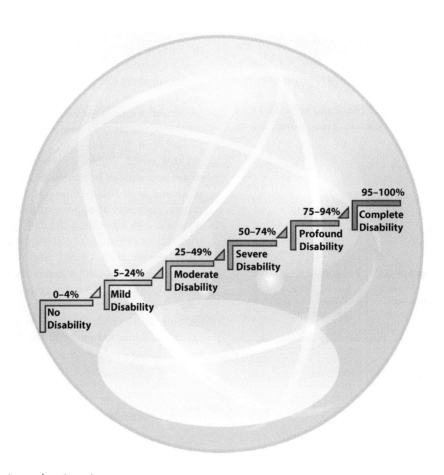

Illustration 4.2 Severity scale—Impairment.

Table 4.1 Sub-grades of severity scale for impairment

No impairment	Mild impairment			Moderate impairment		Severe impairment	Profound impairment		Complete impairment
0%–4%	5%–24%			25%–49%		50%–74%	75%–94%		95%–100%
1% 2.5%	5%	15%	25%	37%	50%	75%	85%	95%	100%

4.3.6 Minimum and maximum impairment—100%

Integrated Evaluation of Disability assigns minimum whole person impairment of 5% for least functional impairment and maximum whole person impairment, 100%, for the permanent vegetative state (Illustration 4.3).

4.3.7 Impairment class

Impairment class is different from the severity scale of impairment (mild, moderate, severe, profound, and complete). The impairment class denotes the gravity or degree of impairment of an individual function/structure. The extent of impairment for each Class 1, Class 2, Class 3, Class 4,

and Class 5 may vary for each function/structure depending on the magnitude of loss of individual function/structure (Table 4.2).

4.3.8 Combining impairments

Formula

$$A + \left[B \frac{100 - A}{100} \right] \tag{4.3}$$

where A = Higher impairment value, B = Lower impairment value (Equation 4.3) integrates the impairment score of individual functions/structure to compute whole person impairment.

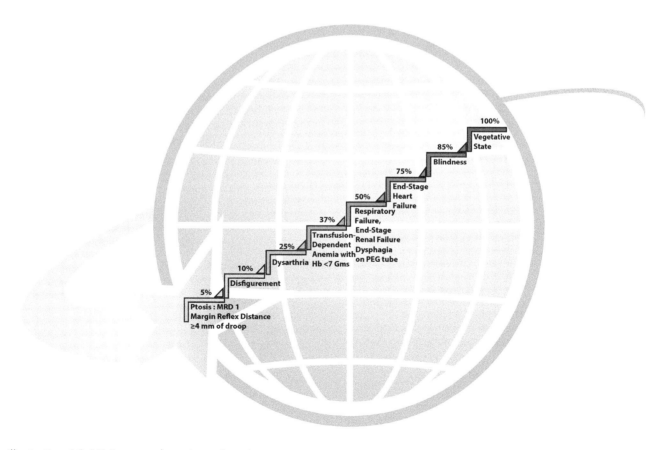

Illustration 4.3 Minimum and maximum impairment.

Table 4.2 Impairment class for specific functions

Clinical functions	Impairment Class 1	Impairment Class 2	Impairment Class 3	Impairment Class 4	Impairment Class 5
Heart failure	15%	25%	50%	75%	
Renal failure	10%	25%	37%	50%	
Neurogenic bladder	5%	15%	25%	37%	50%
Dysarthria	5%	15%	25%		
Disfigurement	2.5%	5%	7.5%	10%	
Ptosis	1.25%	2.5%	5%		

4.4 APPLYING GUIDELINES TO ASSIGN IMPAIRMENT IN *INTEGRATED EVALUATION OF DISABILITY*

4.4.1 Motor impairment

Based on homunculus, total loss of motor function for one upper extremity derives an impairment of 60% and lower extremity 40%. In the upper extremity, the hand derives an impairment of 45%, and in the hand, a thumb derives an impairment of 18%, index finger 9%, middle finger 9%, ring finger 4.5%, and little finger 4.5%. In the lower extremity, the hip derives an impairment of 4%, knee 8%, ankle 16%, foot 8%, and toes 4% based on homunculus.

The motor function comprises of muscle functions namely muscle power, muscle tone and muscle endurance; joint functions namely mobility and stability; and movement functions namely voluntary movement, involuntary movement, the paucity of movement (bradykinesia), and gait—translation movement.

Upper extremity obtains an impairment of 60%, lower extremity 40% and spine 30% for muscle, joint, and movement functions. *Integrated Evaluation of Disability* compares its impairment score with that of the prevailing disability methods and scales around the world. Chapter 5 describes explicitly the methods of validation, namely the "Modified Delphi Process and "Clinical Model" applied in *Integrated Evaluation of Disability*.

4.4.2 Sensory impairment

Total sensory loss of a single upper extremity obtains an impairment of 60%, and lower extremity 40% based on homunculus. In the upper extremity, dermatome representing the hand derives higher impairment, that is, C6—8%, C7—8%, and C8—8%; dermatome-representing arm derives lesser percentage, that is, C5—3% and T1—3%.

Arm receives an impairment of 0.5% for complete loss of sensation over the upper lateral cutaneous nerve of the arm (axillary nerve). It derives an impairment of 0.5% for the lower lateral cutaneous nerve of the arm (radial nerve). It obtains an impairment of 1.0% for the posterior cutaneous nerve of the arm (radial nerve), 0.5% for the medial cutaneous nerve of arm, and 0.5% for the intercostobrachial nerve. In the forearm, complete loss of sensation over the lateral cutaneous nerve of the forearm derives 2%, medial cutaneous nerve of the forearm 2%, and posterior cutaneous nerve of the forearm 2% in the forearm. In the wrist, complete loss of sensation over a lateral cutaneous branch of the forearm, the medial cutaneous nerve of forearm, the posterior cutaneous nerve of forearm, superficial branch of the radial nerve, and dorsal cutaneous branch of ulnar nerve together derives 1%. Complete loss of sensation over median nerve derives 10.5%, ulnar nerve 3.75%, and radial nerve 5.75% in hand.

In the lower extremity, total loss of sensation over thigh derives 4%, leg 4%, and ankle and foot 12%. Boxes 4.11 and 4.12 summarize the impairment of sensory loss over the peripheral nerves in the lower extremity.

BOX 4.11: Sensory impairment: Thigh

Dorsal rami (L1, 2, 3): 0.250%
Dorsal rami (S1, 2, 3): 0.125%
Cutaneous branch of obturator nerve (L2, 3, 4): 0.250%
Iliohypogastric nerve (L1): 0.125%
Subcostal nerve: 0.125%
Ilioinguinal nerve (L1): 0.125%
Femoral branch of genitofemoral (L1, 2): 0.250%
Lateral cutaneous nerve of thigh (L2, 3): 0.750%
Medial and intermediate cutaneous nerve of thigh (L2, 3): 1.00%
Posterior cutaneous nerve of thigh (S1, 2, 3): 1.00%

BOX 4.12: Sensory impairment: Leg

Lateral sural cutaneous nerve: 1.5%
Saphenous nerve: 1.5%
Sural nerve: 0.5%
Superficial peroneal nerve: 0.5%

Sensory Impairment of Ankle and Foot

Medial calcaneal branch: 1.5%
Saphenous nerve: 0.75%
Superficial peroneal nerve: 3.5%
Deep peroneal nerve: 0.5%
Medial plantar nerve: 3.5%
Lateral plantar nerve: 1.5%
Sural nerve: 0.75%

BOX 4.13: Consciousness function

***Integrated Evaluation of Disability*:** Permanent vegetative state—Whole Person Impairment 100%
Belgium BOBI: Severe post-concussion syndrome or coma or prolonged state of confusion following post-traumatic brain injury with or without fracture—40%–60%
French Barema: Vegetative state or coma—100%
US AMA: Persons with irreversible coma on medical management—Maximum Whole Person Impairment—100%
India *Guidelines for Evaluation of Various Disabilities* and Procedure for Certification: Altered sensorium—100%

4.5 COMPARISON OF IMPAIRMENT IN *INTEGRATED EVALUATION OF DISABILITY* WITH THAT OF OTHER COUNTRIES

4.5.1 Consciousness function

Consciousness function refers to a mental state of wakefulness with awareness, attentiveness, and lucidness.

4.5.1.1 VEGETATIVE STATE

Practice parameters describe the vegetative state as persistent when it persists for more than one month and permanent if irreversibility continues with maximum evidence of clinical proof. The definition describes the vegetative state as characterized by lack of awareness of himself/herself and about his/her environment; lack of interpersonal interaction and voluntary response to audiovisual and exteroceptive touch or painful stimulus; and loss of reception, comprehension, and expression of language functions. There is incontinence of bladder and bowel. There is evidence of intermittent wakefulness evinced by the sleep-wake cycle. Further, the definition describes that there may be absence or presence of pupillary, corneal, oculocephalic, vestibulo-ocular, and gag reflexes. The person requires medical and nursing care for survival (35).

Integrated Evaluation of Disability assigns a whole person impairment of 100% for the permanent vegetative state.

In Belgium, the BOBI allocates 40%–60% for a severe post-concussion syndrome, or coma, or prolonged state of confusion following post-traumatic brain injury with or without fracture (16).

The French Barema assigns a disability rate of 100% for vegetative state or coma (16).

AMA *Guides to the Evaluation of Permanent Impairment* assigns maximum whole person impairment of 100% for persons with irreversible coma on complete medical management (36).

Guidelines for Evaluation of Various Disabilities (India) assigns an impairment of 100% for altered sensorium. Box 4.13 summarizes maximum impairment for consciousness function allocated in the *Integrated Evaluation of Disability*, Belgium, French, USA, and India.

4.5.1.2 SEIZURE DISORDERS

A seizure is a brief clinical manifestation of signs and symptoms as a result of the sudden surge of abnormal simultaneous excessive neuronal discharge in the brain (37). Table 4.3 describes the impairment score for seizures in *Integrated Evaluation of Disability*.

AMA *Guides to the Evaluation of Permanent Impairment* assign maximum whole person impairment of 50% for episodic neurological impairments such as syncope, loss of awareness, convulsive disorders and arousal and sleep disorders (17). *Korean Academy of Medical Sciences (KAMS)— Pediatric Impairment Guideline for Brain Lesion* assigns impairment if the seizure disorder refractory to medical management. It grades seizure impairment from 1 to 6 based on the frequency of seizure attacks (38).

The *Guidelines for Evaluation of Various Disabilities* (India), assign a maximum impairment of 75% to more than ten convulsions per month with sufficient medication (19).

In Belgium, the BOBI assigns an impairment of 75%–100% for tonic-clonic seizures occurring daily or frequently (16). The French Barema assigns an impairment of 80% for tonic-clonic seizures occurring daily (16). The Italian Barema assigns 100% to generalized epileptic seizures occurring daily under treatment (16). The German Barema

Table 4.3 Impairment class—Seizure disorders

Impairment class	Severity profile—Seizure disorders	Maximum impairment 50%
Class 1	Focal/generalized seizures under control with mono- or multi-therapy without recurrence (Assigns impairment for burden of treatment compliance, and stigma until the antiepileptic drugs are withdrawn)	5%
Class 2	Focal seizures with preserved consciousness developing recurrence every month with mono/multi-pharmacotherapy	15%
Class 3	Focal seizures with impairment of consciousness, developing recurrence every month with mono/multi-pharmacotherapy	25%
Class 4	Persistent focal seizure occurring every day/week with impairment of consciousness refractory to pharmacotherapy	37%
Class 4	Generalized seizures, developing recurrence every month with mono/multi-pharmacotherapy	37%
Class 5	Persistent generalized seizures with recurrence every day/week refractory to multi-pharmacotherapy	50%

assigns 90%–100% for epilepsy occurring at the minimum weekly interval (16). Box 4.14 compares the impairment for seizure disorders assigned in *Integrated Evaluation of Disability*, Belgium, French, German, India, Italy, and US.

4.5.2 Intellectual function

Intellectual function refers to the ability to comprehend and assimilate various mental functions, such as reasoning, thinking, planning, judging, problem solving, and communication for acquiring life skills. Impairment of intellectual function occurs in mental retardation, and dementia (39). *Integrated Evaluation of Disability* prefers bedside clinical tests to assess intellectual function (Box 4.15).

BOX 4.14: Seizure

Integrated Evaluation of Disability: Maximum impairment of 50%
US AMA: Episodic loss of consciousness or awareness: Maximum whole person impairment 50%
India *Guidelines for Evaluation of Various Disabilities* and Procedure for Certification: Maximum impairment of 75%
Belgium BOBI: Tonic-clonic epileptic seizures occurring almost daily or even more frequently: Impairment of 75%–100%
French Barema: Tonic-clonic Seizures with falls and/or fainting—Impairment greater than 80%
Italian Barema: Generalized epileptic seizures occurring daily under treatment—Impairment of 100%
German Barema: Generalized seizures occurring at least weekly or in bursts—Impairment 90%–100%

BOX 4.15: Bedside clinical tests for intellectual evaluation

1. Aware of the purpose of his/her visit to the doctor
2. Read and understands newspaper
3. Calculations, such as serial addition of 7 from 0 to 50 (or) subtracting 7 from 100
4. Abstraction—Use of proverbs and judgment, such as what to do with a letter found in front of the post box

---

If the bedside clinical tests reveal an impairment of IQ then the person may need an evaluation by a psychologist. The Wechsler Scale (40) and Raven's matrices (41) are widely used to evaluate IQ.

Integrated Evaluation of Disability assigns a median impairment of 4% for IQ score of 71–84, 14% for IQ score of 50–70, 39% for IQ score of 25–49 and 63% for IQ score <25. Further, it combines IQ and activity and participation skill to compute intellectual disability.

The American Psychiatric Association describes the DSM4 classification of IQ (42). An IQ score below two standard deviations from the mean viz. ≤70 signifies a reduction in intellectual functioning (43).

The Government of India's *Guidelines for Evaluation of Various Disabilities* assign maximum 100% for IQ less than 20 (profound mental retardation) (19).

The Italian Barema assigns 41%–100% for mental deficiency (16). Box 4.16 compares an impairment for intellectual function assigned by *Integrated Evaluation of Disability*, India, and Italy.

> **BOX 4.16: Intellectual function**
>
> ***Integrated Evaluation of Disability:*** Maximum whole person impairment of 75%
> **India *Guidelines for Evaluation of Various Disabilities* and Procedure for Certification:** Maximum Impairment of 100%
> **Italian Barema:** Mental Deficiency—Impairment of 41%–100%

4.5.3 Sleep function

Sleep is a physiological state of recurring reversible mental function with the disengagement of one's mind and body from his/her surrounding environment associated with quiescence and closed eyes (44,45). The common sleep functions producing disability are insomnia and sleep apnea.

4.5.3.1 INSOMNIA

Insomnia refers to a disturbance of initiation and maintenance of sleep despite adequate opportunity for sleep with very early waking and impairment of daytime functioning due to the poor quality of sleep (46).

The person falls asleep after a latent period of 15–20 minutes (sleep latency). The person with insomnia exhibits difficulty in falling asleep and difficulty in staying asleep. Further, he/she wakes frequently during sleep. Total Wake Time (TWT) refers to the sum of the duration of each awakening from sleep onset to final awakening. Total sleep time is equal to the total time in bed minus sum of sleep latency and total wake time. It aids to calculates sleep efficiency. Chronic insomnia lasts longer than 1 month, that is, months or years (47,48). It may result in chronic fatigue and sleepiness during the day. Further, it may lead to anxiety, depression, impairment of cognitive function namely attention and memory, increased risk of injury, and difficulty in maintaining family and social relationships. Actigraphy may be necessary to evaluate circadian rhythm pattern and sleep disturbance in chronic insomnia. However, evaluation of insomnia does not require polysomnography and MSLT (Multiple Sleep Latency Test) as a routine investigation in the assessment of chronic insomnia (47).

Integrated Evaluation of Disability evaluates impairment in insomnia using various parameters. These parameters include difficulty in falling asleep, difficulty in staying asleep, early morning awakening, non-restorative sleep, sleep efficiency, daytime fatigue, sleepiness during driving, and associated increased risk of injury, cognitive impairment, depression, and abuse of alcohol and substance.

Integrated Evaluation of Disability assigns Class 1 impairment of 5% for sleep disturbances namely difficulty in falling asleep, difficulty in staying asleep, early morning awakening, non-restorative sleep, sleep efficiency 75%, daytime fatigue, and sleepiness. It assigns Class 2 impairment of 15% for added risk of injury due to sleepiness during driving,

> **BOX 4.17: Sleep functions**
>
> **US AMA:** 50%
> ***Integrated Evaluation of Disability:*** 37%

and sleep efficiency of 50%–74%. It assigns Class 3 impairment of 25% for additional cognitive deficiencies, and sleep efficiency of 25%–49%; and Class 4 impairment of 37% for other features of depression, substance and alcohol abuse, and sleep efficiency less than 25%.

AMA *Guides to the Evaluation of Permanent Impairment* assigns whole person impairment of 50% for sleep and arousal disorders (49). Box 4.17 compares impairment for sleep function assigned by *Integrated Evaluation of Disability* and AMA *Guides to the Evaluation of Permanent Impairment*.

4.5.3.2 SLEEP APNEA/HYPOPNEA SYNDROME

Sleep apnea manifests with disturbed sleep during the night and excessive daytime sleepiness. The Sleep apnea may be either central apnea or obstructive sleep apnea. Obstructive sleep apnea is due to a reduction in airflow due to the occlusion and resistance of the upper airway passage. Respiratory effort accompanies respiratory event in obstructive sleep apnea. In central apnea, there is a reduction in airflow due to decreased ventilatory drive, but there is lack of respiratory effort in central apnea (50).

The criteria for obstructive sleep hypopneas are snoring, drop in positive-airway-pressure device flow signal, or flattening of the nasal pressure from the pre-hypopnea reference level, and thoracoabdominal paradox during hypopnea. Snoring, a drop in positive-airway-pressure device flow signal or flattening of nasal pressure, and thoracoabdominal paradox are absent in central apnea (51).

Central sleep apnea presents without any respiratory effort. Both obstructive and central apnea/hypopnea exhibit multiple events of apnea/hypopnea throughout sleep. Chronic apnea lasts longer than three months (52).

Fifty percent of persons with severe obstructive sleep apnea develop arrhythmias such as bradyarrhythmias, premature ventricular contractions, and atrial fibrillation or flutter. Further being an independent risk factor, individuals with obstructive sleep apnea may also develop pulmonary hypertension and subsequent cor pulmonale (53).

In "Apnea," there is a reduction in airflow by 90% or more of the pre-apnea reference level detected by an oronasal thermal sensor or other recommended sensors, and the decrease in airflow extends for 10 seconds or longer. In "Hypopnea," there is a decline in airflow by 30% or more of the pre-hypopnea reference level detected by nasal pressure sensors or other specified sensors, and the decrease in airflow remains for $\geq$10 seconds, and oxygen desaturation also remains 3% or more from the pre-hypopnea reference level. Respiratory effort-related arousal (RERA) may accompany hypopnea (51). Alpha and theta activity

> ## BOX 4.18: Sleep apnea/hypopnea
>
> **Integrated Evaluation of Disability:** Apnea—Maximum impairment of 50%
> **US AMA:** Sleep and arousal disorders—Maximum whole person impairment of 50%

or waveforms greater than 16 cycles/second in electroencephalography (EEG) detect RERA (50). Respiratory disturbance, or distress, index (RDI) refers to the combined number of respiratory events namely, hypopnea, apnea, and RERA per hour of sleep. RDI is 5–15 events/hour in mild apnea, 15–30/hour in moderate apnea, and more than 30/hour in severe apnea (50).

Integrated Evaluation of Disability assigns an impairment based on disturbed sleep, snoring, daytime sleepiness, impairment of cognition, RDI in obstructive sleep apnea, arrhythmias, cardiac failure, and cor pulmonale. It assigns maximum impairment of 50%.

AMA *Guides to the Evaluation of Permanent Impairment* assigns maximum whole person impairment of 50% for sleep and arousal disorders (49). Box 4.18 compares impairment for apnea awarded by *Integrated Evaluation of Disability* and US AMA *Guides to the Evaluation of Permanent Impairment*.

4.5.4 Cognitive function

Cognitive function is a mental process of attaining knowledge to develop awareness, acquire and comprehend information including ideas through thought, experience, and visual-auditory-gustatory-olfactory-tactile senses. Cognitive function includes orientation, attention, memory, auditory perception, visual perception, olfactory perception, visuospatial perception, thinking, abstraction, organization and planning, judgment, and problem-solving functions.

4.5.4.1 ATTENTION FUNCTION

Attention function is one of the cognitive functions to focus on an external stimulus and internal experience or thoughts. Evaluation of attention includes assessment of attention span, distractibility, vigilance, and mental double tracking. A test of forward-digit-span assesses attention function. The person repeats a series of digits with a span of five to seven at the rate of one digit per second in the same order say, 5664309. A normal person can complete seven ± two digits in one or two attempts. Forward recitation of months, days or alphabets indicates a rough measure of distractibility. Go-No-Go test and serial subtraction are useful tests of vigilance. In Go-No-Go Test, the person keeps his/her hand on the table with all fingers touching the table. The clinician taps the undersurface of the table to avoid visual cues. The person raises one finger in response to one tap and keeps the finger still in response to two taps. Recitation of months, days, or alphabet backward, reverse digit span,

reverse spelling, and so on evaluates the ability of mental double tracking. A normal person can recite in reverse order the months of the year in 20 seconds, or less.

4.5.4.2 MEMORY FUNCTIONS

Memory function is defined as a mental process to register, store and retrieve information (54). Short-term memory refers to a mental process of storing information for about 30 seconds, and vanishes otherwise it consolidates into long-term memory (55). In recent memory (or) short-term memory, the person listens and remembers the given name and address (or) the names of three objects and repeats immediately (registration) and after 3–5 minutes (recall or retrieval). Long-term memory function refers to a mental process of storing information from short-term memory, autobiographical memory and semantic memory in the long-term storage system (55). A long-term memory lasts from weeks to lifetime and contains the memory of personal experience and knowledge. Autobiographical memory refers to the ability of the person to remember his/her background. It includes the capacity to remember whether he/she hails from a rural (or) urban area, childhood—name of the school in which he/she studied, early adult life—the name of the institution and date of the first employment (to be verified by the family members).

4.5.4.3 ORIENTATION FUNCTIONS

Orientation function is a mental function of awareness about person, place, and time. Orientation to time is a mental process of recognizing the day, date, month, and year (56). Person's ability to answer the time of the present moment (or) approximate time of day (morning, afternoon, evening, night), the day of the week, date, month/year evaluates orientation to time. Orientation to place is a mental process of recognizing the surrounding location, town, country (56). Person's ability to answer the location of the hospital, the floor where he/she is, the name of the town, county/district, state, and country judges his/her orientation to place. Orientation to persons is a mental function of awareness of his/her identity, and individuals in his/her close vicinity (56). The ability of the individual to answer the name of the caretaker, his/her relationship and occupation assesses his/her orientation to person.

4.5.4.4 PERCEPTUAL FUNCTIONS

Perceptual function refers to a mental process of recognizing and understanding visual, auditory and tactile stimuli (57). Auditory perception is the ability to comprehend and discriminate sounds and auditory stimulus with its temporal relationship and spectral events such as loudness, pitch. The ability of the person to receive and understand the speech, that is, "can horses fly?" assesses auditory verbal perception; ability to recognize and discriminate non-symbolic sound patterns, such as sirens, dog barks, and thunderclaps, and assesses auditory non-verbal perception. Visual perception function is the mental ability to interpret size, shape, color, and other visual stimuli.

Simple tests such as counting dots, 20 or more, widely scattered over a piece of paper but with an equal number in each quadrant, identifying the correct color of the shirt, and identifying common objects, such as toothbrush, soap, and so on, evaluates visual perception function.

4.5.4.5 VISUOSPATIAL PERCEPTION FUNCTION

Visuospatial perception function is the mental ability to interpret geometry of everyday objects including its spatial relationship in the environment, the spatial relationship of his/her body parts and copying geometrical symbols. Bedside evaluation of visuospatial perception function includes copying a circle, "+," diamond, and cube. The ability to identify the position of the clock either above or below the window also evaluates this function. It also determines the ability of the person to understand the spatial location of the window on his/her left side and then proceed to walk toward the window. It further, assesses the ability to identify body parts namely left hand, left eye, left ear, right hand, identification of examiner's right eye, left leg, left ear, left hand. Visuospatial perception also evaluates body schemes. The body schemes represent right-left discrimination: touching his/her left ear (orientation to own body). It also includes touching his/her right knee with his/her right hand (double uncrossed task), touching his/her right knee with his/her left elbow (double-crossed task), and touch my left hand (orientation to confronting person).

4.5.4.6 CALCULATION FUNCTIONS

The calculation function is a mental process to resolve, estimate, and manipulate mathematical symbols (58). The ability to perform simple calculations, such as addition, subtraction, multiplication, and division, evaluates the calculation function (e.g., addition of 13 and 4, subtraction of 69 from 88 and multiplication of 7 and 6 and division of 84 by 12).

4.5.4.7 ABSTRACTION FUNCTION

Abstraction refers to the mental ability to develop general ideas with essential characteristics from concepts, facts, realities, objects, and real instances. Interpreting proverb such as "Still water runs deep," and "People in the glass houses should not throw stones"; and listening to a story, conceiving, and comprehending important concepts and message discovers abstraction potential: the father gave his three sons a wooden stick each and asked them to break the stick. They could break the stick easily. Then he gave them a bundle of three sticks and asked them to break the bundle. They could not break it. The father said that if all his sons were together, nobody could destroy them. The message is that unity is a strength.

4.5.4.8 ORGANIZATION AND PLANNING

Organization and planning refer to the mental ability to coordinate various functions namely identifying the tasks, developing an orientation to the tasks, arranging tasks in the order of priority, preparing a plan and constructing a system to implement, setting excellent time management, and supervising the project or performing the required task. The ability of a person to manage an emergency when he/she discovers a major fire in his/her house reveals his/her organization and planning potential.

4.5.4.9 JUDGMENT

Judgment refers to a mental ability to develop appropriate and reasonable conclusion/decision by weighing the positive and negative aspects and its future repercussions. The ability of a person to decide when he/she finds a letter on the floor in front of the post box reveals his/her potential for judgment.

4.5.4.10 PROBLEM SOLVING

Problem solving is the mental process to identify a solution for conflicting matters or during tricky situation by collecting evidence and analyzing certitude. The ability of a person to proceed further in an unfamiliar place when stranded in a four-way junction in a high road with dismantled signboard found aside following a storm reveals his/her potential for problem-solving.

Cognitive function derives maximum impairment of 25%. Each cognitive function obtains a weighted score depending on its complexity. *Integrated Evaluation of Disability* assigns 1% for attention function, 2% for memory function, 3% each for orientation function or perceptual function, 4% for visuospatial perception, and 5% for abstraction, or organization and planning. Each function gains a score based on 3 point ordinal scale namely normal, difficulty, and inability.

AMA *Guides to the Evaluation of Permanent Impairment* assigns maximum whole person impairment of 50% for alteration in mental status, cognition, and highest integrative functions (49).

German Barema assigns an impairment of 30%–100% for cognitive disorders (16). Box 4.19 compares impairment for cognitive functions assigned by *Integrated Evaluation of Disability*, AMA *Guides to the Evaluation of Permanent Impairment*, and German Barema.

> **BOX 4.19: Cognitive function**
>
> ***Integrated Evaluation of Disability*:** Maximum impairment of 25%
> **US AMA:** Alteration in mental status, cognition, and highest integrative functions—Maximum WPI of 50%
> **German Barema:** Cerebral disorders with cognitive deficiencies Impairment of 30%–100%

4.5.5 Mental functions of language

Language function is a mental function to communicate formal and informal messages by interpreting signs, symbols, and other means of communication. It includes reception, expression, and integrative functions.

4.5.5.1 APHASIA

In aphasia, there is impairment of comprehension, word finding difficulty, difficulty in naming, and error in spelling and syntax. Receptive aphasia/dysphasia refers to the inability/difficulty to comprehend, name, choosing the correct word, and use correct spelling. Comprehension refers to the ability to follow the conversation. The ability of a person to execute either one step, two steps, or three steps command, that is "raise your hand, take the paper, fold it two times and give it to me," detects receptive aphasia/dysphasia if any.

In receptive aphasia, the person cannot understand either written (or) spoken words/sentences. In receptive dysphasia, the person cannot either understand written/spoken words/sentences or answer inappropriately, but he/she speaks spontaneously without any meaning and sometimes with a neologism.

In *Integrated Evaluation of Disability*, global aphasia obtains an impairment of 50%, receptive aphasia 37%, and receptive dysphasia 25%.

In expressive aphasia, the person understands the questions projected to him/her but unable to express or speak an even single word. In expressive dysphasia, the person understands the questions, struggles to speak a full sentence, and answers in telegraphic style like "yes" or "no" for questions: Is it your name? Is it your age? Are you married? Do you have children? Are you working? Expressive aphasia derives an impairment of 25% and expressive dysphasia 15%.

AMA *Guides to the Evaluation of Permanent Impairment* assigns maximum whole person impairment of 50% for aphasia (17).

Development of Korean Academy of Medical Sciences Guideline Rating the Physical Impairment assigns an impairment of 35% for speaking (20).

The Belgian official disability rating scale, BOBI, attributes an impairment of 40%–100% for aphasia. Italian Barema allocates an impairment of 91%–100% for severe aphasia. German Barema attributes an impairment of 30%–100% for cerebral disorders with aphasia, apraxia, agnosia (16). Box 4.20 compares maximum impairment for aphasia

---

BOX 4.20: Aphasia

Integrated Evaluation of Disability:
  Global Aphasia—Maximum impairment 50%
  Receptive Aphasia—Maximum Impairment 37%
  Expressive Aphasia—Maximum Impairment 25%
US AMA: Aphasia or Dysphasia—Maximum WPI of 50%
Development of Korean Academy of Medical Sciences Guideline Rating the Physical Impairment: Impairment of speaking—35%
Belgium BOBI: Aphasia impairment of 40% to 100%
Italian Barema: Severe aphasia—Impairment of 91% to 100%
German Barema: Cerebral disorders with aphasia—Impairment of 30%–100%

---

awarded by *Integrated Evaluation of Disability*, AMA *Guides to the Evaluation of Permanent Impairment*, *Development of Korean Academy of Medical Sciences Guideline Rating the Physical Impairment*, Belgium BOBI, Italian Barema, and German Barema.

4.5.6 Apraxia

Apraxia is a disorder of skilled movement due to a lesion in the cortical level. Motor weakness does not associate with apraxia. The person with apraxia understands the command and ready to perform the movement but has lost the knowledge, concept, or idea how to perform the skilled movement.

In speech apraxia, the person understands the verbal commands but, he/she has inability (or) difficulty in speaking. He/she can chew and eat. The person with speech apraxia is searching for right sound or word. There is difficulty in putting the sounds and syllables together in the correct order to form words.

Integrated Evaluation of Disability assigns an impairment of 25% for apraxia. A person with apraxia may derive additional disability score for limitation of activity and participation restriction than a person with aphasia.

German Barema assigns an impairment of 30%–100% for aphasia, apraxia, agnosia (16). Box 4.21 compares impairment for speech apraxia awarded by *Integrated Evaluation of Disability* and German Barema.

BOX 4.21: Apraxia

Integrated Evaluation of Disability: Maximum impairment—25%
German Barema: Impairment 30%–100%

4.5.7 Articulation function

Articulation functions refer to a process of generating sounds to produce speech (59). The normal person speaks with clear and distinct sounds and brief speech. In dysarthria, there is defective articulation function resulting in inability/difficulty to use language function. The impairment of articulation includes flaccid dysarthria in lower motor neuron lesion, spastic dysarthria in upper motor neuron lesion, ataxic dysarthria in the cerebellar lesion, hypo/hyperkinetic dysarthria in the extrapyramidal lesion, and mixed dysarthria in combined upper and lower motor neuron lesion. The evaluator directs the person to listen and repeat the underlying words. The examiner identifies any deviation in the articulation of speech sounds. The deviation in the articulation of "Papa" or "Mama" indicates labial dysarthria in the facial nerve lesion, articulation of "La, La, La" indicates lingual dysarthria in the hypoglossal nerve lesion, and articulation of "Ha, Ha, Ha" reveals guttural dysarthria in the vagus nerve lesion. A deviation in pronouncing "British constitution, Westminster street, Baby hippopotamus" indicates ataxic dysarthria in the cerebellar lesion. Monotonous speech while reciting a poem or a verse point to an extrapyramidal lesion, and stiff voice with reduced volume while pronouncing "Ah Ah Ah" continuously for 30 seconds indicates spastic dysarthria in the bilateral pyramidal lesion. The nasal tone of all vowels and oral consonant sounds suggests bulbar and pseudobulbar lesions.

Integrated Evaluation of Disability defines Class 1 impairment for articulation function with a clear speech with less distinct sounds but understandable; Class 2 for articulation function with unclear speech, indistinct sounds, and difficult to understand; and Class 3 for total inability to produce speech. *Integrated Evaluation of Disability* assigns Class 1 impairment of 5%, Class 2 impairment of 15%, and Class 3 impairment of 25%. Box 4.22 compares maximum impairment for articulation function assigned by *Integrated Evaluation of Disability*, AMA *Guides to the Evaluation of Permanent Impairment* (17), *Development of Korean Academy of Medical Sciences Guideline Rating the Physical Impairment* (20), and India *Guidelines for Evaluation of Various Disabilities and Procedure for Certification* (19).

4.5.7.1 STUTTERING

Stuttering refers to a disorder of speech with repetition or prolongation of sounds, syllables, or words disrupting the normal flow of speech (60). Bloodstein classifies stuttering into four grades (61). *Integrated Evaluation of Disability* defines Class 1 impairment of 0% for stuttering occurring occasionally, Class 2 impairment of 5% for stuttering occurring during periods of excitation, and Class 3 impairment of 15% for stuttering occurring all the time.

AMA *Guides to the Evaluation of Permanent Impairment* assigns maximum whole person impairment of 35% for impairment of voice and speech (17).

Development of Korean Academy of Medical Sciences Guideline Rating the Physical Impairment assigns an impairment of 35% for impairment of speech (20).

Government of India's *Guidelines for Evaluation of Various Disabilities* assigns maximum impairment of 50% for severe dysarthria (19).

BOX 4.22: Articulation function

Integrated Evaluation of Disability:
   Dysarthria—Maximum Impairment of 25%
   Stuttering—Maximum Impairment of 15%
US AMA: Maximum WPI of Speech 35%
Development of Korean Academy of Medical Sciences Guideline Rating the Physical Impairment: Impairment of speaking 35%
India *Guidelines for Evaluation of Various Disabilities* and Procedure for Certification: Severe Dysarthria 50%

4.5.8 Voice functions

A passage of air flowing through the larynx vibrates the vocal cord. The vibration of the vocal cord modulates the air to produce sound. Voice has the characteristics of pitch, loudness, resonance, and phonatory quality. The frequency of 300–3400 Hz is important for speech intelligibility and recognition. Vowels infuse power and consonants add intelligibility. The intelligibility is poor with the frequency of 250 Hz, about 12% with 500 Hz, and 57% with 2000–4000 Hz (62). The accuracy of word recognition is increased by 23% when the F_0 (fundamental frequencies) differences between the voices raised by 0–8 semitones. The intelligibility improves with higher fundamental frequency F_0 and fundamental frequency differences (ΔF_0) (63).

Voice evaluation comprises of acoustic assessment namely measurement of frequency, intensity, and resonance; aerodynamic assessment namely measurement of airflow, air pressure and resistance of vocal fold; electroglottography, that is, measurement of vocal fold contact during phonation; and video stroboscopy, that is, measurement of vocal fold movement. Besides instrumental evaluation, a speech and language pathologist performs perceptual evaluation by Grade–Roughness–Breathiness–Asthenia–Strain (GRBAS) (64) using 0–3 severity rating, Consensus Auditory-Perceptual Evaluation of Voice (CAPE-V) (numeric value of 100 mm line). Acoustic assessment, aerodynamic assessment, electroglottography, and video stroboscopy are becoming important in the evaluation of impairment of voice function.

The current facilities for perceptual evaluation or instrumental evaluation in Voice Laboratory are limited in most of the centers due to non-availability of Speech-Language-Pathology services and voice laboratory. Hence, *Integrated Evaluation of Disability* prefers bedside evaluation of dysphonia based on clinical parameters namely pitch, resonance, loudness, and phonatory qualities. It defines Class 1 impairment of 5% for phonatory quality such as flutter, creak, tremor. It defines Class 2 impairment of 10% for resonance such as nasal tone, for example., in cleft palate 10%. It describes Class 3 impairment of 15% for pitch and loudness, and quality of voice namely breathiness or hoarseness, strangled or strained voice; and Class 4 impairment of 25% for aphonia.

AMA *Guides to the Evaluation of Permanent Impairment* assigns maximum whole person impairment of 35% for impairment of voice and speech (17). Box 4.23 compares the impairment of voice function defined by *Integrated Evaluation of Disability* and the AMA *Guides to the Evaluation of Permanent Impairment*.

BOX 4.23: Voice functions

Integrated Evaluation of Disability: Maximum Impairment (Aphonia)—25%
US AMA: Maximum WPI of 35%

4.5.9 Swallowing functions

Dysphagia refers to a subjective feeling of difficulty in swallowing when the food either solid or liquid traverses from mouth to stomach (65).

4.5.9.1 ORAL SWALLOWING FUNCTION

Oral swallowing function refers to the transfer of solid and/or liquid food through the mouth at optimum speed.

Oral dysphagia is due to impairment of motor control of tongue during preparatory and propulsive phases of swallowing. In oral dysphagia, the person has difficulty in chewing solid food, initiating swallowing, (or) difficulty in containing liquid food in oral cavity before swallowing with a tendency for drooling.

4.5.9.2 PHARYNGEAL SWALLOWING FUNCTION

Pharyngeal swallowing function refers to the transfer of either solid and liquid food through the pharynx at optimal speed. In pharyngeal dysphagia, the person develops aspiration of food, nasal penetration of food, nasal quality of voice, the unilateral and bilateral absence of pharyngeal and palatal reflex. Further, there is a lack of upward migration of larynx during attempted swallowing.

4.5.9.3 ESOPHAGEAL SWALLOWING FUNCTION

Esophageal swallowing refers to the transfer of either solid and liquid food through the esophagus at optimum speed. The person with the impaired esophageal function will retain food or liquid in the esophagus after swallowing. In esophageal dysphagia, he/she manifests localized sensation of blockage or discomfort in the retrosternal region, oral and pharyngeal regurgitation and recurrent pneumonia. He/she also exhibits esophageal vomiting, that is, passive vomiting with undigested food, and loss of weight. Video-fluoroscopic imaging can identify stricture esophagus due to corrosive intake, space occupying lesion and esophageal paresis/paralysis. Esophagoscopy and biopsy may confirm space-occupying lesions. Esophageal motility studies may contribute to improving the diagnosis when fluoroscopy and esophagoscopy are unremarkable and noncontributory.

The postural techniques minimize the risk of aspiration, for example, chin-tug, head rotation to the weaker side, side lying position and compensatory maneuvers, for example, Mendelsohn maneuver, effortful swallow, supraglottic swallow, and super-supraglottic swallow (66). Persons with severe dysphagia requires feeding by nasogastric tube or gastrostomy (Percutaneous Endoscopic Gastrostomy) to maintain nutrition.

Integrated Evaluation of Disability defines impairment class by applying the variables namely risk of aspiration, postural techniques and compensatory maneuvers adopted to minimize the possibility of aspiration during swallowing, and alternate feeding methods namely nasogastric feeding,

> ### BOX 4.24: Swallowing functions
>
> ***Integrated Evaluation of Disability:*** Maximum impairment of 50%
> **US AMA:** Maximum WPI of 50%
> **Development of Korean Academy of Medical Sciences Guideline Rating the Physical Impairment:** Maximum impairment of 60%
> **Belgium BOBI:** Acute esophageal stenosis requiring definitive gastrostomy or an esophageal derivation—Impairment of 50%–100%
> **French Barema:** Impairment for Gastrostomy 80%
> **Italian Barema:** Impairment for Gastrostomy 80%

feeding through gastrostomy (percutaneous endoscopic gastrostomy). *Integrated Evaluation of Disability* assigns maximum impairment of 50% for dysphagia.

AMA *Guides to the Evaluation of Permanent Impairment* assigns maximum whole person impairment of 50% for impairment of mastication and deglutition (67).

Development of Korean Academy of Medical Sciences Guideline Rating the Physical Impairment assigns an impairment of 60% for eating (20).

In Belgium, BOBI attributes 50%–100% for acute stenosis in esophagus demanding surgical intervention such as gastrostomy (16). French Barema assigns an impairment of 80% for gastrostomy (16). Italian Barema assigns an impairment of 80% for gastrostomy 80% (16). Box 4.24 compares the impairment of swallowing function defined by *Integrated Evaluation of Disability*, AMA *Guides to the Evaluation of Permanent Impairment*, *Development of Korean Academy of Medical Sciences Guideline Rating the Physical Impairment*, BOBI, and French Barema.

4.5.10 Impairment of functions in upper and lower extremities

In *Integrated Evaluation of Disability*, total loss of motor function in one upper extremity obtains an impairment of 60% and lower extremity 40% based on homunculus. Hand derives an impairment of 45%. In hand, thumb gets an impairment of 18%, index 9%, middle finger 9%, ring finger 4.5% and little finger 4.5%. In the lower extremity, hip derives an impairment of 4%, knee 8%, ankle 16% foot 8% and toes 4%. *Integrated Evaluation of Disability* does not follow stepwise conversion of digit impairment into hand impairment and subsequently hand or wrist or elbow or shoulder into upper extremity impairment and finally into whole person impairment. It assigns impairment directly to each segment of upper or lower extremity to avoid conversion procedure.

4.5.10.1 MOTOR FUNCTIONS

Motor functions comprise muscle functions, joint functions, and movement functions. Muscle functions consist of muscle power, muscle tone, and muscle endurance. Joint functions consist of mobility and stability of the joint. Movement functions consist of control of voluntary movement, involuntary movement, paucity of movement (bradykinesia/akinesia) and gait pattern functions.

4.5.10.1.1 Muscle functions

Muscle power function: Muscle or muscle groups contract to produce a force, that is, muscle power. The Medical Research Council grades muscle power by manual muscle testing (68).

Integrated Evaluation of Disability assigns 100% of maximum specified impairment for grade 0 muscle power of muscle/muscle groups. It allocates 80% of maximum specified impairment for grade 1 muscle power, 60% of maximum specified impairment for grade 2 muscle power, 40% of maximum specified impairment for grade 3 muscle power, and 20% of the maximum specified impairment for grade 4 muscle power.

Muscle tone function: It refers to the resting tension present in the muscle/muscle groups which may offer resistance during passive movement. *Integrated Evaluation of Disability* applies a "Modified Ashworth Scale" to grade hypertonia. *Integrated Evaluation of Disability* developed a method to define hypotonia of the muscle. Grade 0 refers to normal muscle tone; grade 1 to muscle less firm on palpation, diminished resistance during Passive Range of Motion (PROM), and prolonged pendular deep tendon reflexes, for example cerebellar lesion. Grade 2 refers to muscle less firm on palpation, diminished resistance during PROM, and decreased deep tendon reflexes, for example, complete lower motor neuron lesion. Grade 3 refers to abnormally soft muscle, loss of resistance during PROM, absent deep tendon reflexes, and hypermobile joints, for example, anterior horn cell lesion. Grade 4 refers to abnormally soft muscle, loss of resistance during PROM, absent deep tendon reflexes, hypermobile joints, and loss of postural stability. It includes head lag, truncal imbalance and unstable peripheral joints (inability to bear his/her body weight on his lower extremities/upper extremities), for example, progressive anterior horn cell lesion such as spinal muscular atrophy.

Integrated Evaluation of Disability assigns 100% of maximum specified impairment for "Modified Ashworth Scale" (MAS) grade 4 muscle hypertonia. It allocates 80% of maximum specified impairment for MAS grade 3; 60% of maximum specified impairment for MAS grade 2. It allocates 40% of maximum specified impairment for MAS grade 1+; and 20% of the maximum specified impairment for MAS grade 1. Similarly, it assigns 100% of maximum specified impairment for grade 4 hypotonia; 75% of the maximum specified impairment for grade 3 hypotonia; 50% of the maximum specified impairment for grade 2; and 25% of maximum defined impairment for grade 1 hypotonia.

Muscle endurance functions: It refers to the ability of the muscle or muscle groups to sustain its contraction for a longer period.

The strength of the muscle denotes active contraction of the muscle/muscle group with maximum resistance and with few repetitions, whereas endurance of the muscle denotes active contraction of the muscle/muscle group with submaximal resistance and maximum repetitions. The resistance applied in endurance training is either 40%–60% of maximal resistance (69) or about 70% percent of 1 RM or 25% of body weight (70) or thirty repetitions of continuous active contraction of muscle or muscle groups (70,71). Another study applies fatigue test to evaluate endurance of a muscle or muscle groups. It calculates fatigue index by using the formula (72)

$$PT1 - \frac{PT10}{PT1} \times 100 \tag{4.4}$$

Hand dynamometer or isokinetic system also evaluates endurance of the muscle/muscle groups. Hand dynamometer uses sustained muscle contraction. Pinch gauge assesses endurance about the prehensile function of the hand (73). Isometric exercise can increase both systolic and diastolic blood pressure and increase the stress on the left ventricular wall (74). As endurance of the muscle/muscle groups represents the capacity of the aerobic system, sports authority applies these methods to evaluate and institute endurance program for persons in sports.

Still, there is no method described for impairment evaluation of endurance of a muscle or muscle groups. A bedside clinical test is in need to evaluate impairment of endurance of muscle groups. Concentric intermittent muscle contractions are ideal for evaluation of muscle endurance than isometric contraction.

Integrated Evaluation of Disability evolved a clinical bedside method to evaluate impairment of endurance of muscle groups. In Medical Research council's manual muscle testing, grade 3 represents active muscle contraction against gravity, that is, 60% of maximum muscle contraction and grade 5 represents active muscle contraction against gravity with the greatest resistance, that is, 100% of muscle contraction. Forty to sixty percent of maximum concentric intermittent muscle contractions, that is, active muscle contraction against gravity with maximum repetitions limiting to 100, can serve to evaluate impairment of endurance of muscle or muscle groups.

4.5.10.1.2 Joint functions

4.5.10.1.2.1 Mobility of joint functions

Mobility of a joint function refers to a free and full movement of an individual joint. Evaluation of the mobility of a single joint requires a minimum of two measurements to obtain a reliable range without an error. It considers the neutral position of the joint as zero position and the extended anatomic position of the joint as 0° rather than 180°. Total loss of motion in all planes represents ankyloses of the joint. The upper extremity obtains an impairment of 60%. It assigns a weight based on the ankylosis of the joint in functional or non-functional position and limitation of range of movement of joint. Ankylosis of the joint in a non-functional position derives 100% of maximum impairment; ankyloses in functional position 50% of the maximum impairment and limitation of the range of motion (ROM) obtains an impairment based on the actual loss of ROM of the joint.

4.5.10.1.2.2 Stability of joint functions

Stability of joint function refers to adequate functioning of the kinetic chain namely osteoligamentous structure, osteomuscular attachment, and central nervous system (CNS) control system (75). The stability of the joint is essential to transfer weight, permit mobility without injury to the intrinsic and extrinsic structures of the joint. Evaluation of stability of joint functions relates to the stability of both axial joint (spine) and appendicular joints (peripheral joints). Abnormal displacement of a segment of a spine under physiologic loads refers to the instability of the spine (76,77). Instability of the peripheral joints refers to dislocation of the joint in peripheral joints, recurrent dislocation of the joint and complete tear of ligaments/meniscus. *Integrated Evaluation of Disability* assigns impairment for instability of the joint when medical reason(s) defer surgery.

4.5.10.1.3 Movement functions

Movement function comprises voluntary movement functions, involuntary movement functions, the paucity of movement (bradykinesia), and translation of movement—gait.

4.5.10.1.3.1 Voluntary movement function

Voluntary movement functions refer to the process of regulating and harmonizing volitional movement. It includes uniaxial movement, multiaxial/multiplane movement, coordination of movement and stabilization of movement. Uniaxial movement refers to isolated voluntary movements such as flexion of fingers or flexion of elbow or flexion of the shoulder in upper extremity and ankle dorsiflexion or knee flexion or hip flexion in the lower extremity.

Multiaxial/multiplane/multijoint movements include movements such as involved in "Finger Nose Finger Test" and "Heel Knee Shin Test." In the "Finger Nose Finger Test," the person directs the movement of his/her index finger to his/her nose and then to the examiner's outstretched finger in the upper extremity. The examiner moves his/her finger with each repetition and detects any irregularity in amplitude and force of the extremity movement. In the "Heel Knee Shin Test," the person places his/her heel on the contralateral knee and drag his/her heel down the shin to the dorsum of the foot.

Coordination of movement in upper extremity includes "Right-left coordination": the ability to clap with both hands; "Eye-Hand Coordination": the ability to write a few sentences in a paper, and Rhythmic Movement:" dysdiadochokinesia. *Coordination of Movement* in lower extremity also includes "Right-Left Coordination," "Eye-Foot Coordination" and "Rhythmic Movement." Cycling movement of both lower extremities assesses "Right-Left Coordination." An ability to touch the examiner's sudden and fast pointing index finger with his/her big toe while lying down, evaluates "Eye-Foot Coordination." Tapping the floor with the foot by alternate plantar and dorsiflexion of the ankle assess "Rhythmic Movement."

Stabilization of movement refers to pushup, that is, lifting the buttocks with both upper extremities. Stabilization of movement in lower extremity refers to heel-to-toe walking in straight line.

4.5.10.1.3.2 Involuntary movement functions

Involuntary movement function refers to involuntary contractions of a muscle or muscle groups often non-intentional or quasi-purposive or non-purposive. It is easy to identify involuntary movements while taking history while lying still with the eyes gently closed and during ambulation.

Tremors are abnormal involuntary movements that are rhythmical either resting (or) postural (or) intentional.

Chorea is a rapid, jerky non-repetitive involuntary movement. Chorea may involve both proximal, distal muscles and tongue. Respiratory irregularity may coexist with chorea. *Athetosis* is a slow, writhing involuntary movement.

Dystonia is a twisting, repetitive, involuntary movement due to co-contraction of agonist and antagonist. It may be painful.

Ballismus is a violent flinging involuntary movement. It may affect axial and proximal muscles or only one-half of the body.

4.5.10.1.3.3 Bradykinesia or paucity of movement

Bradykinesia refers to a slow movement with a progressive decrement in speed or amplitude (78), and the paucity of spontaneous movement.

The speech is monotone and hypophonic. Facial bradykinesia manifests decreased or complete loss of facial expression, decreased or total loss of eye blinking, mask-like face with or without parted lips. Persons with bradykinesia may present with drooling of saliva due to impairment of spontaneous swallowing of saliva.

Finger Tapping Test: Rapid, and repetitive tapping of the thumb with the index finger, rapid and repetitive hand opening and closing; rapid and repetitive pronation and supination of the forearm, and rapid and repetitive shoulder elevation and depression of shoulder assesses the severity of bradykinesia. The person performs the movement at a slow speed with reduced amplitude in Class 1 impairment, carries out the movement with progressive loss of speed and amplitude resulting in freezing of movement in Class 2 impairment, and inability to perform the movement in Class 3 impairment.

Agility Test: The "Agility Test" assesses bradykinesia in the lower extremity and demonstrates how the person carries out the movement with rapid speed and amplitude. In foot agility test, the person taps the forefoot on the ground with rapid speed and amplitude while the heel is resting on the ground. In the "Leg Agility Test," the person taps heel on the ground and raising the leg as much as 3 inches in rapid succession. In the "Sit to Stand Agility Test," the person gets up repeatedly from sitting to standing position from the chair. In the "Truncal Agility Test," the person performs a repetitive movement from supine position to sitting position. In bradykinesia, the person performs the test at a slow speed with reduced amplitude or loss of progression of speed and amplitude with freezing of the movement. In severe cases, the person may not be able to initiate a movement at all.

Translation of Movement—Gait: The person with bradykinesia walks with short steps (shuffling gait) or sometimes with a faster speed (festinating gait) with decreased arm swing and stooped posture. In moderate severity, there is difficulty in turning, tendency to fall while turning or walking, and freezing of the foot disabling him/her to walk further. In severe cases, there is the inability to initiate walking at all.

4.5.10.1.3.4 Translation movement functions—Gait

Translation movement functions refer to translation of a body from one point to another connected with walking and running, and so on. It includes spastic gait, hemiplegic gait, paraplegic gait, asymmetric gait, limping, and stiff gait pattern. *Integrated Evaluation of Disability* assigns maximum impairment score of 10% for impairment of gait. *Integrated Evaluation of Disability* combines impairment score of motor functions namely muscle functions, joint functions, and movement functions to compute an impairment score of motor function in upper extremity (Table 4.4), lower extremity (Table 4.5).

AMA *Guides to the Evaluation of Permanent Impairment* assigns a maximum whole person impairment of 60% for upper extremity, 54% for hand, 22% for thumb, 11% each for index and middle finger and 5% each for ring and little finger (17). It assigns a whole person impairment of 16%–20% (Upper Extremity Impairment of 26%–34%) for shoulder arthrodesis, whole person impairment of 16%–20% (Upper Extremity Impairment of 26%–34%) for elbow arthrodesis, and whole person impairment of 16%–20% (Upper Extremity Impairment of 26%–34%) for wrist arthrodesis in functional position and higher percentage for arthrodesis in non-optimal position (17). It assigns a maximum whole person impairment of 40% for lower extremity, maximum whole person impairment of 33% (Lower Extremity Impairment 83%) for foot and Ankle, 33% (Lower Extremity Impairment 83%) for knee and 33% (Lower

Table 4.4 Impairment class: Motor functions—Upper extremity: —60%

No	Motor impairments	Reference impairment score	Assigned impairment score
1	Muscle functions—60%		
	Muscle power	20%	
	Muscle tone	20%	
	Muscle endurance	20%	
	Sub-total		
2	Joint Functions—60%		
	Mobility of joint	30%	
	Stability of joint	30%	
	Sub-total		
3	Movement functions—60%		
	Voluntary movement	20%	
	Involuntary movement	20%	
	Movement function—paucity of movement or bradykinesia	20%	
	Sub-total		
	Total		
	Average		

Table 4.5 Impairment class: Motor functions—Lower extremity:—40%

No	Motor functions	Reference impairment score	Assigned impairment score
1	Muscle functions—40%		
	Muscle power	13.33%	
	Muscle tone	13.33%	
	Muscle endurance	13.33%	
	Sub-total		
2	Joint functions—40%		
	Mobility of joint	20%	
	Stability of joint	20%	
	Sub-total		
3	Movement functions—40%		
	Voluntary movement	10%	
	Involuntary movement	10%	
	Movement function—paucity of movement or bradykinesia	10%	
	Gait—translation of movement	10%	
	Sub-total		
	Total		
	Average		

Extremity Impairment 100%) for hip (17). Table 4.6 compares motor impairment of *Integrated Evaluation of Disability*, AMA *Guides to the Evaluation of Permanent Impairment*, *Development of Korean Academy of Medical Sciences Impairment Rating*, and India's *Guidelines for Evaluation of Various Disability*. Table 4.7 compares the impairment score assigned by *Integrated Evaluation of Disability* and guidelines for various disability in India and Europe.

Development of Korean Academy of Medical Sciences Guideline Rating describes whole person impairment of 60% for loss of arms and 60% for loss of legs (20). It assigns very severe impairment of 18–73 points with the residual normal function of 34% in upper extremity, very severe impairment of 10–42 points with residual normal function of 29% in lower extremity in the brain injured and brain diseased persons with motor dysfunction (79). It assigns

20% disability rate of upper limb for the shoulder fixed in 60° without any motion (80). It assigns lower extremity impairment of 50% for ankylosis of the hip joint in optimum position, 67% of lower extremity impairment for ankylosis of knee joint in optimum position, and 25% of lower extremity impairment for ankylosis of ankle joint in optimum position (81).

India's *Guidelines for Evaluation of Various Disabilities* assigns an impairment of 90% for upper extremity, 90% for the lower extremity. It assigns an impairment of 90% for arm component (30% each for shoulder, elbow, and wrist), 90% for hand component in the upper extremity. It combines the impairment by formula

$$A + \frac{B(90 - A)}{90} \tag{4.5}$$

Table 4.6 Comparison of motor impairment between countries

Integrated Evaluation of Disability	AMA—Guides to the Evaluation of Permanent Impairment	Development of Korean Academy of Medical Sciences—Impairment Rating	Guidelines for Evaluation of Various Disabilities—India
Upper extremity—60%	Upper extremity—60%	Loss of arm—60%	Upper extremity impairment—90%
Shoulder—6%	Arthrodesis of	Loss of leg: 60%	Arm—90% (Shoulder 30%,
Elbow—6%	Shoulder/elbow/		Elbow 30%, Wrist 30%)
Wrist—3%	wrist—16%–20%		Hand—90%
Hand—45%	Thumb—22%		
Thumb—18%	Index/Middle—11%		
Index/Middle—9%	Ring/Little—5%		
Ring/Little—4.5%			
Lower extremity—40%	Lower extremity—40%		Lower extremity—90%
Hip—4%	Hip—40%		Mobility component 90%
Knee—8%	Knee—33%		Stability component 90%
Ankle—16%	Ankle and foot—33%		Pain, deformities, contractures,
Foot—8%			loss of sensations and
Toes—4%			shortening—Maximum of 10%

Table 4.7 Comparison of impairment for hemiplegia between countries

Integrated Evaluation of Disability	Guidelines for Evaluation of Various Disabilities—Guidelines for Evaluation of Various Disabilities and Procedure for Certification	Belgium	French Barema	Italian Barema	German Barema
Hemiplegia with hemianesthesia, global aphasia, uninhibited neurogenic bladder, and homonymous hemianopia 94%	Severe Hemiparesis 75%	Hemiplegia non-ambulant or wheelchair ambulant with sphincter impairment 100%	Massive Hemiplegia 80%–90%	Hemiparesia or hemiplegia with sphincter impairment 100%	Hemiplegia 100%

where A = Higher impairment value, B = Lower impairment value (Equation 4.5).

It assigns an impairment of 90% for mobility component (30% each for hip, knee, and ankle and foot) and 90% for stability component and combines by formula (Equation 4.5) in the lower extremity. It assigns maximum physical impairment of 75% for severe hemiparesis (19).

The official Belgian Barema attributes an impairment of 100% for ankylosis of both hips and 45%–55% for ankylosis of knee in flexion of more than 45°. It allocates 100% for hemiplegia non-ambulant or wheelchair ambulant with sphincter impairment and 100% for paraplegia non-ambulant or wheelchair ambulant. It assigns 80%–100% for medullary quadriplegia with complete anesthesia and sphincter impairment, 30%–100% for the bilateral cerebellar syndrome, 60%–100% for a severe parkinsonian syndrome with impairment of speech and mental disorders, and 20%–100% for dyskinesia with spasmodic torsion (16).

French Barema assigns 80%–90% each for dense hemiplegia, complete motor quadriplegia, complete motor paraplegia, severe cerebellar syndromes involving both upper and lower extremities and acute athetosis (16).

Italian Barema assigns 100% for severe hemiparesis or hemiplegia with bladder and bowel impairment, and quadriparesis with severe impairment of muscle power, or quadriplegia with/without sphincter incontinence. It assigns 51%–60% for paraparesis with moderate impairment of muscle power. It allocates 91%–100% each for the severe cerebellar syndrome, severe aphasia, and parkinsonian extrapyramidal syndrome or choreiform or severe chore-athetosis. It assigns 31%–40% for median nerve lesion of the dominant extremity, 21%–30% for sciatic nerve lesion, and 61%–70% for severe impairment of upper extremity on dominant side (16).

German Barema assigns an impairment of 30% for ankylosis of knee in a functional position and 40%–60% for ankylosis of knee in non-functional position, 30%–100% for cerebellar ataxia. It assigns 100% for hemiplegia, 80%–100% for Parkinson's disease with severe functional impairment, and 100% for the incomplete cervical-medullary lesion with quadriplegia, bladder, and bowel disorders (16).

Iceland Barema assigns an impairment of 20% for ankylosis of the hip or knee in a functional position. It allocates 70% for brachial plexus lesion on the right side and 65% for brachial plexus lesion on the left side. It allocates 35% for median nerve lesion on the right side and 30% for median nerve lesion on the left side; 50% for sacral plexus lesion, and 40% for complete sciatic nerve lesion on the right side and 50% for sciatic nerve lesion on the left side (16).

4.5.10.2 SENSORY FUNCTION

Sensory function comprises of exteroceptive sensation wherein external stimulus such as touch, pinprick, thermal stimulus activates corresponding receptors and evokes the perception of sensation. Proprioceptive sensation refers to activation of the receptors located in ligaments, muscles, tendons, joints by the internal stimulus to provide kinesthetic information to the brain. Cortical sensation refers to stereognosis, two-point discrimination and graphesthesia.

The "Three-Point Scale" evaluates sensory modality over a dermatome/nerve distribution and grade the sensory impairment as no impairment for intact sensory function, 50% of assigned impairment for a partial loss, and 100% of designated impairment for a total loss. *Integrated Evaluation of Disability* defines partial impairment if there is a loss of two-point discrimination, joint and position sense or vibration sense with intact touch, pain, and temperature sensation. It also defines partial impairment when complete sensory loss confines only to the digital nerve with intact sensation in proximal segments of the nerve.

Integrated Evaluation of Disability assigns maximum impairment of 60% for the impairment of the sensory function of one upper extremity. It assigns an impairment of 30% for exteroceptive and proprioceptive sensation, 10% for cortical sensation, 10% for sensory perversions and 10% for pain. It assigns maximum impairment of 40% for the sensory function of one lower extremity. It assigns an impairment of 20% for exteroceptive and proprioceptive sensation, 5% for cortical sensation, 5% for sensory perversions, and 10% for pain. It assigns 30% for one-half of neck and trunk in which exteroceptive and proprioceptive sensation obtains 10%, 5% for cortical sensation and 5% for sensory perversions, and 10% for pain.

4.5.10.2.1 Sensory impairment in upper extremity

Integrated Evaluation of Disability assigns an impairment of 8% each for C6, C7, and C8 dermatomes; 3% each for dermatome C5, T1. In hand, area innervated by median nerve receives an impairment of 10.5%; ulnar nerve, 3.75%; and a radial nerve, 5.75%. In the wrist, complete loss of sensation over the posterior, the lateral, and medial cutaneous nerves of the forearm, and, superficial branch of the radial nerve, and dorsal branch of ulnar nerve together get an impairment of 1%. In the forearm, the medial cutaneous nerve of the forearm and lateral cutaneous nerve of the forearm and posterior cutaneous nerve of forearm obtains 2% each. In the arm, area supplied by the upper lateral cutaneous nerve of the arm (axillary nerve) receives an impairment of 0.5%. The area innervated by the lower lateral cutaneous nerve of the arm (radial nerve) gets an impairment of 0.5%, medial cutaneous nerve of arm 0.5%, intercostobrachial nerve 0.5%, and posterior cutaneous nerve of the arm (radial nerve) 1.0% for complete loss of sensation.

4.5.10.2.2 Sensory impairment in lower extremity

In the lower extremity, dermatomes representing L1 receives an impairment of 0.5%; L2, 1.5%; L3, 1.5%; L4, 2%; L5, 6%; S1, 6%; S2, 1.5%; and S3,4,5, C1, 1%.

In the thigh, dorsal rami (L1,2,3) obtains an impairment of 0.25%, dorsal rami (S1,2,3) 0.125%, iliohypogastric nerve (L1) 0.125%, ilioinguinal nerve (L1) 0.125%, subcostal nerve (D12) 0.125%; femoral branch of genitofemoral nerve (L1,2) 0.25%, iliohypogastric nerve (L1) 0.125%, cutaneous branch of obturator nerve (L2,3,4) 0.25%, lateral cutaneous nerve of thigh (L2,3) 0.75%, medial and intermediate cutaneous nerve of thigh (L2,3) 1%, and posterior cutaneous nerve of thigh innervated by S1,2,3 receives 1% for complete loss of sensation.

In the leg, the lateral sural cutaneous nerve gets an impairment of 1.5%, saphenous nerve 1.5%, common peroneal nerve 0.5%, and superficial peroneal nerve 0.5% for complete loss of sensation.

In the ankle and foot, a medial calcaneal branch of tibial nerve obtains an impairment of 1.5%, sural nerve 0.75%, saphenous nerve 0.75%, superficial peroneal nerve 3.5%, deep peroneal nerve 0.5%, medial plantar nerve 3.5%, and lateral plantar nerve 1.5% for complete loss of sensation.

4.5.10.2.3 Sensory ataxia—Romberg

The person stands stationary with the feet together. If he/she can maintain this posture, the person closes the eyes for 5–10 seconds. In positive Romberg, the person tends to sway but is able to keep his/her both feet together, sways markedly, may tend to fall, or tends to keep his/her legs apart for a broader base. *Integrated Evaluation of Disability* assigns a maximum impairment of 10% for positive Romberg.

4.5.10.2.4 Pain

The visual analogue scale assesses the severity of chronic pain (82) and *Integrated Evaluation of Disability* assigns an impairment of 1% if VAS is 1, 2% if VAS is 2, 3% if VAS is 3 and a maximum of 10% impairment if VAS is 10. It assigns maximum impairment of 10% for congenital absence of pain/congenital indifference to pain. It assigns additional impairment for associated amputation of fingers/toes.

AMA *Guides to the Evaluation of Permanent Impairment* assigns a maximum whole person impairment of 2% (upper extremity impairment of 4%) for sensory impairment due to peripheral nerve injury (83). It assigns a maximum lower extremity impairment of 1%–5% each for lateral femoral cutaneous nerve, superficial peroneal, the sural, and saphenous nerve (17).

Development of Korean Academy of Medical Sciences Guideline for Rating Physical Disability in the Upper Extremity assigns a disability of 8% for transverse sensory loss of a thumb, 4% for second or third finger, 2% for fourth and fifth finger in the upper extremity. It assigns 4% for longitudinal sensory loss of a thumb, 2% for second or third finger, 1% for fourth and fifth finger based on two-point discrimination and other sensory examination (80).

India's *Guidelines for Evaluation of Various Disabilities and Procedure for Certification* assign physical impairment of 10% for anesthesia to each limb, and up to 30% for paresthesia depending upon loss of sensation (19). Table 4.8 compares the impairment score assigned by *Integrated Evaluation of Disability*, AMA *Guides to the Evaluation of Permanent Impairment*, *Development of Korean Academy*

Table 4.8 Comparison of sensory impairment between countries

Integrated Evaluation of Disability	AMA—Guides to the Evaluation of Permanent Impairment	Development of Korean Academy of Medical Sciences—Impairment Rating	Guidelines for Evaluation of Various Disabilities—India
Maximum impairment: upper extremity—60% Median nerve—10.5% Ulnar nerve—4% Radial nerve—9.5% Lower extremity—40% Lateral cutaneous nerve of thigh—0.75% Saphenous nerve—1.5% Superficial Peroneal Nerve—3.5% + 0.5% Medial plantar nerve—3.5% Lateral plantar nerve—1.5% Sural nerve—0.75%	Maximum whole person impairment of 2% (upper extremity impairment of 4%) for sensory impairment due to peripheral nerve injury in upper extremity Maximum whole person impairment of 1%–2% (lower extremity impairment of 1%–5%) each for lateral femoral cutaneous nerve, superficial peroneal, sural, and saphenous nerve	Transverse sensory loss of thumb is assigned 8%, second or third finger 4%, fourth and fifth finger 2% Longitudinal sensory loss of thumb 4%, second or third finger 2%, fourth and fifth finger 1%	Assigns physical impairment of 10% for anesthesia to each limb

of Medical Sciences Guideline for Rating Physical Disability, and India's *Guidelines for Evaluation of Various Disabilities and Procedure for Certification.*

4.5.11 Micturition functions

Micturition function refers to storage of urine in the bladder and periodical expulsion of the urine from the bladder mediated by coordinated activation of smooth and striated muscles through neural mechanism residing in the brain, spinal cord, and peripheral ganglia (84). It also includes a sensation of bladder fullness, the sensation of desire to pass urine, and sensation of voiding. *Integrated Evaluation of Disability* defines Class 1 impairment of 5% for the urgency of micturition without incontinence confirmed by decreased bladder compliance with the urodynamic study, or stress incontinence confirmed by Valsalva leak point pressure, urodynamic studies and sphincter electromyography, hesitancy of micturition. It denotes Class 2 impairment of 15% for the urgency of micturition with incontinence confirmed by reduced bladder compliance with the urodynamic study or voiding by abdominal straining (Valsalva Maneuver)/Credé maneuver with no post-void residual urine. It labels Class 3 impairment of 25% for uninhibited neurogenic bladder or reflex voiding, and absence of sensation of desire, fullness. It allocates an impairment of 37% for reflex bladder, detrusor sphincter dyssynergia, and requiring alpha blockers or botulinum toxin injection or transurethral sphincterotomy or endo-urethral stents to eliminate post-void residual urine. It describes Class 4 impairment of 50% for a person with the inability to initiate micturition resulting in retention or inability to hold urine resulting in incontinence. And post-void residual urine persists after abdominal straining or Credé maneuver or sphincter management. Further, he/she manifests the absence of sensation of desire, fullness, and voiding by catheter/requiring diapers. The Urodynamic study confirms neurogenic status.

The AMA *Guides to the Evaluation of Permanent Impairment* assigns a maximum whole person impairment of 30% for total incontinence of bladder (17). Korean Academy of Medical Sciences Guideline Rating the Physical Impairment assigns a maximum body impairment of 30%–39% for loss of voluntary control on micturition or urethral dysfunction requiring permanent urinary diversion (85).

India's *Guidelines for Evaluation of Various Disabilities and Procedure for Certification* assign maximum physical impairment of 100% for very severe bladder disability due to neurogenic involvement (retention/total incontinence) (19).

In Europe, the Official Belgian Barema assigns an impairment of 60%–100% for total urinary incontinence under disorders of the genitourinary system. French Barema attributes 50%–60% for urinary incontinence and 70%–80% for cystostomy. German Barema attributes 50% for impairment of

voiding of the bladder, requiring cystostomy and 50%–70% for urinary incontinence of complex nature (16). Table 4.9 describes the impairment of bladder function assigned by *Integrated Evaluation of Disability*, AMA *Guides to the Evaluation of Permanent Impairment*, Development of Korean Academy of Medical Sciences—Impairment Rating, and *Guidelines for Evaluation of Various Disabilities* in India and Europe.

4.5.12 Bowel: Defecation function

Bowel–Defecation function refers to the process of elimination of wastes and undigested food as feces from the digestive tract by a bowel movement. Impairment of bowel function includes the inability to control bowel movement resulting in incontinence, inability to initiate bowel movement resulting in constipation and loss of sensation of bowel fullness and loss of sensation of bowel movement (neurogenic bowel dysfunction).

Integrated Evaluation of Disability defines Class 1 impairment of 5% for constipation, that is, difficulty to initiate bowel movement and evacuate bowel less than three times per week due to the neurological cause and requiring fiber supplements, and suppositories for evacuation of bowel. It defines Class 2 impairment of 15% for constipation, that is, difficulty to initiate bowel movement and evacuate bowel less than three times per week due to neurological cause refractory to fiber supplements and suppositories and requiring prokinetic agents. It defines Class 3 impairment of 25% for constipation, with difficulty to initiate a bowel movement. He/she evacuates bowel less than three times per week due to neurological cause refractory to fiber supplements, suppositories and prokinetic agents requiring enema for evacuation of the bowel. It defines Class 4 impairment of 37% for inability to control bowel movement resulting in incontinence and lack of sensation of bowel fullness and movement due to the neurological cause and requiring diapers; and Class 5 impairment of 50% for a permanent colostomy.

The AMA *Guides to the Evaluation of Permanent Impairment* assigns maximum whole person impairment of 50% for total incontinence of bowel (17). Korean Academy of Medical Sciences Guideline Rating the Physical Impairment allocates 35% for bowel incontinence (20). In Europe, the Official Belgian Barema attributes an impairment of 30%–100% for incontinence of bowel due to lesions in the anal sphincter. French Barema attributes an impairment of 80%–90% for total fecal incontinence and 70% for colostomy. German Barema assigns minimum impairment of 50% for incontinence of bowel due to lesions in the anal sphincter (16). Table 4.10 compares the impairment of bowel function assigned by *Integrated Evaluation of Disability*, AMA *Guides to the Evaluation of Permanent Impairment*,

Table 4.9 Comparison of impairment of micturition functions between countries

Integrated Evaluation of Disability	AMA—Guides to the Evaluation of Permanent Impairment	Development of Korean Academy of Medical Sciences— Impairment Rating	Official Belgian Barema	French Barema	India—Guidelines for Evaluation of Various Disabilities and Procedure for Certification	German Barema
Inability to hold urine resulting in incontinence (or) inability to initiate micturition resulting in retention (or) persistent post-void residual urine requiring catheterization or diapers; and loss of sensation of desire/ fullness/ voiding Maximum Impairment: 50%	Total incontinence of bladder: Maximum whole person impairment of 30%	Loss of voluntary control of micturition or urethral dysfunction requiring permanent urinary diversion: Impairment: Maximum body impairment 30%–39%	Total urinary incontinence: Impairment of 60%–100%	Urinary incontinence: Impairment 50%–60%, Cystostomy: 70% to 80%	Neurogenic involvement with retention or total incontinence of bladder: Maximum impairment of 100%	Impairment of voiding of urine on cystostomy: Impairment of 50%, Complex urinary incontinence 50%–70%

Table 4.10 Comparison of impairment of defecation function between countries

Integrated Evaluation of Disability	Development of Korean Academy of Medical Sciences— Impairment Rating	American Medical Association—*Guides to the Evaluation of Permanent Impairment*	Official Belgian Barema	German Barema	French Barema
Incontinence of bowel, loss of sensation of bowel fullness and movement or permanent colostomy: Maximum impairment of 50%	Bowel incontinence: Impairment of 35%	Total incontinence of bowel: Maximum whole person impairment of 50%	Incontinence due to impairment of function of the sphincter of the rectum: 30%–100%	Incontinence due to impairment of function of the sphincter of the rectum: 50%	Total fecal incontinence: 80%–90% Colostomy: 70%

Development of Korean Academy of Medical Sciences—Impairment Rating, and Europe.

4.5.13 Genital functions

4.5.13.1 SEXUAL FUNCTION

Sexual functions refer to mental and physical aspects of sexual arousal, sexual act, orgasm, ejaculation, and resolution.

The nocturnal penile tumescence test and serum testosterone and prolactin measurements aid in the assessment of erectile dysfunction along with the International Index of Erectile Function (86). Color Doppler ultrasonography also assists in the evaluation of erectile dysfunction (87).

Integrated Evaluation of Disability describes an impairment of 15% for loss of sexual function, which is the inability to perform sexual intercourse due to erectile dysfunction

even after the maximum medical management (or) anatomical loss of penis and/or testes.

The AMA *Guides to the Evaluation of Permanent Impairment* assigns a whole person impairment of 15% for total loss of sexual function fulfilling their criteria (17).

Development of Korean Academy of Medical Sciences Guideline Rating the Physical Impairment assigns a maximum body impairment of 20%–25% for erectile dysfunction evinced by International Index of Erectile Function, nocturnal penile tumescence test, and vasoactive agents induced color Doppler ultrasonography. It enhances impairment by 50% of score for men younger than 40 years and decreases by 50% of score for men older than 65 years (85). Table 4.11 compares the impairment genital functions assigned by *Integrated Evaluation of Disability*, AMA *Guides to the Evaluation of Permanent Impairment*, and Development of Korean Academy of Medical Sciences—Impairment Rating.

Table 4.11 Comparison of impairment of genital functions between countries

Integrated Evaluation of Disability	Development of Korean Academy of Medical Sciences—Impairment Rating	AMA—*Guides to the Evaluation of Permanent Impairment*
1. Loss of sexual function: Impairment of 15% 2. Menstrual dysfunction namely primary amenorrhea: Impairment of 15% 3. Impairment of procreation function (azoospermia) in men: Impairment of 15%	1. Erectile dysfunction with the inability to penetrate the vagina—maximum body impairment of 20%–25% 2. Total loss of scrotum—maximum body impairment of 11%–15% 3. Anatomical alterations of testis, epididymis or spermatic cord with non-functional semen and hormones— maximum body impairment of 13% 4. Bilateral non-functional ovary before menopause, bilateral tubal agenesis or loss of bilateral tubes or bilateral tubal occlusion before menopause—26%–35%	Total loss of sexual function—whole person impairment of 15%

4.5.13.2 MENSTRUAL FUNCTION

Menstrual function refers to a natural process of cyclic discharge of menstrual fluid. *Integrated Evaluation of Disability* assigns an impairment of 15% for menstrual dysfunction namely primary amenorrhea.

4.5.13.3 PROCREATION FUNCTION

The procreation function refers to the biological potential for fertility, pregnancy, childbirth, and lactation. The impairment of procreation functions in men includes azoospermia. Hormone (or) semen analysis and (or) vasography determines the dysfunction of procreation in men. The impairment of the procreation function in women of reproductive age may be due to primary amenorrhea and cervical/uterine/ovarian/tubal or peritoneal factors, which may result in failure to initiate/continue the pregnancy. Laboratory or imaging studies for cervical/uterine/ovarian/tubal or peritoneal factors confirm the impairment in procreation function in women.

Integrated Evaluation of Disability assigns an impairment of 15% for defective procreation function due to azoospermia in men or structural and functional failure to initiate/continue a pregnancy after maximum medical treatment before 50 years of age in women.

Korean Academy of Medical Sciences Guideline Rating the Physical Impairment assigns maximum body impairment of 11%–15% when there is anatomical or functional impairment of male genital organ including hormones. It assigns maximum body impairment of 26%–35% for bilateral anatomical or functional impairment of ovary, fallopian tubes before menopause, age-related loss of potential for pregnancy in women also modifies the percentage of impairment (85).

4.5.14 Renal excretory function

Urinary excretory functions refer to the filtering function of the kidney; that is, retains the materials needed and expels the toxic metabolic by-products in the urine to store in the bladder for discharge. Glomerular filtration rate serves to classify chronic renal failure into five stages (88). Cockcroft–Gault formula (Equation 4.6) helps to estimate the glomerular filtration rate (GFR) (89).

Creatinine clearance $(\mathrm{mL/min}) =$

$$\frac{(140 - \text{age in year}) \times \text{lean body weight (kg)}}{\text{plasma creatinine} \left(\dfrac{\mathrm{mg}}{\mathrm{dL}} \right) \times 72} (\times 0.85 \text{ in women})$$

$$(4.6)$$

The normal glomerular filtration rate is equal or more than 90 mL/min/1.73 m².

Integrated Evaluation of Disability defines Class 1 impairment of 10% when only one kidney is functioning, or one kidney is congenitally absent for loss of natural safety factor. It defines Class 2 impairment of 25% for non-dialysis dependent chronic renal failure with GFR <60 and ≥30 mL/min/1.73 m². It defines Class 3 impairment of 37% for dialysis-dependent chronic renal failure with GFR <30 mL/min/1.73 m², and Class 4 impairment of 50% for end-stage kidney failure with GFR <15 mL/min/1.73 m² requiring renal transplantation.

The AMA *Guides to the Evaluation of Permanent Impairment* assigns a maximum whole person impairment of 75% for permanent impairment due to upper urinary tract disease (17).

Korean Academy of Medical Sciences Guideline Rating the Physical Impairment assigns maximum body impairment of 90% for the chronic renal disorder with serum creatinine ≥10 mg dL or GFR <15 mL/min/1.73 m² or dialysis for more than 3 months (85).

In Europe, the Official Belgian Barema assigns an impairment of 0%–100% for nephropathy, French Barema 80%–95% for acute renal failure, Italian Barema 100% for nephropathy on continuous dialysis and 25% for nephrectomy with normally functioning another kidney, German Barema 25% for nephrectomy, congenital absence of one kidney, complete unilateral renal failure and 100% for severe renal failure necessitating hemodialysis and Iceland Barema assigns an impairment of 10% for unilateral nephrectomy (16). Table 4.12 compares the impairment of renal function described by *Integrated Evaluation of Disability*, AMA *Guides to the Evaluation of Permanent Impairment*, Development of Korean Academy of Medical Sciences—Impairment Rating and Europe.

4.5.15 Liver function

Liver performs essential functions namely synthesis of albumin, carrier proteins, coagulation factors, growth and hormonal factors, bile acids, cholesterol, lecithin, phospholipids; regulation of nutritive products, such as glucose, glycogen, amino acids, lipids, cholesterol; and metabolism of drugs and other substances.

The serum level of bilirubin indicates the ability of the liver to excrete bile; International Normalized Ratio (INR) measures coagulopathy, that is, the ability of the liver to produce blood clotting factors (90) and is a useful prognostic tool rather than an indicator of bleeding risk in patients with the chronic liver disease. There is associated impairment of renal function in persons with end-stage liver failure, and it is an important predictor of mortality in liver failure (90).

Integrated Evaluation of Disability describes parameters namely serum level of bilirubin, albumin, sodium, INR, and hepatic encephalopathy (impairments of consciousness, sleep, cognition, sensory and motor functions, and personality changes) to define impairment class. *Integrated Evaluation of Disability* assigns an impairment of 25% for Class 1 impairment, 50% for Class 2, 75% for Class 3, and 95% for coma for Class 4.

The AMA *Guides to the Evaluation of Permanent Impairment* assigns maximum whole person impairment

Table 4.12 Comparison of impairment of renal excretory function between countries

Integrated Evaluation of Disability	AMA—Guides to the Evaluation of Permanent Impairment	Korean Academy of Medical Sciences— Impairment Rating	Belgian— BOBI	French Barema	Italian Barema	German Barema
End-stage renal failure requiring renal transplantation: Impairment of 50%	Permanent impairment due to upper urinary tract disease: Maximum WPI of 75%	Chronic renal dysfunction with serum creatinine ≥10 mg dL or GFR <15 mL/min/1.73 m² or dialysis of >3 months: maximum body impairment of 90%	Nephropathy: Impairment of 0%–100%	Acute renal failure: Impairment of 80%–95%	Nephropathy on continuous dialysis: Impairment of 100%	Severe renal failure necessitating hemodialysis: Impairment of 100%

of 65% for impairment for progressive chronic liver diseases due to cirrhosis of the liver or refractory jaundice, or gastric and esophageal varices with bleeding, and hepatic insufficiency (91).

Korean Academy of Medical Sciences, Development of a Rating System for Digestive System Impairments assigns maximum physical impairment above 75% for progressive chronic liver diseases with objective evidence for cirrhosis of the liver, refractory ascites or chronic hepatic encephalopathy or hepatorenal syndrome or hepato-pulmonary syndrome (92).

In Europe, French Barema assigns an impairment of more than 80% for acute hepatic failure, Italian Barema 71%–80% for cirrhosis of the liver with portal hypertension, and German Barema 60%–100% for "liver cirrhosis with ascites (16). Table 4.13 depicts the impairment score of liver function allotted by *Integrated Evaluation of Disability*, AMA *Guides to the Evaluation of Permanent Impairment*,

Development of Korean Academy of Medical Sciences— Impairment Rating, and Europe.

4.5.16 Cardiac function

The heart pumps to move the blood continuously with essential pressure to the whole body. The functions of the heart include sustaining the contractile force of cardiac muscle, maintaining optimum heart rate, rhythm, and cardiac output; valvular functions of the heart; pumping sufficient blood to the pulmonary circulation for the exchange of oxygen and carbon dioxide and providing a continuous supply of blood to the heart. The overall function of the heart is to deliver oxygen and nutrients to all organs and tissues, and transport carbon dioxide and waste products through the venous circulation to the appropriate organs for excretion.

The capacity of a person to perform an aerobic work depends on VO₂max, that is, maximum oxygen consumption.

Table 4.13 Comparison of impairment of liver functions between countries

Integrated Evaluation of Disability	AMA—Guides to the Evaluation of Permanent Impairment	Development of Korean Academy of Medical Sciences— Impairment Rating	French Barema	Italian Barema	German Barema
Hepatic encephalopathy with coma: Maximum impairment of 95%	Progressive chronic liver diseases due to cirrhosis of liver or refractory jaundice, or gastric and esophageal varices with bleeding, and hepatic insufficiency: Maximum WPI of 65%	Progressive chronic liver disease— cirrhosis of liver, hepatic encephalopathy, hepatorenal syndrome, hepato-pulmonary syndrome: >75% of physical impairment	Acute Hepatic Failure: Impairment >80%	Cirrhosis of the liver with portal hypertension: Impairment 71%–80%	Liver of cirrhosis with ascites: Impairment of 60%–100%

Metabolic Equivalent of Task (MET) is an expression of functional capacity of a person. MET is the ratio of an individual's metabolic rate to resting metabolic rate. One MET refers to energy cost required to sit quietly without performing any work and measures 1 kcal/kg/hour or 3.5 mL of oxygen/minute/kg body weight (93,94). The exercise test with or without respiratory gas analysis measures functional capacity. The exercise test with respiratory gas analysis measures VO$_2$max. The exercise test without respiratory gas analysis calculates VO$_2$max from nomograms. The clinician can choose either a motorized treadmill or stationary cycle ergometer and can decide maximal or submaximal exercise depending on the clinical status of the individual (94). Specific Activity Scale of Goldman et al. describes the METs scale based on specific physical activity (95). As per WHO-ICF, function and activity are two different entities. Hence, *Integrated Evaluation of Disability* prefers evaluation of impairment of function without mixing limitation of physical activity. However, it is necessary to derive METs indirectly from the intensity of physical activity only if there is a medical contraindication to performing an exercise test.

The New York Heart Association (NYHA) Functional Classification describes the stages of functional capacity of the heart in persons with heart failure (96).

Echocardiography is one of the clinical tools to evaluate cardiac function. In Echocardiography, "E" velocity refers to peak early filling velocity, and "A" velocity relates to the velocity during atrial contraction. Normally "E" velocity is slightly greater than "A" velocity in middle-aged persons. "E" velocity is low if the rate of ventricular relaxation is slow (97). The measurement of "E" and "A" velocity is useful in evaluating diastolic dysfunction.

Ejection fraction denotes the volume of blood pumped by the ventricle during each heartbeat. The American Heart Association documents that ejection fraction of 55–70 is normal, less than 55 indicates left ventricular dysfunction (98).

Guidelines classify heart failure into four stages based on structural, functional impairment, and response to medical management (99).

4.5.16.1 CORONARY ARTERY DISEASE OR HYPERTENSIVE CARDIOVASCULAR DISEASE OR CARDIOMYOPATHY

In *Integrated Evaluation of Disability*, parameters, namely the severity of cardiovascular symptoms, clinical evidence of cardiac failure, echocardiographic evidence of systolic and diastolic dysfunction, and METs aerobic functional capacity by exercise test with treadmill define impairment class. *Integrated Evaluation of Disability* describes Class 1 impairment of 15%, and Class 2 impairment of 25%. It defines Class 3 impairment of 50%, and Class 4 impairment of 75% for end-stage heart failure refractory to medical management in coronary artery disease or hypertensive cardiovascular disease or cardiomyopathy.

4.5.16.2 DYSRHYTHMIA

The rhythm of heart refers to the regularity of beating of the heart. Dysrhythmia refers to impairment of normal rhythm of the heartbeat. Heart failure can increase the risk of atrial fibrillation. *Integrated Evaluation of Disability* describes parameters namely dysrhythmia, ejection fraction, nature of intervention instituted to define impairment class. *Integrated Evaluation of Disability* represents Class 1 impairment of 5% for isolated dysrhythmia under Guideline-Directed Medical Therapy (GDMT) with normal left ventricular systolic and diastolic function. It defines Class 2 impairment of 10% for isolated dysrhythmia with palpitation requiring or underwent implantation of a pacemaker and/or Automatic Implantable Cardioverter-Defibrillator (AICD) with normal left ventricular systolic and diastolic function. It describes Class 3 impairment of 15% for dysrhythmia with palpitation, missing of a heartbeat, dizziness, sweating, anxiety requiring or underwent implantation of a pacemaker and/or AICD with minimal left ventricular systolic or minimal diastolic dysfunction. It defines Class 4 impairment of 25% for dysrhythmia with palpitation, missing of a heartbeat, dizziness, sweating, anxiety requiring or underwent implantation of a pacemaker and/or AICD with minimal left ventricular systolic and diastolic dysfunction. It defines Class 5 impairment of 37% for dysrhythmia with palpitation, missing of heartbeat, dizziness, sweating, anxiety, dyspnea, chest pain, syncope requiring or underwent implantation of a pacemaker and/or AICD with moderate left ventricular systolic or moderate diastolic dysfunction. It describes Class 6 impairment of 50% for dysrhythmia with palpitation, missing of heartbeat, dizziness, sweating, anxiety, dyspnea, chest pain, syncope requiring or underwent implantation of a pacemaker and/or AICD with moderate left ventricular systolic and diastolic dysfunction. It describes Class 7 impairment of 75% for dysrhythmia with palpitation, missing of heartbeat, dizziness, sweating, anxiety, dyspnea, chest pain, syncope requiring or underwent implantation of a pacemaker, and/or AICD with severe left ventricular systolic and diastolic dysfunction.

4.5.16.3 VALVULAR HEART DISEASE

Evaluation of the person with valvular heart disease entails clinical examination and imaging studies. Echocardiography assesses the impact of the valvular lesions on the size of the atrium and ventricle and its functions besides the severity of valvular lesions.

Guideline for the management of patients with valvular heart disease provides definitions of severity of valve disease based on valve anatomy, hemodynamics, and hemodynamic consequences and symptoms (100).

Integrated Evaluation of Disability defines Class 1 impairment of 5% for Class 1 impairment for asymptomatic valvular heart disease with normal size of the atrium/ventricle, normal systolic and diastolic function and normal pulmonary artery pressure and right ventricular function. It defines Class 2 impairment of 15% for symptomatic valvular heart disease with mild enlargement of atrium/ventricle, minimal systolic dysfunction or minimal diastolic dysfunction, or increased pulmonary artery pressure >20 to ≤30 mm of Hg with normal right ventricular function. It defines Class 3 impairment of 25% for symptomatic valvular heart disease with mild enlargement of atrium/ventricle, minimal systolic dysfunction and minimal diastolic dysfunction, and/or pulmonary hypertension >30 to ≤50 mm of Hg with normal right ventricular function. It defines Class 4 impairment of 37% for symptomatic valvular heart disease with moderate enlargement of atrium/ventricle, moderate systolic dysfunction or moderate diastolic dysfunction, and/or pulmonary hypertension >30 to ≤50 mm of Hg with minimal right ventricular dysfunction. It defines Class 5 impairment 50% for symptomatic valvular heart disease with moderate enlargement of atrium/ventricle, moderate systolic dysfunction and moderate diastolic dysfunction, and pulmonary hypertension >30 to ≤50 mm of Hg with moderate right ventricular dysfunction. It defines Class 6 impairment of 75% for symptomatic valvular heart disease with severe enlargement of atrium/ventricle, severe systolic dysfunction and severe diastolic dysfunction, and/or pulmonary hypertension >50 mm of Hg with severe right ventricular dysfunction.

The AMA *Guides to the Evaluation of Permanent Impairment* assigns maximum whole person impairment of 65% for coronary artery disease, cardiomyopathies, pericardial heart disease and dysrhythmias after fulfilling their criteria (17).

India's *Guidelines for Evaluation of Various Disabilities* defines group 4 as persons who become symptomatic during rest and on minimal exertion due to cardiopulmonary disease with the limitation of his/her daily physical activities by 75%–100% (19).

In Europe, the Official Belgian Barema assigns an impairment of 20%–70% for traumatic valvular lesions of the heart, 10%–40% for coronary artery disease without infarction, 30%–60% for myocardial infarction with ectasia, 50%–100% for decompensated heart following coronary artery disease. French Barema assigns 80%–90% for continuous or intermittent angina pectoris refractory to treatment, 50%–100% for congenital cyanotic heart disease, and 80%–90% for the decompensated heart with congestive heart failure. Italian Barema assigns 25% for aortic valvular heart disease with prosthetic replacement, 100% for severe coronary artery disease, 100% for cardiomyopathy and 100% for valvular heart disease with severe heart failure. German Barema assigns 10%–30% for heart disease with dysrhythmia without permanent deficiency, 90%–100% for valvular heart disease, coronary artery

disease, cardiomyopathies, congenital heart disease developing dyspnea at rest, and pulmonary hypertension (16). Table 4.14 compares the impairment of cardiac functions defined by *Integrated Evaluation of Disability*, AMA *Guides to the Evaluation of Permanent Impairment, Guidelines for Evaluation of Various Disabilities*—India, and Europe.

4.5.17 Pulmonary functions

4.5.17.1 ASTHMA

Asthma is the common cause of pulmonary disability. In asthma, there is hyperresponsiveness of the airway and airway obstruction due to chronic inflammation of the airways (101). Chronic obstruction may lead to occlusion of the small airway with uneven ventilation. It manifests as a cough, expectoration, breathlessness, tightness in chest, wheezing, and expiratory airflow limitation. In asthma, both symptoms and expiratory airflow limitation may vary over a period besides intensity (102). The degree of reversibility, that is, a post-bronchodilator increase in forced expiratory volume in one second (FEV_1) of 12% and more than 200 mL confirms reversible airflow obstruction and thus favors the diagnosis of asthma (103). Peak expiratory flow (PEF) rate refers to the maximum flow rate of exhaled air during forced expiration after maximum inspiration. It assesses the severity of asthma and monitors asthma control. In *Integrated Evaluation of Disability*, clinical and physiological parameters evaluate persons with asthma to assign permanent impairment.

Integrated Evaluation of Disability assigns an impairment of 5% for Class 1 impairment, 25% for Class 2 impairment, 37% for Class 3 impairment, and 50% for Class 4 impairment. Table 4.15 compares the maximum impairment score of the AMA, Belgium, France, and German.

The AMA *Guides to the Evaluation of Permanent Impairment* assigns maximum whole person impairment of 65% for asthma after fulfilling their criteria (17) (Table 4.15).

In Europe, the Official Belgian Barema assigns an impairment of 60%–100% for asthma, French Barema assigns 50%–75% for chronic asthma, Italian Barema assigns 45% for chronic asthma, and German Barema assigns 80%–100% for asthma with severe respiratory failure (16) (Table 4.15).

4.5.17.2 CHRONIC OBSTRUCTIVE PULMONARY DISEASES

Tobacco smoke, occupational dust and chemicals, indoor and outdoor air pollutants predispose to the risk of developing Chronic Obstructive Pulmonary Disease (COPD). Chronic irritants trigger inflammation of airways, parenchyma, and pulmonary vessels. It may lead to a chronic cough, expectoration of sputum, and breathlessness. Persistent non-reversible airflow limitation evinced by

Table 4.14 Comparison of impairment of cardiac functions between countries

Integrated Evaluation of Disability	AMA—Guides to the Evaluation of Permanent Impairment	French Barema	Italian Barema	German Barema	Belgium—BOBI	Guidelines for Evaluation of Various Disabilities—India
End-stage heart failure refractory to medical management: Maximum impairment—75% Dysrhythmia—pacemaker and/or AICD with severe left ventricular systolic and diastolic dysfunction: Maximum impairment—75% Valvular heart disease with severe enlargement of atrium/ventricle, systolic and diastolic dysfunction, and/or pulmonary hypertension > 50 mm of Hg with severe right ventricular dysfunction: Maximum Impairment: 75%	Coronary artery disease, cardiomyopathies, pericardial heart disease and dysrhythmias: Maximum whole person impairment of 65%	Angina pectoris refractory to treatment: Impairment—80%–90% Congenital cyanotic heart disease: Impairment—50%–100% Decompensated congestive heart failure: Impairment—80%–90%	Severe coronary artery disease: Impairment—100% Cardiomyopathy or valvular heart disease with severe heart failure: 100% Aortic valvular heart disease with prosthetic replacement: Impairment—25%	Valvular heart disease, coronary artery disease, cardiomyopathies, congenital heart disease developing dyspnea at rest and pulmonary hypertension: 90%–100% Heart disease with dysrhythmia without permanent deficiency: 10%–30%	Coronary artery disease without infarction: Impairment—10%–40% Myocardial infarction with parietal ectasia: Impairment—30%–60% Coronary artery disease with decompensated heart: Impairment—50%–100% Traumatic Valvular heart Impairment—20%–70%	Group 4 persons with cardiopulmonary disease who becomes symptomatic during rest and on minimal exertion with limitation of everyday physical activities by 75%–100%, and Group 5 Symptomatic intermittently even at rest

Table 4.15 Comparison of impairment of pulmonary functions in asthma between countries

Integrated Evaluation of Disability	AMA—Guides to the Evaluation of Permanent Impairment	Belgium—BOBI	French Barema	Italian Barema	German Barema
Maximum Impairment of 50%	Maximum whole person impairment of 65%	Asthma with secondary cardiac Impairment 60%–100%	Chronic asthma: Impairment 50%–75%	Chronic asthma: Impairment 45%	Asthma with severe respiratory failure: Impairment 80%–100%

Table 4.16 Comparison of impairment in COPD between countries

Integrated Evaluation of Disability	AMA—Guides to the Evaluation of Permanent Impairment	Belgium—BOBI	Italian Barema
Maximum impairment of 50%	Pulmonary dysfunction: Maximum whole person impairment of 65%	Very severe chronic bronchitis: Impairment—70%–100%	Chronic obstructive lung disease: Impairment—75%

the ratio of post-bronchodilator FEV_1 and forced vital capacity (FVC) less than 0.70 suggests COPD (104). Post-bronchodilator FEV_1 serves to classify the severity of airflow limitation (104). The Dyspnea scale from the modified Medical Research Council (mMRC) assesses breathlessness (105,106). The number of exacerbations the person has had within the previous 12 months indicates the gravity of risk associated with COPD.

The WHO's COPD Management states that FEV_1/FVC <70% and FEV_1 < 80% predicted confirms the presence of airflow limitation (107).

The clinical symptoms and signs, respiratory failure and right heart failure, the frequency of exacerbations and post-bronchodilator airflow limitation serve as a parameter to define impairment class for COPD in *Integrated Evaluation of Disability*. *Integrated Evaluation of Disability* describes Class 1 impairment of 5%, Class 2 impairment of 25%, Class 3 impairment of 37% and Class 4 impairment of 50%.

The AMA *Guides to the Evaluation of Permanent Impairment* assigns a maximum whole person impairment of 65% for pulmonary dysfunction after fulfilling their criteria (108).

Belgium assigns an impairment of 70%–100% for very severe chronic bronchitis, and Italian Barema assigns 75% for chronic obstructive lung disease (16). Table 4.16 compares impairment of pulmonary functions in COPD defined by *Integrated Evaluation of Disability*, AMA *Guides to the Evaluation of Permanent Impairment*, and Europe.

4.5.17.3 RESTRICTIVE LUNG DISEASE

Diseases of the lung parenchyma, pleura, chest wall, and neuromuscular apparatus produce restrictive lung diseases. Reduced lung volume suggests restrictive lung disease.

In restrictive lung disease, there is decreased total lung capacity below the fifth percentile of the predicted value, and

reduced FEV_1 and FVC but preserved or increased FEV_1-to-FVC ratio. Care should be taken in interpretation because submaximal inspiratory or expiratory efforts and patchy peripheral airflow obstruction can result in a decrease in vital capacity (VC) and normal or increased FEV_1/VC (109).

The diffusing capacity of the lung for carbon monoxide (D_Lco) the transfer factor decreases in intrinsic restrictive lung disease, whereas it remains normal in extrinsic restrictive lung diseases. It is necessary to interpret D_Lco along with spirometry and lung volumes (body plethysmography) (109). It grades the degree of reduction in diffusing capacity for carbon monoxide as mild: >60% predicted and < lower limit of normal, moderate: 40%–60% predicted, and severe: <40% predicted (109). FEV_1 serves to grade the severity of abnormality in obstructive, restrictive and mixed pulmonary disease. It ranks the impairment as mild (FEV_1 % predicted >70), moderate (FEV_1 % predicted 60–69), moderately severe (FEV_1 % predicted 50–59), severe (FEV_1 % predicted 35–49), and very severe (FEV1 % predicted <35) (109). Table 4.17 compares the impairment score of

Table 4.17 Comparison of impairment—restrictive lung diseases between countries

Integrated Evaluation of Disability	AMA—Guides to the Evaluation of Permanent Impairment	Belgium—BOBI
Maximum impairment of 50%	Maximum whole person impairment of 65% for pulmonary dysfunction	Non-functional parenchymal lesion involving minimum of one-third of pulmonary area: Impairment: 15%–100%

restrictive lung diseases defined by *Integrated Evaluation of Disability*, AMA *Guides to the Evaluation of Permanent Impairment*, and Belgium.

In *Integrated Evaluation of Disability*, FEV_1 defines the severity of spirometric abnormality in extrinsic restrictive ventilatory defect and D_Lco percentage predicted defines the degree of severity in intrinsic lung disease. It classifies Class 1 impairment of 5%, Class 2 impairment of 25%, Class 3 impairment of 37%, and Class 4 impairment of 50% for extrinsic lung diseases. It also classifies Class 1 impairment of 5%, Class 2 impairment of 25%, Class 3 impairment of 37%, and Class 4 impairment of 50% for intrinsic lung diseases.

The AMA *Guides to the Evaluation of Permanent Impairment* assigns maximum whole person impairment of 65% for pulmonary dysfunction after fulfilling their criteria (108).

The Official Belgian Barema assigns an impairment of 15%–100% for non-functional parenchymal lesion involving a minimum of one-third of the pulmonary area (16).

4.5.17.4 CHRONIC RESPIRATORY FAILURE

Respiratory failure is a derangement in gas exchange function, that is, oxygenation and CO_2 elimination. In hypoxemic respiratory failure (type I respiratory failure), PaO_2 is less than 60 mm of Hg and $PaCO_2$ is normal or less than 50 mm of Hg. In hypercapnic respiratory failure (type II respiratory failure), $PaCO_2$ is more than ≥ 45 mm of Hg, and arterial pH <7.45 (110). Persons with severe asthma, COPD, poliomyelitis, cervical spinal cord injury, polyneuropathy, myasthenia gravis, primary muscle disorder, primary alveolar hypoventilation, obesity hypoventilation syndrome, myxedema, and so on, exhibit chronic hypercapnic respiratory failure (type II). Pulmonary hypertension, cor pulmonale, and right ventricular failure may accompany chronic hypercapnic respiratory failure (type II respiratory failure).

Integrated Evaluation of Disability describes an impairment of 50% for type II respiratory failure.

French Barema assigns 85%–90% for acute respiratory failure with secondary right heart failure (16).

4.5.17.5 RESPIRATORY MUSCLE FUNCTIONS

Respiratory muscles comprise intercostal muscles, diaphragm, and accessory muscles of respiration.

The ability of a person to count in single breath 30 and above serves as a bedside clinical test to measure the ventilatory capacity of the individual. If the individual cannot count until 30, the person requires an evaluation of his/her pulmonary function. The pulmonary function tests namely FVC; FEV_1 and peak expiratory flow assesses the ventilation. The level of spinal cord lesion, duration of the lesion, age, respiratory muscle strength, cigarette smoking, and concomitant respiratory conditions influence the pulmonary function (111).

Vital capacity is a simple bedside measure of ventilation. The person inhales maximally and then breathe out as hard, and fast as he/she can into a spirometer. The amount of air expelled by maximal voluntary effort refers to vital capacity.

The measurement of vital capacity is used to decide the person's ability to maintain an adequate gas exchange. Vital capacity is correlating well with FEV_1, inspiratory capacity, expiratory reserve volume, functional residual capacity and ratio of residual volume and total lung capacity (112). The vital capacity serves as a single global measure to assess the ventilatory status of the persons with spinal cord injury because of the good correlation between vital capacity and most of the other pulmonary function tests (113).

Persons with complete spinal cord injury at C1 and C2 require long-term respiratory assistance, either mechanical ventilation or electrophrenic pacing. Depending on the complete or incomplete division of spinal cord in C3–C8 segments, individuals may have varying degrees of respiratory dysfunction and, hence, may or may not need respiratory assistance (112). In complete spinal cord injury below C2 segment, there is a reduction in VC to 20%–50% of predicted, inefficient ventilation, and impairment of a cough due to changes in compliance, chest wall distortion, and impairment of muscles of inspiration and expiration (114). In cervical cord injury, FVC was 32% and FEV_1 was 37%. In high dorsal injuries, FVC was 43.39%, and FEV_1 was 56.74%. In low dorsal injuries, FVC, 47.83% and FEV_1, 44.7%; and FVC, 70% and FEV_1, 58.33% in lumbar injuries (115). Thus, a correlation exists between the level of cord injury and the degree of respiratory dysfunction.

In persons with tetraplegia, vital capacity can increase until ten years post injury even without structured pulmonary rehabilitation program and decline ten years post injury (112).

The vital capacity of a healthy person is about 3000–5000 cc. In unilateral diaphragmatic paralysis, vital capacity is less than 1000–1100 cc. These individuals may require assisted ventilation to restore and maintain alveolar ventilation to meet the metabolic demands as well as to correct arterial hypoxia. The vital capacity in persons with intercostal and abdominal muscle paralysis, intact diaphragm and accessory muscles of respiration are about 2200–2500 cc. In spinal cord injury with complete diaphragmatic paralysis, the vital capacity is very low (C-3: 100 ccs, C-4:670 ccs) (116). Assisted ventilation is essential in persons with a vital capacity less than 500 cc, and when higher vital capacity is rapidly declining (117). The person with bilateral diaphragmatic paralysis remains ventilator dependent during their remaining life.

Integrated Evaluation of Disability defined parameters namely level of spinal cord injury, vital capacity, cough reflex and need for assisted ventilation to assign a percentage of impairment. It assigns impairment of 15%, 25%, 50%, and 75%, respectively, for Class 1, Class 2, Class 3, Class 4 impairment.

4.5.18 Hematologic system functions

4.5.18.1 ANEMIA

In anemia, there is the insufficient oxygen-carrying capacity to meet the physiological needs of the body. Decreased red cell production results in anemia. Nutritional deficiency such as iron, folate, vitamin B12, inherited or acquired disorders affecting hemoglobin synthesis, inflammatory block due to acute and chronic inflammation, or increased destruction due to autoantibodies cause a reduction in red blood cell count. Hemoglobin level in the blood defines the severity of anemia. WHO's Vitamin and Nutrition Information System defines the severity of anemia in men 15 years of age and above as mild: 110–129 g/L, moderate: 80–109 g/L, and severe: lower than 80 g/L. It also defines anemia in non-pregnant women 15 years of age and above as mild: 110–119 g/L, moderate: 80–109 g/L, and severe: lower than 80 g/L (118). A hemoglobin level of 70 g/L serves as a threshold for transfusion of red blood cell (119).

Persons with anemia develop palpitations, dyspnea, tachycardia, angina pectoris, dizziness, syncope. ECG reveals de novo ST depression or elevation on the electrocardiogram and new arrhythmia.

Integrated Evaluation of Disability describes asymptomatic chronic anemia with Hgb 110–129 g/L as Class 1 impairment of 0%, symptomatic chronic anemia without cardiopulmonary limitations and Hgb > 70–109 g/L requiring occasional blood transfusion as Class 2 impairment of 15%. It describes symptomatic chronic anemia with cardiopulmonary limitations, Hgb lower than 70 g/L requiring monthly blood transfusion with transfusion dependence for survival as Class 3 impairment of 37%. *Integrated Evaluation of Disability* assigns impairment for chronic anemia only after having reached maximum medical improvement with maximum medical management.

The AMA *Guides to the Evaluation of Permanent Impairment* assigns maximum whole person impairment of 75% for anemia after fulfilling their criteria (120).

Italian Barema assigns an impairment of 90% for Cooley's anemia and 41% for autoimmune hemolytic anemia (16).

4.5.18.2 LEUKEMIA

4.5.18.2.1 Chronic myeloid leukemia

The discovery of Philadelphia chromosome and abnormal gene BCR-ABL in the blood and bone marrow of persons with chronic myeloid leukemia led to the development of newer drugs Imatinib and later Dasatinib and Nilotinib.

It has improved the management of chronic myeloid leukemia with a prospect of good prognosis (121). The advent of tyrosine kinase inhibitors has completely changed the prognosis, and chronic myeloid leukemia is a curable disease in many persons now (122).

As chronic myeloid leukemia is curable, *Integrated Evaluation of Disability* does not assign any impairment. However, if a person with chronic myeloid leukemia remains under medication for more than the stipulated period, it assigns an impairment of 10% for the burden of treatment compliance.

The AMA *Guides to the Evaluation of Permanent Impairment* assigns a maximum whole person impairment of 85% after fulfilling their criteria for leukemias (17).

French Barema attributes an impairment of 80%–95% for leukemia in an advanced stage and 1%–10% for clinically cured leukemia and reticulocytoses; German Barema allocates 50%–80% for chronic myeloid leukemia (16). Table 4.18 compares the impairment score of *Integrated Evaluation of Disability*, AMA, France, and Germany.

4.5.18.2.2 Chronic lymphoid leukemia

In typical B cell chronic lymphoid leukemia, the circulating lymphocytes are more than 4×10^9/L. *Integrated Evaluation of Disability* assigns Class 1 impairment for persons with asymptomatic chronic lymphoid leukemia with lymphocytosis only in blood and bone marrow. It assigns Class 2 impairment for individuals presenting with lymphocytosis, lymphadenopathy, enlarged spleen or liver; and Class 3 impairment for persons presenting with lymphocytosis, anemia (Hemoglobin $\leq$ 100 g/L) and thrombocytopenia (platelets less than 10,000/μL). *Integrated Evaluation of Disability* assigns an impairment of 0%, 37%, and 50% respectively for Class 1, Class 2 and Class 3 impairment.

The AMA *Guides to the Evaluation of Permanent Impairment* assigns maximum whole person impairment of 85% after fulfilling their criteria for leukemias (17).

French Barema assigns 80%–95% to progressive leukemia and 1%–10% for clinically cured leukemia and reticulocytoses (16). Table 4.19 compares the impairment score of *Integrated Evaluation of Disability*, AMA, and France.

Table 4.18 Comparison of impairment—Chronic myeloid leukemia between countries

Integrated Evaluation of Disability	AMA—*Guides to the Evaluation of Permanent Impairment*	French Barema	German Barema
Maximum impairment 10%	Maximum whole person impairment of 85%	Progressive leukemia: Impairment 80%–95% clinically cured leukemia and reticulocytosis: Impairment 1%–10%	Chronic myeloid leukemia: Impairment: 50%–80%

Table 4.19 Comparison of impairment—Lymphoid leukemia between countries

Integrated Evaluation of Disability	AMA—Guides to the Evaluation of Permanent Impairment	French Barema
Maximum impairment: 50%	Maximum whole person impairment: 85%	Progressive leukemia: Impairment 80%–95% clinically cured leukemia and reticulocytosis: Impairment 1%–10%

4.5.18.3 THROMBOCYTOPENIA

Thrombocytopenia refers to a blood platelet count of less than $150 \times 10^9/L$ and less than $120 \times 10^9/L$ in late pregnancy (123). Thrombocytopenia manifests as skin bruising, petechiae, gum and nasal bleeding, bleeding in gastrointestinal, urinary tracts, and menorrhagia. Platelet count defines the severity of thrombocytopenia. Persons with platelet count over 50,000/µL do not have any significant bleeding diathesis. A platelet count of between 20,000 and 50,000/µL denotes mild thrombocytopenia. These individuals may bleed only on major trauma or surgery. Platelet count of between 10,000 and 20,000/µL refers to moderate thrombocytopenia. In general, there is no severe spontaneous bleeding with a platelet count of above 10,000/µL. Severe thrombocytopenia shows very low platelet count of <10,000/µL with spontaneous bleeding (124).

Integrated Evaluation of Disability assigns Class 1 impairment of 5% for mild impairment, Class 2 impairment of 25% for moderate thrombocytopenia, and 50% for chronic thrombocytopenia refractory to treatment.

The AMA *Guides to the Evaluation of Permanent Impairment* assigns maximum whole person impairment of 65% for individuals with impairment due to platelet disorders after fulfilling their criteria (17).

The Official Belgian Barema allocates 20%–100% for thrombocytopenia or thrombocytopenia due to pathological causes (16). Table 4.20 compares the impairment score of *Integrated Evaluation of Disability*, AMA, and Belgium.

Table 4.20 Comparison of impairment—Thrombocytopenia between countries

Integrated Evaluation of Disability	AMA—Guides to the Evaluation of Permanent Impairment	Belgium—BOBI
Maximum impairment of 50%	Maximum whole person impairment of 65%	Thrombocytopenia or thrombocytopenia due to pathological causes: Impairment—20%–100%

4.5.18.4 HEMOPHILIA

Hemophilia is a bleeding disorder due to deficiency of particular protein necessary for clotting of blood namely "Factor VIII" and "Factor IX." Deficiency of factor VIII produces Hemophilia "A" and deficiency of factor IX produces Hemophilia "B." Hemophilia "A" and "B" are inherited X-linked recessive disorder. Persons with severe hemophilia synthesize less than 1% of normal amount of these factors. Hence, they depend on replacement of factors to prevent bleeding diathesis. A 30%–35% of persons with hemophilia "A" and 1%–3% of persons with hemophilia "B" develop inhibitory antibodies which interfere with the functions of these factors VIII and IX (125). Hemophilia "C" is an autosomal recessive disorder due to deficiency factor XI. The bleeding tendency in "A" and "B" relates mainly to factor level and whereas in "C" the bleeding does not correlate well with the factor levels.

The bleeding/hemorrhage manifests spontaneously or during minor/moderate/severe trauma, and during surgery. The bleeding in hemophilia may be intracranial, hemarthrosis, hematoma in muscles commonly gastrocnemius/iliopsoas/flexor muscles of the arm, and hematuria. If adequate factor replacement is not controlling bleeding, it is necessary to confirm the presence of FVIII or IX antibodies in the blood. The level of coagulation factor serves to classify the severity of hemophilia. Class 1 impairment indicates coagulation factor level of more than 5% and less than 40%, that is, more than 0.05 and less than 0.40 IU/mL and hemorrhage occurs only during major trauma and surgery. Class 2 impairment denotes 1%–5% of normal factor level, that is, 0.01 to 0.05 IU/mL and triggers hemorrhage even with mild to moderate trauma. Class 3 impairment defines less than 1% of normal factor level, that is, less than 0.01 IU/mL and manifests spontaneous hemorrhage and hemarthrosis (124,126).

Integrated Evaluation of Disability assigns Class 1 impairment of 5%, Class 2 impairment of 15%, and Class 3 impairment of 25%. It assigns Class 4 impairment of 50% for hemophilia with hemorrhage and hemarthrosis unresponsive to prophylactic factor replacement due to FVIII inhibitor. Arthropathy due to repeated bleeding often results in a severe limitation of mobility and pain. Furthermore, there is coexisting hemophilia-related nerve lesions, compartment syndrome, the sequel due to intracranial bleeding, and so on. They may derive an additional percentage of impairment.

The AMA *Guides to the Evaluation of Permanent Impairment* assigns maximum whole person impairment of 65% for individuals with impairment due to hemophilia after fulfilling their criteria (17).

4.5.19 Functions of the immune system

4.5.19.1 HIV

Human immunodeficiency virus (HIV) depletes helper T-lymphocytes CD4$^+$ cells and produces a cellular immune deficiency.

The clinical status of the disease, advanced stage of illness, and CD4$^+$ T-lymphocyte counts serve to classify HIV disease into three categories in an adult or adolescent (127).

Category "A" comprises of asymptomatic infection, persistent generalized lymphadenopathy, acute primary infection, or past illness of acute primary infection. Category "B" includes symptomatic infection due to HIV or due to impairment of cell-mediated immunity. Category "C" comprises of clinical conditions included in the 1993 AIDS surveillance definition. CD4$^+$ T cells count subdivides category "A" into A1—$\geq$500/μL, A2—200–499 cell/μL and A3—<200 cell/μL. CD4$^+$ T cells count subdivides category "B" into B1—$\geq$500/μL, B2—200–499 cell/μL and B3—<200 cell/μL and category "C" into C1—$\geq$500/μL, C2—200–499 cell/μL, and C3—<200 cell/μL (127).

AIDS begins with a primary infection with HIV, stays as an asymptomatic chronic disease, and finally emerges as a progressive disease with severe immune deficiency, opportunistic infections, and neoplasms (128).

Persistently low CD4 less than 50 cells/cc; the viral burden remaining 100,000 copies/mL despite combination therapy, and failure of optimized treatment due to multidrug resistance denotes advanced disease. Progressive hepatitis C with hepatic failure, progressive leukoencephalopathy with dementia, unresponsive Kaposi's sarcoma, end-stage renal and cardiac failure, and unresponsive lymphoma/other malignancy accompanies advanced disease (129).

Antiretroviral therapy (ART) decreases the risk of progression of the HIV infection (130). ART is necessary for individuals with the severe and advanced disease, in people with CD4 count $\leq$ 500 cells/mm^3, combined HIV and tuberculosis, combined HIV and Hepatitis B Virus (HBV), and in partners without HIV infection (131).

Integrated Evaluation of Disability assigns Class 1 impairment of 15% for persons with HIV infection (category "A" on ART) for the burden of treatment compliance and stigma associated with HIV infection. It assigns Class 2 impairment of 25% for persons with AIDS disease (category "B"); and Class 3 impairment of 25% + for individuals with advanced AIDS disease (category "C"). Dementia, renal failure, cardiac failure, liver failure, and so forth, add additional impairment score for category "C". Table 4.21 describes the impairment score of HIV/AIDS defined by *Integrated Evaluation of Disability*, AMA, and France.

Table 4.21 Comparison of impairment—HIV/AIDS between countries

Integrated Evaluation of Disability	*AMA—Guides to the Evaluation of Permanent Impairment*	French Barema
Impairment 15%–95%	Maximum whole person impairment of 80%	AIDS: Impairment 80%–95%

The AMA *Guides to the Evaluation of Permanent Impairment* assigns maximum whole person impairment of 80% for persons with HIV disease after fulfilling their criteria (17).

French Barema assigns an impairment of 80%–95% for AIDS (16).

4.5.19.2 SPLEEN—SPLENECTOMY

The spleen plays a significant role in immune functions and removes encapsulated bacteria, foreign matter. Traumatic injuries (blunt injury), idiopathic thrombocytopenic purpura, hereditary spherocytosis, autoimmune hemolytic anemia, thrombocytopenic purpura, Hodgkin and non-Hodgkin lymphoma, chronic lymphocytic leukemia, hemangiomas, idiopathic myelofibrosis, myelodysplastic syndrome, hairy cell leukemia, splenic abscess or cyst, and tuberculosis require a splenectomy (132).

Splenectomy removes 25% of lymphoid tissue and most of the macrophages. Persons with splenectomy are liable for infection with encapsulated bacteria. Vaccines are available to protect them against pneumococcal and Haemophilus Influenza infections. Hence, *Integrated Evaluation of Disability* does not assign any impairment for splenectomy.

German Barema allocates 20% for *Splenectomy before eight years of age* (16).

4.5.20 Visual functions

Visual functions refers to a conglomerate of multiple functions, namely acuity of vision, color vision, acuity of alignment, the perception of movement, and perception of changing luminous intensity or differentiating luminous intensity, that is, contrast (133).

4.5.20.1 ACUITY OF VISION

Acuity of vision refers to the clarity of vision with details of perception such as form and contour of visual stimuli for both distant and near vision.

4.5.20.1.1 Distance vision

The Snellen Chart assesses the acuity of vision in 6 m or 20 ft (134).

ICD-10 Version: 2015 classifies visual impairment into no or mild visual impairment, moderate visual impairment, severe visual impairment, and blindness. It classifies visual impairment into five categories (135).

Persons with total blindness of one eye can function independently with the normal functioning another eye, though there is impairment of depth perception. Hence, *Integrated Evaluation of Disability* assigns maximum impairment of 15% only in persons with total blindness of one eye for lack of depth perception and decreased the level of safety for the normal eye. It assigns maximum impairment of 85% for persons with total blindness of both eyes.

4.5.20.1.2 Near vision

The evaluator uses either reduced Snellen acuity card to evaluate near vision at distance of 16 in. (40 cms) or Jaeger acuity card—20 letter sizes from J1 to J20 or "M" notation (1 "M" unit = 1.454 mm or 1/16") or point system with each point measuring 0.35 mm. It is necessary to evaluate near vision if near vision impairment is severe than distant vision.

Integrated Evaluation of Disability combines both near and distant vision to obtain average impairment of acuity of vision.

4.5.20.2 VISUAL FIELD

Visual field functions refer to the perception of vision outside the macula during fixation of gaze. Accurate evaluation and interpretation of field defect are necessary to classify visual impairment. Confrontation test evaluates visual field at the bedside. Equipment such as Tangent screen/Goldmann Perimetry/standard automated perimetry (SAP) also serves to assess the field of vision (136). Confrontation test identifies only larger defects in the field in four locations in the visual field. Tangent screen evaluates only the central 30° of the visual field. Goldmann Perimetry is a kinetic perimetry in which the stimulus starts from outside the visual field into the visual field. Automated perimetry evaluates the visual field using the computer either by a stationary stimulus or by a kinetic stimulus remaining for about 200 milliseconds. Depending on the visual impairment, the size (0.5°–2° diameter) and intensity of the stimulus (brightest stimulus 0 dB to the dimmest stimulus 51 dB), increases or decreases to the level the person could recognize (133). Goldmann Perimetry applies stimulus size I (0.25 mm²) to V (64 mm²), and Humphrey perimetry uses 4 mm² stimuli (equivalent to Goldmann size III stimulus) (137). The stimulus tests the points in one meridian in a radial or a circular pattern. The visibility of white target in the perimetry depends on the size and the luminous intensity of the spot as well as background illumination. It identifies outer limits or boundaries of the visual field and relative visual acuity. Isopters refers to boundaries or contour lines.

In binocular vision, the disparate two images fuse to form a single image. The binocular fusion also provides depth perception (138). Evaluation of impairment of binocular visual field requires Esterman test in Humphrey Field Analyzer or integrating visual fields by combining right and left visual fields (137).

The central field includes inner 30° of the visual field (139). The visual field extends laterally (temporally) for 100°, medially (nasally) 60°, superiorly 60° and inferiorly 70° from central fixation (137). The absence of vision anywhere in the visual field excepting the blind spot is abnormal. The blind spot is located in the temporal field approximately 12° to 17° from the central fixation and 1.5° below the horizontal meridian (1390).

The visual field in the center is light adapted and have a high acuity of vision with excellent color sensitivity and works efficiently with high illumination (photopic system). The visual field in the periphery is dark adapted and have reduced acuity and poor color sensitivity and works effectively with minimum illumination (scotopic system) (138).

Thus the central field is essential for reading, working on the computer and manipulative tasks involved in domestic, educational, vocational and avocational activities. The peripheral field is vital for activities in the dark as well as during mobility. A defect in the central and inferior field is more disabling than that of the superior field and hence derives more weight for a defect in the central and inferior field.

Integrated Evaluation of Disability assigns an impairment of 42.5% for loss of field of monocular vision. The visual field comprises of central (inner 30°) and peripheral field. The central field receives an impairment of 24% and peripheral field an impairment of 18.50%. The central field consists of four quadrants namely central superior temporal, central superior nasal, central inferior temporal and central inferior nasal fields. Each central field gets an impairment of 6%. *Integrated Evaluation of Disability* divides peripheral field based on vertical and horizontal meridians into vertical superior temporal, vertical superior nasal, horizontal superior temporal, horizontal superior nasal, horizontal inferior temporal, horizontal inferior nasal, vertical inferior temporal, and vertical inferior nasal fields. It assigns an impairment of 2% for vertical superior temporal, 2% vertical superior nasal, 3% vertical inferior temporal, 3% vertical inferior nasal, 2.75% horizontal superior temporal, 2.75% horizontal inferior temporal, 1.50% horizontal superior nasal, and 1.50% horizontal inferior nasal field. If the visual field defect is partial and/or incongruous, it assigns an impairment for the field based on the percentage of the size of the defect, for example, if the size of the vertical superior nasal peripheral is 50%, the impairment is only 0.75% for that field defect. The maximum impairment for visual field defect in both eyes should not exceed 85%.

ICD-10 Version 2015 (135) classifies visual field defects into the enlarged blind spot, generalized contraction of the visual field, (hemianop(s)ia (heteronymous) (homonymous), quadrant anop(s)ia and scotoma: Arcuate, Bjerrum, Central, Ring.

4.5.20.3 CONTRAST SENSITIVITY

Contrast sensitivity refers to the function of discriminating figures from the ground with minimum luminance. It may not impair acuity of vision. The tendency to perceive larger objects with minimum contrast may interfere with activities of daily living (140). Pelli-Robson Contrast Sensitivity Chart measures contrast sensitivity in which the contrast of the capital letters in the successive lines are decreasing without decreasing in size of the letters on white background. Low/poor contrast sensitivity triggers risk of accidents during driving in the night. It derives an impairment of 5% for low contrast sensitivity and 10% for poor contrast sensitivity.

4.5.20.4 LIGHT SENSITIVITY

Light sensitivity refers to visual functions of detecting the minimum amount of light, and discriminate the minimum difference in intensity. It includes functions of dark adaptation, night blindness and photophobia.

4.5.20.4.1 Night blindness

Irreversible night blindness after maximum medical treatment obtains an impairment of 25%.

4.5.20.4.2 Photophobia

Iritis, uveitis, and corneal disease; and flickering lights, and patterns of light with stripes triggers photophobia. The photogenic stimulus of 2–8 cycles/second causes photophobia in persons with a migraine. It assigns an impairment of 10% if photophobia persists even after maximum medical treatment.

4.5.20.5 COLOR VISION

Color vision refers to the visual functions of perception and distinguishing and matching colors. Congenital color blindness is mostly for red and green. Glaucoma and diseases of the optic nerve produce color blindness for blue and yellow (141).

Photoreceptors, that is, "cones" concentrated in the center of the retina mainly fovea, perceive the color of an object. The photoreceptors, that is, long, medium, and short-wavelength sensitive cones recognize primary colors respectively namely red, green, and blue. Color blindness due to deficiencies of photoreceptors namely long and medium cones are sex-linked deficiencies. Color blindness due to a deficiency of small cones is an autosomal inheritance. Protanopia refers to color blindness for red light due to the absence of large cones. Deuteranopia refers to color blindness for green light due to the lack of medium cones. Tritanopia refers to color blindness for blue light due to the lack of small cones. People with anomalous photoreceptors can recognize all colors but with reduced discrimination. Protanomaly refers to reduced sensitivity to red light resulting from the anomaly of large cones, deuteranomaly to reduced sensitivity to green light arising from anomaly of medium cones, and tritanomaly to reduced sensitivity to blue light emerging out of the anomaly of small cones. Normal persons (Trichromats) are sensitive to red, green, and blue light. Dichromates with two photoreceptors can recognize two colors. Most of the dichromats are red and green color deficient. Yellow and blue color–deficient persons are rare. Monochromates with single photoreceptor are color blind as they cannot recognize any color signal. They perceive the only gray scale between black and white. Persons with achromatopsia (140) (monochromats) are deprived of the full experience of color perception in their environment and may interfere with activities of daily living. They may also find difficulty in identifying the color signal in a traffic light and driving only by locating the illumination of upper, middle, or lower lights. Thus, they have the risk of being involved in an accident. Further color discrimination is significantly important in certain occupations requiring critical safety tasks such as in air, marine, road, and train transport systems as well as in certain trades. Hence, they may not be eligible for occupations such as a pilot, train engineer, railroad worker, firefighter, or signalman on railways. In dichromatopsia, and anomalous color vision, there is inaccurate recognition of the actual color, and poor perception of the intensity of color may further augment the difficulty in identifying standard colors at a regular distance or in the presence of mist, smoke, or during rain. Thus, the quality of life is at a low ebb in persons with color vision impairment.

Ishihara, Holmes-Wright lantern tests, FM test (Farnsworth-Munsell 100 hue test), and wire test evaluate color vision (141,142). *Integrated Evaluation of Disability* assigns a maximum of 25% for impairment of color vision based on the degree of impairment of color perception.

4.5.20.6 DOUBLE VISION

Monocular diplopia occurs when there is the defective transmission of light through the eyes to the retina. One of the images is normal quality and the other inferior quality on brightness, contrast, and clarity. Early cataract, corneal opacity, dislocation of the lens, and severe astigmatism may result in monocular diplopia (143).

The normally functioning fovea and synergistic and balanced action of yolked extraocular muscles facilitate the coordinated action of both eyes in creating a single binocular vision. Double vision occurs due to an imbalance of muscle power in the yoked extraocular muscles. Double vision is due to non-fusion of the images resulting in malprojection of the images to the corresponding points on the retina. Double vision becomes severe in the visual field of affected muscles. Horizontal diplopia becomes severe in tasks involving near vision such as reading. Adjustment of the posture may mask the diplopia by movement of the head to the right or left in horizontal diplopia, upward or downward rotation of the head in vertical diplopia and tilting of the head in torsional diplopia.

The Cervical Range of Motion (CROM) and Goldmann Perimetry methods quantify diplopia. CROM is a simple method than Goldmann Perimetry. The CROM method uses a 20/200 "E" target with a head-mounted device in a clinical setting. It uses an "E" target in 10 gaze positions. The gaze positions include a primary position, reading position, 10° upward, 30° upward, 10° downward, 30° downward, 10° rotation to the right, 30° rotation to the right, 10° rotation to the left, 30° rotation to the left, and any position at a 20/200 distance. The CROM method cannot evaluate persons with pacemakers because of the built-in magnet in the CROM device; and individuals with restriction of cervical range of motion. These people require the application of Goldmann Perimetry (144).

The diplopia score evaluated by the CROM method serves as a basis for assigning the percentage of impairment. It assigns maximum impairment of 25% if the diplopia score is between 16 and 25.

The International Council of Ophthalmology recommends visual standards for driving safety namely visual acuity of 20/40 (0.5, 6/12), a binocular visual field of at least 120° horizontal and 40° vertical. The other visual function evaluation includes glare sensitivity, Useful Field of View (UFOV), diplopia, color vision, and night vision.

Persons with monocular vision adapts well within about six months for depth perception (145).

Integrated Evaluation of Disability obtains global impairment of vision by combining acuity of vision, the field of vision, double vision, color vision, night blindness, and photophobia using the formula

$$A + \left[\frac{B(100 - A)}{100} \right] \qquad (4.7)$$

where A = Higher impairment value, B = Lower impairment value (Equation 4.7).

In the *Guides to the Evaluation of Permanent Impairment*—AMA assigns maximum whole person impairment of 85% for impairment of the visual system (17).

Guideline for Rating Physical Impairment—Korea assigns maximum whole person impairment of 85% for loss of vision (20).

The *Guidelines for Evaluation of Various Disabilities*—India assigns 100% for visual disability with counting fingers at one foot to nil or field of vision 10° in the better eye, and counting fingers at one foot to nil in the worse eye (19).

English Barema assigns an impairment of 100% for visual impairment limiting his ability to carry out any work in which vision is essential and 40% for loss of one eye without any complications and normal vision in another eye (16). The official Belgian Barema assigns an impairment of 30% for total loss of vision in one eye and 100% for total blindness with no perception of light (16). French Barema assigns an impairment of 25% for unilateral blindness, 95% for total blindness, 42% for complete hemianopia, 85% (maximum) for complete lateral double hemianopia 85% (16). Italian Barema assigns an impairment of 91%–100% for monocular blindness with the vision of the contralateral eye less than 1/20 and 100% for binocular blindness (16). German Barema assigns an impairment of 30% for total loss of vision in one eye and 100% for total blindness (16). The Federal Ministry of Labour and Social Affairs, German assigns maximum impairment of 100% for complete blindness and 30% for total loss of vision in one eye (16). Iceland Barema allocates 20% for total loss of vision in one eye, 100% for total loss of vision in both eyes and 50% for hemianopia due to brain injury (16). Slovenia assigns an impairment of 90% for 1/10 vision in the right eye and 0.15/10 in the left eye 90% (16). Table 4.22 describes the impairment defined by *Integrated Evaluation of Disability*,

AMA *Guides to the Evaluation of Permanent Impairment*, Development of Korean Academy of Medical Sciences—Impairment Rating, Guidelines for the Evaluation of Various Disabilities, and Europe.

4.5.21 Hearing functions

Hearing function comprises the transformation of sound waves into vibration, and transduction into the electrical impulse for transmission into the brain for interpretation of its location, pitch, loudness, and quality.

The World Health Organization states that treatment of common causes at primary health care level can prevent about 50% of all deafness and resultant hearing impairment (146). Hearing impairment may be sensory neural, conductive, central, and mixed. Sensory neural hearing impairment is due to lesions in the cochlea and injury to the eighth nerve and/or brainstem; conductive hearing impairment due to lesions in the external and/or middle ear; and central due to lesions in the cortex.

Hearing impairment results in difficulty or inability to interpret speech sounds, delay in acquisition of language skills.

4.5.21.1 SOUND

Sound exhibits a series of pressure changes in the air. The frequency and intensity of sound vary depending on the nature of speech. An average person can hear sounds between 20 and 20,000 Hz. The frequency of sound relates to the pitch of the sound. The best hearing exists between the frequency of 3000 and 4000 Hz. Decibel (dB) measures intensity of sound and pressure. The decibel is a logarithmic unit to describe the ratio of a measured value of sound intensity and pressure to a reference value. There is doubling of the intensity of sound for every 6 dB increase in sound pressure level (147). The sound of dropping a pin corresponds to 10 dB, ticking of a watch 20 dB, whisper 30 dB, quiet library 40 dB. The noise of a refrigerator corresponds to 50 dB, normal conversation or sewing machine 60 dB, toilet flushing 70 dB, the vacuum cleaner 80 dB, truck traffic or MRI machine 90 dB, pneumatic drill 100 dB, and a jet engine at takeoff 140 dB.

4.5.21.2 AUDIOMETRY

Pure tone audiometry evaluates hearing impairment. Audiometry delivers sounds of specific frequencies, that is, 125, 250, 500, 1000, 2000, 3000, 4000, 6000, and 8000 Hz

Table 4.22 Comparison of impairment of visual function between countries

Integrated Evaluation of Disability	AMA—Guides to the Evaluation of Permanent Impairment	Development of Korean Academy of Medical Sciences—Impairment Rating	Guidelines for Evaluation of Various Disabilities—India	English Barema	Belgium—BOBI	French Barema	Italian Barema	German Barema	Iceland Barema
85%	85%	85%	100%	100%	100%	95%	100%	100%	100%

at different intensities with earphones for air conduction for measuring hearing thresholds. It delivers 125, 250, 500, 1000, 2000, 3000, 4000 Hz with oscillator held at mastoid or forehead for bone conduction by audiometer for measuring hearing thresholds. The threshold for normal hearing is 0 ± 10 dB.

4.5.21.3 EVALUATION OF HEARING IMPAIRMENT

The World Health Organization defines hearing impairment as the permanent unaided hearing threshold level for the better ear of 41 dB or higher. It recommends average hearing threshold level for four frequencies namely, audiometric ISO value 500, 1000, 2000, and 4000 Hz to evaluate hearing impairment (148). *Integrated Evaluation of Disability* applies the WHO grading of Hearing Impairment (149). Persons with monaural hearing impairment can perform most of his life activities, whereas individuals with binaural hearing impairment cannot perform activities requiring communication.

Hence, *Integrated Evaluation of Disability* describes maximum impairment of 15% for monaural hearing impairment and 50% for binaural hearing impairment.

The AMA *Guides to the Evaluation of Permanent Impairment* assigns maximum whole person impairment of 35% for binaural hearing impairment (17). The labor code of the state of California assigns 60% impairment for complete loss of hearing in both ears (150).

Korea's *Guideline for Rating Physical Impairment* assigns maximum whole person impairment of 60% (20).

India's *Guidelines for Evaluation of Various Disabilities* assigns an impairment of 100% for total deafness (19).

In Europe, the English Barema attributes an impairment of 100% for complete deafness. The official Belgian Barema assigns 80% for a bilateral hearing loss higher than 90 dB in both ears. French Barema assigns 80% for bilateral deafness with 80 dB and more. Italian Barema assigns 65% for a bilateral auditory loss exceeding 275 dB with the better ear. German Barema assigns 70% for hearing loss between 80% and 90% in both ears. Iceland Barema assigns 10% for complete unilateral hearing loss and 75% for complete bilateral hearing loss 75%. Slovenia assigns more than 95% for total hearing loss (16). Table 4.23 compares the hearing impairment defined by *Integrated Evaluation of Disability*, AMA *Guides to the Evaluation of Permanent Impairment*, Development of Korean Academy of Medical Sciences—Impairment Rating, Guidelines for the Evaluation of Various Disabilities—India and Europe.

4.5.22 Impairment of structure

4.5.22.1 AMPUTATIONS

Functional/structural loss of upper extremity derives an impairment of 60% and lower extremity 40% by convention. A person with isolated flaccid motor paralysis involving one lower extremity can walk independently with some gait deviation after stabilization by surgery or by the appliance.

BOX 4.25: Impairment—Amputations

Motor impairment
Sensory impairment
Vascular impairment
Dermal impairment

Combined by

$$A + \left[B\,\frac{100 - A}{100} \right]$$

A person with hip disarticulation/transfemoral amputation has loss of both structure and function. He/she cannot walk without an artificial limb. He/she can walk downhill, climb up the stairs, and run with microprocessor-controlled prosthetic knee joint though with some difficulty. But he/she cannot feel the sensation of his/her leg through the artificial limb.

A person with profound deafness (or) severe hard of hearing can understand speech by a cochlear implant. A series of electrodes in the cochlear implant in the base of the cochlea stimulate the auditory nerve for the perception of sounds by the brain (147,151). Similarly, a pacemaker correct the abnormal heart rhythm and restores the function in a person with severe arrhythmias.

There is no mechanism to interpret the sensation in a person with amputation fitted with an artificial limb. He/she cannot feel the touch sensation through his/her prosthesis. Thus, it is not logical to give the same impairment of motor loss for amputation. Hence, *Integrated Evaluation of Disability* combines impairment score of motor loss, sensory loss, vascular loss, and dermal loss to compute whole person impairment to compute impairment of a person with amputation (Box 4.25).

Based on this concept, forequarter amputation obtains whole person impairment of 80%; shoulder disarticulation derives 79% and elbow disarticulation 72%, wrist disarticulation 65%, and hindquarter amputation 61%, hip disarticulation 60%, knee disarticulation 54%, and ankle disarticulation 45% in *Integrated Evaluation of Disability*. *Integrated Evaluation of Disability* adds additional impairment for stiffness of the proximal joint, phantom pain/sensation. The energy expenditure incurred for ambulation is higher in vascular amputation than in traumatic amputation. Hence, it reduces the endurance of walking with prosthesis in person with vascular amputation. Individuals with congenital amputation adapt very well to the activities, and hence the limitation of activities is less than in people with vascular and traumatic amputation. The "Activity Participation Skill Assessment Scale" evaluates limitation of activities, and "Environmental Factors Measurement Scale" measures environmental barriers/facilitators before computing final percentage of disability.

The AMA *Guides to the Evaluation of Permanent Impairment* assigns whole person impairment of 70% for forequarter amputation, 60% for shoulder disarticulation and 60% for amputation of the arm at or above deltoid insertion, 57% for arm/forearm amputation between deltoid insertion and bicipital insertion (17). It assigns 40% (Lower Extremity Impairment 100%) for hip disarticulation, and above knee proximal amputation. It assigns an impairment of 36%–38% (Lower Extremity Impairment 90%–94%) for

Table 4.23 Comparison of impairment of hearing functions between countries

Integrated Evaluation of Disability	AMA—Guides to the Evaluation of Permanent Impairment	Development of Korean Academy of Medical Sciences—Impairment Rating	Guidelines for Evaluation of Various Disabilities India	English Barema	Belgium BOBI	French Barema	German Barema	Italian Barema	Iceland Barema
Binaural hearing impairment: 50% Monoaural hearing impairment: 15%	Binaural hearing impairment: Maximum whole person impairment 35%	Maximum whole person impairment of 60%	Total deafness—100%	Complete deafness—100%	Loss of hearing >90 dB decibels in both ears: 80%	Bilateral deafness ≥ 80 dB: 80%	Loss of hearing 80%–90% in both ears: Impairment—70%	Hearing loss > 275 dB with better ear: Impairment 65%	Complete hearing loss in one ear: Impairment 10% complete hearing loss in both ears: Impairment 75%

above knee mid-thigh amputation and 32%–34% (Lower Extremity Impairment 80%–84%) for above knee amputation distal amputation, knee disarticulation and below knee amputation less than 3 in. (17).

India's disability guidelines assign 100% impairment for forequarter amputations, 90% for shoulder disarticulation, 85% for above elbow amputation up to upper 1/3 of the arm, and 80% above elbow up to lower 1/3 of the forearm. It assigns 100% for hindquarter amputation, 90% for hip disarticulation, 85% for above knee up to upper 1/3 of the thigh, 80% for above knee up to lower 1/3 of the thigh, 75% for through knee and 70% for below knee amputation up to 8 cm (19).

Korea's Guideline for Rating Physical Disability for the Upper Extremity assigns an impairment of 110% for scapulothoracic amputation, 100% for shoulder disarticulation, and 100% for humeral amputation above the deltoid insertion, 95% for humeral amputation below the deltoid insertion (80).

Korea's Guideline Rating the Physical Impairment assigns the lower extremity impairment for amputations of the lower extremity. It describes 110% for hemipelvectomy, 100% for hip disarticulation, 100% for above knee amputation proximal, 90% for above knee amputation mid-thigh, and 80% for above knee amputation distal amputation. It assigns 80% to knee disarticulation and below knee amputation shorter than 8 cm, and 70% for below knee amputation ≥8 cm (81).

The English Barema assigns 90% for amputation at the shoulder, 80% for amputation below the shoulder with a stump length shorter than 20.5 cm, 100% for loss of both hands and amputations positioned higher up the arm. Further, it assigns 100% for loss of a foot and a hand, 60% for unilateral loss of hand or thumb and all fingers, and 40% for loss of thumb and its metacarpal. It assigns 90% to amputation of hip, 60% for amputation of knee and below with a stump length shorter than 9 cm (16).

The Belgium Barema allocates an impairment of 85% for disarticulation of the shoulder, 75% for disarticulation of the elbow, 65% for disarticulation or amputation of the wrist or above the wrist joint, 90% for total loss of a lower limb, and 50% for total loss of a foot (16).

The French Barema assigns an impairment of 80%–90% for disarticulation of the shoulder, 50–75% for amputation of the forearm, 50%–75% for amputation of the leg or thigh with a prosthesis and 20%–40% for amputation of the ball of the foot (16).

The Italian Barema assigns an impairment of 80% for amputation of the shoulder, 100% anatomical loss of both hands, 85% for disarticulation of the hip, 65% for amputation of the thigh, 65% for disarticulation of the knee and 70% for loss of both feet (16).

The German Barema assigns an impairment of 100% for loss of both arms and hands, 100% for loss of an arm, and a leg. It assigns an impairment of 80% for amputation of the arm below the shoulder with the short stump, 70% for disarticulation of the elbow, 50% for amputation at the forearm, and 50% for complete loss of a hand. It assigns an impairment of 100% for amputation of both legs at the upper thigh, 80% for hip disarticulation or above knee amputation with a

very short stump, and 30% for incomplete unilateral loss of foot at the midtarsal joint (16).

The Iceland Barema assigns an impairment of 70% for amputation of the whole arm on the right side and 65% left side, 60% for elbow disarticulation on the right side and 55% left side. It assigns an impairment of 50% for disarticulation of the wrist on the right side and 45% left, 20% for amputation of thumb in the right hand, and 17% left hand. It assigns an impairment of 50% for total loss of a lower limb on the right and 40% left. It assigns an impairment of 35% for amputation at the knee fitted with an artificial limb on the right/left side and 35% for amputation of the foot at the ankle with poor adaptation to a prosthesis on the right/left side (16). Table 4.24 depicts the impairment due to amputations assigned by various countries.

4.5.22.2 CONGENITAL SKELETAL LIMB DEFICIENCIES

In 1973, the International Society for Prosthetics and Orthotics (ISPO) "Kay" Committee classified the congenital skeletal limb deficiency due to the failure of the formation based on the anatomical and radiological deficiency. It relates to transverse and longitudinal deficiencies. The International Organization for Standardization (ISO) confers it as international standard after minor modification as per ISO 8548-1:1989 "Method of describing limb deficiencies at birth" (152). The transverse deficiencies are like amputations. In transverse deficiency, no skeletal elements are present beyond the normally developed residual limb. Nevertheless, there may be digital buds. In longitudinal deficiency, there is the total or partial absence of skeletal element or elements in the long axis of the limb with preserved distal skeletal elements. It labels the transverse deficiencies by indicating the part at which the extremity ends and further denoting the level within the part distal to it no skeletal structures exist (152). The transverse deficiency is like that of amputation, and hence the whole person impairment is like that of amputation. In longitudinal deficiency, there may be the absence of joint, loss of muscle due to aplasia or hypoplasia of the muscle in the affected segment of the extremity. Due to missing of the skeletal element in the affected segment, there may be a loss of stability of the extremity. As an illustration, there may be a limitation of ROM knee/ankle joint due to the absence of tibia, loss of muscle power in the ankle due to aplasia or hypoplasia of tibial muscles and instability of lower extremity due to the absence of tibia in tibial total longitudinal deficiency. Hence, it computes impairment based on the loss of ROM of a joint, muscle power, stability and shortening. *Integrated Evaluation of Disability* assigns an impairment of 1% for each inch of shortening of the upper/lower extremity.

In the AMA method, ½″ shortening is assigned whole person impairment of 2% (Lower extremity 5%), ½″–1″ is assigned 4% (lower extremity 10%), and 1″–1½″ 6% (lower extremity 15%), 1½″–2″ 8% (lower extremity 20%) (153).

India's Disability Guidelines assign permanent physical impairment of 90% for transverse deficiency arm complete (shoulder disarticulation), and 85% for transverse deficiency

Table 4.24 Comparison of impairment due to amputation between countries

Level of amputation	Integrated Evaluation of Disability	USA AMA	Korea	India	English Barema	Belgium	French Barema	Italian Barema	German Barema	Iceland Barema
Forequarter amputation	80%	70%	110%	100%						
Shoulder disarticulation	79%	60%	100%	90%	90%	85%	80–90%	80%	80%	70%
Transhumera amputation	76%–78%	57%–60%	95%–100%	80%–85%	80%					
Elbow disarticulation	72%	57%		75%		75%			70%	60%
Forearm amputation	66%–70%	57%					50%–75%		50%	
Wrist disarticulation	65%					65%			50%	50%
Loss of thumb and all fingers	55%				60%					
Amputation of thumb	20%–31%				40%					20%
Hemipelvectomy	61%		110%	100%				100%		
Hip disarticulation	60%	40%	100%	90%	90%	90%		85%	80%	50%
Transfemoral amputation	55%–59%	34–40%	80–100%	80–85%			50%–75%	65%		
Knee disarticulation	54%	34%	80%	75%	60%		50%–75%	65%		35%
Trans tibiofibular amputation	47%–53%	32%–34%	70%–80%	60%–70%	60%		50%–75%			
Ankle disarticulation	45%					50%				35%
Loss of both feet	70%							70%		
Amputation of foot— transverse tarsal joint	27% (Chopart)								30%	
Amputation of ball of foot							20%–40%			

proximal upper arm (above elbow amputation). It assigns 75% for transverse deficiency of the whole forearm (elbow disarticulation), 65% for transverse deficiency lower forearm (below elbow amputation), 60% for transverse deficiency carpal complete (wrist disarticulation) and 55% for transverse deficiency metacarpal complete. It assigns 90% to transverse deficiency thigh complete (hip disarticulation). It allocates 80% for transverse deficiency lower thigh (above knee amputation lower third). Loss of ROM, muscle strength, prehensile function/stability of joint, and so on, also derives impairment in addition to the deficient segment in longitudinal deficiencies (19).

4.5.22.3 DWARFISM

Idiopathic Short Stature (ISS) refers to a height below -2 standard deviation score (SDS) based on the science of human growth and development with no evidence for any primary diseases (154). Little People of America defines dwarfism as a medical or genetic condition resulting in an adult height of 4′10″ or shorter (155). The height in dwarfism varies from 2′8″ to 4′8″ (156).

Persons with dwarfism have the limitation of functions such as in overhead operations, limitation of lower-extremity-reach for automobile operations, obstacles to vision during driving, and accessing ATM, gas/petrol pump, and so forth. Americans with Disabilities Act (ADA) states that a person is disabled when his/her physical or mental impairment significantly limit his/her major life activity or activities (157). Thus, the ADA protects the rights of persons with dwarfism. On May 1, 2003, the Republic of Korea included dwarfism under physical disability (158).

Integrated Evaluation of Disability states that a person with a height of 4′10″ (58 in.) or shorter obtains whole person impairment of 1.72% for each inch under 4′10″. Furthermore, impairment of cognition, sensory-motor functions, bladder and bowel function, heart function, pulmonary function, renal function, and limitations of joint functions due to skeletal deformities, and so on, derive additional impairment scores.

The Ministry of Social Justice and Empowerment, Government of India *Guidelines for Evaluation of Various Disabilities and Procedure for Certification* assign 4% permanent physical impairment for every one inch reduction of vertical height. Associated skeletal deformities require separate evaluation for additional impairments (19).

4.5.22.4 IMPAIRMENT OF STRUCTURE OF THE SKIN—BURNS

Impairment of structure of skin includes the total or partial absence of skin (159). Burns per se refers to both total/partial absence of skin and sequel following repair functions of the skin.

In the first-degree burn, injury confined to the epidermis, in second-degree superficial partial thickness burn to the epidermis and papillary dermis, in second-degree deep partial thickness burn to the epidermis, papillary dermis, and deep reticular dermis, and in third degree burns to the epidermis and the full thickness of dermis. First-degree and second-degree superficial burns heal spontaneously. Second degree deep partial thickness burns heal by secondary intention involving epithelization and contraction. Third-degree burns heal only with surgical intervention, usually skin grafting. Hence, it results in scars and deformities (160). Fourth-degree burns also involve muscles and bones (161). Post-burn sequelae comprise loss of hair, loss of the nail, and depigmentation of the skin. It also includes hypertrophic scar, and keloid formation, contracture, and deformities, for example, ectropion of the eyelid. It further includes flexion contracture in the neck, axillary scars, contracture of the joints in the extremities, deformity, or loss of pinna of the ear, scar in the sclera, conjunctiva, cornea and loss of vision. It furthermore includes deformity, scar on the face, microstomia, scarring or loss of breast, scar or loss of genitals, amputations, and disfigurement.

Burns may involve eyelid, conjunctiva, sclera, cornea, lens, and macula. Persons who have sustained high-voltage burns involving eye may develop cataract and maculopathy (162,163). Ocular injury due to fireworks may result in open/globe injury with either partial or total loss of vision (164).

Burns injury to the external ear may result in the bare cartilage of the external ear or amputation of the external ear (165). Burns injury to the ear may also involve tympanic membrane and middle ear (166).

Burns injury to the nose may result in loss of alar lobule or subtotal amputation with complete loss of cartilaginous support or total amputation of the nose (167). Airway occlusion in the nose following burns may produce sleep apnea/hypopnea.

Burns to the perioral tissue may result in microstomia. It may be painful. Microstomia may create an inability to smile, drooling, limitation of feeding only with a straw, restriction of oral hygiene and dental care, and impairment of articulation of speech (168).

Burn injury to the perineum and genitals may present either with partial thickness injury or full thickness injury (169). Full-thickness burns may associate with loss of sensation in the penis. Further, there is discoloration and contracture of the penis (170). Post-burns sequelae of perineum and groin includes perineal obliteration, hidden genitalia, limitation of sexual function, restriction of hip movement, and limitation of perineal hygiene, megarectum, intestinal obstruction, and recurrent ulcerations, in the contracture (171,172).

The acute renal injury is one of the major complications of burns. Among the survivors, majority regains the normal renal function, and few require long-term dialysis (173).

There is severe loss of plasma fluid due to increased capillary permeability. The resultant decreased cardiac output triggers a compensatory increase in heart rate, peripheral vascular resistance, and pulmonary resistance, which may lead to biventricular failure in persons with larger burns.

Loss of elasticity of scar tissue in third-degree burns interferes with respiratory mechanics and ventilation. Smoke inhalation during burns may lead to increased pulmonary artery resistance, pulmonary hypertension and increased right ventricular load (174). In smoke inhalation injury, heat may produce occlusion of the upper respiratory tract and the toxins, particulate matter contained in the smoke may induce inflammation, infection and immunological changes in the lung, hypoxia due to interference with oxygen transport and utilization and ventilation-perfusion mismatch (175,176).

Following burns, there may be impairment of functions and structure, limitation of activities, participation restriction and environmental barriers, fear of rejection by the society and inadequate behavioral adaptation, sometimes with suicidal tendencies.

Integrated Evaluation of Disability assigns an impairment based on disfigurement, loss of structure and loss of function. It allocates combined maximum impairment of 90% for burns affecting head and neck, eye, ear, chest, perineum and genitals, extremities, and sequel of burns affecting renal function, heart function and respiration function.

The *AMA Guides to the Evaluation of Permanent Impairment* assigns maximum whole person impairment of 45% for facial disorder and disfigurement scars after fulfilling their criteria (17).

Korea's *Guideline on the Skin and Related System* evaluates burns under type 2 and 3 skin disorder. It assigns maximum impairment of 51%–60% for unfavorable scar bigger than 60% (3.6%) on the exposed face and neck or unfavorable scar of 30%–60% (8.1%–16.2%) on the exposed limb (177).

India's *Guidelines for Evaluation of Various Disabilities and Procedure for Certification* assign no percentage of mild disfigurement, 2% for moderate disfigurement and 4% for severe disfigurement 4% (19).

The German Barema allocates 50% for disfigurement resulting in visual repulsion (16).

4.6 EXPERT OPINIONS

Integrated Evaluation of Disability developed clinical tools and methods for assigning a percentage of impairment for function/structure. It obtained a global opinion from experts from physical medicine and rehabilitation physicians, orthopedic surgeons, rheumatologist, neurologists, neurosurgeons, cardiologist, pulmonologists, urologists, gastroenterologist, psychiatrists, phoniatrists, plastic surgeons, and psychologists. Furthermore, a "Modified Delphi Process" provided appropriateness of non-standardized clinical methods/tools for evaluation of impairment of function and structure as well as assigning a percentage of impairment of function/structure, limitation of activities, participation restriction, environmental barriers, and behavior of the person with a disability as described in Chapter 5.

REFERENCES

1. McBride ED. Disability evaluation. *J Int Coll Surg.* 1955;24:341–348.
2. McBride ED. Disability evaluation: Principles of treatment of compensable injuries. *Curr Orthop Pract.* 1964;32:5–10.
3. Nordby EJ. Disability evaluation of the neck and back. The McBride system. *Clin Orthop Relat Res.* 1987(221):131–135.
4. Kessler HH, Faber JK. *Disability - Determination and Evaluation.* Philadelphia, PA: Lea & Febiger; 1970.
5. United States. *Physician's Guide: Disability Evaluation Examinations.* Washington, DC: Veterans Administration; 1976.
6. Ustun TB, Saxena S, Rehm J, Bickenbach J. Are disability weights universal? WHO/NIH Joint Project CAR Study Group. *Lancet.* 1999;354(9186):1306.
7. Stouthard MEA, Essink-Bot ML, Bonsel GJ, on behalf of the Dutch Disability Weights (DDW) group. Disability weights for diseases: A modified protocol and results for a Western European region. *Eur J Public Health.* 2000;10(1):24–30.
8. Essink-Bot ML, Bonsel GJ. How to derive disability weights 2002. In: Murray CJL, Salomon JA, Mathers CD, Lopez AD, editors. *Summary Measures of Population Health Concepts, Ethics, Measurement and Applications* [Internet]. Geneva, Switzerland: World Health Organization; 2002. pp. 456–459.
9. *The Global Burden of Disease: 2004 Update.* Geneva, Switzerland: World Health Organization; 2008. pp. 31–33.
10. Essink-Bot ML, Pereira J, Packer C, Schwarzinger M, Burström K, the European Disability Weights Group. Cross-national comparability of burden of disease estimates: the European Disability Weights Project. *Bull World Health Organ.* 2002(80):644–652.
11. Mahapatra P, Salomon JA, Nanda L. *Measuring Health State Values in Developing Countries.* Geneva, Switzerland: World Health Organization; 2002.
12. Christopher JL, Murray ADL. Regional patterns of disability-free life expectancy and disability-adjusted life expectancy: Global Burden of Disease Study. *Lancet.* 1997;349(9062):1347–1352.
13. Prüss-Üstün A, Mathers C, Corvalan C, Woodward A. *Introduction and Methods: Assessing the Environmental Burden of Disease at National and Local Levels.* Geneva, Switzerland: World Health Organization; 2003. pp. 27–40.
14. *The Global Burden of Disease: 2004 Update.* Geneva, Switzerland: World Health Organization; 2008. p. 117.
15. Brandt EN, Pope AM. *Models of Disability and Rehabilitation: Evolution of Models of Disability.* Washington, DC: National Academy Press; 1997. [cited Institute of Medicine].
16. *Assessing Disability in Europe – Similarities and Differences.* Strasbourg, France: Council of Europe Publishing; 2002.
17. *Guides to the Evaluation of Permanent Impairment,* 6th ed. Chicago, IL: American Medical Association; 2007. pp. 19 -24.
18. Rajnes D. Permanent disability social insurance programs in Japan. *Soc Secur Bull.* 2010;70(1):61–84.
19. *Guidelines for Evaluation of Various Disabilities and Procedure for Certification.* In: Ministry of Social Justice and Empowerment GoI, editor. New Delhi, India: Office of the Chief Commissioner for Persons with Disabilities; 2001 and 2009.
20. Lee K-S, Won J-U, Kim S-Y, Sohn M-S, Youm Y-S, Lee Y-S, Kim D-J, Cho S-H, Lee M-J, Choi J-S. Development of the Korean Academy of Medical Sciences guideline for rating physical impairment. *Korean Acad Med Sci.* 2009;24(Suppl 2):S221–S226.
21. *Social Security (Tables for the Assessment of Work-related Impairment for Disability Support Pension) Determination 2011 under subsection 26(1) of the Social Security Act 1991.* In: Ministry for Families, Housing, Community Services and Indigenous Affairs, editor. Australia: I, Jenny Macklin, Minister for Families, Housing, Community Services and Indigenous Affairs; 2011.
22. *Canada Pension Plan Adjudication Framework.* Canada: Employment and Social Development, Canada; 2014.
23. Cassis I, Dupriez K, Burnand B, Vader JP. Quality of work incapacity assessment in the Swiss disability insurance system. *Int J Qual Health Care.* 1996;8(6):567–575.
24. Stucki G, Brage S, Homa D, Escorpizo R. Conceptual framework: Disability evaluation and vocational rehabilitation. In: Escorpizo R, Brage S, Homa D, Stucki G, editors. *Hand Book of Vocational Rehabilitation and Disability Evaluation.* Cham, Switzerland: Springer International Publishing; 2015.

25. *Assessment on Disability Equity in the Public Service*. Republic of South Africa: The Public Service Commission; 2008. p. 64.

26. Fultz E. *Disability Insurance in the Netherlands: A Blueprint for U.S. Reform?* [Internet]. Washington, DC: Center for Budget and Policy Priorities; 2015.

27. Zheng X, Chen G, Song X, Liu J, Yan L, Du W et al. Twenty-year trends in the prevalence of disability in China. *Bull World Health Organ*. 2011;89(11):788–797.

28. *Assessing Disability in Working Age Population: A Paradigm Shift: from Impairment and Functional Limitation to the Disability Approach* [Internet]. Washington, DC: World Bank; 2015.

29. Bartoszek G, Fischer U, von Clarenau SC, Grill E, Mau W, Meyer G et al. Development of an International Classification of Functioning, Disability and Health (ICF)-based standard set to describe the impact of joint contractures on participation of older individuals in geriatric care settings. *Arch Gerontol Geriatr*. 2015;61(1):61–66.

30. Raggi A, Schiavolin S, Leonardi M, Antozzi C, Baggi F, Maggi L, Mantegazza R. Development of the MG-DIS: An ICF-based disability assessment instrument for myasthenia gravis. *Disabil Rehabil*. 2014;36(7):546–555.

31. Penfield W, Rasmussen T, editors. *The Cerebral Cortex of Man: A Clinical Study of Localization of Function*. New York: The Macmillan Company; 1957.

32. Papanicolaou AC, Simos PG, Breier JI, Wheless JW, Mancias P, Baumgartner JE et al. Brain plasticity for sensory and linguistic functions: A functional imaging study using magnetoencephalography with children and young adults. *J Child Neurol*. 2001;16(4):241–252.

33. Roux FE, Boulanouar K, Ibarrola D, Tremoulet M, Chollet F, Berry I. Functional MRI and intraoperative brain mapping to evaluate brain plasticity in patients with brain tumours and hemiparesis. *J Neurol Neurosurg Psychiatry*. 2000;69(4):453–463.

34. Papanicolaou AC, Simos PG, Breier JI, Zouridakis G, Willmore LJ, Wheless JW et al. Magnetoencephalographic mapping of the language-specific cortex. *J Neurosurg*. 1999;90(1):85–93.

35. American Academy of Neurology. Practice parameters: Assessment and management of patients in the persistent vegetative state (summary statement). *Neurology*. 1994;45:1015–1018.

36. *Guides to the Evaluation of Permanent Impairment: The Central and Peripheral Nervous System*. Chicago, IL: American Medical Association; 2007.

37. *Seizure Classification* [Internet]. International League Against Epilepsy; 2014.

38. Jung HY, Ko TS, Kim HD, Yim SY, Kim MO, Hong SK et al. Korean Academy of Medical Sciences pediatric impairment guideline for brain lesion. *J Korean Med Sci*. 2009;24(Suppl 2):S323–S329.

39. *International Classification of Functioning, Disability and Health*. Geneva, Switzerland: World Health Organization; 2001. p. 49.

40. Wechsler DW. *Wechsler Adult Intelligence Scale-III (WAIS - III)*. San Antonio, TX: The Psychological Corporation; 1997.

41. Raven JC. *Standard Progressive Matrices*. London, UK: H. K. Levis; 1958.

42. *IQ Classification in Psychiatric Use Diagnostic and Statistical Manual of Mental Disorders (DSM-IV)* [Internet]. 1994.

43. Trahan LH, Stuebing KK, Fletcher JM, Hiscock M. The Flynn effect: A meta-analysis. *Psychol Bull*. 2014;140(5):1332–1360.

44. Buysse DJ. Sleep health: Can we define it? Does it matter? *Sleep*. 2014;37(1):9–17.

45. *International Classification of Functioning, Disability and Health*. Geneva, Switzerland: World Health Organization; 2001. p. 52.

46. Chronic Insomnia: Final Panel Statement. *NIH State-of-the-Science Conference on Manifestations and Management of Chronic Insomnia in Adults*. NIH Consensus Development Program, Office of Disease Prevention, U.S. Department of Health & Human Services; 2005.

47. Schutte-Rodin S, Broch L, Buysse D, Dorsey C, Sateia M. Clinical guideline for the evaluation and management of chronic insomnia in adults. *J Clin Sleep Med*. 2008;4(5):487–504.

48. Vgontzas AN, Fernandez-Mendoza J, Liao D, Bixler EO. Insomnia with objective short sleep duration: The most biologically severe phenotype of the disorder. *Sleep Med Rev*. 2013;17(4):241–254.

49. *Guides to the Evaluation of Permanent Impairment*. Chicago, IL: American Medical Association; 2007. p. 329.

50. Tsara V, Amfilochiou A, Papagrigorakis MJ, Georgopoulos D, Liolios E. Guidelines for diagnosis and treatment of sleep-related breathing disorders in adults and children. Definition and classification of sleep related breathing disorders in adults: Different types and indications for sleep studies (Part 1). *Hippokratia*. 2009;13(3):187–191.

51. Berry RB, Budhiraja R, Gottlieb DJ, Gozal D, Iber C, Kapur VK et al. Rules for scoring respiratory events in sleep: Update of the 2007 AASM Manual for the Scoring of Sleep and Associated Events. Deliberations of the Sleep Apnea Definitions Task Force of the American Academy of Sleep Medicine. *J Clin Sleep Med*. 2012;8(5):597–619.

52. *The International Classification of Sleep Disorders, Revised: Diagnostic and Coding Manual* [Internet]. Westchester, IL: American Academy of Sleep Medicine; 2001.

53. Adegunsoye A, Ramachandran S. Etiopathogenetic mechanisms of pulmonary hypertension in sleep-related breathing disorders. *Pulm Med*. 2012;2012:273591.

54. *International Classification of Functioning, Disability and Health.* Geneva, Switzerland: World Health Organization; 2001. p. 53.

55. *International Classification of Functioning, Disability and Health.* Geneva, Switzerland: World Health Organization; 2001. p. 54.

56. *International Classification of Functioning, Disability and Health.* Geneva, Switzerland: World Health Organization; 2001. pp. 48–49.

57. *International Classification of Functioning, Disability and Health.* Geneva, Switzerland: World Health Organization; 2001. pp. 55–56.

58. *International Classification of Functioning, Disability and Health.* Geneva, Switzerland: World Health Organization; 2001. p. 60.

59. *International Classification of Functioning, Disability and Health.* Geneva, Switzerland: World Health Organization; 2001. p. 71.

60. Stuttering [Internet]. National Institute on Deaf and other Communication Disorders (NIDCD); 2010. Available from: http://www.nidcd.nih.gov/health/voice/pages/stutter.aspx.

61. Bloodstien O. *A Handbook on Stuttering.* Chicago, IL: National Easter Seal Society; 1987.

62. *Human Speech Spectrum, Frequency Range, Formants* [Internet]. "AV-Info.eu"; 1995.

63. Assmann PF. Fundamental frequency and the intelligibility of competing voices. *14th International Congress of Phonetic Sciences*, San Francisco, CA, August 1–7. Richardson TX: School of Human Development, The University of Texas at Dallas; 1999.

64. Hirano M. *Clinical Examination of the Voice.* New York: Springer Verlag; 1981.

65. *ACR Appropriateness Criteria® dysphagia* [Internet]. American College of Radiology; 2010.

66. Wheeler-Hegland K, Ashford J, Frymark T, McCabe D, Mullen R, Musson N et al. Evidence-based systematic review: Oropharyngeal dysphagia behavioral treatments. Part II—impact of dysphagia treatment on normal swallow function. *J Rehabil Res Dev.* 2009;46(2):185–194.

67. *Guides to the Evaluation of Permanent Impairment.* In: Rondinelli RD, Genovese E, Katz RT, Mayer TG, Mueller K, Ranavaya ML, Brigham BR, editors. Chicago, IL: American Medical Association; 2007. p. 269.

68. Compston A. Aids to the investigation of peripheral nerve injuries. Medical Research Council: Nerve Injuries Research Committee. His Majesty's Stationery Office: 1942; pp. 48 (iii) and 74 figures and 7 diagrams; with aids to the examination of the peripheral nervous system. By Michael O'Brien for the Guarantors of Brain. Saunders Elsevier: 2010; pp. [8] 64 and 94 Figures. *Brain.* 133(10):2838–2844.

69. Radomski MV, Trombly Latham CA. *Occupational Therapy for Physical Dysfunction.* 6th ed. Baltimore, MD: Wolters Kluwer/Lippincott Williams & Wilkins; 2008.

70. Van Cant J, Pineux C, Pitance L, Feipel V. Hip muscle strength and endurance in females with patellofemoral pain: A systematic review with meta-analysis. *Int J Sports Phys Ther.* 2014;9(5):564–582.

71. Demura S, Yamaji S, Goshi F, Nagasawa Y. Lateral dominance of legs in maximal muscle power, muscular endurance, and grading ability. *Percept Motor Skills.* 2001;93(1):11–23.

72. White C, Dixon K, Samuel D, Stokes M. Handgrip and quadriceps muscle endurance testing in young adults. *SpringerPlus.* 2013;2:451.

73. Mathiowetz V, Kashman N, Volland G, Weber K, Dowe M, Rogers S. Grip and pinch strength: Normative data for adults. *Arch Phys Med Rehabil.* 1985(66):69–72.

74. Fielding RA, Bean J. Acute physiological responses to dynamic exercise. In: Frontera WR, Slovik DM, Dawson DM, editors. *Exercise in Rehabilitation Medicine.* Champaign, IL: Human Kinetics Publishers; 2006.

75. Reeves NP, Narendra KS, Cholewicki J. Spine stability: The six blind men and the elephant. *Clin Biomech.* 2007;22(3):266–274.

76. Benzel EC. Chapter 3: Stability and instability of the spine. In: Benzel EC, editor. *Biomechanics of Spine Stabilization.* Rolling Meadows, IL: American Association of Neurological Surgeons; 2001.

77. Torretti JA, Sengupta DK. Cervical spine trauma. *Indian J Orthop.* 2007;41(4):255–267.

78. Massano J, Bhatia KP. Clinical approach to Parkinson's disease: Features, diagnosis, and principles of management. *Cold Spring Harb Perspect Med.* 2012;2(6):a008870.

79. Rah UW, Baik JS, Jang SH, Park DS, Korean Academy of Medical Sciences. Development of the Korean Academy of Medical Sciences Guideline for rating the impairment in the brain injured and brain diseased persons with motor dysfunction. *J Korean Med Sci.* 2009;24(Suppl 2):S247–S251.

80. Park JH, Kim H-C, Lee JH, Kim JS, Roh SY, Yi CH, Kang YK, Kwon BS. Development of Korean Academy of Medical Sciences Guideline for rating physical disability of upper extremity. *J Korean Med Sci.* 2009;24:S288–S298.

81. Kim H-C, Kim J-S, Lee K-H, Lee HS, Choi E-S, Yu J-Y. Development of Korean Academy of Medical Sciences Guideline rating the physical impairment: Lower extremities. *J Korean Med Sci.* 2009;24:S299–S306.

82. Wewers ME, Lowe NK. A critical review of visual analogue scales in the measurement of clinical phenomena. *Res Nurs Health.* 1990;13(4):227–236.

83. *Guides to the Evaluation of Permanent Impairment*, 6th ed. Chicago, IL: American Medical Association; 2007. pp. 341–348.

84. Fowler CJ, Griffiths D, de Groat WC. The neural control of micturition. *Nat Rev Neurosci.* 2008;9(6):453–466.

85. Yu JH, Kim SH, Sohn SH, Paik KH, Lee JZ, Kim JH et al. Development of Korean Academy of Medical Sciences Guideline rating the physical impairment; kidney, bladder, urethra, male and female reproductive systems (preliminary report). *J Korean Med Sci.* 2009;24(Suppl 2):S277–S287.

86. Miller TA. Diagnostic evaluation of erectile dysfunction. *Am Fam Physician.* 2000;61(1):95–104.

87. Bari V, Ahmed MN, Rafique MZ, Ashraf K, Memon WA, Usman MU. Evaluation of erectile dysfunction with color Doppler sonography. *J Pak Med Assoc.* 2006;56(6):258–261.

88. *Clinical Practice Guidelines for Chronic Kidney Disease: Evaluation, Classification and Stratification* [Internet]. New York: National Kidney Foundation Kidney Disease Outcomes Quality Initiative; 2002.

89. Botev R, Mallie JP, Couchoud C, Schuck O, Fauvel JP, Wetzels JF et al. Estimating glomerular filtration rate: Cockcroft-Gault and modification of diet in renal disease formulas compared to renal inulin clearance. *Clin J Am Soc Nephrol.* 2009;4(5):899–906.

90. Asrani SK, Kim WR. Model for end-stage liver disease: End of the first decade. *Clin Liver Dis.* 2011;15(4):685–698.

91. The digestive system. In: Rondinelli RD, Genovese E, Katz RT, Mayer TG, Mueller K, Ranavaya ML, Brigham BR, editor. *AMA Guides to the Evaluation of Permanent Impairment.* Chicago, IL: American Medical Association; 2007. p. 119.

92. Baik SH, Lee KS, Jeong S-Y, Park YK, Kim HS, Lee DH, Oh HJ, Kim BC. Development of a rating system for digestive system impairments: Korean Academy of Medical Sciences Guideline. *Korean Med Sci.* 2009(24):S271–S276.

93. *Global Strategy on Diet, Physical Activity and Health: What is Moderate-Intensity and Vigorous-Intensity Physical Activity?* Geneva, Switzerland: World Health Organization; 2014.

94. Fleg JL, Pina IL, Balady GJ, Chaitman BR, Fletcher B, Lavie C et al. Assessment of functional capacity in clinical and research applications: An advisory from the Committee on Exercise, Rehabilitation, and Prevention, Council on Clinical Cardiology, American Heart Association. *Circulation.* 2000;102(13):1591–1597.

95. Goldman L, Hashimoto B, Cook EF, Loscalzo A. Comparative reproducibility and validity of systems for assessing cardiovascular functional class: Advantages of a new specific activity scale. *Circulation.* 1981;64(6):1227–1234.

96. The Criteria Committee of the New York Heart Association. *Nomenclature and Criteria for Diagnosis of Diseases of the Heart and Great Vessels: Functional Capacity and Objective Assessment of Patients with Diseases of the Heart.* Boston, MA: Little, Brown; 1994. pp. 253–256.

97. Nishimura RA, Tajik AJ. Evaluation of diastolic filling of left ventricle in health and disease: Doppler echocardiography is the clinician's Rosetta Stone. *J Am Coll Cardiol.* 1997;30(1):8–18.

98. Ejection fraction heart failure measurement. The American Heart Association; 2014. Available from: www.heart.org/.

99. Hunt SA, Abraham WT, Chin MH, Feldman AM, Francis GS, Ganiats TG et al. 2009 Focused update incorporated into the ACC/AHA 2005 Guidelines for the Diagnosis and Management of Heart Failure in Adults: A Report of the American College of Cardiology Foundation/American Heart Association Task Force on Practice Guidelines Developed in Collaboration With the International Society for Heart and Lung Transplantation. *J Am Coll Cardiol.* 2009;53(15):e1–e90.

100. Nishimura RA, Otta CM, Bonow RO, Carabello BA, Erwin JP III, Guyton RA et al. 2014 AHA/ACC guideline for the management of patients with valvular heart disease. *J Am Coll Cardiol.* 2014:63:2438–2488.

101. National Asthma Education and Prevention Program. Expert panel report 3 (EPR-3): Guidelines for the diagnosis and management of asthma-summary report 2007. *J Allergy Clin Immunol.* 2007;120(5 Suppl):S94–S138.

102. Reddel HK, Bateman ED, Becker A, Boulet LP, Cruz AA, Drazen JM et al. A summary of the new GINA strategy: A roadmap to asthma control. *Eur Respir J.* 2015;46(3):622–639.

103. Bateman ED, Hurd SS, Barnes PJ, Bousquet J, Drazen JM, FitzGeralde JM et al. Global strategy for asthma management and prevention: GINA executive summary. *Eur Respir J.* 2008;31(1):143–178.

104. Global Initiative for Chronic Obstructive Lung Disease. Global strategy for the diagnosis, management, and prevention of chronic obstructive pulmonary disease (Updated 2013) [Internet]. Global Initiative for Chronic Obstructive Lung Disease; 2013.

105. Kim S, Oh J, Kim Y-I, Ban H-J, Kwon Y-S, Oh I-J, Kim K-S, Kim Y-C, Lim S-C. Differences in classification of COPD group using COPD assessment test (CAT) or modified Medical Research Council (mMRC) dyspnea scores: A cross-sectional analyses. *BMC Pulm Med.* 2013;13:35.

106. Hsu KY, Lin JR, Lin MS, Chen W, Chen YJ, Yan YH. The modified Medical Research Council dyspnoea scale is a good indicator of health-related quality of life in patients with chronic obstructive pulmonary disease. *Singapore Med J.* 2013;54(6):321–327.

107. *Chronic Respiratory Diseases - Chronic Obstructive Pulmonary Diseases (COPD) Management.* Geneva, Switzerland: World Health Organization; 2015.

108. *Guides to the Evaluation of Permanent Impairment.* Chicago, IL: American Medical Association; 2007. p. 88.

109. Pellegrino R, Viegi G, Brusasco V, Crapo RO, Burgos F, Casaburi R et al. Interpretative strategies for lung function tests. *Eur Respir J.* 2005;26(5):948–968.

110. Mokhlesi B, Tulaimat A, Evans AT, Wang Y, Itani AA, Hassaballa HA et al. Impact of adherence with positive airway pressure therapy on hypercapnia in obstructive sleep apnea. *J Clin Sleep Med.* 2006;2(1):57–62.

111. Biering-Sorensen F, Krassioukov A, Alexander MS, Donovan W, Karlsson AK, Mueller G et al. International spinal cord injury pulmonary function basic data set. *Spinal Cord.* 2012;50(6):418–421.

112. Tow AM, Graves DE, Carter RE. Vital capacity in tetraplegics twenty years and beyond. *Spinal Cord.* 2001;39(3):139–144.

113. Roth EJ, Nussbaum SB, Berkowitz M, Primack S, Oken J, Powley S et al. Pulmonary function testing in spinal cord injury: Correlation with vital capacity. *Paraplegia.* 1995;33(8):454–457.

114. Brown R, DiMarco AF, Hoit JD, Garshick E. Respiratory dysfunction and management in spinal cord injury. *Respir Care.* 2006;51(8):853–868;discussion 69–70.

115. Ohry A, Molho M, Rozin R. Alterations of pulmonary function in spinal cord injured patients. *Paraplegia.* 1975;13(2):101–108.

116. Carter RE. Respiratory aspects of spinal cord injury management. *Paraplegia.* 1987;25(3):262–266.

117. Gardner BP, Watt JW, Krishnan KR. The artificial ventilation of acute spinal cord damaged patients: A retrospective study of forty-four patients. *Paraplegia.* 1986;24(4):208–220.

118. *Haemoglobin Concentrations for the Diagnosis of Anaemia and Assessment of Severity.* Vitamin and Mineral Nutrition Information System (VMNIS). Geneva, Switzerland: World Health Organization; 2011.

119. Tobian AA, Heddle NM, Wiegmann TL, Carson JL. Red blood cell transfusion: 2016 clinical practice guidelines from AABB. *Transfusion.* 2016;56(10):2627–2630.

120. *Guides to the Evaluation of Permanent Impairment,* 6th ed. Chicago, IL: American Medical Association; 2007. p. 189.

121. Druker B. *Targeted Therapy for Chronic Myeloid Leukemia.* Washington, DC: American Society of Hematology; 2008.

122. Thiagarajan P. *Expert Opinion on 'WHO - ICF Applied Objective Evaluation of Disability: Chronic Myeloid Leukemia'.* Houston, TX: Department of Hematopathology, Bayer College of Medicine; 2011.

123. Duodecim FMS. Thrombocytopenia. In: *EBM Guidelines. Evidence-Based Medicine* [Internet]. Helsinki, Finland: Wiley Interscience; 2007.

124. Thiagarajan P. *Expert Opinion on 'Integrated Evaluation of Disability: Thrombocytopenia'.* Houston, TX: Department of Hematopathology, Bayer College of Medicine; 2011.

125. Lusher JM. *Hemophilia: From Plasma to Recombinant Factors.* Washington, DC: American Society of Hematology; 2008.

126. White GC 2nd, Rosendaal F, Aledort LM, Lusher JM, Rothschild C, Ingerslev J et al. Definitions in hemophilia. Recommendation of the scientific subcommittee on factor VIII and factor IX of the scientific and standardization committee of the International Society on Thrombosis and Haemostasis. *Thromb Haemost.* 2001;85:560.

127. *1993 Revised Classification System for HIV Infection and Expanded Surveillance Case Definition for AIDS Among Adolescents and Adults.* Atlanta, GA: Morbidity and Mortality Weekly Report, Centers for Disease Control and Prevention, Department of Health and Human Services; 1992.

128. *The Relationship Between the Human Immunodeficiency Virus and the Acquired Immunodeficiency Syndrome.* In: National Institute of Allergy and Infectious Disease - National Institute of Health UDoHaHS, editor. 2010.

129. Anderson JR. *A Guide to the Clinical Care of Women with HIV, 2005 Edition.* Rockville, MD: Department of Health and Human Services, Health Resources and Services Administration, HIV/AIDS Bureau; 2005.

130. Adolescent PoAGfAa. *Guidelines for the Use of Antiretroviral Agents in HIV-1-Infected Adults and Adolescents.* In: Department of Health and Human Services, editor. 2013.

131. Consolidated Guidelines on the use of Antiretroviral Drugs for treating and preventing HIV infection - recommendations for a public health approach. World Health Organization; 2013. p. 28.

132. Gamme G, Birch DW, Karmali S. Minimally invasive splenectomy: An update and review. *Can J Surg.* 2013;56(4):280–285.

133. Visual field testing: From one medical student to another [Internet]. 2014.253. Available from: EYE ROUNDS.ORG.

134. Sue S. Test distance vision using a Snellen chart. *Community Eye Health.* 2007;20(63):52.

135. *ICD-10 Version: 2015 (International Statistical Classification of Diseases and Related Health Problems 10th Revision).* Geneva, Switzerland: World Health Organization.

136. Kedar S, Ghate D, Corbett JJ. Visual fields in neuro-ophthalmology. *Indian J Ophthalmol.* 2011;59(2):103–109.

137. Standard Automated Perimetry [Internet]. EyeWiki. 2014. Available from: http://eyewiki.aao.org.

138. Dragoi V. Chapter 14: Visual processing: Eye and retina. In: *Neuroscience Online* [Internet]. Houston, TX: Department of Neurobiology and Anatomy, University of Texas Medical School; 1997.

139. Spector RH. Chapter 116: Visual fields. In: Walker HK HW, Hurst JW, editor. *Clinical Methods: The History, Physical, and Laboratory Examinations*, 3rd ed. Boston, MA: Butterworths; 1990.

140. Rehabilitation ISfLvRa, editor. GUIDE for the evaluation of VISUAL impairment. *International Low Vision Conference VISION-99*. San Francisco, CA: Pacific Vision Foundation; 1999.

141. Almog Y, Nemet A. The correlation between visual acuity and color vision as an indicator of the cause of visual loss. *Am J Ophthalmol.* 2010;149(6):1000–1004.

142. Colour vision deficiency part 3 – occupational standards [Internet]. *OT CET Continuing Education and Training*, 2014. Available from: http://www.optometry.co.uk/.

143. Spector RH. Chapter 113: Diplopia. In: Walker HK HW, Hurst JW, editor. *Clinical Methods: The History, Physical, and Laboratory Examinations*, 3rd ed. Boston, MA: Butterworths; 1990.

144. Hatt SR, Leske DA, Holmes JM. Comparing methods of quantifying diplopia. *Ophthalmology.* 2007;114(12):2316–2322.

145. (ICO) ICoO, editor. Vision requirements for driving safety—International Council of Ophthalmology—December, 2005. *30th World Ophthalmology Congress*, Sao Paulo, Brazil: International Council of Ophthalmology (ICO); 2006.

146. *Deafness and Hearing Loss.* Geneva, Switzerland: World Health Organization; 2014.

147. Gray L. Section 2 - Sensory systems - Chapter 12: Auditory system: Structure and function. In: *Neurosciences Online.* Houston, TX: Department of Neurobiology and Anatomy, University of Texas Medical School; 1997.

148. *Report of the Informal Consultation on the Economic Analysis of Sensory Disabilities.* Geneva, Switzerland: World Health Organization; 2000.

149. *Prevention of Blindness and Deafness: Grades of Hearing Impairment.* Geneva, Switzerland: World Health Organization; 2014.

150. *Schedule for Rating Permanent Disabilities under Provisions of the Labor Code of the State of California.* In: Department of Industrial Relations DOWC, editor. California, CA: Compiled and Published by Casey L. Young, Administrative Director, Department of Industrial Relations, Division of Workers' Compensation, State of California; 1997.

151. Cochlear Implants. In: (NIDCD) N-NIoDaOCD, editor. Washington, DC: U.S. Department of Health & Human Services; 2014.

152. Day HJB. The ISO/ISPO classification of congenital limb deficiency. *Prosthet Orthot Int.* 1991;15(2):67–69.

153. *Guides to the Evaluation of Permanent Impairment,* 5th ed. Chicago, IL: American Medical Association; 2001. 528 p.

154. Cohen P, Rogol AD, Deal CL, Saenger P, Reiter EO, Ross JL et al. Consensus statement on the diagnosis and treatment of children with idiopathic short stature: A summary of the Growth Hormone Research Society, the Lawson Wilkins Pediatric Endocrine Society, and the European Society for Paediatric Endocrinology Workshop. *J Clin Endocrinol Metab.* 2008;93(11):4210–4217.

155. Dwarfism [Internet]. Little People of America. Available from: http://www.lpaonline.org/.

156. Frequently asked questions: Definition of Dwarfism [Internet]. Little People of America 2008–2011.

157. *A Guide to Disability Rights Laws: Americans with Disabilities Act.* In: U.S. Department of Justice CRD, Disability Rights Section, editor. 2005.

158. *WHO Healthy Cities Jesu: A Need Assessment of Health and Welfare among the Disabled for Community Based Rehabilitation in Jeju.* December 2006. 9 p.

159. *International Classification of Functioning, Disability and Health.* Geneva, Switzerland: World Health Organization; 2001. pp. 103, 4, 5, 22.

160. Tiwari VK. Burn wound: How it differs from other wounds? *Indian J Plast Surg.* 2012;45(2):364–373.

161. Agbenorku P. Burns functional disabilities among burn survivors: A study in Komfo Anokye Teaching Hospital, Ghana. *Int J Burns Trauma.* 2013;3(2):78–86.

162. Faustino LD, Oliveira RA, Oliveira AF, Rodrigues EB, Moraes NS, Ferreira LM. Bilateral maculopathy following electrical burn: Case report. *Sao Paulo Med J.* 2014;132(6):372–376.

163. Reddy SC. Electric cataract: A case report and review of the literature. *Eur J Ophthalmol.* 1999;9(2):134–138.

164. Patel R, Mukherjee B. Crash and burn: Ocular injuries due to fireworks. *Seminars in Ophthalmology.* 2014:1–6.

165. Templer J, Renner GJ. Injuries of the external ear. *Otolaryngol Clin North Am.* 1990;23(5):1003–1018.

166. Lukan N. Burn injuries of the middle ear. *ORL J Otorhinolaryngol Relat Spec.* 1991;53(3):140–142.

167. Taylor HO, Carty M, Driscoll D, Lewis M, Donelan MB. Nasal reconstruction after severe facial burns using a local turndown flap. *Ann Plast Surg.* 2009;62(2):175–179.

168. Maragakis GM, Garcia-Tempone M. Microstomia following facial burns. *J Clin Pediatr Dent.* 1998;23(1):69–74.

169. Rutan RL. Management of perineal and genital burns. *J ET Nurs.* 1993;20(4):169–176.

170. Abdel-Razek SM. Isolated chemical burns to the genitalia. *Ann Burns Fire Disasters.* 2006;19(3):148–152.

171. Sajad W, Hamid R. Outcome of split thickness skin grafting and multiple z-plasties in postburn contractures of groin and perineum: A 15-year experience. *Plast Surg Int.* 2014;2014:358526.

172. Grishkevich VM. Postburn perineal obliteration: Elimination of perineal, inguinal, and perianal contractures with the groin flap. *J Burn Care Res.* 2010;31(5):786–790.

173. Ibrahim AE, Sarhane KA, Fagan SP, Goverman J. Renal dysfunction in burns: A review. *Ann Burns Fire Disasters.* 2013;26(1):16–25.

174. Abu-Sittah GS, Sarhane KA, Dibo SA, Ibrahim A. Cardiovascular dysfunction in burns: Review of the literature. *Ann Burns Fire Disasters.* 2012;25(1):26–37.

175. Jones SW, Zhou H, Ortiz-Pujols SM, Maile R, Herbst M, Joyner BL, Jr. et al. Bronchoscopy-derived correlates of lung injury following inhalational injuries: A prospective observational study. *PLoS One.* 2013;8(5):e64250.

176. Toon MH, Maybauer MO, Greenwood JE, Maybauer DM, Fraser JF. Management of acute smoke inhalation injury. *Crit Care Resusc.* 2010;12(1):53–61.

177. Kim WS, Moon KC, Park MC, Haw CR, Hong IP, Korean Academy of Medical S. Development of Korean Academy of Medical Sciences Guideline on the skin and related system: Impairment evaluation of disfigurement in skin and appearance. *J Korean Med Sci.* 2009;24(Suppl 2):S314–S322.

Validation of clinical methods/scales

5.1 "DELPHI PROCESS"

The Delphi Process verifies the appropriateness of the data from experts by consensus in three rounds by email correspondence. During the first round, the project provides the proposed data to each panelist for interpretation and opinion along with an illustration. The panelist interprets the data and assigns a score between 1 and 9, where the score 1 to 4 is inappropriate; score 5 to 7 is uncertain, and score 8 and 9 is appropriate. During the second round, the project tabulates the survey score of all the panelists from the first round, communicates to all panelists to review the results of the first round, and requests revision of their opinion in their first-round if deemed necessary. The project tabulates the revised score of the panelists from the second round. During the third round, the project sends tabulated revised scores of the second round to each panelist for final approval with further modification if it is essential. The project accepts the results of the third round with a score of 7 and 8 as a final consensus opinion.

In "Modified Delphi Process," the panelists interpret and assign the score to the first two rounds of the Delphi Process. However, in "Modified Delphi Process," during the third round, the project organizes a meeting with the panelists to discuss, analyze. and obtain a consensus opinion. If there is a constraint in having hosted a meeting for discussion, the project can review the results of the second round by personal or email correspondence and finally by trial with a clinical model to conclude.

5.2 "MODIFIED DELPHI PROCESS"

Integrated Evaluation of Disability applied the "Modified Delphi Process" to verify the appropriateness of non-standardized clinical methods/tools as well as assigning disability score for impairment of function/structure, limitation of activities, participation restriction and environmental barriers.

Integrated Evaluation of Disability classifies the severity of disability as mild, moderate, severe, profound, and complete.

The "Modified Delphi Process" included preparation of clinical methods and tools, a guideline for assigning disability, a selection of panelists, a survey in three rounds along with analysis (1,2). Integrated evaluation adopted final trial with the clinical model because of the constraint in field trial after review by senior consultants in respective clinical disciplines (Illustration 5.1).

Integrated Evaluation of Disability selected 50 panelists from physical medicine and rehabilitation, orthopedics, neurology, psychiatry, urologist, and pulmonologist practicing disability evaluation around the world. Thirty-two panelists practicing disability evaluation from Kuwait, Czech Republic, and India consented to participate in the "Modified Delphi Process."

Twenty-eight physicians from physical medicine and rehabilitation, neurology, phoniatry, and psychiatry participated in the Delphi Process (Table 5.1). *Integrated Evaluation of Disability* labeled the panelists as P1, P2, P3, and so on, instead of their names to avoid consultation between them.

During first round, *Integrated Evaluation of Disability* provided model table illustrating the scoring system along with the proposed clinical methods/tools and percentage of impairment to each panelist. Panelists interpreted the proposed clinical method and tools and the percentage of impairment, and furnished the value between 1 and 9, where the score 1 to 4 are inappropriate, score 5 to 7 are uncertain, and 8 and 9 are appropriate (Table 5.2).

During the second round, *Integrated Evaluation of Disability* tabulated the survey score of all the panelists after completion of the first round of the survey and communicated to all panelists without revealing the identity of the individual panelist for their review and revision of their opinion in their first survey, if deemed necessary. It tabulated the revised score from the panelists for analysis.

During the third round, only 11 panelists from physical medicine and rehabilitation and three panelists from neurology participated in the discussion (Table 5.3). During the discussion, *Integrated Evaluation of Disability* (IED) accepted the categories with a score of 8 and 9. IED

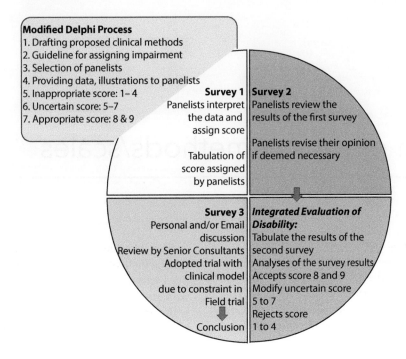

Illustration 5.1 Modified Delphi Process.

Table 5.1 Modified Delphi Process—Panelists

No	Name of the clinical field	Country	Number of participants
1	Physical medicine and rehabilitation	Kuwait (16), India (5), Czech Republic (1)	22
3	Neurology	Kuwait (3)	3
4	Phoniatry	Kuwait (2)	2
5	Psychiatry	India (1)	1

Table 5.2 Modified Delphi Process—Illustration model

	1 least appropriate—9 most appropriate								
Appropriateness scale	1	2	3	4	5	6	7	8	9

Cognitive functions
Orientation to time

(1) What is the present time (or) approximate time of day, for example, morning, afternoon, evening, night?
(2) What is the day of the week?
(3) What is the date, month, and year?
(4) What was your last meal—breakfast/lunch/dinner?
(5) How long have you been in the hospital?

Orientation to place

(1) Can you tell me the location of the hospital?
(2) Can you tell me the floor in which your room exists?
(3) Can you tell me the directions and distance from your house?
(4) Can you tell me your town, county/district, state, and country?

(Continued)

Table 5.2 (*Continued*) Modified Delphi Process—Illustration model

Appropriateness scale	1 least appropriate—9 most appropriate								
	1	2	3	4	5	6	7	8	9

Orientation to the person

(1) What is your name?
(2) How old are you?
(3) What is your date of birth?

Table 5.3 Modified Delphi Process—Panelists/consultants: Discussion

No	Name of the clinical field	Country	Mode of discussion	Number of participants
1	Physical medicine and rehabilitation	Kuwait	Personal	11
2	Neurology	Kuwait	Personal	3

improved uncertain categories with a score of 5 to 7 after valid reason during the discussion. IED rejected most of the categories with a score of 1 to 4 and a modified few with a score of 1 to 4.

Further, consultants in physical medicine and rehabilitation, orthopedic surgery, cardiology, pulmonology, hematology, psychiatry, urology, nephrology, gastroenterology, otorhinolaryngology, ophthalmology, and plastic surgery also reviewed the clinical methods and tools in their respective clinical disciplines during survey 3 and provided their opinion (Tables 5.3 and 5.4).

IED developed "Activity Participation Skill Assessment Scale and Environmental Factor Measurement Scale" for the evaluation of the limitation of activities, participation restriction, and environmental and personal factors. Only a few consultants reviewed these scales in survey 3.

Furthermore, IED subjected the output from survey 3 for trial with a clinical model to establish the appropriateness of the clinical methods/tools and impairment. The "Modified Delphi Process" instituted a pilot study to apply *Integrated Evaluation of Disability* in clinical models and developed a "Ready Reckoner Impairment Table" for about 300 clinical conditions with multiple clinical presentations. The pilot study offered valuable hints to refine further the intricacy of clinical methods/tools, grading of severity of impairment/disability as well as assigning impairment (Tables 5.5 through 5.88).

Clinical methods for evaluation of liver functions, vision functions, hearing functions, dwarfism, burns, and intellectual disability has not undergone the "Modified Delphi Process" but were reviewed by respective specialists.

Table 5.4 Modified Delphi Process—Review by senior consultants

No	Clinical discipline	Country	Mode of discussion	Number of participants
1	Physical medicine and rehabilitation	Austria	Email	1
2	Psychiatry	India	Email and personal discussion	1
3	Cardiology	India	Email and personal discussion	1
4	Pulmonology	Kuwait (1), India (2)	Email and personal discussion	3
5	Hematology	USA	Email and personal discussion	1
6	Orthopedic surgery	India	Email	1
7	Otorhinolaryngology	India	Email and personal discussion	1
8	Ophthalmology	India	Email and personal discussion	2
9	Plastic surgery	India	Email	2
10	Gastroenterology	India	Email	1
11	Urology	India	Email and personal discussion	1
12	Nephrology	India	Email	1

Table 5.5 Clinical methods nervous system—Language, speech, voice

Proposed clinical method	Revision after survey 1 and 2	Revision after survey 3	Revision after trial with clinical model
Performance scale grades language, speech function: "Normal," "Difficulty," "Inability."			
Language - receptive aphasia/dysphasia: Comprehension refers to the ability to follow the conversation by asking to answer questions viz. (a) What is your name? (b) What is your age? (c) Are you married? (d) Do you have children? (e) Are you working? (f) Raise the hand (g) Touch the nose (h) Point to the door (or) look at the door (i) Show me the picture of apple and orange (j) Can you show me the red color		**Receptive aphasia:** The person cannot understand either written (or) spoken words/sentences fully **Receptive dysphasia:** The person cannot understand the question and answer inappropriately, but he/she speaks spontaneously without any meaning and sometimes with a neologism.	

(Continued)

Table 5.5 (Continued) Clinical methods nervous system—Language, speech, voice

Proposed clinical method	Revision after survey 1 and 2	Revision after survey 3	Revision after trial with clinical model
Expressive dysphasia (1) The subject identifies by name the commonly used objects viz. pen, key or body parts (e.g., Semantic error—naming the pen as a pencil). (2) It checks the written matter for spelling mistakes, word order and grammar. (3) Word finding difficulty. (4) Alexia—inability/difficulty in reading written matter. (5) It evaluates "automatic speech" by counting from 1 to 10, reciting the days of the week, months of the year. (6) It assesses spontaneous speech for fluency by asking to read a paragraph, to name the surrounding objects like table/chair/TV and check for ease and rapidity of producing words, some words, initiation of speech, semantic or phonemic errors, word-finding pauses, hesitation or circumlocutions and prosody. (7) It evaluates "dyscalculia," i.e., difficulty/inability to calculate simple addition or subtraction. (8) It evaluates "Repetition" by asking the subject to repeat words, or strings of words or short sentences. **Apraxia** There is no motor weakness. The person with apraxia has lost the knowledge or concept or idea how to perform the skilled movement. Apraxia is identified by inability (or) difficulty to speak, but he (or) she understands the verbal commands. There is difficulty in putting the sounds and syllables together in the correct order to form words. The subject with apraxia are groping for right sound or word and can chew and eat.		**Expressive aphasia:** The person understands the questions projected to him/her but cannot express or speak an even single word. **Expressive dysphasia:** The person comprehends the questions directed to him, struggles to speak a full sentence, and answers the questions in a telegraphic style, for example yes or no only. (a) What is your name? (b) What is your age? (c) Are you married? (d) Do you have children? (e) Are you working **Speech apraxia** The person understands the verbal commands, and he/she has inability (or) difficult to speak. There is difficulty in putting the sounds and syllables together in the correct order to form words. The person with apraxia struggling for right sound or word, and but can chew and eat.	

(Continued)

Table 5.5 (Continued) Clinical methods nervous system—Language, speech, voice

Proposed clinical method	Revision after survey 1 and 2	Revision after survey 3	Revision after trial with clinical model
Dysarthria It evaluates dysarthria at the bedside by asking the subject to repeat simple words, "puh, tuh, Kuh," "puh, puh, puh." prolongation of "aah," reading phrases, reading a paragraph, and counting successively in single breath up to 10. (1) Listen whether the subject pronounces (articulates) clearly (2) Identify any fatigue while counting (3) Whether there is slurring of words and how many sounds are not intelligible (4) Identify any inability or difficulty pronouncing particular sounds, such as /b/,/d/,/p/,/m/ in paralysis of facial muscles; /l/,/d/,/n/,/s/,/t/,/χ/,/z/ in paralysis of the tongue muscles depending upon the demographic (phonemes) pronunciation		**Dysarthria** Normal person speaks clear concise speech with distinct sounds. Observe for any difficulty or deviation in the articulation of speech sounds when the person repeats the following words. (1) Labial dysarthria (Facial nerve): Papa or Mama… (2) Lingual dysarthria (Hypoglossal nerve): La, La, La… (3) Guttural dysarthria (Vagus nerve): Ha, Ha, Ha… (4) Cerebellar dysarthria: Baby hippopotamus, British constitution, Westminster street, and so on. (5) Extrapyramidal - Monotones dysarthria: Observe for monotones when the person recites a poem/song. (6) Spastic dysarthria: (bilateral pyramidal) Observe whether the voice becomes very stiff and muffling when the person repeats Ah, Ah, Ah continuously for 30 seconds. (7) Bulbar and pseudo bulbar lesions: Observe for the nasal tone in all vowels and oral consonant. **Class 1 impairment:** Speech is understandable but initialization difficult, less distinct sounds, impaired stress, or rhythm **Class 2 impairment:** Speech is not clear with indistinct sounds, and poorly understandable **Class 3 impairment:** Speech is unintelligible	

(Continued)

Table 5.5 (Continued) Clinical methods nervous system—Language, speech, voice

Proposed clinical method	Revision after survey 1 and 2	Revision after survey 3	Revision after trial with clinical model
Stuttering is identified by Bloodstien method Grade 1 Grade 2 Grade 3 Grade 4			**Class 1 impairment:** Stuttering occasionally occurring **Class 2 impairment:** Stuttering occurring during periods of excitation **Class 3 impairment:** Stuttering occurring all the time
Perceptive analysis of voice assesses dysphonia – GRBAS. Grade 0 = normal Grade 1 = slight dysphonia Grade 2 = moderate dysphonia Grade 3 = severe dysphonia			**Dysphonia Class 1:** Impairment of phonatory quality such as flutter, creak, tremor **Class 2:** Impairment of resonance, such as nasal tone in cleft palate **Class 3:** Impairment of pitch and loudness, and quality of voice—breathiness or hoarseness, strangled or strained voice **Aphonia - Class 4:** Total loss of voice

Table 5.6 Clinical methods voluntary movement functions—Upper extremity

Proposed clinical method	Revision after survey 1, 2, and 3	Revision after trial with clinical model
Simple movement: Performs isolated movement in individual joints or performs synergic movement pattern. **Dysmetria, dyssynergia and tremor:** *Finger Nose Finger Test* The subject touches his/her index finger to his/her nose and then to the examiner's outstretched finger repetitively. The examiner moves his/her finger with each repetition. There is an irregularity in amplitude and force of the limb movement.	**Multiaxial/ Multiplane/ Multijoint Movement:** *Finger Nose Finger Test* The person directs the movement of his/her index finger to his/her nose and then to the examiner's outstretched finger. The examiner moves his/her finger with each repetition. There is an irregularity in amplitude and force of the extremity movement.	**Uniaxial movement:** **Class 1 impairment** Performs isolated movement limiting to functional range in impairment of joint function or Performs synergic movement in half range in pyramidal lesions or Performs isolated movement with 50% limitation by rigidity in extrapyramidal lesion or Performs isolated movement against gravity only without resistance in impairment of lower motor neuron and muscle functions **Class 2 impairment** Performs isolated movement limiting to non-functional range in impairment of joint function or Performs synergic movement in full range in pyramidal lesion or Performs movement with more than 50% limitation by rigidity in the extrapyramidal lesion or Performs isolated movement only in gravity eliminated plane in impairment of lower motor neuron and muscle functions Performs isolated movement such as raising the arm but overshoot with several bounces in cerebellar lesion **Class 3 impairment** Inability to perform isolated movement or Performs isolated movement such as raising the arm but overshoot wildly with hyperextension of the metacarpophalangeal joint and wrist flexion in cerebellar lesion **Right left coordination:** Ability to clap with both hands. *Mild* - Clumsily clapping with both hands. *Moderate* - Assumes the position of clapping by both hands but could not clap. *Severe* - Inability to take on the position of clapping by both hands and failure to clap. **Eye-hand coordination:** The prehensile function of the hand to hold a pen/pencil and to write a few sentences in a paper. *Mild* - Prehensile function to hold the pen/pencil is effortful, and letters are either micrographic or larger

(Continued)

Table 5.6 (Continued) Clinical methods voluntary movement functions—Upper extremity

Proposed clinical method	Revision after survey 1, 2, and 3	Revision after trial with clinical model
Mild - Overshoot (or) undershoot with few oscillations. *Moderate* - Overshoot (or) undershoot with increased Oscillation. *Severe* - Overshoot (or) undershoot with the gross oscillation of extremity over a distance of more than a foot. **Incoordination (or) Dyssynergia:** **(a) *Tapping in a circle*:** With the pencil tap a series of dots within a circle of 1 cm (In ataxia, dots are spread irregularly over a wider area inside and outside the circle). *Mild* - Taps almost inside the circle and sporadically away from the circle. *Moderate* - Taps unevenly and outside the circle in a wider area. *Severe* - Not able to perform. **(or)** ***Spiral drawing:*** The subject is asked to draw a spiral. *Mild* - Haphazardly draw the spiral. *Moderate* - Difficulty to draw. *Severe* - Not able to draw. **Dysdiadochokinesia:** The person sits with his/her arms flexed at the elbow, holding the forearms vertically with the palms facing inwards, and rotates the hands rapidly at the wrists. The abnormal rhythm refers to a variable rate, velocity or force. *Mild* - Able to perform slowly *Moderate* - Irregular and slow movement *Severe* - Coarse, irregular, and slow movement with the hand dorsiflexed, and the fingers extended with the whole palm shaking rather than wrist rotated **Dysrhythmia:** The back of one hand is tapped rapidly with the fingers of another hand. The tap becomes a rotatory stroking movement in cerebellar lesions. *Mild* - Able to perform slowly. *Moderate* - Irregular and slow movement. *Severe* - Irregular and slow movement with rotatory stroking movement.	*Mild* - Overshoot/undershoot with few oscillations. *Moderate* - Overshoot/undershoot with increased oscillation. *Severe* - Overshoot/undershoot with the gross oscillation of extremity over a distance of more than a foot. or ***Reaching Behind the Back*** - The person reaches contralateral scapula either above the shoulder or below the shoulder with the fingers	*Moderate* - Assumes prehensile position to hold the pen/pencil but could not write *Severe* - Inability to assume the prehensile position to hold the pen/pencil and inability to write. **Rhythmic movement:** ***Dysdiadokokinesia*** - Repetitive alternate pronation and supination of the forearm at an optimum speed of 10 cycles within 10 seconds. *Mild* - Performs partially irregularly in the cerebellar lesion or Performs the movement, but is clumsy in hypertonia or Performs the movement slowly in hypotonia in impairment of muscle function. or Performs the movement only in functional range in impairment of joint function *Moderate* - Performs completely irregularly in cerebellar lesion or Performs the movement slowly and is clumsy in hypertonia or Performs the movement slowly with interruption in hypotonia in impairment of lower motor neuron or muscle function or Performs the movement only in non-functional range in impairment of joint function 1% *Severe* - Inability to perform the movement.

Table 5.7 Clinical methods—Voluntary movement functions: Lower extremity

Proposed clinical method	Revision after survey 1 and 2	Revision after survey 3	Revision after trial with clinical model
Simple movement: Performs isolated movement in individual joints or performs synergic movement pattern			**Uniaxial movement: Class 1 impairment** Performs isolated movement limiting to functional range in impairment of joint function or Performs synergic movement in half range in pyramidal lesions or Performs isolated movement with 50% limitation by rigidity in the extrapyramidal lesion or Performs isolated movement against gravity only without resistance in impairment of lower motor neuron and muscle functions **Class 2 impairment:** Performs isolated movement limiting to non-functional range in impairment of joint function or Performs synergic movement in full range in pyramidal lesion or Performs movement with more than 50% limitation by rigidity in the extrapyramidal lesion or Performs isolated movement only in gravity eliminated plane in impairment of lower motor neuron and muscle functions Performs isolated movement such as raising the leg but overshoot with several bounces in cerebellar lesion **Class 3 impairment:** Inability to perform isolated movement

(Continued)

Table 5.7 (Continued) Clinical methods—Voluntary movement functions: Lower extremity

Proposed clinical method	Revision after survey 1 and 2	Revision after survey 3	Revision after trial with clinical model
Lower extremity dysmetria, dyssynergia and tremor **Heel knee shin test:** The subject places the heel on the contralateral knee and then run the heel down the shin to the dorsum of the foot. He/she performs the same on the other leg. Finally, he/she repeats the maneuver with eyes closed. *Mild* - Side to side oscillation when the heel runs down the shin. *Moderate* - Heel overshoots the knee sideward, and rotatory oscillation as the heel approaches down the shin *Severe* - The Heel overshoots the knee sideward with rotatory oscillation as the heel approaches down the shin and shoots off the foot without control. **Dysrhythmia:** Inability to tap the floor with foot and keep a rhythm. *Mild* - Able to perform slowly. *Moderate* - Irregular and slow movement. *Severe* - Irregular and slow movement with rotatory stroking movement.		**Multiaxial/Multiplane / Multijoint Movement:** **Lower extremity heel knee shin test:** The person places the heel on the contralateral knee and then run the heel down the shin to the dorsum of the foot. *Mild* - There is side to side oscillation when the heel moves down the shin. *Moderate* - Heel overshoots the knee sidewards, and rotatory oscillation as the heel approaches down the shin. *Severe* - The Heel overshoots the knee sidewards with rotatory oscillation and shoots off the foot without control.	**Right left coordination:** Reciprocal movement such as cycling movement of both lower extremities. *Mild* - He/she performs the function, i.e., movement partially. *Moderate* - Initiates the movement but could not continue to perform the movement. *Severe* - Inability to perform the movement. **Eye foot coordination:** Ability to touch the examiner's outstretched hand with his/her big toe by raising his/her one leg while lying down. *Mild* - Performs the movement partially. *Moderate* - Initiates to perform the movement with his/her big toe and the leg bounces several times, and overshoot in cerebellar lesions. *Severe* - Inability to perform the movement.

(Continued)

Table 5.7 (Continued) Clinical methods—Voluntary movement functions: Lower extremity

Proposed clinical method	Revision after survey 1 and 2	Revision after survey 3	Revision after trial with clinical model
Positive Romberg: The subject tends to sway when his/her both feet kept together with the eyes open and sways markedly when he/she closes the eyes. The subject may fall or tends to keep his legs apart for a broader base. *Mild* - The subject stands stationary with the feet together. If he/she maintains the posture, he/she closes eyes for 5–10 seconds. The subject tends to sway. *Moderate* - The subject sways markedly with actual loss of balance when he/she closes the eyes and keeps his/her legs apart for a broader base. *Severe* - The subject cannot stand with feet together. **Tandem walking:** The subject walks heel to toe along a straight line. In "Positive Tandem" he/she tends to sway or fall to one side. *Mild* - He/she performs "Tandem walking," but after few steps, he/she tends to fall. *Moderate* - He/she attempts to perform "Tandem walking" and falls. *Severe* - He/she cannot take the "Tandem position" **Ataxic gait:** The subject keeps his or her legs wide apart for a broader base. *Mild* - He/she walks with broader base support *Moderate* - He/she swings the leg irregularly and reels in several sideward steps *Severe* - He/she attempts to walk, falls and cannot walk further			*Severe* - Inability to perform the movement. ***Rhythmic movement:*** *Mild* - Performs partially irregularly in the cerebellar lesion or Performs the movement, but is clumsy in hypertonia or Performs the movement slowly in impairment of lower motor neuron and muscle function. or Performs the movement only in the functional range in impairment of joint function 0.5%. *Moderate* - Performs completely irregularly in cerebellar lesion or Performs the movement slowly and is clumsy in hypertonia or Performs the movement slowly with interruption in impairment of lower motor neuron and muscle function or Performs the movement only in non-functional range in impairment of joint function 1%

Table 5.8 Clinical methods/tools system—Bradykinesia: Upper extremity

Proposed clinical method	Revision after survey 1, 2, 3	Revision after trial with clinical model

Upper extremity:
  1. Hand movements:
(Rapid successive opening and closing of hand)
Mild - Fatigue with occasional arrest of movement.
Moderate - Hesitation to initiate movement and (or) arrest of ongoing movement.
Severe - Could not perform the movement.
  2. *Finger taps* (Rapid successive tapping with thumb and index finger)
Mild - Fatigue with occasional arrest of movement.
Moderate - Hesitation to initiate movement and (or) arrest of ongoing movement.
Severe - Could not perform the movement.
		Upper extremity:
		Clinical tests:
		  1. Finger-tapping test:
		Rapid and repetitive tapping of the thumb with the index finger.
		  2. Hand:
		Rapid and repetitive hand opening and closing.
		  3. Forearm:
		Rapid and repetitive pronation and supination of the forearm.
		  4. Shoulder:
		Rapid and repetitive shoulder elevation and depression of shoulder.
		Grading of impairment:
		Mild - Slow performance:
		Performs the movement at a slow speed with reduced amplitude
		Moderate - Incomplete performance: Performs the movement but progressive loss of speed and amplitude with freezing of movement.
		Severe - No performance:
		Inability to perform the movement

Table 5.9 Clinical methods/tools system—Bradykinesia: Lower extremity and trunk

Proposed clinical method	Revision after survey 1, 2, 3	Revision after trial with clinical model

Lower extremity:
  1. Leg agility:
Taps heel on the ground and raising the leg as much as 3 inches in rapid succession.
Mild - Fatigue with the occasional arrest of movement.
Moderate - Hesitation to initiate movement and (or) arrest of ongoing movement.
Severe - Could not perform the movement
  2. Rising from the chair
Mild - Pushes the armrest to get up from the chair.
Moderate - Retropulsion with a tendency to fall backward.
Severe - Unable to get up from the chair.
		Lower extremity clinical tests:
		  1. Foot agility test:
		The person taps the forefoot on the ground with rapid speed and amplitude while the heel is resting on the ground.
		  2. Leg agility test:
		The person taps the heel on the ground, and raising the leg as much as 3 inches in rapid succession.
		  3. Sit to stand agility:
		The person's ability to perform the repetitive movement, i.e., getting up from sitting to standing position from the chair.
		Trunk:
		Clinical tests:
		Truncal Agility
		Ability to perform a repetitive sitting movement from a supine position.
		Grading of impairment:
		Mild – Slow performance:
		Performs the function slowly but with difficulty during repetition.
		Moderate – Incomplete performance:
		Progressive difficulty in performing the movement and could not continue the movement.
		Severe – No performance:
		Inability to perform the function.

Table 5.10 Clinical methods—Nervous system: Involuntary movement

Proposed clinical method	Revision after survey 1, 2, 3	Revision after trial with clinical model
Tremor *Mild*: Tremor is mild in amplitude and present occasionally. *Moderate*: Tremor is mild in amplitude and present intermittently. *Severe*: Tremor is moderate in amplitude and present most of the time. *Complete*: Tremor is marked in amplitude and persistent.		**Upper extremity** Tremor, chorea, athetosis, dystonia, hemiballismus **Lower extremity** Chorea, athetosis, dystonia, hemiballismus **Spine** Titubation, dystonia, ballismus
Chorea **Athetosis** **Dystonia** **Hemiballismus** *Mild*: Present in 1%–25% of the day. *Moderate*: Present in 26%–50% of the day. *Severe*: Present in 51%–75% of the day. *Complete*: Present during 76%–100% of the day/painful.		**Impairment** **Grade 1** present <25% of the waking day. **Grade 2** present 25%–50% of the waking day. **Grade 3** present >50% of the waking day **In Cerebellar Dysfunction** **Grade 1** Tremor is present with few oscillations. **Grade 2** Tremor is present with increased oscillations. **Grade 3** Tremor is present with gross oscillations.

Table 5.11 Clinical methods/tools—Nervous system: Swallowing function

Proposed clinical method	Refinement after survey 1 and 2	Refinement after survey 3 discussion	Refinement after hypothetical model
Mild: Occasional choking		**Impairment Class 1:** The person has drooling with occasional choking.	**Impairment Class 1:** Difficulty in swallowing with drooling of saliva or drooling during drinking liquids or accumulation of solid food in the alveoli of mouth.
Moderate: Able to take soft food only		**Impairment Class 2:** The person has limited swallowing ability by modifying food consistency, for example, only liquid food and occasional choking.	**Impairment Class 2:** Difficulty in swallowing with nasal regurgitation and/or occasional choking.
Severe: Nasogastric feeding		**Impairment Class 3:** The person has limited swallowing ability by modifying food consistency, and by minimizing the risk of aspiration with postural techniques and compensatory maneuvers.	**Impairment Class 3:** Difficulty in swallowing with nasal regurgitation and on and off choking. Limited swallowing ability by modifying food consistency.
		Impairment Class 4: The person is not able to swallow, develop significant aspiration on attempted swallowing and require feeding by nasogastric tube or PEG (percutaneous endoscopic gastrostomy).	**Impairment Class 4:** Difficulty in swallowing with frequent nasal regurgitation and choking. Limited swallowing ability by modifying food consistency, and postural techniques and compensatory maneuvers to minimize the risk of aspiration.
			Impairment Class 5: Inability to swallow, develop significant aspiration on attempted swallowing and require feeding by nasogastric tube or PEG (percutaneous endoscopic gastrostomy).

Table 5.12 Clinical methods/tools—Digestive system: Defecation function

Proposed clinical method	Revision after survey 1, 2, 3	Revision after trial with clinical model
1. Inability to control bowel movement resulting in incontinence. 2. Inability to initiate bowel movement resulting in constipation.		**Impairment Class 1:** Constipation – Difficulty in initiating bowel movement and evacuating bowel less than three times per week due to the neurological cause and requiring fiber supplements, and suppositories for evacuation of bowel. **Impairment Class 2:** Constipation – Difficulty in initiating bowel movement and evacuating bowel less than three times per week due to the neurological cause refractory to fiber supplements and suppositories and requiring prokinetic agents. **Impairment Class 3:** Constipation – Difficulty in initiating bowel movement and evacuating bowel one time per week due to the neurological cause and requiring enema for evacuation. **Impairment Class 3:** Constipation – Anismus or dyssynergic constipation, descending perineal syndrome. **Impairment Class 4:** Constipation – Mechanical obstruction due to complete occlusion of the anus, for instance when following burns. **Impairment Class 5:** 1. Inability in controlling bowel movement resulting in incontinence and 2. Lack of sensation of bowel fullness and movement due to the neurological cause and requiring diapers. **Impairment Class 6:** Permanent colostomy.

Table 5.13 Clinical methods/tools—Urinary functions

Proposed clinical method	Revision after survey 1, 2, 3	Revision after trial with clinical model
Bladder: 1. Impairment of urinary function includes inability to hold urine resulting in incontinence, inability to initiate micturition resulting in retention requiring catheterization/diapers. 2. Loss of sensation of desire/fullness/voiding. 3. Urodynamic study confirms motor and sensory impairment of bladder dysfunction. 4. Urgency of micturition – Increased frequency of micturition with low bladder compliance proven by urodynamic study.		**Bladder non-neurogenic lesion:** *Impairment Class 1* Urgency of micturition without incontinence. *Impairment Class 2* Urgency of micturition with incontinence. *Impairment Class 3* Stress incontinence 1. Valsalva leak point pressure measures sphincter weakness. 2. The urodynamic study assesses sphincter dysfunction. 3. Sphincter electromyography ascertains suspected neuropathy. **Neurogenic lesion:** *Impairment Class 2* Voiding by abdominal straining (Valsalva Maneuver)/Credé maneuver with no post-void residual urine.

(Continued)

Table 5.13 (*Continued*) Clinical methods/tools—Urinary functions

Proposed clinical method	Revision after survey 1, 2, 3	Revision after trial with clinical model
		Impairment Class 3 Uninhibited neurogenic bladder. ***Impairment Class 3*** (a) Reflex voiding; (b) No detrusor sphincter dyssynergia; (c) No sensation of desire, fullness, and voiding. ***Impairment Class 4*** (a) Reflex voiding. (b) Detrusor-sphincter dyssynergia. (c) No sensation of desire, fullness, and voiding associated with detrusor dysfunction. (d) Requires alpha blockers or botulinum toxin injection or transurethral sphincterotomy or endourethral stents to eliminate post-void residual urine. ***Impairment Class 5*** (a) Inability to initiate micturition resulting in retention/inability to hold urine resulting in incontinence. (or) Persistent post-void residual urine even after abdominal straining/ Credé maneuver or sphincter management. (b) No sensation of desire, fullness, and voiding. (c) Voiding by catheter/requiring diapers. (d) Neurogenic status confirmed by the urodynamic study.

Table 5.14 Clinical methods/tools—Genital and reproductive functions

Proposed clinical method	Revision after survey 1, 2, 3	Revision after trial with clinical model
Genital and reproductive functions 1. International Index of Erectile Function, nocturnal penile tumescence test, color Doppler ultrasonography, and serum testosterone and prolactin measurements assess erectile dysfunction. 2. The impairment of procreation function in men includes azoospermia. Hormone (or) semen analysis and (or) vasography ascertain azoospermia. 3. The impairment of procreation in women includes primary amenorrhea, structural and (or) functional impairment due to cervical/uterine/ovarian/tubal or peritoneal factors in reproductive age failing to initiate/ continue pregnancy. It requires lab or imaging studies to confirm cervical/uterine/ ovarian/tubal or peritoneal factors.		**Genital and reproductive functions** ***Sexual Function*** 1. Erectile dysfunction - International Index of Erectile Function, nocturnal penile tumescence test, color Doppler ultrasonography, the serum level of testosterone and prolactin assess erectile dysfunction or 2. Anatomical loss of the penis ***Menstrual function*** Primary amenorrhea in reproductive age refractory to medical management. ***Procreation function*** Azoospermia confirmed by hormone or semen analysis and /or vasography before 50 years of age. (or) Structural and/or functional impairment are failing to initiate/continue pregnancy due to cervical/ uterine/ovarian/tubal or peritoneal factors before 50 years of age after maximum medical management.

Table 5.15 Clinical methods—CAD, Hypertensive Cardiovascular, and Cardiomyopathy

Proposed clinical method	Revision after survey 1, 2	Revision after survey 3 and trial with clinical model
Impairment Class 1: (a) American College of Cardiology Foundation/ American Heart Association's Stages of Heart Failure - Stage "A" (b) NYHA Functional Classification – Class I (c) Echocardiographic evidence of systolic and/ or diastolic function: EF 55%–70% E > A (d) METs aerobic capacity by exercise test with treadmill - > 6 METs.		**Impairment Class 1:** (a) Person experiences fatigue, angina and dyspnea during moderate-vigorous-physical exertion (b) Minimal left ventricular systolic dysfunction: EF 45%–55%, or Diastolic dysfunction: E = A (c) ≥3 METs to ≤6 METs.
Impairment Class 2: (a) Heart failure – Stage "B" (b) NYHA – Class II (c) EF 40%–55%, E > A (d) ≥ 3 METs to ≤ 6 METs.		**Impairment Class 2:** (a) Person experiences fatigue, angina, and dyspnea during moderate-vigorous physical exertion (b) Minimal left ventricular systolic dysfunction: EF <45%–55%, and diastolic dysfunction: E = A (c) ≥3 METs to ≤6 METs
Impairment Class 3: (a) Heart failure – Stage "C" (b) NYHA – Class III (c) EF < 40% and/or E = A (d) <3 METs to ≥ 1.5 METs		**Impairment Class 3:** (a) Person experiences fatigue, angina and dyspnea during moderate physical exertion (b) Moderate left ventricular systolic dysfunction: EF ≥ 30%–<45% or diastolic dysfunction: E = A (c) <3 METs to ≥ 1.5 METs
Impairment Class 4: (a) Heart failure – Stage "D" (b) NYHA – Class IV (c) EF < 30% and E < A (d) <1.5 METs		**Impairment Class 4:** (a) Person experiences fatigue, angina and dyspnea during moderate physical exertion (b) Moderate left ventricular systolic dysfunction: EF: ≥30%–<45% and diastolic dysfunction: E = A (c) <3 METs to ≥1.5 METs **Impairment Class 5:** (a) Person experiences fatigue, angina, and dyspnea during minimal physical exertion or at rest. (b) Severe left ventricular systolic dysfunction: EF < 30% and diastolic dysfunction E < A (c) <1.5 METs

Table 5.16 Clinical methods/tools—Cardiovascular system: Valvular heart disease

Proposed clinical method	Revision after survey 1, 2	Revision after survey 3 and trial with clinical model
Aortic Stenosis: *Parameters for grading impairment* 1. Jet velocity 2. Mean gradient 3. Valve area 4. Valve area index		**Impairment Class 1** 1. Asymptomatic valvular heart disease 2. The normal size of atrium/ventricle 3. Normal left ventricular systolic and diastolic function, pulmonary artery pressure, and right ventricular function
Mitral stenosis: *Parameters for grading impairment* 1. Mean gradient 2. Pulmonary artery systolic pressure 3. Valve area		**Impairment Class 2** 1. Symptomatic valvular heart disease - syncope 2. Mild enlargement of atrium/ventricle 3. Minimal left ventricular systolic dysfunction: EF: ≥45 to <55% or diastolic dysfunction: E = A **and/or** Increased pulmonary artery pressure: >20 to ≤30 mm of Hg with normal right ventricular function

(Continued)

Table 5.16 (*Continued*) Clinical methods/tools—Cardiovascular system: Valvular heart disease

Proposed clinical method	Revision after survey 1, 2	Revision after survey 3 and trial with clinical model
Aortic regurgitation: *Parameters for grading impairment* 1. Angiographic grade 2. Color Doppler jet width 3. Doppler vena contracta width 4. Regurgitant volume 5. Regurgitant fraction 6. Regurgitant orifice area 7. Left ventricular size		**Impairment Class 3** 1. Symptomatic valvular heart disease - syncope 2. Mild enlargement of atrium/ventricle 3. Minimal left ventricular systolic dysfunction: EF: ≥45 to <55% and diastolic dysfunction: E = A **and/or** Pulmonary hypertension: >30 to ≤50 mm of Hg with normal right ventricular function
Mitral regurgitation: *Parameters for grading impairment* 1. Angiographic grade 2. Color Doppler jet width 3. Doppler vena contracta width 4. Regurgitant volume 5. Regurgitant fraction 6. Regurgitant orifice area 7. Left atrial size 8. Left ventricular size		**Impairment Class 4** 1. Symptomatic valvular heart disease - syncope, angina, dyspnea 2. Moderate enlargement of atrium/ventricle 3. Moderate left ventricular systolic dysfunction: EF: ≥30% to <45% or diastolic dysfunction: E = A **and/or** Pulmonary hypertension: >30 to ≤50 mm of Hg with minimal right ventricular dysfunction
Tricuspid stenosis: *Parameters for grading impairment* 1. Valve area **Tricuspid regurgitation:** *Parameters for grading impairment* 1. Doppler vena contracta width		**Impairment Class 5** 1. Symptomatic valvular heart disease - syncope, angina, dyspnea 2. Moderate enlargement of atrium/ventricle 3. Moderate left ventricular systolic dysfunction: EF: ≥30% to <45% and diastolic dysfunction: E = A **and/or** Pulmonary hypertension: >30 to ≤50 mm of Hg with moderate right ventricular dysfunction
Pulmonary stenosis: *Parameters for grading impairment* 1. Jet velocity **Pulmonary regurgitation:** *Parameters for classifying impairment* 1. Color Doppler jet width		**Impairment Class 6** 1. Symptomatic valvular heart disease - syncope, angina, dyspnea, decreased exercise tolerance 2. Severe enlargement of atrium/ventricle 3. Severe left ventricular systolic dysfunction: EF: <30% and diastolic dysfunction: E < A **and/or** Pulmonary hypertension: >50 mm of Hg with severe right ventricular dysfunction

Table 5.17 Clinical methods/tools—Cardiovascular system: Dysrhythmia

Proposed clinical method	Revision after survey 1, 2	Revision survey after 3 and trial with clinical model
Impairment Class 1 1. Asymptomatic dysrhythmia 2. LVEF: 55%–70% 3. Requiring or undergoing conventional treatment		**Impairment Class 1** 1. Asymptomatic 2. Isolated dysrhythmia under Guideline-Directed Medical Therapy – GDMT 3. LVEF 55%–70% or E > A
Impairment Class 2 1. Permanent atrial fibrillation 2. LVEF: <40% 3. Requiring or underwent biventricular Pacemaker		**Impairment Class 2** 1. Palpitation 2. Isolated dysrhythmia is requiring or underwent implantation of a pacemaker and/or AICD 3. LVEF 55%–70% or E > A

(Continued)

Table 5.17 (*Continued*) Clinical methods/tools—Cardiovascular system: Dysrhythmia

Proposed clinical method	Revision after survey 1, 2	Revision survey after 3 and trial with clinical model
Impairment Class 3 1. Ventricular fibrillation/ventricular tachycardia 2. LVEF 40%–55% 3. Requiring and/or underwent ICD – Implantable Cardioverter Defibrillator **Impairment Class 4** 1. Ventricular fibrillation/ventricular tachycardia 2. LVEF <40% 3. Requiring and/or underwent ICD – Implantable Cardioverter Defibrillator or biventricular pacemaker		**Impairment Class 3** 1. Palpitation, missing of heartbeat, dizziness, sweating, and anxiety 2. Dysrhythmia is requiring or underwent implantation of a pacemaker and/or AICD 3. LVEF ≥45% to <55% or E = A **Impairment Class 4** 1. Palpitation, missing of heartbeat, dizziness, sweating, and anxiety 2. Dysrhythmia is requiring or underwent implantation of a pacemaker and/or AICD 3. LVEF ≥45% to <55% and E = A **Impairment Class 5** 1. Palpitation, missing of heartbeat, dizziness, sweating, anxiety, chest pain, dyspnea, syncope 2. Dysrhythmia is requiring or underwent implantation of a pacemaker and/or AICD 3. LVEF ≥30% to <45% or E = A **Impairment Class 6** 1. Palpitation, missing of heartbeat, dizziness, sweating, anxiety, chest pain, dyspnea, syncope 2. Dysrhythmia is requiring or underwent implantation of a pacemaker and/or AICD 3. LVEF ≥30% to <45% and E = A **Impairment Class 7** 1. Palpitation, missing of heartbeat, dizziness, sweating, anxiety, chest pain, dyspnea, syncope 2. Dysrhythmia is requiring or underwent implantation of a pacemaker and/or AICD 3. LVEF <30% and E < A

Table 5.18 Clinical methods/tools—Respiratory system: COPD

Proposed clinical method	Revision after survey 1, 2	Revision survey after 3 and trial with clinical model
Impairment Class 1 1. Airflow limitation: FEV_1/FVC <70% 2. Post-bronchodilator FEV_1: $FEV_1 \geq 80\%$ predicted 3. Exacerbations per year: 0–1 4. mMRC score: 0–1 **Impairment Class 2** 1. Airflow limitation: FEV_1/FVC <70% 2. Post-bronchodilator FEV_1: 50% ≤ FEV_1, <80% predicted 3. Exacerbations per year: 0–1 4. mMRC score: ≥2		**Impairment Class 1** 1. History of exposure to risk factors namely tobacco smoke, occupational dust/chemicals, indoor/outdoor air pollutants 2. A chronic cough and sputum 3. No exacerbation 4. Persistent non-reversible airflow obstruction: FEV_1/FVC <70% Post-bronchodilator $FEV_1 \geq 80\%$ predicted **Impairment Class 2** 1. History of exposure to risk factors 2. A chronic cough and sputum, dyspnea 3. Exacerbations: 1–2 per year 4. Persistent non-reversible airflow obstruction: FEV_1/FVC <70% Post-bronchodilator FEV_1 61%–79% predicted

(*Continued*)

Table 5.18 (*Continued*) Clinical methods/tools—Respiratory system: COPD

Proposed clinical method	Revision after survey 1, 2	Revision survey after 3 and trial with clinical model
Impairment Class 3 1. Airflow limitation: FEV_1/FVC <70% 2. Post-bronchodilator FEV_1: 30% ≤ FEV_1, <50% predicted 3. Exacerbations per year: ≥2 4. mMRC score: 0–1		**Impairment Class 3** 1. History of exposure to risk factors 2. A chronic cough and sputum, dyspnea 3. Exacerbations: 3–4 per year 4. Persistent non-reversible airflow obstruction: FEV_1/FVC <70% Post-bronchodilator FEV_1 <30% predicted
Impairment Class 4 1. Airflow limitation: FEV_1/FVC <70% 2. Post-bronchodilator FEV_1: FEV_1 < 30% predicted 3. Exacerbations per year: ≥2 4. mMRC score: ≥2		**Impairment Class 4** 1. History of exposure to risk factors 2. A chronic cough and sputum, dyspnea 3. Exacerbations: >4 per year 4. Persistent non-reversible airflow obstruction: FEV_1/FVC <70% Post-bronchodilator FEV_1 30%–60% predicted 5. Respiratory failure 6. Right heart failure

Table 5.19 Clinical methods/tools—Respiratory system: Asthma

Proposed clinical method	Revision after survey 1 and 2	Revision Survey after 3 and trial with clinical model
Impairment Class 1 Asthma impairment score: 1–4		**Impairment Class 1** 1. Variable symptoms: Wheezing, chest tightness, dry cough 2. Infrequent daytime symptoms with nocturnal episode once a month 3. Post-bronchodilator FEV_1 ≥ 80% predicted 4. Reversible airflow obstruction: Post-bronchodilator increase in FEV_1 of 12% and > 200 mL 5. Asthma control: PEF rate ≥ 80% predicted
Impairment Class 2 Asthma impairment score: 5–8		**Impairment Class 2** 1. Variable symptoms: Wheezing, chest tightness, productive cough 2. Frequent daytime symptoms with nocturnal episode once in two weeks 3. Post-bronchodilator FEV_1 ≥ 70%–79% predicted 4. Reversible airflow obstruction: Post-bronchodilator increase in FEV_1 of 12% and > 200 mL 5. Asthma control: PEF rate 70%–79% predicted
Impairment Class 3 Asthma impairment score: 9–12		**Impairment Class 3** 1. Variable symptoms: Wheezing, chest tightness, productive cough, breathlessness 2. Frequent daytime symptoms with nocturnal episode once a week 3. Post-bronchodilator FEV_1 ≥ 60%–69% predicted 4. Reversible airflow obstruction: Post-bronchodilator increase in FEV_1 of 12% and > 200 mL 5. Asthma control: PEF rate 60%–69% predicted
Impairment Class 4 Asthma impairment score: 12–16		**Impairment Class 4** 1. Persistent symptoms both day and night 2. Post-bronchodilator FEV_1, <60% predicted 3. Refractory to treatment 4. PEF rate <60% predicted

Table 5.20 Clinical methods/tools—Respiratory system: Restrictive lung disease

Proposed clinical method	Revision after survey 1, 2	Revision survey after 3 and trial with clinical model
Extrinsic lung diseases		
Mild: FVC and (or) FEV_1: 70%–79% of predicted		**Impairment Class 1:** Decreased TLC < 5th percentile, FEV_1: ≥80% predicted
Moderate: FVC and (or) FEV_1: 60%–69% of predicted		**Impairment Class 2:** Decreased TLC < 5th percentile, FEV_1: 61%–79% predicted
Severe: FVC and (or) FEV_1: 50%–59% of predicted		**Impairment Class 3:** Decreased TLC < 5th percentile, FEV_1: 31%–60% predicted
Very severe: FVC and (or) FEV_1: 35%–49% of predicted		**Impairment Class 4:** Decreased TLC < 5th percentile, FEV_1: ≤ 30% predicted
Intrinsic lung diseases		**Impairment Class 1:** D_Lco % predicted (Transfer Factor) – >60% and <LLN
		Impairment Class 2: D_Lco % predicted (Transfer Factor) – 51%–60%
		Impairment Class 3: D_Lco % predicted (Transfer Factor) – 41%–50%
		Impairment Class 4: D_Lco % predicted (Transfer Factor) - ≤40%

Table 5.21 Clinical methods—Respiratory system: Hypercapnic respiratory failure

Proposed clinical method	Revision after survey 1 and 2	Revision survey after 3 and trial with clinical model
1. Arterial blood gas – $PaCO_2$ = >50 mm of Hg 2. Arterial blood gas – PaO_2 = <60 mm of Hg 3. Obstructive pulmonary diseases: FEV_1-to-FVC ratio = 0.7 4. Restrictive lung disease: Reduced FEV_1 and FVC but preserved or increased FEV_1-to-FVC ratio 5. Pulmonary hypertension 6. Cor pulmonale 7. Right ventricular failure		1. Arterial blood gas – $PaCO_2$ = >50 mm of Hg 2. Arterial blood gas – PaO_2 = <60 mm of Hg 3. Pulmonary hypertension 4. Cor pulmonale 5. Right ventricular failure

Table 5.22 Clinical methods/tools—Respiratory muscle paralysis

Proposed clinical method	Revision after survey 1, 2, 3	Revision survey after 3 and trial with clinical model
Spinal cord injury – T11: 1. Respiratory dysfunction is minimal Vital capacity is mostly normal 2. A cough is strong **Lower thoracic spinal cord injury:** 1. Respiratory function improves		**Impairment Class 1:** Intercostal muscle paralysis: Rib paradox Abdominal muscle paralysis: Weak cough reflex Vital Capacity: 2000–3000 cc **Impairment Class 2:** Intercostal muscle paralysis: Rib paradox Abdominal muscle paralysis: Ineffective cough reflex Vital Capacity: 1000 to ≤2000 cc
High thoracic spinal cord injury T2 to T4: 1. Vital capacity is 30%–50% of normal 2. A cough is weak		**Impairment Class 3:** Unilateral or bilateral diaphragmatic paralysis: Abdominal and rib paradox, recruitment of accessory muscles of respiration

(Continued)

Table 5.22 (*Continued*) Clinical methods/tools—Respiratory muscle paralysis

Proposed clinical method	Revision after survey 1, 2, 3	Revision survey after 3 and trial with clinical model
Spinal cord injury C3 through C6: 1. Vital capacity is 20% of normal 2. A cough is weak and ineffective		Absence of cough reflex, Recruitment of accessory muscles of respiration Vital Capacity: ≤1000 cc Requiring assisted ventilation
Spinal cord injury C1 or C2: 1. Vital capacity is only 5%–10% of normal 2. A cough is absent		**Impairment Class 4:** Bilateral diaphragmatic paralysis: Abdominal and rib paradox, Recruitment of accessory muscles of respiration Vital capacity ≤500 cc Requiring assisted ventilation

Table 5.23 Clinical methods/tools—Central/obstructive apneas or hypopneas

Proposed clinical method	Revision after survey 1 and 2	Revision survey after 3 and trial with clinical model
Criteria for obstructive sleep apnea: The International Classification of Sleep Disorders, Revised: Diagnostic and Coding Manual of American Academy of Sleep Medicine Criteria for central sleep apnea: The International Classification of Sleep Disorders, Revised: Diagnostic and Coding Manual of American Academy of Sleep Medicine		**Impairment Class 1:** 1. Disturbed sleep, snoring, daytime sleepiness, impaired cognition 2. RDI: 5–15/hour in OSA **Impairment Class 2:** 1. Disturbed sleep, snoring, daytime sleepiness, impaired cognition 2. RDI: 15–30/hour in OSA 3. Asymptomatic cardiac arrhythmias **Impairment Class 3:** 1. Disturbed sleep, snoring, daytime sleepiness, impaired cognition 2. RDI: >30/hour in OSA 3. Symptomatic cardiac arrhythmias: Bradyarrhythmias, PVC, Atrial fibrillation, Atrial flutter **Impairment Class 4:** 1. Disturbed sleep, snoring, daytime sleepiness, impaired cognition 2. RDI: >30/hour in OSA 3. Cardiac arrhythmias 4. Cardiac failure and/or 5. Cor pulmonale

Table 5.24 Clinical methods/tools—Chronic liver failure

Proposed clinical method	Revision after survey 1, 2, 3	Revision survey after 3 and trial with clinical model
Impairment Class 1: 1. Encephalopathy 2. Increased serum bilirubin 3. Prolonged INR 4. Prolonged prothrombin time 5. Ascites 6. 90% chance of survival more than 5 years without transplantation		**Impairment Class 1:** 1. Encephalopathy: Anxiety or euphoria 2. Serum bilirubin: 1–2 mg/dL 3. INR: 1.1–2.0 4. Serum albumin: >3.5 gm/dL 5. Serum sodium: 136–140 mMol/L

(Continued)

Table 5.24 (*Continued*) Clinical methods/tools—Chronic liver failure

Proposed clinical method	Revision after survey 1, 2, 3	Revision survey after 3 and trial with clinical model
Impairment Class 2: 1. Encephalopathy 2. Increased serum bilirubin 3. Prolonged INR 4. Prolonged prothrombin time 5. Ascites 6. 80% chance of surviving 5 years		**Impairment Class 2:** 1. Encephalopathy – Lethargy, and minor impairment of awareness; impairment of cognition: poor attention span, difficulty in orientation for time and place, difficulty in calculation for addition, subtraction; asterixis (flapping tremor); inappropriate behavior 2. Serum bilirubin: 2.1–3.0 mg/dL 3. INR: 2.1–3.0 4. Serum albumin: 3.1–3.5 gm/dL 5. Serum sodium: 131–135 mMol/L
Impairment Class 3: 1. Encephalopathy 2. Increased serum bilirubin 3. Prolonged INR 4. Prolonged prothrombin time 5. Ascites 6. Chance of dying within one year		**Impairment Class 3:** 1. Encephalopathy – Somnolent but arousable, lack of orientation for place/time/person, asterixis, hyperreflexia and plantar extensor response, bizarre behavior 2. Serum bilirubin: 3.1–4 mg/dL 3. INR: 3.1–4.0 4. Serum albumin: 2.6–3.0 gm/dL 5. Serum sodium: 126–130 mMol/L
		Impairment Class 4: 1. Encephalopathy – Coma not responding to verbal or painful stimuli 2. Serum bilirubin: >4 mg/dL 3. INR: >4 4. Serum albumin: ≤2.5 gm/dL 5. Serum sodium: ≤125 mMol/L

Table 5.25 Clinical methods/tools—Hematological systems: Anemia

Proposed clinical method	Revision after survey 1, 2	Revision after survey 3	Revision after trial with clinical model
Impairment Class 1 1. No symptoms 2. No cardiopulmonary/cerebrovascular manifestations 3. Hgb: 10–12 g/dL 4. NYHA functional Class I 5. Does not require blood transfusion		**Impairment Class 1** 1. No symptoms 2. No cardiopulmonary limitations 3. Hgb: 110–129 g/L 4. Transfusion not required	
Impairment Class 2 1. Symptoms of hypoxia 2. Cardiopulmonary/cerebrovascular manifestations: syncope, angina 3. Hgb: 7–10 g/dL 4. NYHA functional Class II 5. Require occasional blood transfusion		**Impairment Class 2** 1. Symptomatic anemia without cardiopulmonary limitations 2. Hgb: 70–109 g/L 3. Requires occasional transfusion	
Impairment Class 3 1. Symptoms of hypoxia 2. Cardiopulmonary/cerebrovascular manifestations: syncope, angina, and heart failure 3. Hgb: <7 g/dL 4. NYHA functional Class III 5. Requires monthly blood transfusion or transfusion dependent for survival		**Impairment Class 3** 1. Symptomatic anemia with cardiopulmonary limitations 2. Hgb: <70 g/L 3. Requires monthly blood transfusion or transfusion dependent for survival	

Table 5.26 Clinical methods—Hematological systems: Chronic myeloid leukemia

Proposed clinical method	Revision after survey 1, 2	Revision after survey 3	Revision after trial with clinical model
The prognosis has been completely changed since the advent of tyrosine kinase inhibitors and CML is a curable disease now. Hence it does not assign impairment for chronic myeloid leukemia.		Discovery of Philadelphia chromosome and abnormal gene BCR-ABL in the blood and bone marrow of persons with chronic myeloid leukemia and advent of newer drugs - Tyrosine kinase inhibitors improved the management of CML with a prospect of good prognosis. CML is a curable disease in many patients now. Hence a person with chronic myeloid leukemia does not require any impairment.	*Integrated Evaluation of Disability* assigns an impairment for the burden of treatment compliance if chronic myeloid leukemia remains uncured and under medication for more than the stipulated period.

Table 5.27 Clinical methods—Hematological systems: Chronic lymphoid leukemia

Proposed clinical method	Revision after survey 1 and 2	Revision after survey 3	Revision after trial with clinical model
Impairment Class 1: There is a low risk in persons with lymphocytosis only in blood and bone marrow with median survival of more than 10 years		**Impairment Class 1:** No symptoms Lymphocytosis only in blood and bone marrow	
Impairment Class 2: Intermediate risk in persons with lymphocytosis, lymphadenopathy, splenomegaly and with or without hepatomegaly with the median survival of 7 years		**Impairment Class 2:** Lymphocytosis, Lymphadenopathy Enlarged spleen or liver	
Impairment Class 3: There is a high risk in persons with lymphocytosis, anemia, and thrombocytopenia with median survival of 1.5 years		**Impairment Class 3:** Lymphocytosis, Anemia (Hemoglobin $\leq$ 100 g/L) and Thrombocytopenia (platelets less than 10,000/μL)	

Table 5.28 Clinical methods—Hematological systems: Thrombocytopenia

Proposed clinical method	Revision after survey 1, 2	Revision after survey 3	Revision after trial with clinical model
Mild: Platelet count of 20,000–50,000/μL		**Impairment Class 1:** Platelet count of between 20,000 and 50,000/μL Bleed only on major trauma or surgery Respond well to prophylactic therapy/blood transfusion	
Moderate: Platelet count of 10,000–20,000/μL		**Impairment Class 2:** Platelet count of between 10,000 and 20,000/μL No severe spontaneous bleeding. Responding to therapy/blood transfusion	
Severe: Platelet count of less than 10,000/μL		**Impairment Class 3:** Platelet count less than 10,000/μL, Frequent spontaneous bleeding, Refractory to treatment	

Table 5.29 Clinical methods—Hematological systems: Hemophilia

Proposed clinical method	Revision after survey 1, 2	Revision after survey 3	Revision after trial with clinical model
Mild: More than 5%–40% normal factor level i.e., more than 0.05–0.40 IU/mL triggers hemorrhage only during major trauma and surgery		**Class 1 impairment:** Coagulation factors >5% to <40% Triggers hemorrhage only during major trauma or surgery	
Moderate: 1%–5% normal factor level, i.e., 0.01–0.05 IU/mL Manifests hemorrhage even with mild to moderate trauma		**Class 2 impairment:** Coagulation factors 1%–5% Manifests hemorrhage even with mild to moderate trauma Replacement of factor controls hemorrhage	
Severe: Less than 1% of normal factor level, i.e., less than 0.01 IU/mL Manifests spontaneous hemorrhage and hemarthrosis		**Class 3 impairment:** Coagulation factors <1% Develops spontaneous hemorrhage and hemarthrosis Replacement of factor controls hemorrhage and hemarthrosis	
		Class 4 impairment: Factor replacement could not control hemorrhage and hemarthrosis due to VIII factor inhibitor	

Table 5.30 Clinical methods—Immunological systems—HIV/AIDS

Proposed clinical method	Revision after survey 1, 2	Revision after survey 3	Revision after trial with clinical model
Asymptomatic HIV infection: Generalized lymphadenopathy and steady decline in CD4+ T-cell (200–500). During asymptomatic stage person also requires antiretroviral therapy.		**Impairment Class 1:** 1. HIV infection under category "A" on ART 2. Asymptomatic infection 3. Persistent generalized lymphadenopathy 4. History of acute primary HIV infection	
AIDS disease: US surveillance guidelines use the CD4+ T-cell count less than 200/μL for diagnosing AIDS. A person is also on antiretroviral therapy.		**Impairment Class 2:** 1. Category "B" AIDS disease 2. Symptomatic infection due to HIV or due to impairment of cell-mediated immunity.	
Advanced disease: There is persistently low CD4 less than 50 cells/cc, the viral burden remains 100,000 copies/mL despite combination therapy. There is a failure of optimized therapy due to multidrug resistance. There is progressive hepatitis C with hepatic failure, progressive leukoencephalopathy with dementia, unresponsive Kaposi's sarcoma, end-stage renal, cardiac failure, and unresponsive lymphoma/other malignancy.		**Impairment Class 3:** Category "C" - advanced AIDS disease with 1. Dementia 2. Renal failure 3. Hepatic failure 4. Cardiac failure 5. Kaposi's sarcoma 6. Lymphoma etc.	

Table 5.31 Amputations

Proposed clinical method	Revision after survey 1, 2 and 3	Revision after trial with clinical model
Upper extremity derives an impairment of 60% and lower extremity 40% for functional, or structural loss by convention.		In amputations, there is a combined motor loss, sensory loss, vascular loss, and dermal loss. Hence, it combines impairment of motor loss, sensory loss, vascular loss, and dermal loss to compute whole person impairment.

Table 5.32 "Activity Participation Skill Assessment Scale"—Learning-applying knowledge

Proposed questionnaire	Revision after survey 1, 2	Revision after survey 3 and trial with clinical model
Basic Learning 1. *Whether the subject can copy an alphabet, rehearse a poem, learn a lesson/read and write (or) including Braille/calculate such as addition or subtraction, acquiring skills such as in games?* 1. Failure to learn: 4 2. Learn with maximum personal assistance: 3 3. Difficulty/increased effort in basic learning or learn only some of the learning items: 2 4. Takes longer time to learn: 1		**Learning-Applying Knowledge-Acquiring Skills** 1. *Can he/she copy an alphabet, learn a lesson, read, and write, calculate such as addition or subtraction* 2. *Can a person with blindness use Braille?* 3. *Can he/she rehearse a song?* 4. *Can he/she acquire skills such as using a spoon and fork for eating food?* 5. *Can he/she able to learn playing games such as football?* 1. Cannot learn: 5 2. Can learn with maximum personal assistance: 4 3. Can learn only some of the items: 3 4. Can learn with difficulty/increased effort: 2 5. Can learn at slow pace: 1 6. Can normally learn: 0

Table 5.33 "Activity Participation Skill Assessment Scale"—Task management

Proposed questionnaire	Revision after survey 1, and 2	Revision after survey 3 and trial with clinical model
Purposeful sensory experience *Whether the subject can watch the movie or sport event in the television, listen to news in the radio or music and comprehend?* 1. Total inability to watch television (or) listen radio and comprehend: 4 2. Watch, listen but needs personal assistance to interpret and understand (or) persons with blindness able to listen and comprehend but not able to visualize the events (or) persons with deafness able to visualize the event and comprehend partially/not able to hear the music (or) news: 3 3. Difficulty/increased effort to understand, and needs hearing aids/visual aids/assistive devices to overcome (or) reduce the difficulty/comprehend only some of the activities: 2 4. Delay in understanding: 4		**Task management—Performing isolated single task** *Can he/she and perform a single task such as identifying the books for his/her class or writing a letter?* 1. Cannot perform the task: 5 2. Can perform the task with assistance: 4 3. Can perform only part of the task: 3 4. Can perform the task with difficulty or increased effort: 2 5. Can perform the task at slow pace: 1 6. Can perform the task normally: 0 **Task management—Performing multiple tasks** *Can he/she plan, organize, and execute tasks at outstation independently? Can he/she locate the place of personal/official work, identifying time and date of travel, mode of travel – bus/train/air, purchasing a ticket, collecting travel kits, clothes, keeping the necessary money – cash or check or credit/debit card and work-related materials?* 1. Cannot perform the task: 5 2. Can perform the task with assistance: 4 3. Can perform only part of the task: 3 4. Can perform the task with difficulty or increased effort: 2 5. Can perform the task at slow pace: 1 6. Can perform the task normally: 0

Table 5.34 "Activity Participation Skill Assessment Scale"—Performing daily activities

Proposed questionnaire	Revision after survey 1, and 2	Revision after survey 3 and trial with clinical model
		Performing daily activities *Can he/she plan, manage, and complete daily activities namely getting up early from bed, toileting, washing his/her body/body parts, dressing, eating, and drinking, traveling and reaching the school/workplace?* *or* *Can he/she plan, organize, cook, serve food, clean cooking and dining area, and clean utensils?* 1. Cannot perform the task: 5 2. Can perform the task with assistance: 4 3. Can perform only part of the task: 3 4. Can perform the task with difficulty or increased effort: 2 5. Can perform the task at slow pace: 1 6. Can perform the task normally: 0

Table 5.35 "Activity Participation Skill Assessment Scale"—Managing responsibilities

Proposed questionnaire	Revision after survey 1, and 2	Revision after survey 3 and trial with clinical model
		Managing responsibilities, stress, and emergency *Can he/she coordinate, control psychological demands to accomplish the task namely driving to reach the airport during heavy road traffic?* *or* *Can he/she cope up with the stress while accompanying his wife/her husband with chest pain to come to an emergency service in the hospital?* 1. Cannot perform the task: 5 2. Can perform the task with personal assistance: 4 3. Can perform only part of the task: 3 4. Can perform the task with difficulty: 2 5. Can perform the task with moral support by accompanying person: 1 6. Can cope up and perform the task normally: 0

Table 5.36 "Activity Participation Skill Assessment Scale"—Communication: Reception

Proposed questionnaire	Revision after survey 1, 2	Revision after survey 3 and trial with clinical model
Communication—Receiving spoken/ nonverbal/sign language/written messages *Whether the subject understands news in a TV/reading and understands newspapers/ understands the traffic signs?* 1. Cannot understand: 4 2. Can understand only partially with maximum personal assistance: 3 3. Difficulty or increased effort to understand (or) needs hearing aids/visual aids to overcome (or) reduce the difficulty (or) comprehend only some of the messages: 2		**Communication—Reception** 1. *Can he/she understand news on a TV?* 2. *Can he/she read and understand a newspaper?* 3. *Can he/she understand traffic signs?* 4. *Can he/she visualize or interpret bus numbers?* 5. *Can he/she visualize or interpret street numbers/name?* 6. *Can he/she hear the safety alarm?* 7. *Can he/she understand messages by sign language?* 8. *Can he/she read and understand a news by Braille?* 9. *Can he/she follow safe lane by tactile surface?* 1. Cannot understand: 5 2. Can understand only partially with maximum personal assistance: 4 3. Can communicate or understand with hearing aids or visual aids or tactile surface: 3 or

(Continued)

Table 5.36 (*Continued*) "Activity Participation Skill Assessment Scale"—Communication: Reception

Proposed questionnaire	Revision after survey 1, 2	Revision after survey 3 and trial with clinical model
4. Takes longer time to understand: 1		Can understand the telephone voice with captioned telephone which displays every character in the conversation, or by TTY—device for communication by typing message forth and back: 3
		or
		Can understand by hearing aid with amplifiers, or understand by speech recognition system: 3
		or
		Can understand Braille language: 3
		or
		Can use the joystick to open the computer and view the email or comprehend only some of the messages: 3
		4. Can understand with difficulty or increased effort: 2
		or
		Can understand traffic lights/signals with difficulty due to color blindness: 2
		5. Can take longer time to understand: 1
		6. Can normally understand the verbal, non-verbal, written messages: 0

Table 5.37 "Activity Participation Skill Assessment Scale"—Communication: Expression

Proposed questionnaire	Revision after survey 1, 2	Revision after survey 3 and trial with clinical model
Communication – producing speaking/non-verbal messages/sign language/written messages 1. Not able to express by verbal message (or) not able to express by a written message (or) not able to use sign language (or) not able to communicate by telephone (or) not able to use the computer for communicating by email: 4 2. Expresses or writes both verbal/non-verbal/sign language with maximum personal assistance: 3 3. Difficulty or increased effort to express or write (or) needs aids such as voice amplifier/assistive devices/modified equipment (or) perform only some of the communication activities: 2 4. Expresses or writes both verbal/non-verbal/sign language but takes more than the normal duration/uses the left hand for writing if right hand is dominant: 1		**Communication expression** 1. *Can he/she express a fact in a spoken message?* 2. *Can he/she send a message by writing a letter to a friend?* 3. *Can he/she express a message by gesture?* 4. *Can he/she convey a message by electronic devices?* 1. Cannot express by verbal message or written message or by gesture: 5 2. Can communicate a message only with the assistance of a person: 4 or Can write a letter only with the assistance of a person: 4 3. Can express a verbal message with voice amplifier: 3 Can use Braille writer to express: 3 Can use the computer with joystick to reply to an email: 3 4. Can express a message with difficulty or increased effort: 2 or Can write a letter with difficulty or increased effort: 2 5. Can write or express verbal, and non-verbal messages at slow pace: 1 or Can use only the left hand for writing if right hand is dominant: 1 Can use verbal, and non-verbal communication normally: 0

Table 5.38 "Activity Participation Skill Assessment Scale"—Mobility: Posture and transfer

Proposed questionnaire	Revision after survey 1, 2	Revision after survey 3 and trial with clinical model
Mobility—Changing basic body positions/maintaining a body position/transferring oneself *Whether the subject can lie down?* *Whether the subject can sit?* *Whether the subject can stand?* *Whether the subject can squat?* *Whether the subject can kneel?* 1. Cannot maintain/change position or transfer by hoist: 4 2. Can change position/transfer only with personal help/maintain position with restraints: 3 3. Can change position and/or transfer with difficulty (or) increased effort (or) needs (orthosis/mobility aids) to overcome (or) reduce the difficulty (or) perform only some of the activities: 2 4. Change position but takes more than normal duration: 1		**Mobility—Changing posture** 1. *Can he/she lie down?* 2. *Can he/she sit?* 3. *Can he/she stand?* 4. *Can he/she squat?* 5. *Can he/she kneel?* 6. *Can he/she bend down and pick up a coin from the floor?* 7. *Can he/she change positions from lying down, from squatting, kneeling, from sitting or standing, bending?* 1. Cannot change and/or maintain position: 5 2. Can change position only with personal help: 4 3. Can change position only with tools or equipment such as overhead sling, orthosis, or mobility aids and maintain position with restraints or perform just some of the activities: 3 4. Can change position with difficulty or increased effort: 2 5. Can change position but takes more than normal duration: 1 6. Can perform all activities normally: 0 **Mobility—Transfer** *Can he/she transfer from a bed to a chair?* 1. Cannot transfer: 5 2. Can transfer only with personal help: 4 3. Can transfer using equipment such as hoist or overhead sling, orthosis, or mobility aids: 3 4. Can transfer with difficulty or increased effort: 2 5. Can transfer but takes more than normal duration: 1 6. Can normally transfer: 0

Table 5.39 "Activity Participation Skill Assessment Scale"—Mobility: Lifting and carrying

Proposed questionnaire	Revision after survey 1, 2	Revision after survey 3 and trial with clinical model
Mobility—Lifting and carrying objects *Whether the subject can lift an object?* *Whether the subject can carry an object in the hands/arms/shoulder/hip/back/head?* *Whether the subject can put down an object on a surface or place?* 1. Cannot perform an activity: 4 2. Performs with personal help: 3 3. Performs with difficulty (or) increased effort, and needs assistive devices/performs only some of the activities: 2 4. Performs completely but takes more than normal duration: 1		**Mobility—Lifting and carrying objects** 1. *Can he/she lift a suitcase weighing more than 20 kg (6 METs) and put the suitcase in a weighing machine or remove the suitcase from the conveyer belt and put it in the trolley?* 2. *Can he/she carry a briefcase weighing 7 kg in the hands/arms/shoulder/hip/back/head?* 3. *Can he/she able to put down an object on the surface or place?* 1. Cannot lift and put down an object weighing ≥23 kg, and cannot carry an object weighing about 7 kg: 5 2. Cannot lift and put down an object weighing ≥23 kg including object weighing about 7 kg and requires personal help: 4 3. Can lift, use trolley to carry an object and can put down an object weighing ≥23 kg, and carry an object weighing about 7 Kg: 3 4. Can lift, carry, and put down an object weighing ≥23 kg with difficulty: 2 5. Can lift, carry with intermittent rest, and put down an object weighing ≥23 kg: 1 6. Can lift, carry, and put down an object weighing ≥23 kg without difficulty: 0

Table 5.40 Activity Participation Skill Assessment Scale—Mobility: Fine hand function

Proposed questionnaire	Revision after survey 1, 2	Revision after survey 3 and trial with clinical model
Mobility—Fine hand use *Whether the subject can pick up a coin from the purse and pay it to the cashier?* *Whether the subject can dial the telephone?* *Whether the subject can turn the doorknob?* 1. Cannot perform the activity: 4 2. Can perform with personal help or environmental control systems – remote control for operating doors (or) windows (or) electronic equipment: 3 3. Can perform with difficulty (or) increased effort (or) need assistive devices or modified objects such as large diameter pen (or) perform only some of the activities: 2 4. Can perform but takes longer time than normal: 1		**Mobility—Fine hand function** 1. *Can he/she write?* *Can he/she turn the pages of a book?* 2. *Can he/she pick up a coin from the purse and pay it to the cashier?* 3. *Can he/she dial the telephone or press the key or swipe across a touchscreen in the cellphone?* 4. *Can he/she turn the doorknob?* 5. *Can he/she operate the computer keyboard/touchscreen?* 6. *Can he/she screw/unscrew a cap of a bottle?* 1. Cannot perform any activity: 5 2. Can perform with personal help 4 3. Can perform with assistive devices/remote control for opening doors or windows or operating electronic equipment or perform only some of the activities: 3 4. Can perform with difficulty (or) increased effort: 2 5. Can perform but takes longer time than normal: 1 6. Can normally perform all the activities: 0

Table 5.41 Activity Participation Skill Assessment Scale—Mobility: Gross hand function

Proposed questionnaire	Revision after survey 1, 2	Revision after survey 3 and trial with clinical model
Mobility—Hand and arm use *Whether the subject can push the door/pull the door?* *Whether the subject can reach across a table for the book? Whether the subject can throw a ball/catch a ball?* 1. Cannot perform the activity: 4 2. Can perform with personal help/environmental control systems – remote control for operating doors (or) windows (or) electronic equipment: 3 3. Can perform with difficulty (or) increased effort (or) perform only some of the activities: 2 4. Can perform but takes longer time than normal: 1		**Mobility—Gross actions of the hand and arm** 1. *Can he/she push the door/pull the door?* 2. *Can he/she reach across the table for a book?* 3. *Can he/she throw a ball/catch a ball?* 1. Cannot perform any activity: 5 2. Can perform with personal help for opening doors or windows: 4 3. Can perform with remote control for opening doors or windows or perform only some of the activities: 3 4. Can perform with difficulty or increased effort: 2 5. Can perform but takes longer time than normal: 1 6. Can normally perform all the activities: 0

Table 5.42 Activity Participation Skill Assessment Scale—Mobility: Walking

Proposed questionnaire	Revision after survey 1, 2	Revision after survey 3 and trial with clinical model
Mobility—Walking *Whether the subject can walk short distance?* *Whether the subject can walk a long distance—1 km?* *Whether the subject can walk around the marketplace?* *Whether the subject can walk through traffic?* 1. Cannot walk: 4 2. Can walk with personal assistance: 3 3. Can walk with difficulty (or) increased effort (or) reduced endurance (or) perform only some of the activities: 2 4. Can walk but takes longer time than normal: 1		**Mobility—Walking** 1. *Can he/she walk inside the house/office?* 2. *Can he/she walk outside the house on different terrains or uneven surfaces?* 3. *Can he/she walk long distance at his/her own pace continuously in open space/treadmill for about 30 minutes?* 4. *Can he/she walk around the marketplace?* 5. *Can he/she walk through traffic?* 1. Cannot walk: 5 2. Can walk with personal assistance: 4 3. Can walk with cane/crutch: 3 4. Can walk with difficulty or increased effort or may fall: 2 5. Can walk but takes longer time than normal: 1 6. Can walk long distance: 0

Table 5.43 Activity Participation Skill Assessment Scale—Mobility: Wheelchair/walker

Proposed questionnaire	Revision after survey 1, 2	Revision after survey 3 and trial with clinical model
Mobility—Moving around using equipment *Whether the subject can move inside the house (or) move down the street in a wheelchair?* *Whether the subject can move inside the house (or) move down the street with a walker?* 1. Cannot use wheelchair and can move only by stretcher: 8 2. Can move in wheelchair propelled by the caregiver/motorized wheelchair: 7 3. Can move with difficulty or increased effort with wheelchair/walker by himself or herself indoor: 6 4. Can move with walker indoor without difficulty but cannot move with walker/wheelchair in the street: 5 5. Can move with difficulty (or) increased effort with walker in the street: 4 6. Can move down the street in a walker/wheelchair without difficulty: 3 7. Can move down the street with a crutch: 2 8. Can move down the street with a cane: 1		**Mobility with wheelchair/walker** 1. *Can he/she move inside the house in a wheelchair?* 2. *Can he/she move on the street in a wheelchair?* 3. *Can he/she move inside the house with a walker?* 4. *Can he/she move on the street with a walker?* 1. Cannot ambulate in a wheelchair and move only by stretcher: 5 2. Can ambulate in a wheelchair propelled by the caregiver: 4 3. Can ambulate in a motorized wheelchair: 3 4. Can propel the wheelchair/walker with difficulty or with increased effort for indoor mobility: 5 5. Can propel wheelchair/walk with walker indoor without difficulty but cannot move with walker or wheelchair in the street: 1 6. Can ambulate in the street in a wheelchair/walker by himself/herself without difficulty: 0

Table 5.44 Activity Participation Skill Assessment Scale—Mobility in and around

Proposed questionnaire	Revision after survey 1, 2	Revision after survey 3 and trial with clinical model
Mobility—Moving from one place to another Whether the subject can climb the stairs? *Whether the subject can run/jog/jump/swim?* 1. Cannot perform any activity: 4 2. Can perform with personal assistance, for instance, climbing: 3 3. Can perform with difficulty (or) increased effort (or) perform using tools/equipment (or) perform only some of the activities: 2 4. Can perform independently with deviation or can take more than normal duration: 1		**Mobility in and around** 1. *Can he/she climb in a mountainous terrain/slope to reach his/her house or workplace?* 2. *Can he/she climb the stairs?* 3. *Can he/she run/jog/jump/swim?* 1. Cannot perform any activity (or) can swim (or) restricted due to seizures: 5 2. Can perform with assistance from a person, for example, climbing: 4 3. Can perform with mobility aids (e.g., crutches, cane)/equipment or perform only some of the activities: 3 4. Can perform with difficulty or increased effort: 2 5. Can perform independently but with deviation (e.g., run with abnormal pattern): 1 or Can perform independently at slow pace: 1 6. Can perform all activities normally: 0

Table 5.45 Activity Participation Skill Assessment Scale—Mobility: Transportation

Proposed questionnaire	Revision after survey 1, 2	Revision after survey 3 and trial with clinical model
Mobility—Moving around using transportation *Whether the subject can travel by bus/taxi/train?* *Whether the subject can travel in a boat?* *Whether the subject can travel in an aircraft?* 1. Cannot travel in any transport independently: 4 2. Can travel with personal assistance: 3 3. Can travel with difficulty (not able to sit for a long time) (or) can travel only by train with facility to lie during travel: 2 4. Can travel but takes longer time to get in/get out of the transport: 1		**Mobility using transportation** 1. *Can he/she travel in a bus/taxi/train?* 2. *Can he/she travel in a boat?* 3. *Can he/she travel in an aircraft?* 1. Cannot travel in any transport independently: 5 2. Can travel only with personal assistance: 4 3. Can travel in vehicles, such as a train or airplane, with the facility to lie and sleep: 3 4. Can travel with difficulty because of difficulty to sit for a long time: 2 5. Can travel but takes longer time to get in and get out of the vehicle: 1 6. Can travel normally using a bus/taxi/train/boat/aircraft: 0

Table 5.46 Activity Participation Skill Assessment Scale—Mobility: Driving

Proposed questionnaire	Revision after survey 1, 2	Revision after survey 3 and trial with clinical model
Mobility—Driving *Whether the subject can drive a car/motorbike/motorboat?* *Whether the subject can bicycle?* *Whether the subject can row a boat?* *Whether the subject can drive a horse-drawn cart?* 1. Cannot drive any vehicle: 4 2. Can bicycle/row a boat with difficulty (or) with increased effort (or) drive only modified hand-controlled car: 3 3. Can drive a modified car such as hand-controlled car: 2 4. Can bicycle or drive slowly: 1		**Mobility—Driving** *Can he/she drive a car/motorbike/motorboat?* *Can he/she bicycle?* *Can he/she row a boat?* *Can he/she drive a horse-drawn cart/bullock cart?* *Applicable only to those who have already been trained to drive a vehicle and to use them* 1. Cannot drive any vehicle or can drive but restriction due to seizures: 5 2. Can drive only in the presence of caregiver for want of moral support as well as to assist him/her to get in/out of the vehicle: 4 3. Can drive a car after modification with hand control: 3 4. Can drive a car only for less than 30 minutes because of difficulty in sitting or can drive with difficulty or increased effort to bicycle/row a boat: 2 5. Can bicycle or drive slowly: 1 6. Can normally drive – bicycling fast/driving a car/driving a boat/driving a vehicle powered by animals such as horse-drawn cart or bullock cart: 0

Table 5.47 Activity Participation Skill Assessment Scale—Self-care: Washing

Proposed questionnaire	Revision after survey 1, 2	Revision after survey 3 and trial with clinical model
Self-care—Washing whole body *Whether the subject can take bath or shower using soap and dry the body?* 1. Cannot take bath and dry the body: 4 2. Can take bath, dry the body with personal assistance: 3 3. Can take bath, dry the body with difficulty (or) increased effort: 2 4. Can take bath, dry the body but takes more time than normal duration: 3		**Self-care—Washing** 1. *Can he/she take a bath/shower using soap?* 2. *Can he/she dry the body after bath/shower?* 1. Cannot take a bath, and dry the body: 5 2. Cannot take a bath, and dry the body without personal assistance: 4 or Can take a bath independently but requires supervision due to seizures: 4 3. Can take a bath with supportive or safety devices such as raised shower stool and grab bar, and dry the body: 3 4. Can take a bath, and dry the body with difficulty or increased effort: 2 5. Can take a bath, and wipe the body but takes more time than normal: 1

Table 5.48 Activity Participation Skill Assessment Scale—Self-care: Caring of body parts

Proposed questionnaire	Revision after survey 1, 2	Revision after survey 3 and trial with clinical model
Self-care—Caring of body parts *Whether the subject can brush teeth/comb hair/trim nails/moisturize the skin?* 1. Cannot brush teeth, comb hair, and cut nails: 4 2. Cannot brush teeth, comb hair, and trim nails without personal assistance: 3 3. Can brush teeth, comb hair and trim nails with difficulty (or) increased effort, with (or) without assistive devices, (or) adapting the unaccustomed hand to brushing teeth, combing hair and trimming nails, (or) perform some of the activities: 2 4. Can brush teeth, comb hair, and trim nails but takes more time than normal duration: 1		**Self-care—Taking care of body parts** *Can he/she brush teeth/comb hair/trim nails/moisturize the skin?* 1. Cannot brush teeth, comb hair, and trim nails: 5 2. Cannot brush teeth, comb hair, and trim nails without personal assistance: 4 3. Can brush teeth, comb hair, and trim nails with assistive devices or perform only some of the activities: 3 4. Can brush teeth, comb hair, and trim nails with difficulty or increased effort: 2 or Can brush teeth, comb hair, and trim nails with unaccustomed hand: 2 5. Can brush teeth, comb hair, and trim nails but takes time than normal: 1 6. Can caring for the body parts normally: 0

Table 5.49 Activity Participation Skill Assessment Scale—Self-care: Toileting

Proposed questionnaire	Revision after survey 1, 2	Revision after survey 3 and trial with clinical model
Self-care—Toileting *Whether the subject can coordinate and manage – proper position and manipulate clothes before and after urination and cleaning after urination?* *Whether the subject can organize and manage – correct position and manipulate clothes before and after defecation and cleaning after defecation?* *Whether the subject can organize and manage – correct position and manipulate clothes to maintain hygiene during menstruation?* 1. Cannot carry out toileting: 4 2. Cannot toilet using commode or bedpan or urinal or carryout intermittent catheterization safely without personal assistance: 3 3. Can toilet with increased effort (or) with difficulty (or) adapting the unaccustomed hand for cleaning (or) perform only some of the activities, e.g., able to get into proper position but not able to adjust clothes (or) not able to clean: 2 4. Can carry out toileting but takes more time than normal duration: 1		**Self-care—Toileting** 1. *Can he/she adjust clothes and position before and after urination and cleaning after urination?* 2. *Can he/she adjust clothes and position before and after defecation and cleaning after defecation?* 3. *Can he/she adjust clothes, and position and clean to maintain hygiene during menstruation?* 1. Cannot carry out toileting by himself/herself: 5 2. Cannot toilet and needing personal assistance or nursing assistance to put indwelling catheter or safely perform intermittent catheterization or apply condom or clean and change diaper: 4 3. Can carry out toileting with raised toilet sheet, toilet frame and grab bar: 3 4. Can toilet with increased effort or with difficulty or adapt unaccustomed hand for cleaning: 2 5. Can toilet but takes more time than normal duration: 1 6. Can toilet normally: 0

Table 5.50 Activity Participation Skill Assessment Scale—Self-care: Dressing

Proposed questionnaire	Revision after survey 1, 2	Revision after survey 3 and trial with clinical model
Self-care—Dressing *Whether the subject can put on /take off clothes?* *Whether the subject can put on/take off socks, stockings, and footwear?* *Whether the subject can choose clothes based on the dress codes and climatic conditions?* 1. Cannot carry out dressing: 4 2. Cannot dress without personal assistance: 3 3. Can dress with increased effort (or) assistive devices (or) modified garments to overcome (or) reduce the difficulty (or) can perform only some of the activities, for example, able to dress but not able to put on (or) take of footwear (or) carry out either upper (or) lower body dressing only: 2 4. Can dress but takes more time than normal duration: 1		**Self-care—Dressing** 1. *Can he/she choose appropriate clothes as per the dress codes and climatic conditions?* 2. *Can he/she put on/take off socks, stockings, and footwear?* 1. Cannot dress himself/herself: 5 2. Can carry out dressing with personal assistance: 4 3. Can dress with assistive devices/modified garments with Velcro tabs instead of buttons or perform only some of the activities, for example, can dress but cannot put on or take of footwears or carry out either upper or lower body dressing: 3 4. Can dress with increased effort: 2 5. Can carry out dressing but takes more time than normal duration: 1 6. Can normally dress: 0

Table 5.51 Activity Participation Skill Assessment Scale—Self-care: Eating and drinking

Proposed questionnaire	Revision after survey 1, 2	Revision after survey 3 and trial with clinical model
Self-care—Eating and drinking *Whether the subject can perform the coordinated tasks and actions of eating/drinking?* Cannot carry out the tasks and actions of eating/drinking: 4 Can eat and drink only with personal help: 3 Can eat and drink with difficulty (or) with increased effort adopt a safe posture of the neck for safe drinking/eating (or) assistive devices to overcome (or) reduce difficulty (or) adapting the unaccustomed hand (or) perform either drinking (or) eating: 2 Can eat/drink but takes more time than normal duration: 1		**Self-care—Eating and drinking** *Can he/she perform the act of eating food and drinking?* 1. Cannot perform the act of eating and drinking: 5 2. Can eat and drink only with personal help: 4 3. Can use only straw, for instance, microstomia following burns or adopt safe posture of the neck for safe drinking and eating or use assistive devices or perform only either drinking or eating: 3 4. Can eat and drink with difficulty or require increased effort or adopt an unaccustomed hand: 2 5. Can eat/drink but takes more time than normal duration: 1 6. Can eat/drink normally: 0

Table 5.52 Activity Participation Skill Assessment Scale—Looking after one's health

Proposed questionnaire	Revision after survey 1, 2	Revision after survey 3 and trial with clinical model
		Looking after one's health
		1. *Can he/she eat a nutritious diet, perform an appropriate physical activity, received immunizations, avoid drug, and abstain from unsafe sexual practice (AIDS)?*
		2. *Can he/she recognize an illness/injury, seek medical advice, and adhere to medical management?*
		1. Cannot understand to maintain his/her body and mind in good health: 5
		2. Can keep his/her body and mind in good health only with personal assistance: 4
		3. Can take care of his/her health only during illness: 3
		4. Can take intermittent care to maintain his/her body and mind in good health after counseling: 2
		5. Can take adequate care to keep his/her body and mind in good health after counseling: 1
		6. Can take proper care to keep his/her body and mind in good health without counseling: 0

Table 5.53 Activity Participation Skill Assessment Scale—Household activities

Proposed questionnaire	Revision after survey 1, 2	Revision after survey 3 and trial with clinical model
Acquisition of goods and services		**Household activities—Purchasing goods and services**
Whether the subject can perform shopping and gather daily needs such as cereals, crockery, vegetables, fruits, clothes, cleaning material by comparing quality and price?		*Can he/she perform shopping and gather daily needs such as cereals, crockery, vegetables, fruits, clothes, and cleaning material by comparing quality and price?*
Whether the subject can reattach buttons, iron clothes, polish footwear?		1. Cannot perform shopping and gather daily needs by himself/herself: 5
1. Cannot perform the activities: 4		2. Can perform with personal help: 4
2. Cannot perform the activities without personal assistance: 3		3. Can perform only some of the activities: 3
3. Can perform with difficulty (or) with increased effort (or) perform only some of the activities: 2		4. Can perform with difficulty or increased effort: 2
4. Can perform at slow pace and takes more time than normal duration: 1		5. Can perform at slow pace and takes more time than normal: 1
		6. Can normally perform: 0

Table 5.54 Activity Participation Skill Assessment Scale—Preparing food

Proposed questionnaire	Revision after survey 1, 2	Revision after survey 3 and trial with clinical model
Preparing meals *Whether the subject can plan, organize, cook, and serve simple and/or complex meals?* 1. Cannot prepare meal: 4 2. Can prepare with personal help if provided with ingredients: 3 3. Can plan, prepare, and serve with difficulty (or) increased effort (or) perform only some of the activities: 2 4. Can plan, prepare, serve at slow pace, and takes more time than normal duration: 1		**Preparing food** *Can he/she select ingredients, arrange cooking utensils, cook, and serve food?* *Applicable only to those who have experience in cooking* 1. Cannot prepare food: 5 2. Can prepare food with personal help: 4 3. Can prepare food if provided with ingredients or perform only some of the activities: 3 4. Can plan, prepare, and serve with difficulty or increased effort: 2 5. Can plan, prepare, serve at slow pace, and takes more time than normal duration: 1 6. Can normally perform: 0

Table 5.55 Activity Participation Skill Assessment Scale—Cleaning household appliances

Proposed questionnaire	Revision after survey 1, 2	Revision after survey 3 and trial with clinical model
Doing household work *Whether the subject can clean cooking area and utensils?* *Whether the subject can clean living area?* *Whether the subject can wash and dry clothes and garments?* *Whether the subject can use household appliances such as washing machine, driers, irons, vacuum cleaners, and dishwashers?* 1. Cannot do household work: 4 2. Can perform it only with personal help: 3 3. Can perform with difficulty (or) increased effort (or) perform only some of the activities: 2 4. Can perform at slow pace and takes more time than normal duration: 1		**Household activities—Cleaning the house and using household appliances?** *Can he/she clean cooking and dining area and utensils?* *Can he/she clean living area?* *Can he/she wash, dry, and iron clothes and garments?* *Can he/she polish footwear?* *Can he/she household appliances such as washing machine, driers, irons, vacuum cleaners, and dishwashers?* Applicable only to those who have already experienced to do the earlier work 1. Cannot perform any activity: 5 2. Can perform with personal help: 4 3. Can perform only some of the activities: 3 4. Can perform with difficulty or increased effort: 2 5. Can perform at slow pace and takes more time than normal duration: 1 6. Can perform it normally: 0

Table 5.56 Activity Participation Skill Assessment Scale—Social interactions

Proposed questionnaire	Revision after survey 1, 2	Revision after survey 3 and trial with clinical model
		Interpersonal skills—Social interactions
		1. *Can he/she create and maintain mutual esteem relationship with friends?*
		2. *Can he/she create an informal relationship with neighbors and acquaintances?*
		3. *Can he/she maintain an informal relationship with colleagues?* (In comparison to pre-morbid levels of interactions)
		1. Cannot create and maintain appropriate relationship with friends, neighbors, acquaintances, and peer because of the unsociable attitude following disability: 5
		2. Cannot create and sustain appropriate relationship with friends, neighbors, acquaintances, and peer due to fear of neglect and inhibition.: 4
		3. Can sustain limited interaction with friends only after counseling: 3
		4. Can interact with neighbors, acquaintances, and peer after initial hesitation: 2
		5. Can sustain interaction with neighbors, acquaintances, and peer in slow pace: 1
		6. Can create and maintain always normal relationship with friends, neighbors, acquaintances, and peer: 0

Table 5.57 Activity Participation Skill Assessment Scale—Interaction with family

Proposed questionnaire	Revision after survey 1, 2	Revision after survey 3 and trial with clinical model
Interpersonal interactions and relationships— Family relationship		**Interpersonal skills—Interaction with family**
Whether the subject can maintain a parent-child relationship and provide physical, intellectual, emotional nurture?		1. *Can he/she maintain a parent-child relationship and provides physical, intellectual, emotional nurture?*
Whether the subject can create and maintain child-parent relationship such as obeying his parents and taking care of his/her elderly parents?		2. *Can he/she create and sustain child-parent relationship such as obeying his/her parents and taking care of his/her elderly parents?*
Whether the subject can maintain brotherly (or) sisterly relationship with his (or) her siblings?		3. *Can he/she maintain a brotherly or sisterly relationship with his or her siblings?*
Whether the subject can create and maintain with members of the extended family such as cousins, aunts, uncles, and grandparents?		4. *Can he/she create and sustain a relationship with members of the extended family such as cousins, aunts, uncles, and grandparents?*
Cannot create, and maintain specified role or poor interpersonal adjustment: 4		(In comparison to pre-morbid levels of interactions)
Cannot perform the specified role, only accept affection, guidance and support from family members and could not reciprocate and limited interpersonal adjustment: 3		1. Cannot create and maintain specified role: 5
		2. Cannot accomplish the role even after guidance by the caregiver: 4
Can perform the role of parent /sibling/child, fair interpersonal adjustment, and satisfied with his/her performance partially: 2		3. Can accept love and affection, and support from family members on advice and cannot reciprocate: 3
Can perform the role of parent/sibling /child in slow pace, good interpersonal adjustment, and happy with his/her performance: 1		4. Can attempt to perform the role of parent/ sibling/child, and exhibit limited interpersonal adjustment with on and off arguments: 2
		5. Can perform the role of parent/sibling/child at slow pace, and maintain fair interpersonal adjustment with occasional tension: 1
		6. Can perform the role of parent/sibling/child normally and retain good interpersonal adjustment: 0

Table 5.58 Activity Participation Skill Assessment Scale—Intimate interactions

Proposed questionnaire	Revision after survey 1, 2	Revision after survey 3 and trial with clinical model
Interpersonal interactions and relationships— Intimate relationships *Whether the subject can maintain a spousal relationship?* *Whether the subject can maintain a sexual relationship with a spouse or another partner?* Cannot create and maintain specified role/ intimate relations: 4 Can attempt to perform the specified role only by guidance with limited interpersonal adjustment: 3 Can perform the role of spouse in slow pace and clumsy or qualitatively inadequate in intimate relations: 2 Can perform the role of spouse with fair interpersonal adjustment partially and satisfy his/her partner in sexual relationship: 1		**Interpersonal skills—Intimate interactions** *Can he/she maintain a sexual relationship with a spouse or another partner? (In comparison to pre-morbid levels of intimacy)* 1. Cannot participate in sexual life: 5 2. Can participate passively in sexual life: 4 3. Can participate in sexual life but clumsy or qualitatively inadequate and cannot satisfy his/ her partner: 3 4. Can participate in sexual life with excessive effort and cannot completely satisfy his/her partner 5. Can satisfy his/her partner in sexual life: 1 6. Can maintain normal sexual relationship (Happy as both a pleasure-receiver and pleasure-giver to the partner): 0

Table 5.59 Activity Participation Skill Assessment Scale—Education

Proposed questionnaire	Revision after survey 1, 2	Revision after survey 3 and trial with clinical model
Major life areas—Education *Whether the subject can pursue education if undergoing education—Preschool/School/ Higher Education?* Cannot continue education: 4 Can continue education in school for special needs: Learning with braille/ alternative script/ augmentative or alternative models/sign language: 3 Can learn facilitated by peer support and mentoring/learn with difficulty (or) increased effort: 2 Can learn only at slow pace: 1		**Education and employment—School education** *Can he/she pursue school education or higher education?* 1. Cannot continue/pursue education: 5 2. Can learn by peer support and mentoring: 4 3. Can study only in school for special needs or learn only with braille or learn sign language or learn by "Augmentative and Alternative Communication": 3 4. Can learn with difficulty or increased effort: 2 5. Can learn slowly (slow learner): 1 6. Can pursue education normally: 0

Table 5.60 Activity Participation Skill Assessment Scale—Employment

Proposed questionnaire	Revision after survey 1, 2	Revision after survey 3 and trial with clinical model
Remunerative employment Whether the subject can pursue self-employment? (or) Whether the subject can pursue part-time employment? (or) Whether the subject can pursue full-time employment? 1. Cannot work: 4 2. Can perform sheltered employment: 3 3. Can perform full-time employment with increased effort (or) return to alternate employment with less strenuous work: 2 4. Can return to original employment but with reduced working hours: 1		**Employment** *Can he/she perform sedentary work/ light work/ medium work/heavy work/very heavy work?* *(in comparison to pre-morbid level of occupation)* 1. Cannot pursue any employment: 5 2. Can perform only sheltered employment: 4 3. Can return to alternate employment with less strenuous work with less salary: 3 4. Can obtain full-time new employment or previous full-time employment for the first time and perform the work with increased effort: 2 or cannot work at height or work involving fire or work involving unguarded machinery because of restriction due to seizures: 2 5. Can perform/obtain employment with less salary for the first time or can return to original employment/alternate employment but with reduced working hours: 1 6. Can return to original employment or better full-time employment: 0

Table 5.61 Activity Participation Skill Assessment Scale—Economic skill

Proposed questionnaire	Revision after survey 1, 2	Revision after survey 3 and trial with clinical model
Major life areas—Economic transactions *Whether the subject can use the money to purchase food?* *Whether the subject can perform bank transaction?* 1. Cannot perform economic transaction: 4 2. Can perform transaction with personal assistance: 3 3. Can perform transaction with difficulty (or) increased effort: 2 4. Can perform transaction but takes more time than normal duration: 1		**Economic transactions and management** Can he/she transact money from ATM? Can he/she perform bank transaction? Can he/she purchase goods using money/credit cards/debit cards? *(in comparison to pre-morbid level of functioning)* 1. Cannot transact money from ATM/Bank, purchase goods using money/credit cards/debit cards: 5 2. Cannot transact money from ATM/Bank, purchase goods using money/credit cards/debit cards without personal assistance: 4 3. Cannot transact money from ATM/Bank, but purchase goods using money only and cannot use credit cards/debit cards: 3 4. Can transact money from ATM/Bank, use money/credit cards/debit cards for purchasing goods with difficulty or increased effort: 2 5. Can transact money from ATM/Bank, use money/credit cards/debit cards for purchasing goods but takes more time than normal duration: 1 Can transact money from ATM/Bank, use money/ debit cards/credit cards for buying goods: 0

Table 5.62 Activity Participation Skill Assessment Scale—Community life

Proposed questionnaire	Revision after survey 1, 2	Revision after survey 3 and trial with clinical model
Community life *Whether the subject can participate in local social clubs/social groups?* *Whether the subject can participate in his/her professional academies or exclusive social groups?* *Whether the subject can participate in marriage functions, funeral functions, initiation functions?* 1. Cannot participate community meetings/ functions: 4 2. Cannot participate community meetings/ functions without personal assistance: 3 3. Can participate community meetings/ functions with increased effort: 2 4. Can participate community meetings/ functions less frequently: 1		**Community life** *Can he/she participate in local social clubs/social groups?* *Can he/she participate in his/her professional academies or exclusive social groups?* *Can he/she participate in marriage functions, initiation functions, funeral functions?* *(In comparison to pre-morbid level of participation in community)* 1. Cannot participate in any community meetings/ functions: 5 2. Can participate community meetings/functions assisted by caregiver: 4 3. Can participate community meetings/functions only with mobility aids or assistive devices: 3 4. Can participate community meetings/functions only with difficulty or increased effort: 2 5. Can participate community meetings/functions less frequently: 1 6. Can normally participate in informal and formal community meetings/functions: 0

Table 5.63 Activity Participation Skill Assessment Scale—Social life: Recreation

Proposed questionnaire	Revision after survey 1, 2	Revision after survey 3 and trial with clinical model
Social life *Whether the subject can engage in games/ sports?* *Whether the subject can engage in fine arts (or) culture events such as cinema, museum, and a musical instrument?* *Whether the subject can engage in hobbies?* *Whether the subject can visit friends, relatives, or meeting informally in public places?* 1. Cannot participate: 4 2. Can participate in personal support under compulsive situations: 3 3. Can participate with difficulty (or) increased effort: 2 4. Can participate less frequently at slow pace: 1		**Social life: Recreation** *Can he/she participate in games/sports?* *Can he/she attend fine arts or cultural events such as cinema, museum, and musical shows?* *Can he/she dance?* *Can he/she participate in hobbies?* *Can he/she able to visit friends, relatives, or meeting informally in public places? (in comparison to pre-morbid level of functioning)* 1. Cannot participate or attend leisure and recreational activity: 5 2. Can participate or attend recreational and leisure activity only with the assistance of trainer or caregiver: 4 3. Can participate or attend recreational and leisure activity only with mobility aids/assistive devices if facility for wheelchair accessibility exists: 3 4. Can participate or attend recreational and leisure activity only with increased effort: 2 5. Can participate or attend recreational and leisure activity at slow pace: 1 6. Can participate or attend recreational and leisure activity normally: 0

Table 5.64 Activity Participation Skill Assessment Scale—Social life: Religion

Proposed questionnaire	Revision after survey 1, 2	Revision after survey 3 and trial with clinical model
Religion and spirituality *Whether the subject can participate in religious ceremonies in church/ mosque/temple?* *Whether the subject can engage in religious (or) spiritual activities in church/mosque/temple/ spiritual contemplation?* 1. Cannot participate in religious ceremonies/ activities: 4 2. Can participate in religious ceremonies/ activities with personal assistance: 3 3. Can participate in religious activities /perform religious ceremonies with increased effort (or) in an alternate way (or) in personally non-gratifying manner: 2 4. Can participate in religious activities /perform religious ceremonies in slow pace (or) infrequently: 1		**Social life: Religious functions and activities** 1. *Can he/she participate in religious ceremonies in church/mosque/temple?* 2. *Can he/she participate in religious or spiritual activities in church/mosque/temple/spiritual contemplation?* (in comparison to pre-morbid levels) 1. Cannot participate in religious ceremonies/ activities: 5 2. Can participate in religious activities/perform ceremonies only with the help of caregiver: 4 3. Can participate in religious activities/perform ceremonies with mobility aids or assistive devices: 3 4. Can participate in religious activities/perform religious ceremonies only in alternate way or personally non-gratifying manner: 2 5. Can attend religious activities/perform ceremonies in slow pace (or) less frequently: 1 6. Can normally participate: 0

Table 5.65 Activity Participation Skill Assessment Scale—Civic life

Proposed questionnaire	Revision after survey 1, 2	Revision after survey 3 and trial with clinical model
Political life and citizenship *Whether the subject can engage in the political and governmental life of a citizen?* *Whether the subject can franchise vote?* 1. Cannot participate in political/ governmental life and franchise vote: 4 2. Can participate or perform in political/ governmental life and franchise vote with personal assistance. Independent decision-making may not be possible: 3 3. Can take part in political and/or governmental life, franchise vote independently and yet indecisive: 2 4. Can take part partially in political/ governmental life and franchise vote in an alternate way but independent, decisive, and yet, clumsy in decision-making		**Community-social-civic life: Activity in political system and citizenship** 1. *Can he/she participate in political and governmental life as a citizen?* 2. *Can he/she franchise vote?* 1. Cannot participate in political/governmental life and franchise vote: 5 2. Can take part in political/governmental life and franchise vote with the help of a caregiver. Independent decision-making may not be possible: 4 3. Can take part in political/governmental life and franchise vote with mobility aids and assistive devices: 3 4. Can participate in political/governmental life with increased effort and franchise vote. Independent and yet indecisive: 2 5. Can participate partially in political/ governmental life and franchise vote in an alternate way but independent, decisive, and yet, clumsy in decision-making: 1 6. Can normally participate in political/ governmental life and franchise vote: 0

Table 5.66 Environmental Factors Measurement Scale—Assistive technology

Proposed questionnaire	Revision after survey 1, 2, 3	Revision after trial with clinical model
Assistive technology for personal use in daily living *Whether cardiac pacemaker, neural prosthesis is available in his/her immediate environment?* 1. Assistive products and technology not available in the environment in which the individual lives: 4 2. Assistive products and technology available in the environment in which the individual lives but available only at high cost, and with no government support: 3 3. Assistive products and technology available in the environment in which the individual lives but available only at high cost, but with partial government support (subsidy): 2 4. Assistive products and technology available in the environment in which the individual lives and available at affordable cost: 1		**Vital organ impairment** 1. Does a facility exist to avail CPAP – Continuous Positive Airway Pressure or BiPAP-Bilevel Positive Airway Pressure devices or phrenic nerve stimulation device to assist respiration in his/her immediate 2. Does a facility exist to undergo pacing (placement of cardiac pacemaker) in his/her immediate environment? **Impairment of bladder and bowel** 3. Does a facility exist to avail sacral neuromodulation therapy to control bladder and bowel movement in his/her immediate environment?

Table 5.67 Environmental Factors Measurement Scale—Assistive technology: Motor

Proposed questionnaire	Revision after survey 1, 2, 3	Revision after trial with clinical model
1. *Whether the prosthetic device is available in his/her immediate environment?* 2. *Whether the Orthotic device is available in his/her immediate environment?* 3. *Whether walking aids is available in the environment in which he/she lives?* 4. *Whether special cars/van is available in the environment in which he/she lives?* 5. *Whether assistive technology for modification of the vehicles is available in the environment in which he/she lives?* 6. *Whether wheelchair is available in the environment in which he/she lives?* 7. *Whether transfer devices are available in the environment in which he/she lives?*		**Motor impairment** 4. Does a service exist to avail artificial limb in his/her immediate environment? 5. Does a service exist to avail appliances in his/her immediate environment? 6. Does a service exist to avail transfer equipment, such as a hoist, in his/her immediate environment? 7. Does a service exist to avail assistive devices namely walking aids in his/her immediate environment? 8. Does a service exist to avail mobility aids namely manual wheelchair/motorized wheelchair in his/her immediate environment? 9. Does a service exist to avail special cars/van/scooters or modified vehicles in his/her immediate environment to commute from one place to another? 10. Does a facility exist to avail "Typing System" to enter, retrieve data in the computer, Robotic Arm, Environmental Control System, 'Phone System' to communicate over extended distance?

Table 5.68 Environmental Factors Measurement Scale—Assistive technology: Vision

Proposed questionnaire	Revision after survey 1, 2, 3	Revision after trial with clinical model
Impairment of vision		**Visual impairment**
1. *Whether glasses and contact lenses are available for a person with low vision in the environment in which he/she live?*		11. Is there a facility to avail assistive technology services namely "type reader" or TTS – Text to Speech for converting text to speech using synthesized speech in his/her immediate environment?
2. *Whether signaling systems for persons with blindness and specialized computer software and hardware is available in the environment in which he/she lives?*		12. Is there any facility to avail assistive technology services namely orientation system to locate a geographical location in his/her immediate surroundings?
1. Assistive products and technology not available: 4		13. Is there any service to avail assistive technology services namely recording system for transcribing and retrieving in his/her immediate surroundings?
2. Assistive products and technology available at high-cost with no government support: 3		14. Is there any service to avail assistive technology services namely intraocular lens in his/her immediate surroundings?
3. Assistive products and techniques available only at high-cost, but with partial government support (subsidy): 2		
4. Assistive products and technology available at affordable cost: 1		

Table 5.69 Environmental Factors Measurement Scale—Assistive technology: Hearing

Proposed questionnaire	Revision after survey 1, 2, 3	Revision after trial with clinical model
Hearing impairment		**Hearing impairment**
Whether cochlear implants, hearing aids, FM auditory trainers for persons with hard of hearing is available in the environment in which he/she lives?		15. Does a service exist to avail assistive technology services namely cochlear implants, hearing aids, FM auditory trainers in his/her immediate environment?
1. Assistive products and technology not available in the environment in which the individual lives: 4		16. Does a service exist to avail assistive technology services namely "Alert System" using lights or vibration in his/her immediate surroundings?
2. Assistive products and technology available in the environment in which the individual lives but available only at high-cost, no government support: 3		17. Does a service exist to avail assistive technology services namely telecommunication display devices/text telephones exist in his/her immediate surroundings? Text telephones transfer coded signals through a telephone network for interactive text-based communication.
3. Assistive products and techniques available in the environment in which the individual lives but available only at high cost, but with partial government support (subsidy): 2		18. Does a facility exist to avail assistive technology services namely "Speech Recognition System" in his/her immediate environment? Speech recognition system is a device with a software program to convert words or phrases in a speech into a readable format.
4. Assistive products and technology available in the environment in which the individual lives and available at affordable cost: 1		

Table 5.70 Environmental Factors Measurement Scale—Assistive technology language: Language, daily living

Proposed questionnaire	Revision after survey 1, 2, 3	Revision after trial with clinical model
Impairment of language function 1. *Whether special writing devices, drawing or handwriting devices, is available in the environment in which he/she lives?* 2. *Whether communication boards are available?* 1. Assistive products and technology not available: 4 2. Assistive products and technology available at high cost with no government support: 3 3. Assistive products and techniques available at high cost, but with partial government support (subsidy): 2 4. Assistive products and technology available at affordable cost: 1		**Impairment of language function** 19. Is there any facility to avail augmentative alternative communication technology such as alphabet or picture symbol boards, a computer-based system for synthesis of speech in his/her immediate environment? **Assistive technology for daily living** 20. Does a facility exist for environmental control systems such as electronic devices to operate air conditioner, television, computers, and other appliances exist in his/her home/workplaces?

Table 5.71 Environmental Factors Measurement Scale—Architectural design: Signage, ramps, doors

Proposed questionnaire	Revision after survey 1, 2, 3	Revision after trial with clinical model
Signage, ramps, doors 1. *Whether signage, in Braille or writing, size of corridors, floor surfaces, accessible kiosks are available in the environment in which he/she works?* 2. *Whether portable and stationary ramps, power assisted doors, lever door handle and level door thresholds are available in the environment in which he/she works?* 1. Architectural design and technology not available: 4 2. Architectural design and technology partially available (25%): 3 3. Architectural design and technology partially available (50%): 2 4. Architectural design and technology partially available (75%): 1		**Signage, ramps, and doors** 21. Is there signage visible, simple without glare even at night in the entrance and inside building? 22. Is an international symbol of accessibility displayed inside and outside the building? 23. Does ramp with sufficient width, the hard and non-slippery surface including tactile marking strips, a slope with a gradient of 1:20, landing at the place of change of direction and the bottom and top of a ramp, and handrails on both sides of the entire length of ramp exist? 24. Does ramp with a maximum width of 1000 mm and slip-resistant surface for wheelchair mobility exist? 25. Do the exterior and interior door have adequate width, and level thresholds in the doorway for wheelchair access exist? 26. Do power assisted doors with increased opening interval or sliding doors or swinging doors with outward opening hinges with a mechanism for easy opening, and lever-style door handle exist? 27. Do low-set windows exist to enable a person in a wheelchair to open and close the window without effort? 28. Do low-set electrical fixtures are in place to enable an individual in a wheelchair for operating controls with minimum force exist?

Table 5.72 Environmental Factors Measurement Scale—Architectural design: Floors and corridors

Proposed questionnaire	Revision after survey 1, 2, 3	Revision after trial with clinical model
Floors and corridors 1. *Whether size of corridors, floor surfaces, accessible for persons with motor impairment?* 1. Architectural design and technology not available: 4 2. Architectural design and technology (25%): 3 3. Architectural design and technology partially available (50%): 2 4. Architectural design and technology partially available (75%): 1		**Steps and stairs, and corridors** 29. Do steps and stairs with adequate width for one-way traffic or two-way traffic exist? Do slip-resistant surface, uniform risers and tread without nosing for indoor stairs, intermediate landing for the difference in the level of more than 2.5 m, handrails on both sides of the stairs, landing extending beyond the stairs at bottom and top of the stairs, tactile strip with contrasting color exist? 30. Do round handrails fix firmly to the wall/supporting structure at a suitable height above the floor level of the step and ramp with adequate space between the wall and handrail? A tactile strip of 900 mm with contrasting color incorporated at the bottom and top edge of the handrails? 31. Do public corridors with an unobstructed width allowing two wheelchairs and full maneuvering of a wheelchair, and slip-resistant floor with drinking fountains, public telephone housed in a recess outside the pathway exist?

Table 5.73 Environmental Factors Measurement Scale—Architectural design: Lifts or elevators, escalators

Proposed questionnaire	Revision after survey 1, 2, 3	Revision after trial with clinical model
Lifts or elevators, escalators 1. *Whether lifts or elevators, escalators are available?* 1. Architectural design and technology not available: 4 2. Architectural design and technology partially available (25%): 3 3. Architectural design and technology partially available (50%): 2 4. Architectural design and technology partially available (75%): 1		**Elevators** 32. Do the elevators with adequate dimension, sufficient door opening for wheelchair access and maneuver, handrails on three sides, slip-resistant floor surface, maximum stop precision, control panel at an accessible height with numerals embossed in the control buttons for tactile selection of levels exist? 33. Do the call buttons located at a convenient height from the floor, provision for minimum door opening interval of 5 seconds, and audio signal and visual display to forecast arrival of the elevator for each floor exist? 34. Do the entrance and exit of the escalators have two flat steps and steps of the escalator identifiable by yellow guide strip along the sides and back of the steps?

Table 5.74 Environmental Factors Measurement Scale—Architectural design: Kitchen

Proposed questionnaire	Revision after survey 1, 2, 3	Revision after trial with clinical model
		Kitchen 35. Does the "U"-shaped kitchen have an adequate work area, wide door with lever-type handle for wheelchair access and maneuverability? 36. Do the countertop or height adjustable counter, sinks with clear space underneath for knee clearance, single-lever faucet, sliding drawers on either side of the sink, detachable cabinetry under the kitchen work surface, kitchen wall cabinet either power adjusted cabinets or pull-down shelves exist? Do insulation of underside of the cooktop to prevent burns, electric burner or oven with controls fixed on the front panel, the minimum operating force of the controls for the appliances, or touchpad or tactile controls with raised buttons and low-set electrical fixtures exist? 37. Do dishwasher and bottom-drawer freezer type refrigerator with a clear floor area from the center of the kitchen exist? **Dining, reading, and working surfaces** 38. Does the reading/work/dining table exist with clear space underneath for knee clearance for wheelchair accessibility?

Table 5.75 Environmental Factors Measurement Scale—Architectural design: Washroom

Proposed questionnaire	Revision after survey 1, 2, 3	Revision after trial with clinical model
Washroom 1. *Whether washroom facilities are available in the environment in which he/she works?* 1. Architectural design and technology not available: 4 2. Architectural design and technology partially available (25%): 3 3. Architectural design and technology partially available (50%): 2 4. Architectural design and technology partially available (75%): 1		**Rest Room** 39. Does the restroom have sufficient space for maneuvering wheelchair with slip resistant floor, self-closing pivoted doors open outward? Is the toilet seat at a convenient height from the floor with adequate space from the midline of the toilet seat to the adjacent wall? Do grab bar fixed behind the water closet and adjacent walls of the water closet, flush controls either automatic or hand operating with minimum effort set on the open side of the water closet and toilet paper dispenser mounted at an accessible height above the floor? 40. Does the washbasin with its top edge at a convenient height from the floor and lever type handle for faucets exist? 41. Does the bathtub with specified dimension exist with provision for permanent bath seat or a detachable in-tub seat at the head end of the tub and with two grab bars on the back wall above the brim of the tub and one at the head end and another at the control end of the tub? Do shower stalls with adequate dimension with shower seat, shower head with a long hose, and horizontal grab bar in the back and side walls away from the entrance? 42. Does full-length urinal or urinal with the protruding lip at the optimum height from the floor with sufficient space on either side, urine shield, grab bars and automatic or hand-operated flush control exist? 43. Do hot water pipes have insulation?

Table 5.76 Environmental Factors Measurement Scale—Architectural design: Public places

Proposed questionnaire	Revision after survey 1, 2, 3	Revision after trial with clinical model
Public places 1. *Whether accessible kiosks are available in the environment in which he/she lives/works?* 2. *Whether thermostats and dispersed accessible seating in auditoriums or stadiums are available in the environment in which he/she works?* 1. Architectural design and technology not available: 4 2. Architectural design and technology partially available (25%): 3 3. Architectural design and technology partially available (50%): 2 4. Architectural design and technology partially available (75%): 1		**Public utility services** 44. Does drinking water fountain fixed at the optimum height from the floor and control with effortless operation exist? 45. Does a public dealing counters exist at optimum height with clear underneath space and depth for wheelchair accessibility? 46. Do accessible open book stacks, equipment, and other facilities in the library for wheelchair users, and a separate room for assistance for reading exist? 47. Is there a provision of seats with detachable or flip-up armrests located in a level floor area at the end of the row in a conference hall, movie theatre, sports auditorium? 48. Does thermostat exist to protect persons with impaired thermoregulation? 49. Do minimum slope of the boarding and alighting areas at the bus stop, and rail platform exist for wheelchair access, and maneuverability, provision for accessible seating and other facilities exist in the bus, aircraft, and train as well as in bus/train stations and air terminals? 50. Does cantilevered tables or tables without central pedestal exist in restaurants, and a minimum of one room with restroom, etc., designed for wheelchair users exist on the ground floor of the hotel? 51. Does the public telephone booth with folding seats for wheelchair accessibility, low set phones with elevated touch buttons, coin slot fixed at optimum height exist? 52. Does the letter slot in the mailbox exist at optimum height? 53. Does provision of fire alarm systems in public use areas, employee work areas, lodging and residential facilities with audible alarm signals exist to indicate emergency situations?

Table 5.77 Environmental Factors Measurement Scale—Architectural design: Parking area

Proposed questionnaire	Revision after survey 1, 2, 3	Revision after trial with clinical model
		Parking area 58. Whether parking space of sufficient width including an access aisle between two common parking areas, minimum height clearance for indoor parking, near accessible elevator or exit, and near the entrance with guiding signs and international symbol toward parking area exist? 59. Whether textured tactile marking strip is in place to separate the pathway from vehicular area to caution transition zone during crossing? 60. Whether drop-off area of sufficient width including aisle at bus stops exists nearby from the entrance to pick up or drop off persons with impairment of function as well as to unload and upload luggage?

Table 5.78 Environmental Factors Measurement Scale—Architectural design: Vision

Proposed questionnaire	Revision after survey 1, 2, 3	Revision after trial with clinical model
Architectural design and technology: Signage, lifts 1. Whether lifts or elevators, escalators are available? 2. Whether signage, in Braille or writing, size of corridors, floor surfaces accessible for persons with visual impairment exist? 1. Architectural design and technology not available: 4 2. Architectural design and technology partially available (25%): 3 3. Architectural design and technology partially available (50%): 2 4. Architectural design and technology partially available (75%): 1		**Signage, door, ramp, stairs, elevator** 61. Whether any signage in Braille or embossed or text with bold color contrasted letter exists in the entrance of the building? 62. Whether there is the provision of international symbols of accessibility in a contrasting color? 63. Whether the entrance door painted with contrasting color to assist persons with low vision? 64. Whether tactile markings on the handrails of exit and around the knob of the exit door exist? 65. Whether ramp exist with slip-resistant surface and tactile marking strips? 66. Whether tactile marking strip of specified width extending over the whole stairs along with tactile strip incorporated at the bottom and top edge of the handrails exist? 67. Whether the lifts/elevator has a control panel with the button of sufficient diameter, and numerals embossed in the control buttons for tactile selection of floors? 68. Whether the provision of audio signals namely bell exist to indicate the arrival of the elevator for each floor? 69. Whether door frame of the elevator/lift painted with a contrasting color to assist persons with low vision?

Table 5.79 Environmental Factors Measurement Scale—Architectural design: Vision

Proposed questionnaire	Revision after survey 1, 2, 3	Revision after trial with clinical model
Architectural design and technology: Public places 1. *Whether thermostats and dispersed accessible seating in auditoriums or stadiums are available in the environment in which he/she works?* 2. *Whether signage, in Braille or writing, size of corridors, floor surfaces, accessible kiosks are available in the environment in which he/she works?* 1. Architectural design and technology not available: 4 2. Architectural design and technology partially available (25%): 3 3. Architectural design and technology partially available (50%): 2 4. Architectural design and technology partially available (75%): 1		**Pathways and public utility services** 70. Whether a path with guide strip with contrasting color exist? 71. Whether tactile surfaces with line-type blocks indicating the correct path, dot-type blocks exist to indicate hazards or rubber tiles with both tactile and acoustic guidance in the pathway exist? 72. Whether tactile marking strips or signage in bright color or alarm signals exist around obstruction? 73. Whether pedestrian guide strip toward traffic light pole with push button, tactile tile, or rubber tile incorporated in the pedestrian crossing, provision of audio signals at the beginning of the pedestrian crossing, and provision of sufficient time for crossing the road exist? 74. Whether tactile marking strips exist in places of change of route or direction sign in bright and contrasting color letters to orient and reach a place of destination? 75. Whether tactile marking strips exist in places of change of route or direction sign in bright and contrasting color letters to orient and reach a place of destination? 76. Whether there is the provision of a minimum of one push-button type telephone with raised numbers/letters in public telephone booth? 77. Whether "Text to Speech" TTS synthesis system or assistance for reading exist in a separate room in a library? 78. Whether the letter slot in the mailbox exists at optimum height?

Table 5.80 Environmental Factors Measurement Scale—Architectural design-hearing

Proposed questionnaire	Revision after survey 1, 2, 3	Revision after trial with clinical model
Architectural design and technology: Lifts/elevators 1. *Whether lifts or elevators, escalators are available in the environment in which he/she lives/works?* 1. Architectural design and technology not available: 4 2. Architectural design and technology partially available (25%): 3 3. Architectural design and technology partially available (50%): 2 4. Architectural design and technology partially available (75%): 1		**Signage, elevator, pathway, and public utility services** 79. Whether there is provision for signage with contrasting color and bold letter? 80. Whether there is provision for indication of the arrival of the elevator by flashlight for each floor? 81. Whether there is provision for flashing of emergency light in the door or elevator? 82. Whether visual signals exist in pedestrian? 83. Whether assistance for reading exist in a separate room in a library? 84. Whether the public telephone booths exist with a minimum of one phone with hearing aid and amplifiers to improve the perception of hearing? (Assistive listening system with transmitter, receiver and coupling devices for transmitting audio signals to hearing aid by eliminating or decreasing background noise for better perception by induction loop, radio frequency, infrared system, or direct-wired equipment in public telephone) 85. Whether speech recognition system exists in conference hall?

Table 5.81 Environmental Factors Measurement Scale—Social security and health services

Proposed questionnaire	Revision after survey 1, 2, 3	Revision after trial with clinical model
Social security services, systems, and policies 1. *Whether the person with a disability obtain disability-related benefits such as pension, priority in education and employment, in travel, tax benefits, construction of barrier-free houses?* 1. Disability benefit scheme not available: 4 2. Disability benefit scheme such as pension available with 25% assistance to meet basic needs: 3 3. Disability benefit scheme such as pension available with 50% assistance to meet basic needs: 2 4. Disability benefit schemes such as pension available with 75% assistance to meet basic needs: 1 **Health services** *Whether health services for providing medical rehabilitation intervention is available to persons with a disability?* 1. Health services not available free of cost: 4 2. Health services available free of cost only for acute care rehabilitation: 3 3. Health services available free of cost only for acute care rehabilitation and short-term rehabilitation care: 2 4. Health services available free of cost only for acute care rehabilitation and one-time long-term rehabilitation care: 1		**Social security and health services, systems, and policies** 86. Does disability-related pension subsist for the person with a disability? 87. Does subsidy exist for assisted technology related equipment/devices? 88. Does priority for admission in educational courses exist for the person with a disability? 89. Does provision for suitable employment exist for the person with a disability? 90. Is tax exemption available to the person with a disability? 91. Is subsistence for the construction of barrier-free house available to the person with a disability? 92. Do health services provide facilities for medical rehabilitation free of cost or by insurance?

Table 5.82 Environmental Factors Measurement Scale—Attitudinal environment

Proposed questionnaire	Revision after survey 1, 2, 3	Revision after trial with clinical model
Support and relationships? 1. *Whether acquaintances, peers, colleagues, neighbors extend physical and emotional support?* 2. *Whether community members continue physical and emotional support?* 3. *Whether people in authority, subordinate continue physical and emotional support?* 4. *Whether personal care providers, personal assistants continue physical and emotional support?* 5. *Whether health professionals provide physical and emotional support?* 1. Person with disability does not receive physical and emotional support: 4 2. Person with disability occasionally receive physical and emotional support: 3 3. Person with disability infrequently receive physical and emotional support: 2 4. Person with disability receive physical and emotional support most of the time: 1		**Attitude of immediate and extended family members, friends, employers, and society** 93. Immediate family members exhibit inhibitory attitude to spend time and money toward rehabilitation management because of loss or limitation of productivity of the person with disability to support his/her family 94. Extended family members and friends ignore the person with disability because of disability 95. Lack of supportive attitude of the employers to provide reasonable accommodation in the workplace for persons with disability 96. Inhibition of the employers to recruit eligible individuals because of underestimation of the potential of the person with disability 97. Society has a stereotyped attitude of feeling different and inferior to other individuals about persons with disability 98. Society attach stigma to the person with disability 99. Society has a prejudice that persons with disability are docile 100. Society judge that persons with disability have abilities at a low ebb, and cannot perform the task like a person without a disability

Table 5.83 Personal Factors Measurement Scale—Behavior toward health

Proposed questionnaire	Revision after survey 1, and 2	Revision after survey 3 and trial with clinical model
Adaptive behavior of the person with disability toward health *Does the person with disability cooperate for feeding himself/herself to maintain nutrition? Does the person with disability cooperate for initial treatment and further rehabilitation programs?* 1. The person with disability does not accept his/her disability, develops aggressive behavior and/or suicidal tendency, and rejects food, initial treatment, and further rehabilitation program: 4 2. The person with disability develops depression and does not cooperate for feeding to maintain nutrition and rehabilitation program to regain function: 3 3. The person with disability cooperates partially for eating and drinking and undergo rehabilitation management irregularly after counseling: 2 4. The person with disability cooperates fully for eating and drinking and undergoes rehabilitation programs regularly after counseling: 1 5. The person with disability cooperates for eating and drinking and undergoes rehabilitation management even without counseling: 0		**Behavior of the person with disability toward health** *Does the person with disability cooperate for feeding himself/herself to maintain nutrition? Does the person with disability cooperate for initial treatment and further rehabilitation programs?* 1. The person with disability does not accept his/her disability, develops aggressive behavior and suicidal tendency, and rejects food, initial treatment, and further rehabilitation programs: 5 2. The person with disability develops depression and does not cooperate for feeding to maintain nutrition and rehabilitation program to regain function: 4 3. The person with disability does not cooperate in feeding to maintain nutrition and rehabilitation program to restore function: 3 4. The person with disability cooperates partially for eating and drinking and undergo rehabilitation management irregularly after counseling: 2 5. The person with disability cooperates fully for eating and drinking and undergoes rehabilitation programs regularly after counseling: 1 6. The person with disability cooperates for eating and drinking and undergoes rehabilitation management even without counseling: 0

Table 5.84 Personal Factors Measurement Scale—Behavior toward self-care

Proposed questionnaire	Revision after survey 1, and 2	Revision after survey 3 and trial with clinical model
Adaptive behavior of the person with disability toward self-care Is the person with disability performs or cooperates for washing and drying whole body/caring body parts in the presence of preserved skills for self-care? Does the person with disability care for or cooperate for caring skin, face, teeth, scalp, nails, and genitals in the presence of preserved skills for self-care? Does the person with a disability perform or cooperate for toileting in the presence of preserved skills for self-care? Does the person with a disability perform or cooperate for dressing in the presence of preserved skills for self-care? 1. The person with disability does not cooperate for self-care and exhibits aggressive behavior and/or suicidal tendency: 4 2. The person with disability does not cooperate for self-care and/or exhibits depression: 3 3. The person with disability cooperates partially for self-care after counseling: 2 4. The person with disability cooperates fully for self-care after counseling: 1 5. The person with disability cooperates normally all activities relating to self-care: 0		**Behavior of the person toward self-care** Does the person with a disability perform or cooperate for washing and drying whole body/caring body parts in the presence of preserved skills for self-care? Does the person with disability care for or cooperate for caring skin, face, teeth, scalp, nails, and genitals in the presence of preserved skills for self-care? Does the person with a disability perform or cooperate for toileting in the presence of preserved skills for self-care? Does the person with a disability perform or cooperate for dressing in the presence of preserved skills for self-care? 1. The person with disability does not cooperate for self-care and exhibits aggressive behavior and suicidal tendency: 5 2. The person with disability does not cooperate for self-care and exhibits depression: 4 3. The person with disability does not cooperate for self-care: 3 4. The person with disability cooperates partially for self-care after counseling: 2 5. The person with disability cooperates fully for self-care after counseling: 1 6. The person with disability normally cooperates with all activities relating to self-care: 0

Table 5.85 Personal Factors Measurement Scale—Behavior toward communication

Proposed questionnaire	Revision after survey 1, and 2	Revision after survey 3 and trial with clinical model
Adaptive behavior of the person with disability during communication Does the person with disability communicate in the presence of preserved communication skills? 1. The person with disability does not communicate in the presence of preserved communication skills and exhibits aggressive behavior and/or suicidal tendency: 4 2. The person with disability avoids communication and/or exhibits depression in the presence of preserved communication skills: 3 3. The person with disability communicates only with his family members and friends after counseling: 2 4. The person with disability communicates after counseling with everyone after counseling: 1 5. The person with disability communicates normally with everyone even without counseling: 0		Does the person with disability communicate in the presence of preserved communication skills? 1. The person with a disability has preserved communication. He/she does not communicate because of elective mutism and exhibits aggressive behavior and suicidal tendency: 5 2. The person with a disability has preserved communication and exhibited a paucity of communication. He/she answers only in monosyllables or by gestures: 4 3. The person with a disability has preserved communication, but answers only to questions directed at him/her. There is no spontaneity of communication: 3 4. The person with disability has preserved communications and exchanges with limited audience such as family members and friends only after counseling: 2 5. The person with disability had preserved communications and communicated with everyone after counseling: 1 6. The person with disability normally communicates with everyone even without counseling: 0

Table 5.86 Personal Factors Measurement Scale—Behavior toward education

Proposed questionnaire	Revision after survey 1, and 2	Revision after survey 3 and trial with clinical model
Adaptive behavior of the person with disability toward learning—Education Whether the person with disability accepts learning or resumes education in the presence of preserved mental faculty? 1. The person with disability does not cooperate for continuing education and exhibits aggressive behavior and/or suicidal tendency: 4 2. The person with disability has depression and does not cooperate for continuing education: 3 3. The person with disability has a fear of social acceptance and inhibition and resumes education only irregularly: 2 4. The person with disability resumes learning/education regularly only after counseling: 1 5. The person with disability resumes education without counseling: 0		**Behavior of the person with disability toward learning** Whether the person with disability accepts learning or resumes education in the presence of preserved mental faculty? 1. The person with disability does not cooperate for continuing education and exhibits aggressive behavior and suicidal tendency: 5 2. The person with a disability does not refuse but lacks motivation for continuing to learn: 4 3. The person with a disability cooperate for continuing education but only sporadically: 3 4. The person with disability has lack of spontaneity but continues to cooperate in learning: 2 5. The person with disability resumes learning/education regularly only after counseling: 1 6. The person with disability continues education without counseling: 0

Table 5.87 Personal Factors Measurement Scale—Behavior in work and employment

Proposed questionnaire	Revision after survey 1, 2	Revision after survey 3 and trial with clinical model
Adaptive behavior of the person with disability toward work and employment Does the person with disability accept and resume work or training in the presence of preserved occupational or work skills? 1. The person with disability does not cooperate for continuing his/her work or training and exhibits aggressive behavior and/or suicidal tendency: 4 2. The person with disability has depression and does not cooperate for continuing his/her work or training and develops alcohol or substance abuse: 3 3. The person with disability attends to his/her work or training irregularly and develops conflicts with peer workers requiring intervention by the superior officers or change of placement: 2 4. The person with disability accepts and resumes employment regularly only after counseling: 1 5. The person with disability agrees and continues work even without counseling: 0		**Behavior of the person—Work and employment** Does the person with disability accept and resume work or training in the presence of preserved occupational or work skills? 1. The person with disability does not cooperate for continuing his/her work or training and exhibits aggressive behavior and suicidal tendency: 5 2. The person with disability does not refuse but has inadequate motivation/executive skills in pursuing his/her occupation: 4 3. The person with disability continues to cooperate but is unable to sustain his/her motivation/execution: 3 4. The person with a disability can sustain his/her motivation/execution only under supervision. He/she lacks spontaneous plan and execution: 2 5. The person with disability has adequate motivation, execution, and spontaneity but only after counseling and under supervision: 1 6. The person with disability accepts and resumes employment even without counseling or supervision: 0

Table 5.88 Personal Factors Measurement Scale—Behavior toward social life

Proposed questionnaire	Revision after survey 1, and 2	Revision after survey 3 and trial with clinical model
Adaptive behavior of the person with disability in relation to social life Is the person with disability able to maintain normal social relationship? 1. The person with disability exhibits physical and verbal aggressive behavior in social life: 4 2. The person with disability has a fear of social acceptance and prefers to live in isolation: 3 3. The person with disability remains reserved and expresses his/her affection and desire only to his/her family members after counseling: 2 4. The person with disability maintains social relationship with everyone after counseling: 1 5. The person with disability maintains normal social relationship with everyone even without counseling: 0		Is the person with a disability able to maintain normal social relationship? 1. The person with disability exhibits physical and verbally aggressive cum disruptive behavior in social life: 5 2. The person with a disability remains withdrawn. Though willing he/she is unable to participate in social life: 4 3. The person with disability attempts to sustain a social life but only with the inner circle of family/known members: 3 4. The person with disability can maintain a social interaction but without any spontaneity and on continued efforts by others and counseling: 2 5. The person with disability maintains spontaneous social relationship with everyone only on positive intervention by others and after counseling: 1 6. The person with disability continues normal social relationship with everyone even without counseling: 0

REFERENCES

1. K. Cuhls. *Delphi Method*. Karlsruhe, Germany: Fraunhofer Institute for Systems and Innovation Research.

2. ACR Appropriateness Criteria® dysphagia [Internet]. American College of Radiology; 2010.

3. *A Guide to the Clinical Care of Women with HIV*. 2005 ed. Rockville Department of Health and Human Services, Health Resources and Services Administration, HIV/AIDS Bureau; 2005.

Impairment of functions of the nervous system

6.1 CONSCIOUSNESS FUNCTION

Consciousness function refers to the mental state of wakefulness with awareness, attentiveness, and lucidness (1).

6.1.1 Vegetative state

Practice parameters for persistent vegetative state define persistent vegetative state when it persists for more than one month and permanent vegetative state if irreversibility persists with maximum evidence of clinical proof (2). Box 6.1 describes clinical profile of the vegetative state. The permanent vegetative state derives maximum whole person impairment of 100%.

BOX 6.1: Vegetative state

1. Lack of awareness of himself/herself and about his/her surroundings
2. No voluntary response to audiovisual and exteroceptive touch or painful stimulus
3. Loss of reception, comprehension, and expression of language functions
4. Evidence of sleep-wake cycle on and off suggesting wakefulness
5. Intact cardiopulmonary functions
6. Incontinence of bladder and bowel
7. Pupillary, corneal, oculocephalic, vestibulo-ocular, and gag reflexes may be present or absent
8. Requires medical and nursing care for survival

6.1.2 Episodic loss of consciousness, uncontrolled seizure

A seizure is a brief clinical manifestation of signs and symptoms because of a sudden surge of abnormal simultaneous excessive neuronal discharge in the brain (3). Simple focal seizure refers to focal seizure with preservation of consciousness. Complex focal seizure refers to focal seizure with impairment of consciousness. Generalized-onset seizure has sub-classes, namely, absence seizure, myoclonic seizures, tonic seizures, clonic seizures, primary generalized tonic-clonic seizures, and atonic seizures. In absence seizures, there is a brief period of impairment of consciousness. Myoclonic seizures manifest arrhythmic jerking movements lasting less than one second. Clonic seizures display rhythmic jerking movements. Impairment of consciousness may accompany clonic seizures. Tonic seizures present as sudden onset tonic extension or flexion of head, neck and extremities lasting for several seconds. Generalized tonic-clonic seizures or grand mal epilepsy manifests clonic jerking movements of the extremity preceded by tonic extension of extremities lasting for several seconds and may manifest post-seizure confusion. An atonic seizure is a sudden onset brief loss of postural tone resulting in loss of balance and fall.

Persons with seizures may sustain laceration, facial injuries, tongue bite, hematomas, dislocation of shoulder and burns during seizures. EEG evidence of epileptiform abnormalities forecasts the risk of recurrence of seizures. Besides clinical evaluation, seizure disorders require imaging studies such as CT, MRI in persons with the first seizure (4).

About 0.5%–1% of the population in the world suffers from epilepsy. Epilepsy persists in one-third of people

Table 6.1 Impairment class—Seizure disorders

Impairment class	Severity profile—Seizure disorders	Maximum impairment 50%
Class 1	Focal/generalized seizures under control with mono- or multi-therapy without recurrence (Assigns impairment for burden of treatment compliance, and stigma until the antiepileptic drugs are withdrawn)	5%
Class 2	Focal seizures with preserved consciousness developing recurrence every month with mono/multi-pharmacotherapy	15%
Class 3	Focal seizures with impairment of consciousness, developing recurrence every month with mono/multi-pharmacotherapy	25%
Class 4	Persistent focal seizure occurring everyday/week with impairment of consciousness refractory to pharmacotherapy	37%
Class 4	Generalized seizures, developing recurrence every month with mono/multi-pharmacotherapy	37%
Class 5	Persistent generalized seizures with recurrence everyday/week refractory to multi-pharmacotherapy	50%

despite appropriate treatment. Furthermore, 1 in 150 persons with refractory epilepsy develop sudden, unexpected and unexplained death, and it is more common with uncontrolled tonic-clonic seizures (5).

If the person with a seizure disorder is free from a seizure at least for 2 years, they can discontinue the antiepileptic drug slowly over a period of 2–3 months. At first, one drug is withdrawn and followed by weaning of the second drug (6).

It is necessary to impose restrictions on activities like driving, swimming, and bathing without supervision, and restriction of participation in work such as working at heights, using power tools, and working with fire in persons with epileptic seizures. Table 6.1 describes the severity profile and impairment class for seizure disorders.

6.2 SLEEP FUNCTION

Sleep is a physiological state of recurring reversible mental function with the disengagement of one's mind and body from his/her surrounding environment associated with quiescence and closed eyes (7,8). The common sleep function posing disability is insomnia and sleep apnea.

6.2.1 Insomnia

Insomnia refers to a disturbance of sleep in initiation and maintenance with poor quality despite adequate opportunity for sleep with very early waking and impairment of daytime functioning (9). Normally, the person falls asleep after a latent period of 15–20 minutes (sleep latency). The person with insomnia has difficulty in falling asleep and difficulty in staying asleep. Further, he/she wakes frequently during sleep. Total Wake Time (TWT) refers to the sum of the duration of each awakening from sleep onset to final awakening. Total sleep time is equal to the total time in bed minus sum of sleep latency and total wake time. Formula

$$\frac{\text{Total sleep time}}{\text{Total time in bed}} * 100 \qquad (6.1)$$

computes the percentage of sleep efficiency. Chronic insomnia lasts longer than one month, that is, months or years (10,11). Section 4.5.3.1 in Chapter 4 describes the clinical profile of chronic insomnia. Insomnia with a short duration of sleep is associated with activation of both the limbs of stress system namely hypothalamic pituitary adrenal (HPA) axis and sympatho-adrenal-medullary axis (11). Fatal familial insomnia manifests broad spectrum of clinical symptoms and signs. It includes organic sleep disturbance, loss of weight, hyperthermia, hyperhidrosis, pruritus, obstipation, tachycardia; and psychiatric manifestations such as anxiety, depression, personality impairment, hallucinations, aggressiveness, disinhibition, and listlessness. It also includes cognitive or amnestic impairment, double vision, husky voice, dysarthria, bulbar speech, dysphagia, fasciculation of tongue, ataxia, pyramidal and extrapyramidal signs, myoclonus, and vegetative state (12). Table 6.2 describes impairment class for insomnia. Chapters 20 and 21 describes "Activity Participation Skill

Table 6.2 Impairment class—Sleep functions: Chronic insomnia

Impairment class	Severity profile of chronic insomnia	Maximum impairment 37%
Class 1	1. Difficulty in falling asleep 2. Difficulty in staying asleep 3. Final early awakening 4. Non-restorative sleep with feeling of unrefreshed after early morning 5. Sleep efficiency 75% 6. Day time fatigue, and sleepiness	5%
Class 2	1. Difficulty in falling asleep 2. Difficulty in staying asleep 3. Final early awakening 4. Non-restorative sleep with feeling of unrefreshed after early morning 5. Sleep efficiency 50%–74% 6. Daytime fatigue, sleepiness during driving and increased risk of injury	15%
Class 3	1. Difficulty in falling asleep 2. Difficulty in staying asleep 3. Final early awakening 4. Non-restorative sleep with feeling of unrefreshed after early morning 5. Sleep efficiency 25%–49% 6. Daytime fatigue, increased risk of injury during driving and cognitive deficiencies	25%
Class 4	1. Difficulty in falling asleep 2. Difficulty in staying asleep 3. Final early awakening 4. Non-restorative sleep with feeling of unrefreshed after early morning 5. Sleep efficiency <25% 6. Daytime fatigue, sleepiness during driving with increased risk of injury and cognitive deficiencies 7. Depression 8. Abuse of alcohol and substance	37%

Note: If there is associated cognitive impairment, needs evaluation under cognitive function.

Assessment Scale" and "Personal Factors Measurement Scale" to evaluate restriction of social or limitation of occupational functioning.

6.3 COGNITIVE FUNCTION

Cognitive function is a mental process of attaining knowledge to develop awareness, acquire and comprehend information including ideas through thought, experience, and visual–auditory–gustatory–olfactory–tactile senses. Cognitive function includes orientation, attention, memory, auditory perception, visual perception, olfactory perception, visuospatial perception, abstraction, organization and planning, judgment, and problem-solving functions. Section 4.5.4 in Chapter 4 describes the clinical profile and evaluation of cognitive function.

Cognitive function derives maximum impairment of 25%. Each cognitive function obtains a weighted score of 1% for attention function, 2% for memory function, 3% each for orientation function and visual/auditory perceptual function, 4% for visuospatial perception, and 5% each for high-level cognitive functions such as abstraction, and organization and planning. Each function derives a score based on "Three-Point Scale," that is, normal, difficulty, and inability (Table 6.3).

Table 6.3 Impairment class—Cognitive functions

Clinical tools	Normal	Difficulty	Inability	Maximum impairment 25%
Attention	0%	0.5%	1%	
Tests of attention span				
Forward digit span test				
The ability to listen and repeat series of digits in the same order (span of five to seven digits 5664309) at the rate of one digit per second. The normal person can complete 7 ± 2 digits in one or two attempts.				
Distractibility				
Forward recitation of months, days, or alphabets.				
Test of vigilance—Go-No-Go test				
The person keeps his/her hand on the table with all fingers touching the table. The clinician taps the undersurface of the table to avoid visual cues. The person raises one finger in response to one tap and keeps the finger still in response to two taps.				
Mental double tracking				
Ability to recite the month of the year, days of the week and alphabet in reverse order (a normal person can recite in reverse order the months of the year in 20 seconds or less).				
Memory function	0%	1%	2%	
Recent/short-term memory				
Registration				
Ability to listen; remember the given name and address (or) the names of three objects; ability to repeat immediately				
Recall				
Repeat after 3–5 minutes				
Long-term memory				
Ability to remember his/her childhood memories namely whether he/she hails from a rural (or) urban area, the name of the school in which he/she studied, *early adult life*—the name of the institution and date of the first employment (to be verified by the family members)				
Orientation function	0%	1.5%	3%	
Orientation to time				
Ability of the person to answer				
(1) What is the present time (or) approximate time of day, e.g., morning, afternoon, evening, night?				
(2) What is the day of the week, and date?				
(3) What are the month and year?				
Orientation to person				
Ability of the person to answer				
What is the name of the caretaker, his/her occupation, and his/her relationship with you?				
Orientation to place				
Ability of the person to answer				
(1) What is the location of the hospital?				
(2) What is the floor in which he/she is staying?				
(3) What is your town, county, and district?				
(4) What is your state and country?				

(Continued)

Table 6.3 (*Continued*) Impairment class—Cognitive functions

Clinical tools	Normal	Difficulty	Inability	Maximum impairment 25%
Auditory perception function	0%	1.5%	3%	
Auditory verbal perception				
Ability to receive and comprehend the speech				
Whether horse can fly?				
Auditory non-verbal perception				
Ability to recognize and discriminate non-symbolic sound patterns				
Whether he/she can recognize sirens, dog barks, and				
thunderclaps?				
Visual perception	0%	1.5%	3%	
Ability to recognize familiar faces, identifying a common object				
Whether he/she can identify a pen, toothbrush, soap, and identify				
color of a shirt				
Visuospatial perception	0%	2%	4%	
Ability to understand the spatial location				
Whether he/she can identify the location of the window on his/her				
left side and then proceeds to walk toward the window?				
(Or)				
Ability to identify body parts namely left hand, left eye, left ear,				
right hand, identification of examiners right eye, left leg, left ear,				
left hand				
The body schemes				
Right-left discrimination: Touching his/her left ear (orientation to				
own body)				
Double-uncrossed task: Touching his/her right knee with his/her				
right hand				
Double-crossed task: Touching his/her right knee with his/her left				
elbow				
Orientation to confronting person: Touch my left hand				
Abstraction	0%	2.5%	5%	
Story test				
Ability to abstract well the concepts and message:				
The father gave his three sons a wooden stick each and asked				
them to break the stick. They could break the stick easily. Then				
he gave them a bundle of three sticks and asked them to break				
the bundle. They could not break it. The father said that if all his				
sons were together, nobody could destroy them. The message is				
that unity is a strength.				
Organization and planning	0%	2.5%	5%	
The ability how he/she would manage when he/she discovers a				
major fire in his/her house.				
Judgment	0%	2.5%	5%	
The ability to decide what he/she would do if he/she finds a letter				
on the ground in front of the post box.				
Problem-solving	0%	2.5%	5%	
The ability to proceed further in an unfamiliar place when stranded				
in a four-way junction in a high road with dismantled signboard				
found aside following a storm.				
Sum of the impairment				

Notes: In cognitive dysfunction, the minimum score is 5%, and maximum impairment is 25%. If minimum summated score is between 1 and 4, it assigns 5%.

6.4 LANGUAGE FUNCTIONS

Language function is a mental function for communicating formal and informal messages by interpreting signs, symbols, and other means of language. It includes reception, expression, and integrative functions (13).

The mental process of interpreting and understanding verbal messages refers to reception of spoken language function; written messages to reception of written language function; and signs to reception of sign language. The mental process of constructing an expression of verbal messages refers to the expression of spoken language function; and written messages to written language function (13).

6.4.1 Receptive aphasia

In aphasia, there is impairment of comprehension, word finding difficulty, difficulty in naming, error in spelling and syntax. Receptive aphasia/dysphasia refers to the inability/difficulty to comprehend, naming, choosing the correct word, and using correct spelling. Comprehension denotes the ability to follow the conversation. Evaluation of comprehension involves the person to execute a command either in one-step, or two steps or three steps namely stretch your hand, take the paper and fold it two times, and give it to me.

In receptive aphasia, the person cannot understand either written (or) spoken words/sentences. In receptive dysphasia, the person cannot either understand written/spoken words/sentences but answer them inappropriately or speaks spontaneously without any meaning and sometimes with a neologism.

6.4.2 Expressive aphasia

In expressive aphasia, the person understands the questions projected to him but is unable to express or speak even single word. In expressive dysphasia, the person understands the questions, struggles to speak a full sentence, and answers in telegraphic style like "yes" or "no" for questions: Is it your name? Is it your age? Are you married? Do you have children? Are you working?

Receptive aphasia derives an impairment of 37%, and receptive dysphasia 25%; expressive aphasia 25%, expressive dysphasia 15%, and global aphasia 50% (Table 6.4).

6.4.3 Speech apraxia

One of the mental functions of sequencing complex movements is speech apraxia (14). Apraxia is a disorder of skilled movement due to a lesion in the cortex. There is no motor

Table 6.4 Impairment class—Language functions

Clinical tools	Normal	Difficulty	Total inability	Maximum impairment 50%
Receptive aphasia The person cannot understand either written (or) spoken words/ sentences fully.	—	—	37%	
Receptive dysphasia The person cannot understand the question and answer inappropriately, but he/she speaks spontaneously without any meaning and sometimes with a neologism.	—	25%	—	
Expressive aphasia The person understands the questions projected to him/her but cannot express or speak an even a single word.	—	—	25%	
Expressive dysphasia The person understands the questions, struggles to speak a full sentence, and answers the questions in a telegraphic style, e.g., yes, or no only. (a) What is your name? (b) What is your age? (c) Are you married? (d) Do you have children? (e) Are you working?	—	15%	—	
Speech apraxia The person understands the verbal commands, and he/she has inability (or) difficulty to speak. There is difficulty in putting the sounds and syllables together in the correct order to form words. The person with apraxia is struggling for right sound or word, and but can chew and eat.	—	—	25%	

weakness linked with apraxia. The person with apraxia understands the command, is ready to perform the movement, but has lost the knowledge, concept, or idea of how to perform the skilled movement.

In speech apraxia, the person understands the verbal commands, but has an inability (or) difficulty to speak. There is difficulty in putting the sounds and syllables together in the correct order to form words. The person with apraxia is struggling for the right sound or word, but can chew and eat. Apraxia derives an impairment of 25% (Table 6.4). A person with apraxia will gain additional score for limitation of activity and participation restriction and environment barrier than the person with aphasia.

6.5 ARTICULATION FUNCTIONS

Articulation functions refer to a process of generating sounds related to speech (15). A normal person speaks with clear and distinct sounds and concise speech.

6.5.1 Dysarthria

Section 4.5.7 in Chapter 4 describes the classification and clinical profile of dysarthria. Table 6.5 defines the

impairment class for articulation function and maximum impairment does not exceed 25%.

6.5.2 Stuttering

Stuttering refers to a disorder of speech with repetition or prolongation of sounds, syllables, or words disrupting the normal flow of speech. Tremor of the lips and blinking of the eyes may accompany stuttering during excitation (16). Stuttering derives maximum impairment of 15% (Table 6.6).

Table 6.6 Impairment class—Articulation functions: Stuttering

Clinical tools—Stuttering	Impairment score
Impairment Class 1: Occurring occasionally	0%
Impairment Class 2: Occurring during periods of excitation	5%
Impairment Class 3: Occurring all the time	15%

Table 6.5 Impairment class—Articulation functions

Clinical tools	Class 1	Class 2	Class 3
Normal speech Clear concise with distinct sounds. Observe for any difficulty or deviation in the articulation of speech sounds, when the person repeats the following words	Speech is understandable but with initialization difficulty, less distinct sounds, and impaired stress or rhythm	Speech is not clear with indistinct sounds and poorly understandable	Speech is unintelligible
Labial dysarthria (Facial nerve) Papa or Mama…	5%	15%	25%
Lingual dysarthria (Hypoglossal nerve) La, La, La…	5%	15%	25%
Guttural dysarthria (Vagus nerve) Ha, Ha, Ha	5%	15%	25%
Cerebellar dysarthria Baby hippopotamus, British constitution, West-minster street, etc.	5%	15%	25%
Extrapyramidal monotones dysarthria Observe for monotones when the person recites a poem/song	5%	15%	25%
Spastic dysarthria (bilateral pyramidal) Observe whether the voice becomes very stiff and volume reduced when the person repeats Ah, Ah, Ah continuously for 30 seconds	5%	15%	25%
Bulbar and pseudobulbar lesions Observe for nasal tone in all vowels and oral consonant	5%	15%	25%

6.6 VOICE FUNCTIONS

A passage of air flowing through the larynx vibrates the vocal cord. The vibration of the vocal cord modulates the air to produces sound. Voice has the characteristics of pitch, loudness, resonance, and phonatory quality.

Aphonia is a loss of voice due to an organic or functional disturbance of the vocal organs. Laryngectomy/paralysis of vocal cord, and so on, may cause aphonia. The vocal cord paralysis may be unilateral (or) bilateral, and it may be in abduction (or) adduction. The bilateral vocal cord paralysis in abduction produces aphonia. The unilateral vocal cord paralysis in abduction may produce dysphonia. Dysphonia may also be due to tracheostomy. Both unilateral and bilateral paralysis in abduction has a potential risk of aspiration. The bilateral vocal cord paralysis in adduction is an acute emergency mainly with respiratory compromise demanding tracheostomy. The unilateral vocal cord paralysis in adduction produces mostly respiratory insufficiency.

Section 4.5.8 in Chapter 4 illustrates the evaluation methods of voice functions. The current facilities for perceptual evaluation, or instrumental evaluation in Voice laboratory, are limited in most of the centers because of non-availability of Speech-Language-Pathology services and voice lab. Hence, *Integrated Evaluation of Disability* has developed a bedside evaluation of dysphonia based on clinical parameters. Class 1 dysphonia derives an impairment of 5%; Class 2, 10%; Class 3, 15%; and aphonia, 25% (Table 6.7).

Table 6.7 Impairment class—Voice function

Impairment class	Description	Impairment score
Class 1 Dysphonia	Impairment of phonatory quality such as flutter, creak, tremor	5%
Class 2 Dysphonia	Impairment of resonance such as nasal tone, e.g., in cleft palate	10%
Class 3 Dysphonia	Impairment of pitch, loudness and quality of voice—breathiness or hoarseness strangled or strained voice	15%
Class 4 Aphonia	Total loss of voice	25%

6.7 CRANIAL NERVE FUNCTIONS

6.7.1 Olfactory functions

Olfactory perception is a mental function to perceive and discriminate variations in smell (17). Before evaluation, the physician ascertains that the nasal passages are clear. Evaluation of olfactory function requires the person to occlude each nostril separately by digital pressure to evaluate the perception of smell by another nostril. The person should close the eyes and sniff the substance one after the other, that is, peppermint, almond oil, coffee, clove, soap, and distinguish the differences in smell. It is important to avoid irritating substances like ammonia as it may stimulate the trigeminal nerve. Hyposmia derives an impairment of 2.5% and anosmia 5%.

6.7.2 Visual function

Chapter 13 describes the evaluation of impairment of visual function.

6.7.3 Oculomotor function

A lesion in the oculomotor nerve results in oculomotor nerve palsy. The oculomotor nerve palsy manifests as diplopia due to paralysis of extraocular muscle namely superior rectus, inferior rectus, and inferior oblique muscles, ptosis due to paralysis of levator palpebrae superioris, and dilatation of the pupil due to paralysis of ciliary muscles and constrictor papillae.

Ptosis refers to dropping of the upper eyelid 1.5–2.0 mm below the upper limbus. The ptosis may be due to slippage of the aponeurosis; impairment of muscle function viz., levator palpebrae superioris in myasthenia gravis, muscular dystrophy, myopathy, and so on; neurogenic lesion in oculomotor nerve or sympathetic nerve; prolapse of the orbital fat, tumor of the eyelid; traumatic disinsertion of the levator palpebrae superioris. *Integrated Evaluation of Disability* defines impairment of ptosis based on margin reflex distance (18) (Table 6.8). *Integrated Evaluation of Disability*

Table 6.8 Impairment class—Ptosis

Class 1	Ptosis: Distance between the center of the upper lid margin and light reflex in primary gaze (Margin reflex distance—MRD1): 2 mm of droop	1.25%
Class 2	Ptosis: Distance between the center of the upper lid margin and light reflex in primary gaze (Margin reflex distance—MRD1): 3 mm of droop	2.5%
Class 3	Ptosis: Distance between the center of the Upper lid margin and light reflex in primary gaze (Margin reflex distance—MRD1): ≥4 mm of droop	5%

Table 6.9 Impairment class—Diplopia

Class 1	Diplopia score 1–5	5%
Class 2	Diplopia score 6–10	10%
Class 3	Diplopia score 11–15	15%
Class 4	Diplopia score 16–20	20%
Class 5	Diplopia score 21–25	25%

assigns impairment only when medical/surgical management does not restore the function.

Oculomotor nerve palsy manifests as diplopia due to paralysis of extraocular muscle, namely superior rectus, inferior rectus, and inferior oblique muscles. Trochlear and abducent nerve supply superior rectus and lateral rectus. The lesion of trochlear and abducent nerves also produce diplopia. *Integrated Evaluation of Disability* assigns impairment for diplopia based on diplopia score measured by Cervical Range of Motion (CROM) method and Goldmann perimetry. Section 13.7 of Chapter 13 describes in detail about the method of measuring diplopia (Table 6.9).

6.7.4 Trigeminal nerve

Evaluation of trigeminal nerve includes assessment of sensory function and muscle function. Sensory function includes touch, pain, and temperature sensation. In general, the touch function identifies hard/soft surfaces, texture, or quality. The temperature sensitivity function detects cold and hot sensation. Pain refers to uncomfortable sensation to a noxious stimulus. Muscle power functions relate to the force produced by the muscle (19). Muscle function includes chewing. The chewing function comprises of mastication, crushing, and grinding of food (20).

Ophthalmic division supplies cornea, iris, conjunctiva, the skin of the forehead, eyelid, eyebrows, nose, mucous membrane of the nasal cavity, and lacrimal gland. The maxillary division supplies skin and conjunctiva of the lower eyelid, the external side of the nose and upper lip, and mucous membrane of the mouth. The mandibular division distributes sensory fibers to teeth and gums of the mandible, temporal region, auricle, lower lip, the lower part of the face, and mucous membrane of the anterior two-thirds of the tongue.

Impairment includes numbness, anesthesia, tingling, paresthesia and hyperesthesia, painful sensation, and impairment of mastication with a deviation of the jaw to the side of paralysis. Complete impairment of sensory and motor functions of trigeminal nerve derives 15% and partial impairment 5%. If there is visual impairment due to corneal opacity secondary to anesthesia of the cornea, the percentage of impairment is as per visual impairment.

6.7.5 Facial nerve

Evaluation of facial nerves includes motor, sensory, and gustatory functions. Motor function comprises of blinking of the eyelid, which is a protective reflex to protect the eye from foreign matters and bright light (21) as well as to spread the tears to moisten the eye. It also includes facial expression and sucking, which is the process of drawing liquid into the mouth by a suction force created by the muscles of cheek, lips, and tongue (20). Gustatory function detects and differentiates various taste stimuli, namely sweet, sour, salt, and bitter by the tongue (17).

A facial nerve lesion may produce lagophthalmos, facial asymmetry, hyperacusis, dysarthria, impairment of sucking, and impairment of taste sensation. The evaluator requests the person to abstain from speaking during evaluation of taste function, as the tongue may retract and dissipate the test substance to the opposite side or posterior third of the tongue. The person protrudes the tongue, and the evaluator gently holds the tongue and places the test substance (strong solution of sugar, common salt, weak solutions of citric acid and quinine) one after the other over the anterior two-thirds of the tongue. The person needs to identify the substance by pointing to the appropriate word written on a card.

Complete unilateral facial paralysis due to lower motor neuron lesion derives an impairment of 15% and partial paralysis, 7.5%. If there is visual impairment due to corneal opacity secondary to exposure of the cornea, the percentage of impairment is as per visual impairment. Articulation and swallowing dysfunction if any adds additional impairment. Complete unilateral facial paralysis due to upper motor neuron lesion derives 10% and partial paralysis 5% (Table 6.10).

6.7.6 Hearing function

Chapter 14 describes the evaluation of impairment of hearing function.

6.7.7 Swallowing functions

Dysphagia refers to a subjective feeling of difficulty in swallowing when the solid or liquid food traverses from mouth to stomach at optimum speed (22,23). Section 4.5.9 in Chapter 4 provides description about impairment of oral, pharyngeal, and esophageal swallowing functions.

Integrated Evaluation of Disability defines impairment class based on multiple variables. It includes drooling, accumulation of solid food in the alveoli of mouth, need for modification of food consistency, the risk of aspiration, postural techniques and compensatory maneuvers adopted to minimize the risk of aspiration during swallowing, and alternate feeding methods namely nasogastric feeding, feeding through gastrostomy (Table 6.11).

Table 6.10 Impairment of facial nerve functions

Clinical tests/scales	Normal function	Partial loss of function	Total loss of function	Maximum impairment of 30%
Lagophthalmos	0%	2.5%	5%	
Facial asymmetry	0%	2.5%	5%	
Hyperacusis	0%	0%	2.5%	
Taste sensation	0%	2.5%	5%	
Dysarthria—(Impairment of bilabial consonants, pot, boy, nasal semivowel—"may," labiodental sounds—fright, vase)	Speech is intact 0%	Speech sounds are less distinct, but one can understand 5%	Speech is not clear with indistinct sounds, and one can understand with difficulty 15%	
Oral swallowing	Intact		Difficulty in swallowing with drooling of saliva or drooling during drinking liquids or accumulation of solid food in the alveoli of mouth 2.5%	

Table 6.11 Impairment class—Oral, pharyngeal, and esophageal swallowing

Impairment class	Criteria	Reference impairment score
Class 1	Difficulty in swallowing with drooling of saliva or drooling during drinking liquids or accumulation of solid food in the alveoli of mouth.	2.5%
Class 2	Prolonged duration of the meal with the sensation of holding of food in the throat. Difficulty in swallowing with nasal regurgitation and/or occasional choking.	5.0%
Class 3	Difficulty in swallowing with nasal regurgitation and on-and-off choking or Limited swallowing ability by modifying food consistency.	15%
Class 4	Difficulty in swallowing with frequent nasal regurgitation and choking or Limited swallowing ability by modifying food consistency, and postural techniques and compensatory maneuvers to minimize the risk of aspiration.	25%
Class 5	Inability to swallow and develops significant aspiration on attempted swallowing requiring feeding by nasogastric tube or PEG (percutaneous endoscopic gastrostomy).	50%

6.7.8 Spinal accessory nerve

Impairment of the spinal accessory nerve produces weakness of the sternomastoid and trapezius muscles. Motor function also includes evaluation of impairment of muscle power of trapezius and sternomastoid.

6.7.9 Hypoglossal nerve

The hypoglossal nerve innervates the muscles of the tongue. The tongue deviates to the side of paralysis on the protrusion. Impairment of the hypoglossal nerve produces slurring of speech, drooling, or aspiration of food due to impairment of control of the muscles of the tongue. Complete unilateral lesion with dysarthria and dysphagia with drooling derives an impairment of 15%. Incomplete unilateral lesion with dysphagia and dysarthria derives an impairment of 7.5%. Section 6.5.1 describes impairment due to articulation and 6.7.7 describes the evaluation of impairment due to swallowing dysfunction.

6.8 MOTOR FUNCTIONS

Motor functions comprise muscle functions, joint functions, and movement functions. Muscle functions consist of muscle power, muscle tone, and muscle endurance.

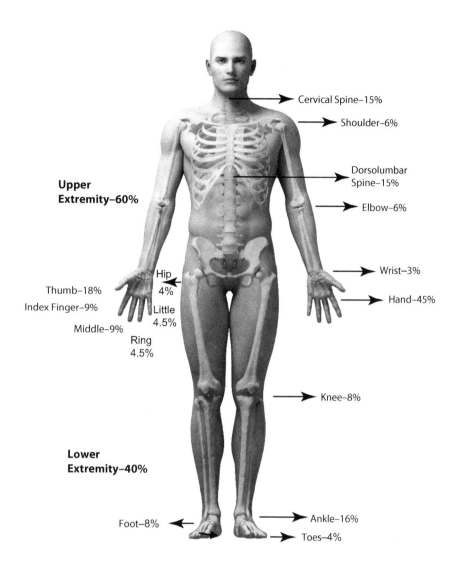

Upper Extremity–60%

Cervical Spine–15%

Shoulder–6%

Dorsolumbar Spine–15%

Elbow–6%

Wrist–3%

Hand–45%

Thumb–18%

Index Finger–9%

Middle–9%

Hip 4%

Little 4.5%

Ring 4.5%

Knee–8%

Lower Extremity–40%

Foot–8%

Ankle–16%

Toes–4%

Figure 6.1 Motor impairment.

Joint functions consist of mobility and stability of individual joints. Movement functions consist of voluntary movement, involuntary movement, the paucity of movement (brady-kinesia) and translation movement—gait. Section 4.5.10.1 in Chapter 4 explicates clinical methods for impairment evaluation of motor function. Complete loss of motor function of one upper extremity derives an impairment of 60%, and lower extremity 40%. In the upper extremity, shoulder derives 6%, elbow 6%, wrist 3%, and hand 45%. In hand, thumb obtains 18%, index 9%, middle finger 9%, and ring finger 4.5% and little finger 4.5%. In the lower extremity, hip derives 4%, knee 8%, ankle 16%, and foot 12% (Figure 6.1).

Integrated Evaluation of Disability integrates impairment of muscle functions, joint functions, and movement functions to compute an impairment of motor functions (Illustration 6.1).

6.8.1 Muscle functions

Integrated Evaluation of Disability adds impairment of muscle power, tone, and endurance functions to arrive an impairment of muscle function and does not exceed 60% in the upper extremity, 40% in the lower extremity, and 30% in the spine.

6.8.1.1 MUSCLE POWER FUNCTION

Muscle power assessment is done either about muscle or muscle groups. *Integrated Evaluation of Disability* prefers myotome assessment in spinal cord lesion and brachial plexus lesion. In the upper extremity, shoulder derives maximum impairment of 2%, elbow 2%, wrist 1%, thumb 6%, index 3%, middle finger 3%, ring finger 1.5%, and little finger 1.5% for complete loss of muscle power (Table 6.12).

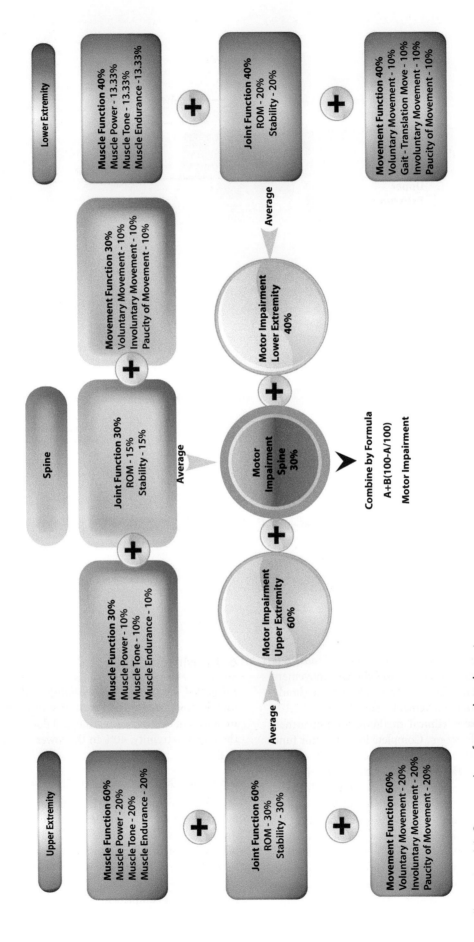

Illustration 6.1 Computation of motor impairment.

Table 6.12 Impairment evaluation—Muscle power function: Upper extremity

Muscle groups	Reference score	Weightage muscle power	Assigned impairment	Maximum impairment 20%
(Shoulder, elbow, and wrist: Hand = 1:3)				
Shoulder, elbow, and wrist	**5.000%**			
Shoulder girdle	**0.800%**	MRC 0 = 0.200% MRC 1 = 0.160% MRC 2 = 0.120% MRC 3 = 0.080% MRC 4 = 0.040%		
Elevators	0.200%			
Depressors	0.200%			
Protractors	0.200%			
Retractors	0.200%			
Shoulder	**1.200%**	MRC 0 = 0.200% MRC 1 = 0.160% MRC 2 = 0.120% MRC 3 = 0.080% MRC 4 = 0.040%		
Flexors	0.200%			
Extensors	0.200%			
Adductors	0.200%			
Abductors	0.200%			
Internal rotators	0.200%			
External rotators	0.200%			
Elbow and forearm	**2.000%**	MRC 0 = 0.500% MRC 1 = 0.400% MRC 2 = 0.300% MRC 3 = 0.200% MRC 4 = 0.100%		
Flexors	0.500%			
Extensors	0.500%			
Pronators	0.500%			
Supinator	0.500%			
Wrist	**1.000%**	MRC 0 = 0.500% MRC 1 = 0.400% MRC 2 = 0.300% MRC 3 = 0.200% MRC 4 = 0.100%		
Palmar flexor	0.500%			
Dorsiflexor	0.500%			
Hand 15%				
Thumb—6% (IP:MCP = 1:2)				
MCP joint	5.000%	MRC 0 = 1.000% MRC 1 = 0.800% MRC 2 = 0.600% MRC 3 = 0.400% MRC 4 = 0.200%		
Flexor	1.000%			
Extensor	1.000%			
Adductor	1.000%			

(Continued)

Table 6.12 (*Continued*) Impairment evaluation—Muscle power function: Upper extremity

Muscle groups	Reference score	Weightage muscle power	Assigned impairment	Maximum impairment 20%
Abductor	1.000%			
Opponens pollicis	1.000%			
IP joint	1.000%	MRC 0 = 0.500%		
		MRC 1 = 0.400%		
		MRC 2 = 0.300%		
		MRC 3 = 0.200%		
		MRC 4 = 0.100%		
Flexors	0.500%			
Extensors	0.500%			
Index finger—3% (DIP:PIP:MCP = 1:2:3)				
MCP joint	**1.500%**	MRC 0 = 0.375%		
		MRC 1 = 0.300%		
		MRC 2 = 0.225%		
		MRC 3 = 0.150%		
		MRC 4 = 0.075%		
Flexors	0.375%			
Extensors	0.375%			
Adductors	0.375%			
Abductors	0.375%			
PIP joint	**1.000%**	MRC 0 = 0.500%		
		MRC 1 = 0.400%		
		MRC 2 = 0.300%		
		MRC 3 = 0.200%		
		MRC 4 = 0.100%		
Flexors	0.500%			
Extensors	0.500%			
DIP joint	**0.500%**	MRC 0 = 0.250%		
		MRC 1 = 0.200%		
		MRC 2 = 0.150%		
		MRC 3 = 0.100%		
		MRC 4 = 0.050%		
Flexors	0.25%			
Extensors	0.25%			
Middle finger—3% (DIP:PIP:MCP = 1:2:3)				
MCP joint	**1.500%**	MRC 0 = 0.500%		
		MRC 1 = 0.400%		
		MRC 2 = 0.300%		
		MRC 3 = 0.200%		
		MRC 4 = 0.100%		
Flexors	0.500%			
Extensors	0.500%			
Abductors	0.500%			
PIP joint	**1.000%**	MRC 0 = 0.500%		
		MRC 1 = 0.400%		
		MRC 2 = 0.300%		
		MRC 3 = 0.200%		
		MRC 4 = 0.100%		

(*Continued*)

Table 6.12 (*Continued*) Impairment evaluation—Muscle power function: Upper extremity

Muscle groups	Reference score	Weightage muscle power	Assigned impairment	Maximum impairment 20%
Flexors	0.500%			
Extensors	0.500%			
DIP joint	**0.500%**	MRC 0 = 0.250%		
		MRC 1 = 0.200%		
		MRC 2 = 0.150%		
		MRC 3 = 0.100%		
		MRC 4 = 0.050%		
Flexors	0.250%			
Extensors	0.250%			
Ring finger—1.5% (DIP:PIP:MCP = 1:2:3)				
MCP joint	**0.750%**	MRC 0 = 0.187%		
		MRC 1 = 0.149%		
		MRC 2 = 0.112%		
		MRC 3 = 0.074%		
		MRC 4 = 0.037%		
Flexors	0.187%			
Extensors	0.187%			
Adductors	0.187%			
Abductors	0.187%			
PIP joint	**0.500%**	MRC 0 = 0.250%		
		MRC 1 = 0.200%		
		MRC 2 = 0.150%		
		MRC 3 = 0.100%		
		MRC 4 = 0.050%		
Flexors	0.250%			
Extensors	0.250%			
DIP joint	**0.250%**	MRC 0 = 0.125%		
		MRC 1 = 0.100%		
		MRC 2 = 0.075%		
		MRC 3 = 0.050%		
		MRC 4 = 0.025%		
Flexors	0.125%			
Extensors	0.125%			
Little finger—1.5% (DIP:PIP:MCP = 1:2:3)				
MCP joint	**0.750%**	MRC 0 = 0.150%		
		MRC 1 = 0.120%		
		MRC 2 = 0.090%		
		MRC 3 = 0.060%		
		MRC 4 = 0.030%		
Flexors	0.150%			
Extensors	0.150%			
Adductors	0.150%			
Abductors	0.150%			
Opponens digiti minimi	0.150%			
PIP joint	**0.500%**	MRC 0 = 0.250%		
		MRC 1 = 0.200%		
		MRC 2 = 0.150%		
		MRC 3 = 0.100%		
		MRC 4 = 0.050%		

(*Continued*)

Table 6.12 (*Continued*) Impairment evaluation—Muscle power function: Upper extremity

Muscle groups	Reference score	Weightage muscle power	Assigned impairment	Maximum impairment 20%
Flexors	0.250%			
Extensors	0.250%			
DIP joint	**0.250**%	MRC 0 = 0.125%		
		MRC 1 = 0.100%		
		MRC 2 = 0.075%		
		MRC 3 = 0.050%		
		MRC 4 = 0.025%		
Flexors	0.125%			
Extensors	0.125%			

Regarding myotome, C5 myotome derives maximum impairment of 3%, C6—2%, C7—5%, C8—5%, and T1—5% for complete loss of muscle power (Table 6.13).

In the lower extremity, the hip derives maximum impairment of 1.33%, knee 2.66%, ankle 5.33%, foot 2.66%, and toes 1.33% for complete loss of muscle power (Table 6.14). Regarding myotome, L2 derives 1%, L2—2%, L3—4%, L5—1%, S1—4%, and S2,3,4—1.33% (Table 6.15). The maximum impairment of muscle power for one lower extremity does not exceed 13.33%.

Table 6.13 Impairment evaluation—Muscle power function: Upper extremity myotome

Myotomes	Reference score	Weightage muscle power	Assigned impairment score	Maximum impairment 20%
C5 Myotome:	3.000%	MRC 0 = 3.000%		
Deltoid (middle fibers)		MRC 1 = 2.400%		
Movements:		MRC 2 = 1.800%		
Shoulder abductors		MRC 3 = 1.200%		
		MRC 4 = 0.600%		
C6 Myotome:	2.000%	MRC 0 = 2.000%		
Brachioradialis, extensor carpi radialis longus		MRC 1 = 1.600%		
Movements:		MRC 2 = 1.200%		
Elbow flexors, and wrist extensors		MRC 3 = 0.800%		
		MRC 4 = 0.400%		
C7 Myotome:	5.000%	MRC 0 = 5.000%		
Triceps, extensor digitorum		MRC 1 = 4.000%		
Movements:		MRC 2 = 3.000%		
Elbow extensors; finger extensors		MRC 3 = 2.000%		
		MRC 4 = 1.000%		
C8 Myotome:	5.000%	MRC 0 = 5.000%		
Flexor pollicis longus, flexor digitorum profundus		MRC 1 = 4.000%		
		MRC 2 = 3.000%		
Movements:		MRC 3 = 2.000%		
Flexors of IP joint of thumb and finger flexors of DIP joint		MRC 4 = 1.000%		
T1 Myotome:	5.000%	MRC 0 = 5.000%		
Abductor pollicis brevis and dorsal interossei		MRC 1 = 4.000%		
Movements:		MRC 2 = 3.000%		
Palmar abductors of thumb, and abductors of fingers		MRC 3 = 2.000%		
		MRC 4 = 1.000%		

Table 6.14 Impairment evaluation—Muscle power function: Lower extremity

Muscle groups	Reference score	Weightage muscle power	Assigned impairment score	Maximum impairment 13.333%
(Hip:Knee:Ankle:Foot:Toes = 1:2:4:2:1)				
Hip	**1.333%**	MRC 0 = 0.222% MRC 1 = 0.177% MRC 2 = 0.133% MRC 3 = 0.088% MRC 4 = 0.044%		
Flexors	0.222%			
Extensors	0.222%			
Adductors	0.222%			
Abductors	0.222%			
Internal rotators	0.222%			
External rotators	0.222%			
Knee	**2.666%**	MRC 0 = 1.333% MRC 1 = 1.066% MRC 2 = 0.799% MRC 3 = 0.533% MRC 4 = 0.266%		
Flexors	1.333%			
Extensors	1.333%			
Ankle	**5.333%**	MRC 0 = 2.666% MRC 1 = 2.132% MRC 2 = 1.599% MRC 3 = 1.066% MRC 4 = 0.533%		
Plantar flexors	2.666%			
Dorsiflexor	2.666%			
Foot	**2.666%**	MRC 0 = 1.333% MRC 1 = 1.066% MRC 2 = 0.799% MRC 3 = 0.533% MRC 4 = 0.266%		
Invertors	1.333%			
Evertors	1.333%			
Toes	**1.33%**			
Big toe	**0.533%**	MRC 0 = 0.133% MRC 1 = 0.106% MRC 2 = 0.079% MRC 3 = 0.053% MRC 4 = 0.026%		
Flexors	0.133%			
Extensors	0.133%			
Abductors	0.133%			

(Continued)

Table 6.14 (*Continued*) Impairment evaluation—Muscle power function: Lower extremity

Muscle groups	Reference score	Weightage muscle power	Assigned impairment score	Maximum impairment 13.333%
Adductor	0.133%			
Other toes	**0.800%**	MRC 0 = 0.200%		
		MRC 1 = 0.160%		
		MRC 2 = 0.120%		
		MRC 3 = 0.080%		
		MRC 4 = 0.040%		
Flexors	0.200%			
Extensors	0.200%			
Abductors	0.200%			
Adductors	0.200%			

Table 6.15 Impairment evaluation—Muscle power function: Lower extremity myotomes

Myotomes	Reference score	Weightage muscle power	Assigned impairment score	Maximum impairment 13.333%
L2 Myotome:	1.000%	MRC 0 = 1.000%		
Psoas major, iliacus, pectineus		MRC 1 = 0.800%		
Movements:		MRC 2 = 0.600%		
Hip flexors		MRC 3 = 0.400%		
		MRC 4 = 0.200%		
L3 Myotome:	2.000%	MRC 0 = 2.000%		
Quadriceps		MRC 1 = 1.600%		
Movements:		MRC 2 = 1.200%		
Knee extensors		MRC 3 = 0.800%		
		MRC 4 = 0.400%		
L4 Myotome:	4.000%	MRC 0 = 4.000%		
Quadriceps, tibialis anterior		MRC 1 = 3.200%		
Movements:		MRC 2 = 2.400%		
Knee extensors, ankle dorsiflexors		MRC 3 = 1.600%		
		MRC 4 = 0.800%		
L5 Myotome:	1.000%	MRC 0 = 1.000%		
Extensor digitorum longus, tibialis anterior, extensor hallucis longus		MRC 1 = 0.800%		
		MRC 2 = 0.600%		
Movements:		MRC 3 = 0.400%		
Dorsiflexors of ankle and toes, extensor of big toe		MRC 4 = 0.200%		
S1,2 Myotome:	5.333%	MRC 0 = 5.333%		
Gastrocnemius		MRC 1 = 4.266%		
Movements:		MRC 2 = 3.199%		
Ankle plantar flexors		MRC 3 = 2.133%		
		MRC 4 = 1.066%		

The impairment of muscle power for cervical spine derives 5% and dorsolumbar spine 5%. The maximum impairment of muscle power of spine does not exceed 10% (Table 6.16).

6.8.1.2 MUSCLE TONE FUNCTION

Muscle tone refers to the tension present in the muscle during rest and the resistance offered during passive movement (24).

The descending input from the motor cortex modulates the intrinsic circuit existing in the spinal cord. The input from the intrinsic circuit either exerts an excitatory or inhibitory effect on alpha and gamma motor neurons. Interruption of these descending inputs results in increased activation of alpha and gamma motor neurons causing an increase in resting muscle tone. Alpha motor neurons activate the extrafusal muscle fibers, and any lesion in the alpha motor neurons results in decrease or loss of muscle

Table 6.16 Impairment evaluation of muscle power—Spine

Muscle groups	Reference value	Weightage Muscle power	Assigned power	Maximum impairment 10%
Cervical spine	5.000%	MRC 0 = 0.833%		
		MRC 1 = 0.665%		
		MRC 2 = 0.499%		
		MRC 3 = 0.333%		
		MRC 4 = 0.166%		
Flexors	0.833%			
Extensors	0.833%			
Lateral flexors—right	0.833%			
Lateral flexors—left	0.833%			
Rotators—right	0.833%			
Rotators—left	0.833%			
Dorsolumbar spine	5.000%	MRC 0 = 0.833%		
		MRC 1 = 0.665%		
		MRC 2 = 0.499%		
		MRC 3 = 0.333%		
		MRC 4 = 0.166%		
Flexors	0.833%			
Extensors	0.833%			
Lateral flexors—right	0.833%			
Lateral flexors—right	0.833%			
Rotators—right	0.833%			
Rotators—left	0.833%			

tone (25). The "Modified Ashworth Scale" describes grading of hypertonia (26). *Integrated Evaluation of Disability* has developed a method to grade hypotonia of the muscle (Illustration 6.2).

The impairment of muscle tone does not exceed 20% for upper extremity (Tables 6.17 and 6.18), 13.33% for lower extremity (Tables 6.19 and 6.20), and 10% for the spine (Table 6.21).

6.8.1.3 MUSCLE ENDURANCE FUNCTION

Muscle endurance functions refer to the ability of the muscle or muscle groups to sustain its contraction for longer period (24). Section 4.5.10.1.1 in Chapter 4 reviewed studies on VO$_2$ max; endurance and slow twitch, fast twitch fatigue resistant and fast twitch fatigable muscle fibers; fatigue test, and endurance exercise/training in sports (27–35). Finally, *Integrated Evaluation of Disability* explicated and evolved a clinical method to assess endurance of muscle groups for impairment evaluation. In the Medical Research Council's (MRC) manual muscle testing, grade 3 represents active muscle contraction against gravity, that is, 60% of maximum muscle contraction and grade 5 represents active muscle contraction against gravity with maximum resistance, that is, 100% of muscle contraction. Forty to sixty percent of maximum concentric muscle contractions, that is, submaximal active muscle contraction against gravity for maximum repetitions can serve to evaluate impairment of endurance of muscle or muscle groups.

Illustration 6.3 describes the principle of clinical grading of muscle endurance. The impairment does not exceed 20% for complete loss of endurance in upper extremity (Table 6.22), 13.33% in lower extremity (Table 6.23), and 10% in spine (Table 6.24).

6.8.2 Movement functions

The integrated function of upper motor neurons, basal ganglia, cerebellum, and lower motor neuron with its skeletal muscles create a spectrum of voluntary movement from fine prehensile function of hand, through smooth fluid movement to rigid stabilizing movement. Disorders of upper motor neurons, basal ganglia, cerebellum, and lower motor neurons produces impairment of voluntary movement functions: that is, uniaxial movement, multiaxial/multiplane/multijoint movement, coordination of movement, stabilization of movement, and gait translation movement; involuntary movement functions, and paucity of movement (bradykinesia). *Integrated Evaluation of Disability* adds up the impairment of voluntary movement, involuntary movement paucity of movement (bradykinesia), and gait translation movement to arrive at impairment of movement functions. It does not exceed 60% in upper extremity, 40% in lower extremity, and 30% in spine.

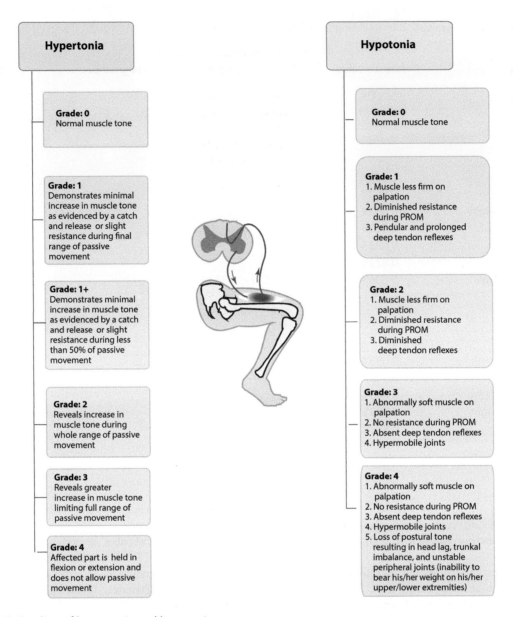

Illustration 6.2 Grading of hypertonia and hypotonia.

Table 6.17 Impairment evaluation—Muscle tone functions: Upper extremity

Muscle groups	Reference score	Weightage Hypertonia	Weightage Hypotonia	Assigned score	Maximum impairment 20%
(Shoulder, elbow, and wrist: Hand = 1:3)					
Shoulder, elbow, and wrist	5.000%				
Shoulder	2.000%	MAS 1 = 0.066%	Hypotonia 1 = 0.083%		
		MAS 1+ = 0.133%	Hypotonia 2 = 0.166%		
		MAS 2 = 0.199%	Hypotonia 3 = 0.249%		
		MAS 3 = 0.266%	Hypotonia 4 = 0.333%		
		MAS 4 = 0.333%			
Flexors	0.333%				
Extensors	0.333%				
Adductors	0.333%				
Abductors	0.333%				

(Continued)

Table 6.17 (*Continued*) Impairment evaluation—Muscle tone functions: Upper extremity

Muscle groups	Reference score	Weightage Hypertonia	Weightage Hypotonia	Assigned score	Maximum impairment 20%
Internal rotators	0.333%				
External rotators	0.333%				
Elbow and forearm	2.000%	MAS 1 = 0.100%	Hypotonia 1 = 0.125%		
		MAS 1+ = 0.200%	Hypotonia 2 = 0.250%		
		MAS 2 = 0.300%	Hypotonia 3 = 0.375%		
		MAS 3 = 0.400%	Hypotonia 4 = 0.500%		
		MAS 4 = 0.500%			
Flexors	0.500%				
Extensors	0.500%				
Pronators	0.500%				
Supinator	0.500%				
Wrist	1.000%	MAS 1 = 0.100%	Hypotonia 1 = 0.125%		
		MAS 1+ = 0.200%	Hypotonia 2 = 0.250%		
		MAS 2 = 0.300%	Hypotonia 3 = 0.375%		
		MAS 3 = 0.400%	Hypotonia 4 = 0.500%		
		MAS 4 = 0.500%			
Palmar flexor	0.500%				
Dorsiflexor	0.500%				

Hand: 15%
Thumb:Index, middle, ring, and little fingers = 4:6
MCP:PIP:DIP = 3:2:1

Muscle groups	Reference score	Weightage Hypertonia	Weightage Hypotonia	Assigned score	Maximum impairment 20%
Thumb	6.000%				
CMC and MCP:IP = 2:1					
CMC and MCP joints	5.000%	MAS 1 = 0.200%	Hypotonia 1 = 0.250%		
		MAS 1+ = 0.400%	Hypotonia 2 = 0.500%		
		MAS 2 = 0.600%	Hypotonia 3 = 0.750%		
		MAS 3 = 0.800%	Hypotonia 4 = 1.000%		
		MAS 4 = 1.000%			
Flexor	1.000%				
Extensor	1.000%				
Adductor	1.000%				
Abductor	1.000%				
Opponens	1.000%				
IP joint	**1.000%**	MAS 1 = 0.100%	Hypotonia 1 = 0.125%		
		MAS 1+ = 0.200%	Hypotonia 2 = 0.250%		
		MAS 2 = 0.300%	Hypotonia 3 = 0.375%		
		MAS 3 = 0.400%	Hypotonia 4 = 0.500%		
		MAS 4 = 0.500%			
Flexor	0.500%				
Extensor	0.500%				
Fingers	**9.000%**				
MCP:	4.500%	MAS 1 = 0.225%	Hypotonia 1 = 0.281%		
Index		MAS 1+ = 0.450%	Hypotonia 2 = 0.562%		
Middle		MAS 2 = 0.675%	Hypotonia 3 = 0.843%		
Ring		MAS 3 = 0.900%	Hypotonia 4 = 1.125%		
Little		MAS 4 = 1.125%			
Flexors	1.125%				
Extensors	1.125%				
Adductors	1.125%				

(*Continued*)

Table 6.17 (*Continued*) Impairment evaluation—Muscle tone functions: Upper extremity

Muscle groups	Reference score	Weightage Hypertonia	Weightage Hypotonia	Assigned score	Maximum impairment 20%
Abductors	1.125%				
PIP	3.000%	MAS 1 = 0.300%	Hypotonia 1 = 0.375%		
Index		MAS 1+ = 0.600%	Hypotonia 2 = 0.750%		
Middle		MAS 2 = 0.900%	Hypotonia 3 = 1.125%		
Ring		MAS 3 = 1.200%	Hypotonia 4 = 1.500%		
Little		MAS 4 = 1.500%			
Flexors	1.500%				
Extensors	1.500%				
DIP	1.500%	MAS 1 = 0.150%	Hypotonia 1 = 0.187%		
Index		MAS 1+ = 0.300%	Hypotonia 2 = 0.375%		
Middle		MAS 2 = 0.450%	Hypotonia 3 = 0.562%		
Ring		MAS 3 = 0.600%	Hypotonia 4 = 0.750%		
Little		MAS 4 = 0.750%			
Flexors	0.750%				
Extensors	0.750%				
Sum of impairment					

Table 6.18 Impairment evaluation—Muscle tone functions upper extremity: Myotome

Myotomes	Reference score	Weightage Hypertonia	Weightage Hypotonia	Assigned score	Maximum impairment 20%
C5 Myotome:	3.000%	MAS 1 = 0.600%	Hypotonia 1 = 0.750%		
Rhomboids, deltoid, supraspinatus, infraspinatus, teres minor, biceps		MAS 1+ = 1.200%	Hypotonia 2 = 1.500%		
Movements:		MAS 2 = 1.800%	Hypotonia 3 = 2.250%		
Retractors, shoulder—abductors, flexors, extensors, external rotators; elbow flexors and supinators		MAS 3 = 2.400% MAS 4 = 3.000%	Hypotonia 4 = 3.000%		
C6 Myotome:	2.000%	MAS 1 = 0.400%	Hypotonia 1 = 0.500%		
Serratus anterior, latissimus dorsi, subscapularis, teres major, pectoralis major, biceps, coracobrachialis, brachialis, brachioradialis, supinator, extensor carpi radialis longus		MAS 1+ = 0.800% MAS 2 = 1.200% MAS 3 = 1.600% MAS 4 = 2.000%	Hypotonia 2 = 1.000% Hypotonia 3 = 1.500% Hypotonia 4 = 2.000%		
Movements:					
Protractors, shoulder adductors, shoulder internal rotators, **Elbow flexors**, forearm supinator, and wrist extensors					
C7 Myotome:	5.000%	MAS 1 = 1.000%	Hypotonia 1 = 1.250%		
Serratus anterior, latissimus dorsi, pectoralis major, pectoralis minor, triceps, pronator teres, flexor carpi radialis, flexor digitorum superficialis, extensor carpi radialis longus and brevis, extensor digitorum, extensor digiti minimi		MAS 1+ = 2.000% MAS 2 = 3.000% MAS 3 = 4.000% MAS 4 = 5.000%	Hypotonia 2 = 2.500% Hypotonia 3 = 3.750% Hypotonia 4 = 5.000%		
Movements:					
Protractors, shoulder adductors, **Elbow extensors**; forearm pronators; wrist extensors, flexors; finger flexors (proximal joint), finger extensors					

(Continued)

Table 6.18 (*Continued*) Impairment evaluation—Muscle tone functions upper extremity: Myotome

Myotomes	Reference score	Weightage Hypertonia	Weightage Hypotonia	Assigned score	Maximum impairment 20%
C8 Myotome: Pectoralis major, pectoralis minor, triceps, pronator quadratus, flexor pollicis longus, flexor digitorum superficialis, flexor digitorum profundus, flexor carpi ulnaris, extensor carpi ulnaris, abductor pollicis longus, extensor pollicis longus, extensor pollicis brevis, extensor indicis, abductor pollicis brevis, flexor pollicis brevis, opponens pollicis **Movements:** Shoulder adductors, elbow extensors, forearm pronators, **Finger flexors**, thumb—flexors, extensors, opponens, adductors, and abductors (palmar)	5.000%	MAS 1 = 1.000% MAS 1+ = 2.000% MAS 2 = 3.000% MAS 3 = 4.000% MAS 4 = 5.000%	Hypotonia 1 = 1.250% Hypotonia 2 = 2.500% Hypotonia 3 = 3.750% Hypotonia 4 = 5.000%		
T1 Myotome: Flexor digitorum profundus, lumbricals, and interossei **Movements:** **Finger abductors**, finger flexors	5.000%	MAS 1 = 1.000% MAS 1+ = 2.000% MAS 2 = 3.000% MAS 3 = 4.000% MAS 4 = 5.000%	Hypotonia 1 = 1.250% Hypotonia 2 = 2.500% Hypotonia 3 = 3.750% Hypotonia 4 = 5.000%		

Table 6.19 Impairment evaluation—Muscle tone function: Lower extremity

Muscle groups	Reference score	Weightage Hypertonia	Weightage Hypertonia	Assigned score	Maximum impairment 13.333%
(Hip:Knee:Ankle:Foot:Toes = 1:2:4:2:1)					
Hip	1.333%	MAS 1 = 0.044% MAS 1+ = 0.088% MAS 2 = 0.133% MAS 3 = 0.177% MAS 4 = 0.222%	Hypotonia 1 = 0.055% Hypotonia 2 = 0.111% Hypotonia 3 = 0.166% Hypotonia 4 = 0.222%		
Flexors	0.222%				
Extensors	0.222%				
Adductors	0.222%				
Abductors	0.222%				
Internal rotators	0.222%				
External rotators	0.222%				
Knee	2.666%	MAS 1 = 0.266% MAS 1+ = 0.533% MAS 2 = 0.799% MAS 3 = 1.066% MAS 4 = 1.333%	Hypotonia 1 = 0.333% Hypotonia 2 = 0.666% Hypotonia 3 = 0.999% Hypotonia 4 = 1.333%		
Flexors	1.333%				
Extensors	1.333%				

(Continued)

Table 6.19 (*Continued*) Impairment evaluation—Muscle tone function: Lower extremity

Muscle groups	Reference score	Weightage Hypertonia	Weightage Hypertonia	Assigned score	Maximum impairment 13.333%
Ankle	5.333%	MAS 1 = 0.533% MAS 1+ = 1.066% MAS 2 = 1.599% MAS 3 = 2.132% MAS 4 = 2.666%	Hypotonia 1 = 0.666% Hypotonia 2 = 1.333% Hypotonia 3 = 1.999% Hypotonia 4 = 2.666%		
Plantar flexors	2.666%				
Dorsiflexor	2.666%				
Foot	2.666%	MAS 1 = 0.266% MAS 1+ = 0.533% MAS 2 = 0.799% MAS 3 = 1.066% MAS 4 = 1.333%	Hypotonia 1 = 0.333% Hypotonia 2 = 0.666% Hypotonia 3 = 0.999% Hypotonia 4 = 1.333%		
Invertors	1.333%				
Evertors	1.333%				
Toes	1.333%				
Big toe	0.533%	MAS 1 = 0.026% MAS 1+ = 0.053% MAS 2 = 0.079% MAS 3 = 0.106% MAS 4 = 0.133%	Hypotonia 1 = 0.033% Hypotonia 2 = 0.066% Hypotonia 3 = 0.099% Hypotonia 4 = 0.133%		
Flexors	0.133%				
Extensors	0.133%				
Adductors	0.133%				
Abductors	0.133%				
Toes	0.800%	MAS 1 = 0.040% MAS 1+ = 0.080% MAS 2 = 0.120% MAS 3 = 0.160% MAS 4 = 0.200%	Hypotonia 1 = 0.050% Hypotonia 2 = 0.100% Hypotonia 3 = 0.150% Hypotonia 4 = 0.200%		
Flexors	0.200%				
Extensors	0.200%				
Adductors	0.200%				
Abductors	0.200%				

Table 6.20 Impairment evaluation—Muscle tone function—Lower extremity: Myotome

Myotomes	Reference score	Weightage Hypertonia	Weightage Hypertonia	Assigned score	Maximum impairment 13.333%

L2 Myotome:
Psoas major, iliacus, sartorius,
   gracilis, pectineus, adductor
   longus, adductor brevis
Movements:
Hip flexors, hip adductors
	1.000%	MAS 1 = 0.200%
		MAS 1+ = 0.400%
		MAS 2 = 0.600%
		MAS 3 = 0.800%
		MAS 4 = 1.000%
			Hypotonia 1 = 0.250%
			Hypotonia 2 = 0.500%
			Hypotonia 3 = 0.750%
			Hypotonia 4 = 1.000%		

L3 Myotome: Quadriceps, adductor magnus, adductor longus, adductor brevis **Movements:** *Knee extensors*, hip adductors	2.000%	MAS 1 = 0.400% MAS 1+ = 0.800% MAS 2 = 1.200% MAS 3 = 1.600% MAS 4 = 2.000%	Hypotonia 1 = 0.500% Hypotonia 2 = 1.000% Hypotonia 3 = 1.500% Hypotonia 4 = 2.000%		

(Continued)

Table 6.20 (*Continued*) Impairment evaluation—Muscle tone function—Lower extremity: Myotome

Myotomes	Reference score	Weightage Hypertonia	Weightage Hypertonia	Assigned score	Maximum impairment 13.333%
L4 Myotome: Tibialis anterior, quadriceps, tensor fasciae latae, adductor magnus, obturator externus, tibialis posterior **Movements:** *Ankle dorsiflexors*, knee extensors, hip adductors	4.000%	MAS 1 = 0.800% MAS 1+ = 1.600% MAS 2 = 2.400% MAS 3 = 3.200% MAS 4 = 4.000%	Hypotonia 1 = 1.000% Hypotonia 2 = 2.000% Hypotonia 3 = 3.000% Hypotonia 4 = 4.000%		
L5 Myotome: Extensor hallucis longus, gluteus medius, gluteus minimus, obturator internus, semimembranosus, semitendinosus, extensor digitorum longus, peroneus tertius, popliteus **Movements:** *Extensor of big toe*, knee flexor, hip abductor, toe extensor	1.000%	MAS 1 = 0.200% MAS 1+ = 0.400% MAS 2 = 0.600% MAS 3 = 0.800% MAS 4 = 1.000%	Hypotonia 1 = 0.250% Hypotonia 2 = 0.500% Hypotonia 3 = 0.750% Hypotonia 4 = 1.000%		
S1 Myotome: Biceps femoris, gluteus maximus, obturator internus, piriformis, popliteus, gastrocnemius, soleus, peronei, extensor digitorum brevis, semitendinosus **Movements:** *Ankle plantar flexors, knee flexors*, hip extensor, Foot evertors	4.000%	MAS 1 = 0.800% MAS 1+ = 1.600% MAS 2 = 2.400% MAS 3 = 3.200% MAS 4 = 4.000%	Hypotonia 1 = 1.000% Hypotonia 2 = 2.000% Hypotonia 3 = 3.000% Hypotonia 4 = 4.000%		
S2/3 Myotome: Intrinsic muscles of foot, piriformis, biceps femoris, gastrocnemius, soleus, flexor digitorum longus, flexor hallucis longus **Movements:** *Intrinsic movements of foot*, ankle plantar flexor, knee flexor, flexor of toes and big toe	1.333%	MAS 1 = 0.266% MAS 1+ = 0.533% MAS 2 = 0.799% MAS 3 = 1.065% MAS 4 = 1.331%	Hypotonia 1 = 0.333% Hypotonia 2 = 0.666% Hypotonia 3 = 0.999% Hypotonia 4 = 1.333%		

Table 6.21 Impairment evaluation—Muscle tone: Spine

Muscle groups	Assigned impairment	Weightage Hypertonia	Weightage Hypotonia	Assigned impairment	Maximum impairment 10%
Cervical spine	5.000%	MAS 1 = 0.166% MAS 1+ = 0.333% MAS 2 = 0.499% MAS 3 = 0.666% MAS 4 = 0.833%	Hypotonia 1 = 0.208% Hypotonia 2 = 0.416% Hypotonia 3 = 0.624% Hypotonia 4 = 0.833%		

(Continued)

Table 6.21 (*Continued*) Impairment evaluation—Muscle tone: Spine

Muscle groups	Assigned impairment	Weightage Hypertonia	Weightage Hypotonia	Assigned impairment	Maximum impairment 10%
Flexors	0.833%				
Extensors	0.833%				
Lateral flexors—right	0.833%				
Lateral flexors—left	0.833%				
Rotators—right	0.833%				
Rotators—left	0.833%				
Dorsolumbar spine	5%	MAS 1 = 0.166% MAS 1+ = 0.333% MAS 2 = 0.499% MAS 3 = 0.666% MAS 4 = 0.833%	Hypotonia 1 = 0.208% Hypotonia 2 = 0.416% Hypotonia 3 = 0.624% Hypotonia 4 = 0.833%		
Flexors	0.833%				
Extensors	0.833%				
Lateral flexors—right	0.833%				
Lateral flexors—left	0.833%				
Rotators—right	0.833%				
Rotators—left	0.833%				

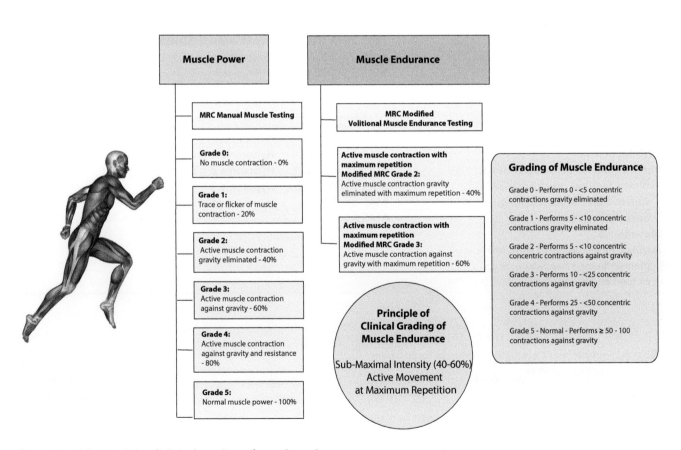

Illustration 6.3 Principle of clinical grading of muscle endurance.

Table 6.22 Impairment evaluation—Endurance of muscle: Upper extremity

Muscle groups	Reference impairment score	Weightage Muscle endurance	% of endurance score—right	% of endurance score—left	Maximum impairment 20%
(Shoulder, elbow, and wrist:Hand = 1:3)					
Shoulder girdle	**0.800**%	Endurance 0 = 0.200%			
		Endurance 1 = 0.160%			
		Endurance 2 = 0.120%			
		Endurance 3 = 0.080%			
		Endurance 4 = 0.040%			
Elevators	0.200%				
Depressors	0.200%				
Protractors	0.200%				
Retractors	0.200%				
Shoulder	**1.200**%	Endurance 0 = 0.200%			
		Endurance 1 = 0.160%			
		Endurance 2 = 0.120%			
		Endurance 3 = 0.080%			
		Endurance 4 = 0.040%			
Flexors	0.200%				
Extensors	0.200%				
Adductors	0.200%				
Abductors	0.200%				
Internal rotators	0.200%				
External rotators	0.200%				
Elbow and forearm	**2.000**%	Endurance 0 = 0.500%			
		Endurance 1 = 0.400%			
		Endurance 2 = 0.300%			
		Endurance 3 = 0.200%			
		Endurance 4 = 0.100%			
Flexors	0.500%				
Extensors	0.500%				
Pronators	0.500%				
Supinator	0.500%				
Wrist	**1.000**%	Endurance 0 = 0.500%			
		Endurance 1 = 0.400%			
		Endurance 2 = 0.300%			
		Endurance 3 = 0.200%			
		Endurance 4 = 0.100%			
Palmar flexors	0.500%				
Dorsiflexor	0.500%				
Hand: 15%					
Thumb:Index, middle, ring, and little fingers = 4:6					
MCP:PIP:DIP = 3:2:1					
Thumb	**6.000**%				
CMC and MCP joints	**5.000**%	Endurance 0 = 1.000%			
		Endurance 1 = 0.800%			
		Endurance 2 = 0.600%			
		Endurance 3 = 0.400%			
		Endurance 4 = 0.200%			
Flexor	1.000%				
Extensor	1.000%				
Adductor	1.000%				

(Continued)

Table 6.22 (*Continued*) Impairment evaluation—Endurance of muscle: Upper extremity

Muscle groups	Reference impairment score	Weightage Muscle endurance	% of endurance score—right	% of endurance score—left	Maximum impairment 20%
Abductor	1.000%				
Opponens	1.000%				
IP joint	**1.000%**	Endurance 0 = 0.500%			
		Endurance 1 = 0.400%			
		Endurance 2 = 0.300%			
		Endurance 3 = 0.200%			
		Endurance 4 = 0.100%			
Flexor	0.500%				
Extensor	0.500%				
MCP	**4.500%**	Endurance 0 = 1.125%			
Index		Endurance 1 = 0.900%			
Middle		Endurance 2 = 0.675%			
Ring		Endurance 3 = 0.450%			
Little		Endurance 4 = 0.225%			
Flexors	1.125%				
Extensors	1.125%				
Adductors	1.125%				
Abductors	1.125%				
PIP	**3.000%**	Endurance 0 = 1.500%			
Index		Endurance 1 = 1.200%			
Middle		Endurance 2 = 0.900%			
Ring		Endurance 3 = 0.600%			
Little		Endurance 4 = 0.300%			
Flexors	1.500%				
Extensor	1.500%				
DIP	**1.500%**	Endurance 0 = 0.750%			
Index		Endurance 1 = 0.600%			
Middle		Endurance 2 = 0.450%			
Ring		Endurance 3 = 0.300%			
Little		Endurance 4 = 0.150%			
Flexors	0.75%				
Extensor	0.75%				

Note: Muscle Endurance assessment is applicable only in Myasthenia Gravis, Myopathy, and Muscular Dystrophy.

Table 6.23 Impairment evaluation—Endurance of muscle: Lower extremity

Muscle groups	Reference impairment score	Weightage Muscle endurance	Endurance score—right	Endurance score—left	Maximum impairment should not exceed 13.333%
(Hip:Knee:Ankle:Foot:Toes = 1:2:4:2:1)					
Hip	1.333%	Endurance 0 = 0.222%			
		Endurance 1 = 0.177%			
		Endurance 2 = 0.133%			
		Endurance 3 = 0.088%			
		Endurance 4 = 0.044%			
Flexors	0.222%				
Extensors	0.222%				

(*Continued*)

Table 6.23 (*Continued*) Impairment evaluation—Endurance of muscle: Lower extremity

Muscle groups	Reference impairment score	Weightage Muscle endurance	Endurance score—right	Endurance score—left	Maximum impairment should not exceed 13.333%
Adductors	0.222%				
Abductors	0.222%				
Internal rotators	0.222%				
External rotators	0.222%				
Knee	2.666%	Endurance 0 = 1.333%			
		Endurance 1 = 1.066%			
		Endurance 2 = 0.799%			
		Endurance 3 = 0.533%			
		Endurance 4 = 0.266%			
Flexors	1.333%				
Extensors	1.333%				
Ankle	5.333%	Endurance 0 = 2.666%			
		Endurance 1 = 2.132%			
		Endurance 2 = 1.599%			
		Endurance 3 = 1.066%			
		Endurance 4 = 0.533%			
Plantar flexors	2.666%				
Dorsiflexor	2.666%				
Foot	2.666%	Endurance 0 = 1.333%			
		Endurance 1 = 1.066%			
		Endurance 2 = 0.799%			
		Endurance 3 = 0.533%			
		Endurance 4 = 0.266%			
Invertors	1.333%				
Evertors	1.333%				
Toes	1.333%				
Big toe:2nd:3rd:4th:5th toes = 4:2:2:1:1					
Big toe	0.533%	Endurance 0 = 0.266%			
		Endurance 1 = 0.212%			
		Endurance 2 = 0.159%			
		Endurance 3 = 0.106%			
		Endurance 4 = 0.053%			
Flexors	0.266%				
Extensors	0.266%				
2nd toe	0.266%	Endurance 0 = 0.133%			
		Endurance 1 = 0.106%			
		Endurance 2 = 0.079%			
		Endurance 3 = 0.053%			
		Endurance 4 = 0.026%			
Flexors	0.133%				
Extensors	0.133%				
3rd toe	0.266%	Endurance 0 = 0.133%			
		Endurance 1 = 0.106%			
		Endurance 2 = 0.079%			
		Endurance 3 = 0.053%			
		Endurance 4 = 0.026%			

(*Continued*)

Table 6.23 (*Continued*) Impairment evaluation—Endurance of muscle: Lower extremity

Muscle groups	Reference impairment score	Weightage Muscle endurance	Endurance score—right	Endurance score—left	Maximum impairment should not exceed 13.333%
Flexors	0.133%				
Extensors	0.133%				
4th toe	0.133%	Endurance 0 = 0.066%			
		Endurance 1 = 0.053%			
		Endurance 2 = 0.039%			
		Endurance 3 = 0.026%			
		Endurance 4 = 0.013%			
Flexors	0.066%				
Extensors	0.066%				
5th toe	0.133%	Endurance 0 = 0.066%			
		Endurance 1 = 0.053%			
		Endurance 2 = 0.039%			
		Endurance 3 = 0.026%			
		Endurance 4 = 0.013%			
Flexors	0.066%				
Extensors	0.066%				

Table 6.24 Impairment evaluation—Muscle endurance: Spine

Muscle groups	Reference impairment score	Weightage Muscle power	Impairment score right	Impairment score left	Maximum impairment 10%
Cervical spine	5.000%	Endurance 0 = 0.833%			
		Endurance 1 = 0.666%			
		Endurance 2 = 0.499%			
		Endurance 3 = 0.333%			
		Endurance 4 = 0.166%			
Flexors	0.833%				
Extensors	0.833%				
Lateral flexors—right	0.833%				
Lateral flexors—left	0.833%				
Rotators—right	0.833%				
Rotators—left	0.833%				
Dorsolumbar spine	5%	Endurance 0 = 0.833%			
		Endurance 1 = 0.666%			
		Endurance 2 = 0.499%			
		Endurance 3 = 0.333%			
		Endurance 4 = 0.166%			
Flexors	0.833%				
Extensors	0.833%				
Lateral flexors—right	0.833%				
Lateral flexors—left	0.833%				
Rotators—right	0.833%				
Rotators—left	0.833%				

6.8.2.1 VOLUNTARY MOVEMENT FUNCTION

The upper extremity derives maximum impairment of 20% for complete loss of voluntary movement (Table 6.25), lower extremity 10% (Table 6.26), and spine 10% (Table 6.27).

6.8.2.2 INVOLUNTARY MOVEMENT

Involuntary movement refers to a spontaneous sustained or intermittent contraction of a muscle or muscle groups without voluntary effort. It is often non-intentional or

Table 6.25 Impairment evaluation—Voluntary movement: Upper extremity

Clinical tools	Ability to perform the function partially	Assumes functional position and performs movement only within functional range	Inability to perform the function	Maximum impairment 20%
Uniaxial movement: Isolated voluntary movement—flexion of fingers or dorsiflexion of wrist or supination of forearm or flexion of elbow or flexion of shoulder	Performs isolated movement limiting to functional range in impairment of joint function or Performs synergic movement in half range in pyramidal lesions or Performs isolated movement with 50% limitation by rigidity in extrapyramidal lesion or Performs isolated movement against gravity only without resistance in impairment of lower motor neuron and muscle functions or Performs isolated movement such as raising the arm but overshoot in cerebellar lesion 0.25%	Performs isolated movement limiting to non-functional range in impairment of joint function or Performs synergic movement in full range in pyramidal lesion or Performs movement with more than 50% limitation by rigidity in extrapyramidal lesion or Performs isolated movement only in gravity eliminated plane in impairment of lower motor neuron and muscle functions or Performs isolated movement such as raising the arm but overshoot with several bounces in cerebellar lesion 0.50%	Inability to perform isolated movement or Performs isolated movement such as raising the arm but overshoot wildly with hyperextension of the metacarpophalangeal joint and wrist flexion in cerebellar lesion 1.00%	
Multiaxial/multiplane/multijoint movement: *Reaching behind the back:* The person reaches contralateral scapula either above the shoulder or below the shoulder with the fingers or *Finger nose finger test:* The person directs the movement of his/her index finger to his/her nose and then to the examiner's outstretched finger in the upper extremity. The examiner moves his/her finger with each repetition and observe for irregularity in amplitude and force of the extremity movement	Performs the movement partially or Overshoot/Undershoot with few oscillations in cerebellar lesion 1.50%	Initiates the movement but could not continue to perform the movement or Overshoot/ Undershoot with increased oscillation in cerebellar lesion 3.00%	Inability to perform the movement or Overshoot/ Undershoot with gross oscillation of extremity over more than a foot in cerebellar lesion 6.00%	

(Continued)

Table 6.25 (Continued) Impairment evaluation—Voluntary movement: Upper extremity

Clinical tools	Ability to perform the function partially	Assumes functional position and performs movement only within functional range	Inability to perform the function	Maximum impairment 20%
Coordination of movement				
Right left coordination: Ability to clap with both hands	Clapping with both hands in a clumsy way 0.50%	Takes up the position of clapping by both hands but could not clap 1%	Inability to perform the function 2%	
Eye-hand coordination: Prehensile function of the hand to hold the pen/pencil and to write a few sentences in a paper	Prehensile function to hold the pen/pencil is effortful, and letters are either micrographic or larger or letters are in irregular trajectory 1.00%	Assumes prehensile position to hold the pen/pencil but could not write 2.00%	Inability to perform the function 4.00%	
Rhythmic movement: Dysdiadochokinesia—Rapid repetitive alternate pronation and supination of the forearm at an optimum speed of 10 cycles within 10 seconds. In Cerebellar lesion, it is slow, irregular, coarse and trembling. In hypertonia, it is slow and clumsy. In Hypotonia and impairment of muscle function, it is slow with interruption. In impairment of joint function, the movement is limited.	Performs partially irregularly in the cerebellar lesion or Performs the movement, but is clumsy in hypertonia or Performs the movement slowly with impairment of lower motor neuron or muscle function 0.50%	Performs completely irregularly in cerebellar lesion or Performs the movement slowly and is clumsy in hypertonia or Performs the movement slowly with interruption in impairment of lower motor neuron or muscle function 1.00%	Inability to perform the movement 2.00%	
Stabilization of movement: ***Pushup:*** Lift the buttocks with both upper extremities while sitting and sustain for ten counts	Performs the movement partially 1.25%	Initiates the movement but could not continue to perform the movement 2.5%	Inability to perform the movement 5%	

Table 6.26 Impairment evaluation—Voluntary movement: Lower extremity

Clinical tools	Ability to perform the function slowly	Assumes functional position and/or performs isolated movement within the functional range	Inability to perform the function	Maximum impairment 10%
Uniaxial movement: Isolated voluntary movements—dorsiflexion of ankle, flexion of knee, abduction of hip	Performs isolated movement limiting to functional range or Performs synergic movement in half range in pyramidal lesions or Performs isolated movement with 50% limitation by rigidity in extrapyramidal lesion or Performs isolated movement against gravity only without resistance in impairment of lower motor neuron and muscle functions 0.25%	Performs isolated movement limiting to non-functional range or Performs synergic movement in full range in pyramidal lesion or Performs isolated movement with more than 50% limitation by rigidity in extrapyramidal lesion or Performs isolated movement only in gravity eliminated plane in impairment of lower motor neuron and muscle functions 0.5%	Inability to perform isolated movement 1%	
Multiaxial/multiplane/multijoint movement: Heel Knee Shin Test—The person, places the heel on the contralateral knee and then runs the heel down the shin of the tibia to the dorsum of the foot.	Performs the movement partially or side to side oscillation when the heel runs down the shin in cerebellar lesion 0.75%	Initiates the movement but could not continue to perform the movement or Heel overshoots the knee sideward, and rotatory oscillation as the heel approaches down the shin in cerebellar lesion 1.50%	Inability to perform the movement or Heel overshoots the knee sideward, and rotatory oscillation as the heel approaches down the shin and shoots off the foot without control in cerebellar lesion 3.00%	
Coordination of movement: *Right left coordination:* Reciprocal movement such as cycling movement of both lower extremities	Performs the movement partially 0.25%	Initiates the movement but could not continue to perform the movement 0.50%	Inability to perform the movement 1.00%	

(Continued)

Table 6.26 (Continued) Impairment evaluation—Voluntary movement: Lower extremity

Clinical tools	Ability to perform the function slowly	Assumes functional position and/or performs isolated movement within the functional range	Inability to perform the function	Maximum impairment 10%
Eye foot coordination: Ability to touch the examiner's outstretched hand with his/her big toe by raising his/her one leg while lying down	Performs the movement partially 0.25%	Initiates to perform the movement with his/her big toe and the leg bounces several times, and overshoot in cerebellar lesions 0.50%	Inability to perform the movement 1.00%	
Rhythmic movement: Tapping the floor with the foot by rapid alternate plantar and dorsiflexion of ankle	Performs the movement but clumsy or performs partially irregularly 0.25%	Performs the movement slowly and is clumsy or performs completely irregularly 0.5%	Inability to perform the movement 1%	
Stabilization of movement: Able to stabilize the body without staggering or fall during heel to toe walking—Tandem walking: The person is asked to walk keeping the heel touching big toe of the rear foot in straight line for ten steps, turn and walk another ten steps toward the initial point (Also evaluates cerebellar lesions)	Performs the function but staggers during turning 0.750%	Performs the function with staggering and tends to fall or seeks the support of a person or wall 1.500%	Inability to perform the function 3.000%	

Table 6.27 Impairment evaluation—Voluntary movement: Spine

Clinical tools	Ability to perform the function partially	Initiates the function but could not continue to perform the movement	Inability to perform the function	Maximum impairment 10%
Uniaxial movement *Cervical Spine:* Flexion/extension or *Dorsolumbar Spine:* Flexion/extension	Performs isolated movement limiting to functional range Or Performs the movement partially 0.25%	Performs isolated movement limiting to non-functional range or Initiates the movement but could not continue to perform the movement 0.5%	Inability to perform the movement 1%	
Multiaxial/multiplane movement *Cervical Spine:* Spurling Maneuver or *Dorsolumbar Spine:* Hyperextension and Rotation Maneuver	Performs the movement partially 0.75%	Initiates the movement but could not continue to perform the movement 1.5%	Inability to perform the movement 3%	
Coordination of movement Ability to sit without staggering: Evaluate impairment of cerebellar function—truncal ataxia	Able to sit without staggering but staggers when pushed aside 0.750%	Able to sit with a tendency to stagger 1.500%	Unable to sit due to staggering with a fall 3.000%	
Stabilization of movement *Cervical Spine:* Cervical spine serves to support the weight of the head (about 5 kg) as well as to tolerate minimum head load of 7 kg *Dorsolumbar Spine:* Ability to sit without any hand support	*Cervical Spine:* Ability to hold the head and finding difficult to carry minimum head load of about 7 kg or *Dorsolumbar Spine:* Sitting upright with one hand support 0.75%	*Cervical Spine:* Ability to hold the head and but inability to carry minimum head load of about 7 kg or *Dorsolumbar Spine:* Sitting upright with both hand support 1.5%	*Cervical Spine:* Inability to hold the head resulting in head lag or *Dorsolumbar Spine:* Inability to sit upright even with both hand support 3%	

quasi-purposive or non-purposive (24). Involuntary movements are best identified while taking history, while lying still with the eyes gently closed and during ambulation.

Tremors are abnormal involuntary movements that are rhythmical either resting (or) postural (or) intentional. Chorea is a rapid, jerky non-repetitive involuntary movement. Chorea may involve both proximal, distal muscles and tongue. Respiratory irregularity may accompany chorea. Athetosis is a slow, writhing involuntary movement. Dystonia is a twisting, repetitive, involuntary movement due to co-contraction of agonist and antagonist. It may be painful. Ballismus is a violent flinging involuntary movement. It may affect axial and proximal muscles or one-half of the body. Involuntary movement derives maximum impairment of 20% for upper extremity (Table 6.28) and 10% for lower extremity (Table 6.29) and 10% for spine (Table 6.30).

6.8.2.3 BRADYKINESIA—PAUCITY OF MOVEMENT

Bradykinesia, or paucity of movement, manifests slowing of movement with a progressive decrement in speed or amplitude (36), and the paucity of spontaneous movement. The speech is monotone and hypophonic. Decreased or loss of facial expression, decreased or loss of eye blinking, and mask-like face with or without parted lips present with facial bradykinesia. Persons with bradykinesia may present with drooling of saliva due to impairment of spontaneous swallowing of saliva. Section 4.5.10.1.3.3 in Chapter 4 describes clinical tests to evaluate the severity of bradykinesia. The upper extremity derives maximum impairment of 20% for bradykinesia (Table 6.31) and lower extremity 10% (Table 6.32) and spine 10% (Table 6.33).

Table 6.28 Impairment class—Involuntary movement functions: Upper extremity

Involuntary movement	Class 1 present in <25% of the waking day	Class 2 present in 25%–50% of the waking day	Class 3 present in >50% of the waking day	Maximum impairment 20%
Tremor	0.50%	1.0%	2%	
Chorea	0.75%	1.5%	3%	
Athetosis	0.75%	1.5%	3%	
Dystonia	1%	2%	4%	
Hemiballismus	2%	4%	8%	

Table 6.29 Impairment class—Involuntary movement functions: Lower extremity

Involuntary movement	Class 1 present in <25% of the waking day	Class 2 present in 25%–50% of the waking day	Class 3 present in >50% of the waking day	Maximum impairment score 10%
Chorea	0.375%	0.750%	1.500%	
Athetosis	0.375%	0.750%	1.500%	
Dystonia	0.750%	1.500%	3.000%	
Hemiballismus	1.000%	2.000%	4.000%	

Table 6.30 Impairment class—Involuntary movement functions: Spine

Involuntary movement	Class 1 present in <25% of the waking day	Class 2 present in 25%–50% of the waking day	Class 3 present in >50% of the waking day	Maximum impairment score 10%
Titubation	0.5%	1%	2%	
Dystonia	0.75%	1.5%	3%	
Ballismus	1.25%	2.5%	5%	

Table 6.31 Impairment evaluation—Paucity of movement/bradykinesia: Upper extremity

Clinical tools	Slow performance	Incomplete performance	No performance	Maximum impairment 20%
	Performs the movement at a slow speed with reduced amplitude	Performs the movement but progressive loss of speed and amplitude with freezing of movement	Inability to perform the movement	
Finger tapping test: Rapid and repetitive tapping of the thumb with index finger	1.25%	2.5%	5%	
Rapid and repetitive hand opening and closing	1.25%	2.5%	5%	
Rapid and repetitive pronation and supination of forearm	1.25%	2.5%	5%	
Rapid and repetitive shoulder elevation and depression of shoulder	1.25%	2.5%	5%	

Table 6.32 Impairment evaluation—Paucity of movement/bradykinesia: Lower extremity

Clinical tests	Slow performance	Incomplete performance	No performance	Maximum impairment 10%
Foot agility test: The person taps the forefoot on the ground with rapid speed and amplitude while heel is resting on the ground	Performs the movement at a slow speed with reduced amplitude 0.75%	Performs the movement but progressive loss of speed and amplitude with freezing of movement 1.5%	Inability to perform the movement 3%	
Leg agility test: The person taps heel on the ground and raising the leg as much as 3 inches in rapid succession	Performs the movement at slow speed and with reduced amplitude 0.75%	Performs the movement but progressive loss of speed and amplitude with freezing of movement 1.5%	Inability to perform the movement 3%	
Sit to stand agility: Ability to perform repetitive movement, i.e., getting up from sitting to standing position from the chair	Performs repetitive movement slowly and with difficulty 1%	Progressive difficulty in performing repetitive movement and could not continue the movement 2%	Inability to perform the movement 4%	

Table 6.33 Impairment evaluation of paucity of movement/bradykinesia—Spine

Clinical tools	Slow performance Ability to perform the function slowly	Incomplete performance Perform the function with difficulty	No performance Inability to perform the function	Assigned impairment
Truncal agility: Ability to perform repetitive movement from supine to sitting position	Performs the function slowly but with difficulty during repetition 2.5%	Progressive difficulty in performing the movement and could not continue the movement 5%	Inability to perform the function 10%	

Table 6.34 Impairment evaluation of gait—Translation movement

Gait translation of movement	Independent ambulation with specified gait deviation	Abnormal gait and ambulant with cane	Abnormal gait and ambulant with orthosis or prosthesis and crutch	Abnormal gait and ambulant with orthosis or prosthesis and Walker	Non-ambulant even with orthosis or prosthesis and Walker	Maximum impairment
Percentage of impairment	1.25%	2.5%	5%	7.5%	10%	10%

6.8.2.4 TRANSLATION OF MOVEMENT FUNCTIONS—GAIT

Gait pattern movement relates to translation of a body from one point to another. It is connected with walking and running, and so on (37). In hemiplegia, the person presents with circumduction gait with adduction at the shoulder, flexion of elbow, wrist and fingers and extension of hip, knee, and ankle. Table 6.34 describes impairment classes for gait pattern functions. Persons with paraplegia walk with scissoring gait with stiff lower extremities. Persons with apraxia walks with short shuffling gait with stooped posture with the delay in the initiation and often interrupted by freezing. Persons with parkinsonism walk with shuffling gait with short steps decreased arm swing and stooped posture or festinating gait with faster steps and often associated with propulsion and retropulsion or tremor or walking interrupted by difficulty in turning or freezing with a tendency to fall or associated with fall. Persons with ataxia walk with wide-based gait with irregular speed and step. The person spreads his or her legs apart to widen the base of support to compensate for the imbalance while walking. In severe cases, the person swings the leg irregularly and tends to reel in several sideward steps. Persons with choreoathetosis walk with a gait with disruption of normal pattern with a pelvic lurch, and flexion and extension of the hip and intermittent irregular choreoathetoid movement. In waddling gait, the person walks with bilateral pelvic lift and rotation. In high stepping gait, the person walks with foot drop and high stepping. In antalgic gait, the person walks with painful limp while walking.

6.9 SENSORY FUNCTIONS

Sensory function comprises of exteroceptive sensation, proprioceptive sensation, and cortical sensation. In exteroceptive sensation, an external stimulus such as touch, pinprick, thermal stimulus activates corresponding receptors and evokes the perception of sensation. In proprioceptive sensation, internal stimulus activates the receptors located in ligaments, muscles, tendons, and joints to provide kinesthetic information to the brain. In cortical sensation, parietal lobe analyses interpret and discriminate individual sensory stimulus.

6.9.1 Exteroceptive sensation

A wisp of cotton evokes a touch sensation with the person's eyes closed. Hot water at a temperature of about 110°F and chilly water at 45°F in a test tube evokes the perception of temperature sensation. A pinprick with both sharp end and smooth head differentially evokes the perception of pain sensation.

6.9.2 Proprioceptive sensation

Evaluation of proprioceptive sensation comprises of joint and position sense, and vibration sense. During evaluation of joint position sense, the examiner holds the extremity laterally distal to the joint and passively moves the joint with minimal movement and the examinee responds about the sensation of joint movement as well as the position of the joint. The examiner uses tuning fork with a frequency of 128 Hz to elicit vibration sense and compares the response in proximal and distal segments.

6.9.3 "Three-Point Scale"

The "Three-Point Scale" evaluates sensory modality over a dermatome/nerve distribution and grade intact sensory function as no impairment, partial loss as partial impairment, and total loss as complete impairment. *Integrated Evaluation of Disability* defines partial impairment if there is a loss of "Two-Point" discrimination, joint and position sense or vibration sense with intact touch, pain, and temperature sensation. It also defines partial impairment when complete sensory loss confines only to the digital nerve with intact sensation in proximal segments of the nerve.

6.9.4 Pain

The visual analogue scale (VAS) assesses the severity of chronic pain (38). *Integrated Evaluation of Disability* assigns an impairment of 1% if VAS is 1, 2% if VAS is 2, 3% if VAS is 3, and a maximum of 10% impairment if VAS is 10. Alternatively, the following guideline can serve to grade the pain. It assigns grade 0 for no pain, grade 2 for annoying minimal pain, and grade 4 for uncomfortable resting pain eased out by activity. It also assigns grade 6 for dreadful pain and performs an activity with discomfort, grade 8 for severe, persistent pain and cannot perform any activity, and grade 10 for maximum pain and cannot bear it. It assigns maximum impairment of 10% for congenital absence of pain/congenital indifference to pain (Table 6.35).

6.9.5 Sensory ataxia—Rombergism

The person stands stationary with the feet together. If he/she can maintain this posture, the person closes the eyes for 5–10 seconds. In positive Romberg, the person tends to sway, but able to keep his/her both feet together, or sway markedly, or may tend to fall or tends to keep his/her legs apart for a broader base. *Integrated Evaluation of Disability* assigns maximum impairment of 10% for positive Romberg.

6.9.6 Cortical sensation

Cortical sensation consists of stereognosis, "Two-Point" discrimination, and graphesthesia. Stereognosis refers to the ability of a person to recognize known objects, such as a coin, key, or pen, with their eyes closed. Astereognosis indicates the inability of a person to recognize objects by touch sensation with the eyes closed. "Two-Point" discrimination represents the ability to perceive the double stimuli applied simultaneously by a pair of calipers with blunt ends. If the person is unable to discriminate and recognize two points, they are deemed to have an impairment of "Two-Point" discrimination. In graphesthesia, a person can recognize either the alphabet or numbers written on their skin by the perception of touch (Tables 6.36 through 6.38).

6.9.7 Sensory perversions

Sensory perversions comprise paresthesia and dysesthesia. Paresthesia is abnormal sensation evoked without any stimulus. It may be a tactile or thermal or burning sensation. Dysesthesia is a painful sensation evoked by a light touch over the affected area (Tables 6.39 through 6.41).

Table 6.35 Impairment evaluation of sensory functions—Pain

Pain	VAS 1	VAS 2	VAS 3	VAS 4	VAS 5	VAS 6	VAS 7	VAS 8	VAS 9	VAS 10	Max 10

Table 6.36 Impairment of sensory functions—Cortical sensation: Upper extremity

Cortical sensation	Normal function	Difficulty in perception	Inability in perception	Maximum impairment 10%
Stereognosis: Stereognosis represents the ability to recognize the known objects such as coin, key, pen with eyes closed. Astereognosis indicates the inability to recognize the objects eyes closed with touch sensation.	0%	2.5%	5%	
Two-point discrimination: The two-point discrimination represents the ability to perceive the double stimuli applied using a pair of calipers. A normal person could discriminate and recognize simultaneously applied double stimuli at a distance 1 mm in tongue, 2 mm in fingertips, 4–6 mm in the dorsal aspect of the fingers, 8–12 mm in palmar surface of the hand, 20–30 mm in the dorsal surface of the hand.	0%	1.25%	2.5%	
Graphesthesia: In graphesthesia, a person can recognize the letters or numerical written over his/her skin by the perception of touch.	0%	1.25%	2.5%	

Table 6.37 Impairment of sensory functions—Cortical sensation: Lower extremity

Cortical sensation	Normal function	Difficulty in perception	Inability in perception	Maximum impairment 5%
Two-point discrimination: The two-point discrimination represents the ability to perceive the double stimuli applied using a pair of calipers. Normal person could discriminate and recognize simultaneously applied double stimuli at a distance 1 mm in tongue, 2 mm in finger tips, 4–6 mm in dorsal aspect of the fingers, 8–12 mm in palmar surface of the hand, 20–30 mm in dorsal surface of the hand.	0%	1.25%	2.5%	
Graphesthesia: In graphesthesia, a person can recognize the letters or numerical written over his/her skin by the perception of touch.	0%	1.25%	2.5%	

Table 6.38 Impairment of sensory functions—Cortical sensation: Neck and trunk

Cortical sensation	Normal function	Difficulty in perception	Inability in perception	Maximum impairment 5%
Two-point discrimination: The two-point discrimination represents the ability to perceive the double stimuli applied using a pair of calipers.	0%	1.25%	2.5%	
Graphesthesia: In graphesthesia, a person can recognize the letters or numerical written over his/her skin by the perception of touch.	0%	1.25%	2.5%	

Table 6.39 Impairment of sensory functions—Sensory perversions: Upper extremity

Sensory perversions	Normal sensation	Intermittent manifestation	Persistent whole day	Maximum impairment 10%
Paresthesia: Paresthesia are abnormal sensation evoked without any stimulus. It may be tactile, thermal, and burning.	0%	2.5%	5%	
Dysesthesia: Dysesthesia is painful stimulation evoked by a light touch over the affected area.	0%	2.5%	5%	

Table 6.40 Impairment of sensory functions—Sensory perversions: Lower extremity

Sensory perversions	Normal sensation	Intermittent manifestation	Persistent whole day	Maximum impairment 5%
Paresthesia: Paresthesia are abnormal sensation evoked without any stimulus. It may be tactile, thermal, and burning.	0%	2.5%	5%	
Dysesthesia: Dysesthesia is painful stimulation evoked by a light touch over the affected area.	0%	2.5%	5%	

Table 6.41 Impairment of sensory functions—Sensory perversions: Neck and trunk

Sensory perversions	Normal sensation	Intermittent manifestation	Persistent whole day	Maximum impairment 5%
Paresthesia: Paresthesia are abnormal sensation evoked without any stimulus. It may be tactile, thermal, and burning.	0%	2.5%	5%	
Dysesthesia: Dysesthesia is painful stimulation evoked by a light touch over the affected area.	0%	2.5%	5%	

6.9.8 Impairment of sensory function

The upper extremity derives an impairment of 30% for exteroceptive and proprioceptive sensation, 10% for cortical sensation, 10% for sensory perversions, and 10% for pain in upper extremity with a maximum of 60%. The lower extremity derives an impairment of 20% for exteroceptive and proprioceptive sensation, 5% for cortical sensation, 5% for sensory perversions, and 10% for pain with a maximum of 40%. One-half of the neck and trunk derive an impairment of 10% for exteroceptive and proprioceptive sensation, 5% for cortical sensation, 5% for sensory perversions, and 10% for pain with a maximum of 30%. Figures 6.2 through 6.4 depict dermatome distribution of upper extremity, lower extremity, and spine.

The upper extremity dermatome representing C6 derives 8%, C7—8% and C8—8%, C5—3% and T1—3% for exteroceptive sensation (Table 6.42). In lower extremity, dermatomes representing L1 derives 0.5%, L2—1.5%, L3—1.5%, L4—2%, L5—6%, S1—6%, S2—1.5%, and S3,4,5, Cx1—1% for exteroceptive sensation (Table 6.43). In neck and trunk, each dermatome derives maximum impairment of 0.75% for C2–C4 and 0.70% for T1–T12 for exteroceptive sensation (Table 6.44). The evaluators should make sure that there are positive correlating neurological findings before assigning impairment to the sensory deficit as it is a subjective symptom (Illustration 6.4).

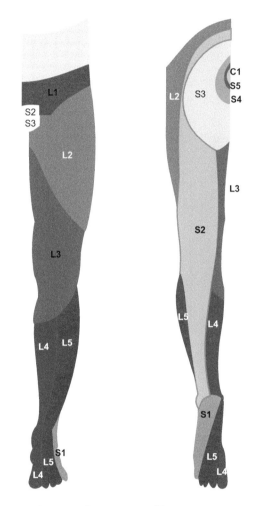

Figure 6.3 Sensory dermatome of lower extremity.

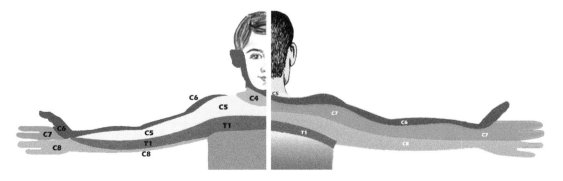

Figure 6.2 Sensory dermatome of upper extremity.

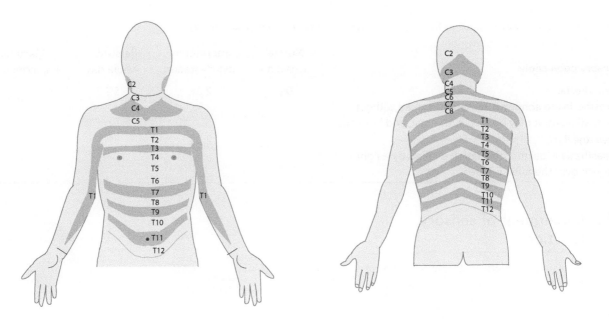

Figure 6.4 Spine—Sensory dermatome spine.

Table 6.42 Impairment evaluation—Sensory functions: Upper extremity (dermatome)

Dermatome	Reference impairment score	Weightage	Sensory loss— Touch total or partial	Sensory loss— Pain total or partial	Sensory loss— Thermal total or partial	Sensory loss— Vibration total or partial	Maximum impairment 30%
C5 dermatome	3%	Touch total loss = 0.75% Touch partial loss = 0.375% Pain total loss = 0.75% Pain partial loss = 0.375% Thermal total loss = 0.75% Thermal partial loss = 0.375% Vibration total loss = 0.75% Vibration partial loss = 0.375%					
C6 dermatome	8%	Touch total loss = 2% Touch partial loss = 1% Pain total loss = 2% Pain partial loss = 1% Thermal total loss = 2% Thermal partial loss = 1% Vibration total loss = 2% Vibration partial loss = 1%					
C7 dermatome	8%	Touch total loss = 2% Touch partial loss = 1% Pain total loss = 2% Pain partial loss = 1% Thermal total loss = 2% Thermal partial loss = 1% Vibration total loss = 2% Vibration partial loss = 1%					

(Continued)

Table 6.42 (*Continued*) Impairment evaluation—Sensory functions: Upper extremity (dermatome)

Dermatome	Reference impairment score	Weightage	Sensory loss— Touch total or partial	Sensory loss— Pain total or partial	Sensory loss— Thermal total or partial	Sensory loss— Vibration total or partial	Maximum impairment 30%
C8 dermatome	8%	Touch total loss = 2% Touch partial loss = 1% Pain total loss = 2% Pain partial loss = 1% Thermal total loss = 2% Thermal partial loss = 1% Vibration total loss = 2% Vibration partial loss = 1%					
T1 dermatome	3%	Touch total loss = 0.75% Touch partial loss = 0.375% Pain total loss = 0.75% Pain partial loss = 0.375% Thermal total loss = 0.75% Thermal partial loss = 0.375% Vibration total loss = 0.75% Vibration partial loss = 0.375%					

Table 6.43 Impairment evaluation—Sensory functions: Lower extremity (dermatome)

Dermatome	Reference impairment score	Weightage	Sensory loss— Touch partial or total	Sensory loss— Pain partial or total	Sensory loss— Thermal partial or total	Sensory loss— Vibration partial/total	Maximum impairment 20%
L1 dermatome	0.500%	Touch total loss = 0.1250% Touch partial loss = 0.0625% Pain total loss = 0.1250% Pain partial loss = 0.0625% Thermal total loss = 0.1250% Thermal partial loss = 0.0625% Vibration total loss = 0.1250% Vibration partial loss = 0.0625%					
L2 dermatome	1.500%	Touch total loss = 0.3750% Touch partial loss = 0.1875% Pain total loss = 0.3750% Pain partial loss = 0.1875% Thermal total loss = 0.3750% Thermal partial loss = 0.1875% Vibration total loss = 0.3750% Vibration partial loss = 0.1875%					

(Continued)

Table 6.43 (*Continued*) Impairment evaluation—Sensory functions: Lower extremity (dermatome)

Dermatome	Reference impairment score	Weightage	Sensory loss— Touch partial or total	Sensory loss— Pain partial or total	Sensory loss— Thermal partial or total	Sensory loss— Vibration partial/total	Maximum impairment 20%
L3 dermatome	1.500%	Touch total loss = 0.3750% Touch partial loss = 0.1875% Pain total loss = 0.3750% Pain partial loss = 0.1875% Thermal total loss = 0.3750% Thermal partial loss = 0.1875% Vibration total loss = 0.3750% Vibration partial loss = 0.1875%					
L4 dermatome	2.000%	Touch total loss = 0.50% Touch partial loss = 0.25% Pain total loss = 0.50% Pain partial loss = 0.25% Thermal total loss = 0.50% Thermal partial loss = 0.25% Vibration total loss = 0.50% Vibration partial loss = 0.25%					
L5 dermatome	6.000%	Touch total loss = 1.5% Touch partial loss = 0.75% Pain total loss = 1.5% Pain partial loss = 0.75% Thermal total loss = 1.5% Thermal partial loss = 0.75% Vibration total loss = 1.5% Vibration partial loss = 0.75%					
S1 dermatome	6.000%	Touch total loss = 1.5% Touch partial loss = 0.75% Pain total loss = 1.5% Pain partial loss = 0.75% Thermal total loss = 1.5% Thermal partial loss = 0.75% Vibration total loss = 1.5% Vibration partial loss = 0.75%					
S2 dermatome	1.500%	Touch total loss = 0.3750% Touch partial loss = 0.1875% Pain total loss = 0.3750% Pain partial loss = 0.1875% Thermal total loss = 0.3750% Thermal partial loss = 0.1875% Vibration total loss = 0.3750% Vibration partial loss = 0.1875%					
S3,4,5, C1 dermatome	1.000%	Touch total loss = 0.250% Touch partial loss = 0.125% Pain total loss = 0.250% Pain partial loss = 0.125% Thermal total loss = 0.250% Thermal partial loss = 0.125% Vibration total loss = 0.250% Vibration partial loss = 0.125%					

Table 6.44 Impairment evaluation—Sensory functions: Right/left neck and trunk

Spinal segment	Reference impairment score	Weightage	Sensory loss—Touch partial or total	Sensory loss—Pain partial or total	Sensory loss—Thermal partial or total	Sensory loss—Vibration partial or total	Maximum impairment score—10%
C2 dermatome	0.75%	Touch total loss = 0.187% Touch partial loss = 0.094% Pain total loss = 0.187% Pain partial loss = 0.094% Thermal total loss = 0.187% Thermal partial loss = 0.094% Vibration total loss = 0.187% Vibration partial loss = 0.094%					
C3 dermatome	0.75%	Touch total loss = 0.187% Touch partial loss = 0.094% Pain total loss = 0.187% Pain partial loss = 0.094% Thermal total loss = 0.187% Thermal partial loss = 0.094% Vibration total loss = 0.187% Vibration partial loss = 0.094%					
C4 dermatome	0.75%	Touch total loss = 0.187% Touch partial loss = 0.094% Pain total loss = 0.187% Pain partial loss = 0.094% Thermal total loss = 0.187% Thermal partial loss = 0.094% Vibration total loss = 0.187% Vibration partial loss = 0.094%					
T2 dermatome	0.70%	Touch total loss = 0.175% Touch partial loss = 0.088% Pain total loss = 0.175% Pain partial loss = 0.088% Thermal total loss = 0.175% Thermal partial loss = 0.088% Vibration total loss = 0.175% Vibration partial loss = 0.088%					
T3 dermatome	0.70%	Touch total loss = 0.175% Touch partial loss = 0.088% Pain total loss = 0.175% Pain partial loss = 0.088% Thermal total loss = 0.175% Thermal partial loss = 0.088% Vibration total loss = 0.175% Vibration partial loss = 0.088%					
T4 dermatome	0.70%	Touch total loss = 0.175% Touch partial loss = 0.088% Pain total loss = 0.175% Pain partial loss = 0.088% Thermal total loss = 0.175% Thermal partial loss = 0.088% Vibration total loss = 0.175% Vibration partial loss = 0.088%					

(Continued)

Table 6.44 (*Continued*) Impairment evaluation—Sensory functions: Right/left neck and trunk

Spinal segment	Reference impairment score	Weightage	Sensory loss—Touch partial or total	Sensory loss—Pain partial or total	Sensory loss—Thermal partial or total	Sensory loss—Vibration partial or total	Maximum impairment score—10%
T5 dermatome	0.70%	Touch total loss = 0.175% Touch partial loss = 0.088% Pain total loss = 0.175% Pain partial loss = 0.088% Thermal total loss = 0.175% Thermal partial loss = 0.088% Vibration total loss = 0.175% Vibration partial loss = 0.088%					
T6 dermatome	0.70%	Touch total loss = 0.175% Touch partial loss = 0.088% Pain total loss = 0.175% Pain partial loss = 0.088% Thermal total loss = 0.175% Thermal partial loss = 0.088% Vibration total loss = 0.175% Vibration partial loss = 0.088%					
T7 dermatome	0.70%	Touch total loss = 0.175% Touch partial loss = 0.088% Pain total loss = 0.175% Pain partial loss = 0.088% Thermal total loss = 0.175% Thermal partial loss = 0.088% Vibration total loss = 0.175% Vibration partial loss = 0.088%					
T8 dermatome	0.70%	Touch total loss = 0.175% Touch partial loss = 0.088% Pain total loss = 0.175% Pain partial loss = 0.088% Thermal total loss = 0.175% Thermal partial loss = 0.088% Vibration total loss = 0.175% Vibration partial loss = 0.088%					
T9 dermatome	0.70%	Touch total loss = 0.175% Touch partial loss = 0.088% Pain total loss = 0.175% Pain partial loss = 0.088% Thermal total loss = 0.175% Thermal partial loss = 0.088% Vibration total loss = 0.175% Vibration partial loss = 0.088%					
T10 dermatome	0.70%	Touch total loss = 0.175% Touch partial loss = 0.088% Pain total loss = 0.175% Pain partial loss = 0.088% Thermal total loss = 0.175% Thermal partial loss = 0.088% Vibration total loss = 0.175% Vibration partial loss = 0.088%					

(*Continued*)

Table 6.44 (*Continued*) Impairment evaluation—Sensory functions: Right/left neck and trunk

Spinal segment	Reference impairment score	Weightage	Sensory loss— Touch partial or total	Sensory loss— Pain partial or total	Sensory loss— Thermal partial or total	Sensory loss— Vibration partial or total	Maximum impairment score—10%
T11 dermatome	0.70%	Touch total loss = 0.175% Touch partial loss = 0.088% Pain total loss = 0.175% Pain partial loss = 0.088% Thermal total loss = 0.175% Thermal partial loss = 0.088% Vibration total loss = 0.175% Vibration partial loss = 0.088%					
T12 dermatome	0.70%	Touch total loss = 0.175% Touch partial loss = 0.088% Pain total loss = 0.175% Pain partial loss = 0.088% Thermal total loss = 0.175% Thermal partial loss = 0.088% Vibration total loss = 0.175% Vibration partial loss = 0.088%					

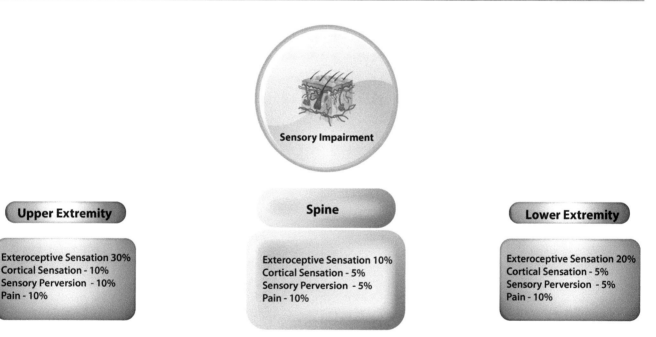

Illustration 6.4 Sensory impairment.

6.10 COMBINING IMPAIRMENTS

In upper motor neuron lesions, evaluation includes only muscle tone functions, movement functions, mobility of joint functions, gait pattern functions, and sensory functions. However, evaluation does not include muscle power and endurance functions, and stability of joint functions.

Formula

$$A + B\left[\frac{100 - A}{100}\right] \tag{6.2}$$

combines motor and sensory impairments of extremities; and impairments of visual, language, articulation, swallowing, and urination functions, if any, to arrive at the whole person impairment score.

6.11 "READY RECKONER IMPAIRMENT TABLE"

Integrated Evaluation of Disability developed a "Ready Reckoner Impairment Table" (see Chapter 23) for common clinical conditions based on a clinical model for easy reference by the audience.

REFERENCES

1. *International Classification of Functioning, Disability and Health.* Geneva, Switzerland: World Health Organization; 2001. pp. 48–49.
2. American Academy of Neurology. Practice parameters: Assessment and management of patients in the persistent vegetative state (summary statement). American Academy of Neurology Quality Standards Subcommittee. *Neurology.* 1994;45:1015–1018.
3. *Seizure Classification* [Internet]. International League Against Epilepsy; 2014.
4. Krumholz A, Wiebe S, Gronseth G, Shinnar S, Levisohn P, Ting T et al. Practice parameter: Evaluating an apparent unprovoked first seizure in adults (an evidence-based review): Report of the Quality Standards Subcommittee of the American Academy of Neurology and the American Epilepsy Society. *Neurology.* 2007;69(21):1996–2007.
5. Hirsch LJ, Donner EJ, So EL, Jacobs M, Nashef L, Noebels JL et al. Abbreviated report of the NIH/NINDS workshop on sudden unexpected death in epilepsy. *Neurology.* 2011;76(22):1932–1938.
6. *The Epilepsies: The Diagnosis and Management of the Epilepsies in Adults and Children in Primary and Secondary Care: Pharmacological Update of Clinical Guideline 20.* London, UK: National Institute for Health and Clinical Excellence; 2012.
7. Buysse DJ. Sleep health: Can we define it? Does it matter? *Sleep.* 2014;37(1):9–17.
8. *International Classification of Functioning, Disability and Health.* Geneva, Switzerland: World Health Organization; 2001. p. 52.
9. Chronic Insomnia: Final Panel Statement. *NIH State-of-the-Science Conference on Manifestations and Management of Chronic Insomnia in Adults.* NIH Consensus Development Program, Office of Disease Prevention, U.S. Department of Health & Human Services; 2005.
10. Schutte-Rodin S, Broch L, Buysse D, Dorsey C, Sateia M. Clinical guideline for the evaluation and management of chronic insomnia in adults. *J Clin Sleep Med.* 2008;4(5):487–504.
11. Vgontzas AN, Fernandez-Mendoza J, Liao D, Bixler EO. Insomnia with objective short sleep duration: The most biologically severe phenotype of the disorder. *Sleep Med Rev.* 2013;17(4):241–254.
12. Krasnianski A, Sanchez Juan P, Ponto C, Bartl M, Heinemann U, Varges D et al. A proposal of new diagnostic pathway for fatal familial insomnia. *J Neurol Neurosurg Psychiatry.* 2014;85(6):654–659.
13. *International Classification of Functioning, Disability and Health.* Geneva, Switzerland: World Health Organization; 2001. pp. 57–59.
14. *International Classification of Functioning, Disability and Health.* Geneva, Switzerland: World Health Organization; 2001. p. 60.
15. *International Classification of Functioning, Disability and Health.* Geneva, Switzerland: World Health Organization; 2001. p. 71.
16. Stuttering [Internet]. National Institute on Deaf and other Communication Disorders (NIDCD); 2010. Available from: http://www.nidcd.nih.gov/health/voice/pages/stutter.aspx.
17. *International Classification of Functioning, Disability and Health.* Geneva, Switzerland: World Health Organization; 2001. pp. 55–56.
18. Burkat CN, Oh D. Margin to reflex distance 1,2,3. American Academy of Ophthalmology; 2018. Available from: http://eyewiki.aao.org/.
19. *International Classification of Functioning, Disability and Health.* Geneva, Switzerland: World Health Organization; 2001. p. 96.
20. *International Classification of Functioning, Disability and Health.* Geneva, Switzerland: World Health Organization; 2001. p. 81.
21. *International Classification of Functioning, Disability and Health.* Geneva, Switzerland: World Health Organization; 2001. p. 64.
22. *International Classification of Functioning, Disability and Health.* Geneva, Switzerland: World Health Organization; 2001. p. 82.
23. ACR Appropriateness Criteria® dysphagia [Internet]. American College of Radiology; 2010.
24. *International Classification of Functioning, Disability and Health.* Geneva, Switzerland: World Health Organization; 2001. pp. 98–99.
25. Knierim J. Section 3: Motor system, Chapter 6: Disorders of the motor system. In: *Neuroscience Online* [Internet]. Department of Neurobiology and Anatomy, University of Texas Medical School; 1997. Available from: http://neuroscience.uth.tmc.edu/.
26. Bohannon RW, Smith MB. Interrater reliability of a modified Ashworth scale of muscle spasticity. *Phys Ther.* 1987;67(2):206–207.

27. Hoffman MD. Adaptations to endurance exercise training. In: Frontera WR, Dawson DM, Slovik DM, editors. *Exercise in Rehabilitation Medicine*, 2nd ed. Champaign, IL: Human Kinetics; 2006.

28. Knierim J. Section 3: Motor system, Chapter 1: Motor units and muscle receptors. In: *Neuroscience Online* [Internet]. Houston, TX: Department of Neurobiology and Anatomy, University of Texas Medical School; 1997.

29. Radomski MV, Latham CAT. *Occupational Therapy for Physical Dysfunction*, 6th ed. Philadelphia, PA: Lippincott Williams & Wilkins; 2008.

30. Fielding RA, Bean J. Acute physiological responses to dynamic exercise. In: *Exercise in Rehabilitation Medicine*. Champaign, IL: Human Kinetics; 2006.

31. Mazurek K, Krawczyk K, Zmijewski P, Norkowski H, Czajkowska A. Effects of aerobic interval training versus continuous moderate exercise programme on aerobic and anaerobic capacity, somatic features and blood lipid profile in collegate females. *Ann Agric Environ Med.* 2014;21(4):844–849.

32. Van Cant J, Pineux C, Pitance L, Feipel V. Hip muscle strength and endurance in females with patellofemoral pain: A systematic review with meta-analysis. *Int J Sports Phys Ther.* 2014;9(5):564–582.

33. Demura S, Yamaji S, Goshi F, Nagasawa Y. Lateral dominance of legs in maximal muscle power, muscular endurance, and grading ability. *Percept Motor Skills.* 2001;93(1):11–23.

34. White C, Dixon K, Samuel D, Stokes M. Handgrip and quadriceps muscle endurance testing in young adults. *SpringerPlus.* 2013;2:451.

35. Mathiowetz V, Kashman N, Volland G, Weber K, Dowe M, Rogers S. Grip and pinch strength: Normative data for adults. *Arch Phys Med Rehabil.* 1985(66):69–72.

36. Massano J, Bhatia KP. Clinical approach to Parkinson's disease: Features, diagnosis, and principles of management. *Cold Spring Harb Perspect Med.* 2012;2(6):a008870.

37. *International Classification of Functioning, Disability and Health.* Geneva, Switzerland: World Health Organization; 2001. p. 102.

38. Wewers ME, Lowe NK. A critical review of visual analogue scales in the measurement of clinical phenomena. *Res Nurs Health.* 1990;13(4):227–236.

39. Bigley GK. Chapter 67: Sensation. In: Walker HK, Hall WD, Hurst JW, editors. *Clinical Methods: The History, Physical, and Laboratory Examinations*, 3rd ed. Boston, MA: Butterworths; 1990.

Impairment of functions in the neuromusculoskeletal system

Evaluation of neuro-musculoskeletal system includes motor and sensory functions.

7.1 MOTOR FUNCTIONS

Motor functions comprise muscle functions, joint functions, and movement functions. Muscle functions consist of muscle power, muscle tone, and muscle endurance. Joint functions consist of mobility of joint and stability of joint. Movement functions consist of voluntary movement and gait—translation of movement. Total loss of motor functions of one upper extremity derives an impairment of 60%, one lower extremity 40%, and spine 30%. In the upper extremity, the shoulder derives 6%, elbow 6%, wrist 3%, and hand 45%. In the hand, thumb obtains 18%, index finger 9%, middle finger 9%, ring finger 4.5%, and little finger 4.5%. In the lower extremity, the hip derives 4%, knee 8%, ankle 16%, and foot 12%. *Integrated Evaluation of Disability* combines impairment of muscle functions, joint functions, and movement functions to compute impairment of motor functions (Illustration 7.1). Section 6.9 in Chapter 6 describes in detail the impairment evaluation of motor function.

7.1.1 Muscle functions—Tendon

Tendon is a collagen tissue comprising mostly of tenoblasts, tenocytes, and chondrocytes, which mainly are at the bony insertion. Tendon possesses enormous tensile strength (1). Tendon serves to transmit the force from the muscle to the bone for creating a movement at the joint, adds flexibility to the joint, and extensibility to the muscle. It also serves

as a shock absorber to avert or minimize the injury to the muscle. Furthermore, it stores elastic energy gained during the stretching phase of the muscle to transfer it for the elastic recoil required during the gait cycle (2). Flexor tendon injuries are confined to five zones in the hand. Zone 1 refers to the segment distal to the insertion of flexor digitorum superficialis, Zone 2 refers to the segment between (annular) the A1 pulley and insertion of flexor digitorum superficialis. Zone 3 refers to the segment between the distal margin of transverse carpal ligament and A1 pulley. Zone 4 refers to the segment of the carpal tunnel, and zone 5 is proximal to the carpal tunnel (1). Reconstructive surgery combined with hand rehabilitation restores the function to the greater extent of tendon injuries. Zone 2 derives a discredit that is "No-mans-land" due to poor prognosis. In the lower extremity, most of the tendon injuries relate to sports and include adductor tendon, gluteus medius, hamstrings, Achilles tendon, and peronei. In addition to an isolated tendon injury, muscle tears are also prevalent in sports injury (3–7). Wrist flexion strength is 40% higher than wrist extensors as measured by hand dynamometer (8). *Integrated Evaluation of Disability* prefers assigning equal impairment to flexors and extensors because of the complex role of extensors in the release function of fingers, stabilization of finger joints, and intrinsic function of the hand. *Integrated Evaluation of Disability* assigns only impairment for tendon injuries or rupture of the tendon when medical reason(s) defer surgery to regain function (9) (Tables 7.1 through 7.4).

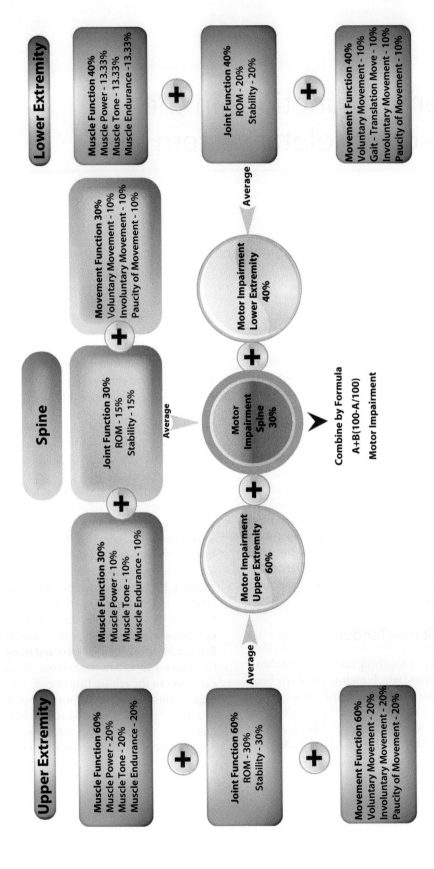

Illustration 7.1 Computation of motor impairment.

Table 7.1 Impairment of tendon functions—Upper extremity: Shoulder, elbow, and wrist

Region—Shoulder, elbow, and wrist	Reference impairment score	Maximum impairment 15%
Shoulder girdle—2.4%		
Shoulder elevators—trapezius, levator scapulae, rhomboids	0.600%	
Shoulder depressors—pectoralis minor, latissimus dorsi, lower fibers of trapezius, serratus anterior	0.600%	
Shoulder protractors—serratus anterior	0.600%	
Shoulder retractors—rhomboids major, rhomboids minor, and trapezius	0.600%	
Shoulder—3.6%		
Full-thickness rupture of the rotator cuff tendons	3.600%	
Elbow—4.000%		
Cut injury or rupture of long head of biceps	1.500%	
Cut injury or rupture of short head of biceps	0.500%	
Cut injury or rupture of triceps at the osseous insertion of olecranon/musculotendinous junction	2.000%	
Cut injury or rupture of medial head of triceps	1.000%	
Cut injury or rupture of lateral head of triceps	0.500%	
Cut injury or rupture of long head of triceps	0.500%	
Forearm—2%		
Rupture of supinator	1.000%	
Rupture of pronator	1.000%	
Wrist—3%		
Cut injury or rupture of flexor carpi radialis	0.750%	
Cut injury or rupture of flexor carpi ulnaris	0.750%	
Cut injury or rupture of extensor carpi radialis longus and brevis	0.750%	
Cut injury or rupture of extensor carpi ulnaris	0.750%	

Note: Assigns impairment only if medical reason(s) defer surgery to restore function.

Table 7.2 Impairment of tendon functions—Upper extremity: Palm

Region—Palm	Reference impairment score	Maximum impairment 20%
Palm—20.000%		
Cut injury of tendon of flexor digitorum superficialis to index finger (zones 4 and 3) in the palm	2.000%	
Cut injury of flexor digitorum profundus tendon to index finger (zones 4 and 3) in the palm	2.000%	
Cut injury or rupture of extensor digitorum tendon to index finger in the dorsum of hand	2.000%	
Cut injury or rupture of extensor digitorum indicis tendon to index finger in the dorsum of hand	1.000%	
Cut injury of flexor digitorum superficialis tendon to middle finger (zones 4 and 3) in the palm	2.000%	
Cut injury of flexor digitorum profundus tendon to middle finger (zones 4 and 3) in the palm	2.000%	
Cut injury or rupture of extensor tendon to middle finger in the dorsum of hand	2.000%	
Cut injury of flexor digitorum superficialis tendon to ring finger (zones 4 and 3) in the palm	1.000%	
Cut injury of flexor digitorum profundus tendon to ring finger (zones 4 and 3) in the palm	1.000%	
Cut injury or rupture of tendon of extensor digitorum to ring finger in the dorsum of hand	1.000%	
Cut injury of flexor digitorum superficialis tendon to little finger (zones 4 and 3) in the palm	1.000%	
Cut injury of flexor digitorum profundus tendon to little finger (zones 4 and 3) in the palm	1.000%	
Cut injury of tendon of extensor digitorum to little finger in the dorsum of hand	1.000%	
Cut injury of tendon of extensor digiti minimi to little finger in the dorsum of hand	0.500%	

Note: Assigns impairment only if medical reason(s) defer surgery to restore function.

Table 7.3 Impairment of tendon functions—Upper extremity: Fingers

Region—Fingers	Reference impairment score	Maximum impairment 25%
Thumb—10%		
Cut injury tendon of flexor pollicis longus	0.750%	
Cut injury of tendon of flexor pollicis brevis	1.500%	
Cut injury of tendon of extensor pollicis longus	0.750%	
Cut injury of tendon of extensor pollicis brevis	1.500%	
Cut injury of tendon of abductor pollicis longus	1.500%	
Cut injury of tendon of abductor pollicis brevis	1.500%	
Cut injury of tendon of adductor pollicis	1.500%	
Cut injury of tendon of opponens pollicis	1.500%	
Index finger—5%		
Cut injury of tendon of flexor digitorum superficialis (zone 2)	1.500%	
Cut injury of flexor digitorum profundus tendon (zone 2)	1.500%	
Cut injury of flexor digitorum profundus tendon (zone 1)	0.750%	
Cut injury of extensor digitorum tendon in the finger	1.500%	
Cut injury of extensor digitorum indicis tendon in the finger	0.500%	
Middle finger—5%		
Cut injury of flexor digitorum superficialis tendon (zone 2)	1.500%	
Cut injury of flexor digitorum profundus tendon (zone 2)	1.500%	
Cut injury of flexor digitorum profundus tendon (zone 1)	0.750%	
Cut injury of extensor digitorum tendon in the finger	1.500%	
Ring finger—2.500%		
Cut injury of tendons of flexor digitorum superficialis (zone 2)	0.750%	
Cut injury of flexor digitorum profundus tendon (zone 2)	0.750%	
Cut injury of flexor digitorum profundus tendon (zone 1)	0.375%	
Cut injury of extensor digitorum tendon in the finger	0.750%	
Little finger—2.500%		
Cut injury of tendons of flexor digitorum superficialis (zone 2)	0.750%	
Cut injury of flexor digitorum profundus tendon (zone 2)	0.750%	
Cut injury of flexor digitorum profundus tendon (zone 1)	0.375%	
Cut injury of extensor digitorum tendon in the finger	0.750%	
Cut injury of extensor digiti minimi tendon in the finger	0.250%	

Note: Assigns impairment only if medical reason(s) defer reconstructive surgery to restore function.

Table 7.4 Impairment of tendon functions—Lower extremity

Region—Tendons	Reference impairment score	Maximum impairment 40%
Hip—4.000%		
Tear of adductor tendons	1.000%	
Tear of gluteus medius tendon	1.000%	
Knee—8.000%		
Tear of hamstring tendon	4.000%	
Tear of quadriceps tendon	4.000%	

(Continued)

Table 7.4 (*Continued*) Impairment of tendon functions—Lower extremity

Region—Tendons	Reference impairment score	Maximum impairment 40%
Ankle—16.000%		
Tear of Achilles tendon	8.000%	
Tear of the tendon of the extensor digitorum longus	4.000%	
Tear of the tendon of the tibialis anterior	2.000%	
Tear of the tendon of the tibialis posterior	2.000%	
Foot—8.000%		
Tear of tendon of tibialis anterior	2.000%	
Tear of tendon of the tibialis posterior	2.000%	
Tear of the peronei tendon	4.000%	
Big toe—1.500%		
Tear of the tendon of flexor hallucis longus	0.750%	
Tear of the tendon of extensor hallucis longus	0.750%	
Toes—2.500%		
Tear of flexor tendons at the level of the sole	2.500%	

Note: Assigns impairment only if medical reason(s) defer reconstructive surgery to restore function.

7.2 FUNCTIONS OF THE JOINTS

Integrated Evaluation of Disability combines impairment of mobility and stability functions to assign impairment of joint function. The impairment of joint function does not exceed 60% in the upper extremity, 40% in the lower extremity, and 30% in the spine.

7.2.1 Mobility of joint function

The mobility of joint function refers to a free and full movement of an individual joint. The examiner uses a goniometer or inclinometer to measure a passive range of motion of a joint. Evaluation of mobility of the joint requires a minimum of two measurements to obtain a reliable range without error. It considered the neutral position of the joint as zero position and extended anatomic position of the joint as 0° rather than 180°. The Cobb angle measures the degree of scoliosis in the anteroposterior view of a plain X-ray of the dorsolumbar spine, and the degree of kyphosis in a lateral view of the dorsolumbar spine. It is the angle formed between the parallel lines drawn along the superior endplate of the normal upper vertebra and inferior endplate of the normal lower vertebra (Figure 7.1).

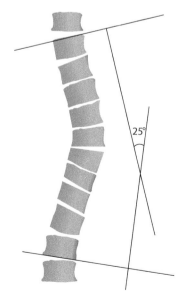

25°

Scoliosis - Cobb angle

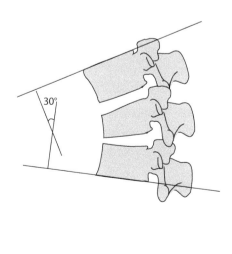

30°

Kyphosis - Cobb angle

Figure 7.1 Cobb angle.

Ankyloses of the joint refers to total loss of motion in all planes. Ankylosis of the joint in a non-functional position derives 100% of impairment of a deformity; ankyloses in functional position 50% of the impairment of a deformity and limitation of range of motion (ROM) obtains impairment according to the actual loss of ROM of joint. The upper extremity derives maximum impairment of 30% for mobility of joint function (Table 7.5), 20% for lower extremity (Table 7.6), and 15% for spine (Table 7.7).

Table 7.5 Evaluation of impairment—Mobility of joint function: Upper extremity

Joints	Reference impairment score	Weightage	Right upper extremity maximum impairment 30%	Left upper extremity maximum impairment 30%
Shoulder, elbow, and wrist:Hand = 1:3				
Shoulder	**3.000%**			
Shoulder Joint ROM: Flexion 0°–180°ª + Extension 0°–60°ª = 0°–240° Functional position (20°–40° flexion)	1.000%	% of limitation of ROM = 240-Existing ROM/240*100 % of Impairment = 1/100* % limitation of ROM		
Adduction 0°–75°ª + Abduction 0°–180°ª = 0°–255° Functional position (20°–50° abduction)	1.000%	% of limitation of ROM = 255-Existing ROM/255*100 % of impairment = 1/100* % limitation of ROM		
Internal rotation 70°ª + External rotation 90°ª = 160° with arm in 90° abduction Functional position (30°–50° internal rotation)	1.000%	% of limitation of ROM = 160-Existing ROM/160*100 % of impairment = 1/100* % limitation of ROM		
Elbow	**3.000%**			
Elbow Joint Flexion–Extension: 0°–150°ª Functional position (80°)	2.000%	% of limitation of ROM = 150-Existing ROM/150*100 % of impairment = 2/100* % limitation of ROM		
Forearm Pronation 80°ª + Supination 80°ª = 160° Functional position (20° of Pronation)	1.000%	% of limitation of ROM = 160-Existing ROM/160*100 % of impairment = 1/100* % limitation of ROM		
Wrist	**1.500%**			
Palmar Flexion 80°ª + Dorsiflexion 70°ª = 150° Functional position (Dorsiflexion 10°)	1.000%	% of limitation of ROM = 150-Existing ROM/150*100 % of impairment = 1/100* % limitation of ROM		
Ulnar deviation 0°–30° + radial deviation 0°–20° = 50° Functional position (0°–10° of ulnar deviation) (10)	0.500%	% of limitation of ROM = 50-Existing ROM/50*100 % of impairment = 0.5/100* % limitation of ROM		
Hand 22.5% (Thumb:Index:Middle:Ring:Little = 4:2:2:1:1)				
Thumb—9.000% (CMC:MCP:IP = 3:2:1)				
CMC Flexion: 0°–15°ª	1.000%	% of limitation of ROM = 15-Existing ROM/15*100 % of impairment = 1/100* % limitation of ROM		

(Continued)

Table 7.5 (*Continued*) Evaluation of impairment—Mobility of joint function: Upper extremity

Joints	Reference impairment score	Weightage	Right upper extremity maximum impairment 30%	Left upper extremity maximum impairment 30%
CMC Radial Abduction: 0°–50°	1.000%	% of limitation of ROM = 50-Existing ROM/50*100 % of impairment = 1/100* % limitation of ROM		
CMC Palmar Abduction: 0°–70°a	1.000%	% of limitation of ROM = 70-Existing ROM/70*100 % of impairment = 1/100* % limitation of ROM		
CMC Opposition: 0–8 cm (10) The tip of the thumb touches the tip of the little finger/the base of the fifth fingera or the linear distance from the flexor crease of the interphalangeal joint of thumb to distal palmar crease of the metacarpophalangeal joint near the middle finger (10)	1.500%	% of limitation of ROM = 8-Existing ROM/8*100 % of impairment = 1.5/100* % limitation of ROM		
MCP Flexion: 0°–50°a = 50° Functional position (20° flexion)	3.000%	% of limitation of ROM = 50-Existing ROM/50*100 % of impairment = 3/100* % limitation of ROM		
IP Flexion: 0°–80°a = 80° Functional position (20° of flexion)	1.500%	% of limitation of ROM = 80-Existing ROM/80*100 % of impairment = 1.5/100* % limitation of ROM		
Index—4.500% (MCP:PIP:DIP = 3:2:1)				
MCP Flexion 0°–90°a + Extension 0°–45°a = 0°–135° Functional position (30° of flexion)	2.250%	% of limitation of ROM = 135-Existing ROM/135*100 % of impairment = 2.25/100* % limitation of ROM		
PIP Flexion 0°–100°a = 0°–100° Functional position (40° of flexion)	1.500%	% of limitation of ROM = 100-Existing ROM/100*100 % of impairment = 1.5/100* % limitation of ROM		
DIP Flexion 0°–90°a + Extension 0°–10°a = 0°–100° Functional position (20° of flexion)	0.750%	% of limitation of ROM = 100-Existing ROM/100*100 % of impairment = 0.75/100* % limitation of ROM		
Middle finger—4.500% (MCP:PIP:DIP = 3:2:1)				
MCP Flexion 0°–90°a + Extension 0°–45°a = 0°–135° Functional position (30° of flexion)	2.250%	% of limitation of ROM = 135-Existing ROM/135*100 % of impairment= 2.25/100* % limitation of ROM		
PIP Flexion 0°–100°a = 0°–100° Functional position (40° of flexion)	1.500%	% of limitation of ROM = 100-Existing ROM/100*100 % of impairment = 1.5/100* % limitation of ROM		

(*Continued*)

Table 7.5 (*Continued*) Evaluation of impairment—Mobility of joint function: Upper extremity

Joints	Reference impairment score	Weightage	Right upper extremity maximum impairment 30%	Left upper extremity maximum impairment 30%
DIP Flexion 0°–90°[a] + Extension 0°–10°[a] = 0°–100° Functional position (20° of flexion)	0.750%	% of limitation of ROM = 100-Existing ROM/100*100 % of impairment = 0.75/100* % limitation of ROM		
Ring finger—2.250% (MCP:PIP:DIP = 3:2:1)				
MCP Flexion 0°–90°[a] + Extension 0°–45°[a] = 0°–135° Functional position (30° of flexion)	1.125%	% of limitation of ROM = 135-Existing ROM/135*100 % of impairment = 1.25/100* % limitation of ROM		
PIP Flexion 0°–100°[a] = 0°–100° Functional position (40° of flexion)	0.750%	% of limitation of ROM = 100-Existing ROM/100*100 % of impairment = 0.75/100* % limitation of ROM		
DIP Flexion 0°–90°[a] + Extension 0°–10°[a] = 0°–100° Functional position (20° of flexion)	0.375%	% of limitation of ROM = 100-Existing ROM/100*100 % of impairment = 0.375/100* % limitation of ROM		
Little finger—2.250% (DIP:PIP:MCP = 1:2:3)				
MCP Flexion 0°90°[a] + Extension 0°–45°[a] = 0°–135° Functional position (30° of flexion)	1.125%	% of limitation of ROM = 135-Existing ROM/135*100 % of impairment = 1.25/100* % limitation of ROM		
PIP Flexion 0°–100°[a] = 0°–100° Functional position (40° of flexion)	0.750%	% of limitation of ROM = 100-Existing ROM/100*100 % of impairment = 0.75/100* % limitation of ROM		
DIP Flexion 0°–90°[a] + Extension 0°–10°[a] = 0°–100° Functional position (20° of flexion)	0.375%	% of limitation of ROM = 100-Existing ROM/100*100 % of impairment = 0.375/100* % limitation of ROM		

[a] Joint motion—Method of measuring and recording, American Academy of Orthopedic Surgeons 1965.

Table 7.6 Evaluation of impairment—Mobility of joint function: Lower extremity

Joints—lower extremity	Reference impairment score	Weightage	Right lower extremity maximum impairment 20%	Left lower extremity maximum impairment 20%
Hip:Knee:Ankle:Foot:Toes = 1:2:4:2:1				
Hip joint	2%			
Flexion 0°–120°[a] + Extension 0°–30°[a] = 0°–150° Functional position (25°–40° of flexion)	0.666%	% of limitation of ROM = 150-Existing ROM/150*100 % of impairment = 0.666/100* % limitation of ROM		

(Continued)

Table 7.6 (*Continued*) Evaluation of impairment—Mobility of joint function: Lower extremity

Joints—lower extremity	Reference impairment score	Weightage	Right lower extremity maximum impairment 20%	Left lower extremity maximum impairment 20%
Adduction 0°–30°[a] + Abduction 0°–45°[a] = 0°–75° Functional position (Neutral)	0.666%	% of limitation of ROM = 75-Existing ROM/75*100 % of impairment = 0.666/100* % limitation of ROM		
Internal Rotation 0°–45°[a] + External Rotation 0°–45°[a] = 0°–90° Functional position (Neutral)	0.666%	% of limitation of ROM = 90-Existing ROM/90*100 % of impairment = 0.666/100* % limitation of ROM		
Knee joint: Flexion-Extension: 0°–135°[a] Functional position (10°–15° of flexion)	**4.000%**	% of limitation of ROM = 135-Existing ROM/135*100 % of impairment = 4/100* % limitation of ROM		
Ankle joint: Plantar Flexion 0°–50°[a] + Dorsiflexion 0°–20°[a] = 0°–70° Functional position (Neutral)	**8.000%**	% of limitation of ROM = 70-Existing ROM/70*100 % of impairment = 8/100* % limitation of ROM		
Foot: Subtalar Inversion 0°–35°[a] + Eversion 0°–15°[a] = 0°–50° Functional position (Neutral)	**4.000%**	% of limitation of ROM = 50-Existing ROM/50*100 % of impairment = 4/100* % limitation of ROM		
Toes	**2%**			
Big toe: MTP:IP = 1:2	**0.800%**			
MTP: Flexion 0°–45°[a] + Extension 0°–70°[a] = 0°–115°	0.533	% of limitation of ROM = 115-Existing ROM/115*100 % of impairment = 0.533/100* % limitation of ROM		
Big toe—IP: Flexion 0°–90°[a]	0.266	% of limitation of ROM = 90-Existing ROM/90*100 % of impairment = 0.266/100* % limitation of ROM		
2nd toe: MTP:PIP:DIP = 1:2:3	**0.400%**			
MTP: Flexion 0°–40°[a] + Extension 0°–40°[a] = 0°–80°	0.199	% of limitation of ROM = 80-Existing ROM/80*100 % of impairment = 0.199/100* % limitation of ROM		
PIP: Flexion 0°–35°[a] + Extension 0°–40°[a] = 0°–75°	0.133	% of limitation of ROM = 75-Existing ROM/75*100 % of impairment = 0.133/100* % limitation of ROM		
DIP: Flexion 0°–60°[a] + Extension 0°–40°[a] = 0°–100°	0.066	% of limitation of ROM = 100-Existing ROM/100*100 % of impairment = 0.066/100* % limitation of ROM		

(*Continued*)

Table 7.6 (*Continued*) Evaluation of impairment—Mobility of joint function: Lower extremity

Joints—lower extremity	Reference impairment score	Weightage	Right lower extremity maximum impairment 20%	Left lower extremity maximum impairment 20%
3rd toe: MTP:PIP:DIP = 1:2:3	**0.400%**			
MTP: Flexion 0°–40°[a] + Extension 0°–40°[a] = 0°–80°	0.199	% of limitation of ROM = 80-Existing ROM/80*100 % of impairment = 0.199/100* % limitation of ROM		
PIP: Flexion 0°–35°[a] + Extension 0°–40°[a] = 0°–75°	0.133	% of limitation of ROM = 75-Existing ROM/75*100 % of impairment = 0.133/100* % limitation of ROM		
DIP: Flexion 0°–60°[a] + Extension 0°–40°[a] = 0°–100°	0.066	% of limitation of ROM = 100-Existing ROM/100*100 % of impairment = 0.066/100* % limitation of ROM		
4th toe: MTP:PIP:DIP = 1:2:3	**0.200%**			
MTP: Flexion 0°–40°[a] + Extension 0°–40°[a] = 0°–80°	0.099	% of limitation of ROM = 80-Existing ROM/80*100 % of impairment = 0.099/100* % limitation of ROM		
PIP: Flexion 0°–35°[a] + Extension 0°–40°[a] = 0°–75°	0.066	% of limitation of ROM = 75-Existing ROM/75*100 % of impairment = 0.066/100* % limitation of ROM		
DIP: Flexion 0°–60°[a] + Extension 0°–40°[a] = 0°–100°	0.033	% of limitation of ROM = 100-Existing ROM/100*100 % of impairment = 0.033/100* % limitation of ROM		
5th toe: MTP:PIP:DIP = 1:2:3	**0.200%**			
MTP: Flexion 0°–40°[a] + Extension 0°–40°[a] = 0°–80°	0.099	% of limitation of ROM = 80-Existing ROM/80*100 % of impairment = 0.099/100* % limitation of ROM		
PIP: Flexion 0°–35°[a] + Extension 0°–40°[a] = 0°–75°	0.066	% of limitation of ROM = 75-Existing ROM/75*100 % of impairment = 0.066/100* % limitation of ROM		
DIP: Flexion 0°–60°[a] + Extension 0°–40°[a] = 0°–100°	0.033	% of limitation of ROM = 100-Existing ROM/100*100 % of impairment = 0.033/100* % limitation of ROM		

[a] Joint motion—method of measuring and recording, American Academy of Orthopedic Surgeons 1965.

Table 7.7 Evaluation of impairment—Mobility of joint function: Spine

Spine	Reference impairment score	Weightage	Maximum impairment 15%
Atlanto-occipital joint: Nodding (Flexion—Extension: 25° + Rotation 5°)	**1.500**%	% of limitation of ROM = 25-Existing ROM/25*100 % of impairment = 1.5/100* % limitation of ROM	
Cervical spine	**6.000**%		
Flexion 0°–45°ª Functional Position—(Neutral)	1.000%	% of limitation of ROM = 45-Existing ROM/45*100 % of impairment = 1.0/100* % limitation of ROM	
Extension 0°–45°ª Functional Position—(Neutral)	1.000%	% of limitation of ROM = 45-Existing ROM/45*100 % of impairment = 1.0/100* % limitation of ROM	
Lateral flexion to right 0°–45°ª Functional Position—(Neutral)	1.000%	% of limitation of ROM = 45-Existing ROM/45*100 % of impairment = 1.0/100* % limitation of ROM	
Lateral flexion to left 0°–45°ª Functional Position—(Neutral)	1.000%	% of limitation of ROM = 45-Existing ROM/45*100 % of impairment = 1.0/100* % limitation of ROM	
Rotation to right 0°–60°ª	1.000%	% of limitation of ROM = 60-Existing ROM/60*100 % of impairment = 1.0/100* % limitation of ROM	
Rotation to left 0°–60°ª	1.000%	% of limitation of ROM = 60-Existing ROM/60*100 % of impairment = 1.0/100* % limitation of ROM	
Dorsolumbar spine	**7.500**%		
Flexion 0°–80°ª Functional Position—(Neutral)	1.500%	% of limitation of ROM = 80-Existing ROM/80*100 % of impairment = 1.5/100* % limitation of ROM	
Extension 0°–30°ª Functional Position—(Neutral)	1.000%	% of limitation of ROM = 30-Existing ROM/30*100 % of impairment = 1.0/100* % limitation of ROM	
Rotation to right: 0°–45°ª Functional Position—(Neutral)	1.500%	% of limitation of ROM = 45-Existing ROM/45*100 % of impairment = 1.5/100* % limitation of ROM	
Rotation to left 0-45°ª Functional Position—(Neutral)	1.500%	% of limitation of ROM = 45-Existing ROM/45*100 % of impairment = 1.5/100* % limitation of ROM	

(Continued)

Table 7.7 (*Continued*) Evaluation of impairment—Mobility of joint function: Spine

Spine	Reference impairment score	Weightage	Maximum impairment 15%
Lateral Flexion to right 0°–35°a Functional Position—(Neutral)	1.000%	% of limitation of ROM = 35-Existing ROM/35*100 % of impairment = 1.0/100* % limitation of ROM	
Lateral Flexion to left 0°–35°a Functional Position—(Neutral)	1.000%	% of limitation of ROM = 35-Existing ROM/35*100 % of impairment = 1.0/100* % limitation of ROM	

a Joint motion—Method of measuring and recording, American Academy of Orthopedic Surgeons 1965.

7.2.2 Stability of joint function

Stability of joint function depends on adequate functioning of the kinetic chain, namely the osteoligamentous structure, osteomuscular attachment, and central nervous system (CNS) control system (11). The stability of the joint is a vital requirement to transfer weight, and permit mobility without injury to the intrinsic and extrinsic structures of the joint. Impairment of stability may be either at the axial joint (spine) or at appendicular joints (peripheral joints). Abnormal displacement of a segment of the spine under physiologic loads denotes instability of the spine (12,13). Incongruity of the joint surface, loss of structural integrity of ligaments/meniscus (such as a tear of meniscus or rupture of ligaments), and abnormal displacement of a joint leads to instability of the peripheral joints (14–17). *Integrated Evaluation of Disability* assigns impairment for instability of the joint when medical reason(s) defer surgery (Tables 7.8 and 7.9).

Table 7.8 Evaluation of impairment of instability of peripheral joints—Upper extremity

Joints	Instability of peripheral joints	Reference impairment score	Maximum impairment 30%
Shoulder 3%	Persistent instability of shoulder following flaccid paralysis, recurrent dislocation	3.000%	
Elbow 3%	Ligamentous injury with complete tear of the medial/lateral collateral ligament/s	3.000%	
Wrist 1.5%	Ligamentous injury with complete tear	1.500%	
Thumb 9%	1. Instability due to MCP collateral ligament injury, dorsal capsule, and palmar plate laxity	6.000%	
	2. Instability due to IP collateral ligament injury, dorsal capsule, and palmar plate laxity	3.000%	
Index finger 4.5%	1. Instability due to MCP collateral ligament injury, dorsal capsule, and palmar plate laxity	2.250%	
	2. Instability due to PIP collateral ligament injury, dorsal capsule, and palmar plate laxity	1.500%	
	3. Instability due to DIP collateral ligament injury, dorsal capsule, and palmar plate laxity	0.750%	
Middle finger 4.5%	1. Instability due to MCP collateral ligament injury, dorsal capsule, and palmar plate laxity	2.250%	
	2. Instability due to PIP collateral ligament injury, dorsal capsule, and palmar plate laxity	1.500%	
	3. Instability due to DIP collateral ligament injury, dorsal capsule, and palmar plate laxity	0.750%	

(*Continued*)

Table 7.8 (*Continued*) Evaluation of impairment of instability of peripheral joints—Upper extremity

Joints	Instability of peripheral joints	Reference impairment score	Maximum impairment 30%
Ring finger 2.25%	1. Instability due to MCP collateral ligament injury, dorsal capsule, and palmar plate laxity	1.125%	
	2. Instability due to PIP collateral ligament injury, dorsal capsule, and palmar plate laxity	0.750%	
	3. Instability due to DIP collateral ligament injury, dorsal capsule, and palmar plate laxity	0.375%	
Little finger 2.25%	1. Instability due to MCP collateral ligament injury, dorsal capsule, and palmar plate laxity	1.125%	
	2. Instability due to PIP collateral ligament injury, dorsal capsule, and palmar plate laxity	0.750%	
	3. Instability due to DIP collateral ligament injury, dorsal capsule, and palmar plate laxity	0.375%	

Note: Assigns impairment only if medical reason(s) defer surgery to restore the function.

Table 7.9 Impairment evaluation of instability of peripheral joints—Lower extremity

Joints	Instability of peripheral joints	Reference impairment score	Maximum impairment 20%
Hip	Tom Smith arthritis, labral tears, ligament tears, tear of the ligamentum teres, dysplasia of the hip joint, femoro acetabular impingement, capsular, and ligamentous laxity	2.000%	
Knee	Recurrent dislocation/subluxation of patella; tear of anterior cruciate ligament, posterior cruciate ligament, medial collateral ligament, lateral collateral ligament, and meniscus injury	4.000%	
Ankle	Instability due to Charcot's joint, ligamentous injury with partial or complete tear	8.000%	
Foot	Charcot's joint, and subtalar instability	4.000%	
Toes	Subluxation/ligamentous instability	2.000%	
	Big toe—subluxation/ligamentous instability of MTP joint	0.440%	
	Big toe—subluxation/ligamentous instability of IP joint	0.220%	
	2nd toe—subluxation/ligamentous instability of MTP joint	0.199%	
	2nd toe—subluxation/ligamentous instability of PIP joint	0.133%	
	2nd toe—subluxation/ligamentous instability of DIP joint	0.066%	
	3rd toe—subluxation/ligamentous instability of MTP joint	0.199%	
	3rd toe—subluxation/ligamentous instability of PIP joint	0.133%	
	3rd toe—subluxation/ligamentous instability of DIP joint	0.066%	
	4th toe—subluxation/ligamentous instability of MTP joint	0.132%	
	4th toe—subluxation/ligamentous instability of PIP joint	0.088%	
	4th toe—subluxation/ligamentous instability of DIP joint	0.044%	
	5th toe—subluxation/ligamentous instability of MTP joint	0.132%	
	5th toe—subluxation/ligamentous instability of PIP joint	0.088%	
	5th toe—subluxation/ligamentous instability of DIP joint	0.044%	

Note: Assigns impairment only if medical reason(s) defer surgery.

White and Panjabi define the stability of the spine as the ability of the spine to limit abnormal displacement between vertebral segments under physiologic loads without producing damage and irritation of the spinal cord/nerve roots and without developing structural changes resulting in deformity and pain. Instability of the spine indicates the abnormal displacement of a segment of the spine under physiologic loads (12,13).

Occipito-cervical dissociation, fracture of the occipital condyle, fracture of the atlas, fracture of the dens, and disruption of the alar ligament and transverse ligament may result in instability of the upper cervical spine. It is obligatory to apply the Harris Rule of 12s to ascertain occipito-cervical dissociation. In the Harris Rule of 12's, basion-axial interval refers to the distance from the basion to the posterior axial line; and basion-dens interval refers to a distance from the basion to the tip of the dens. The optimum basion-axis interval and basion-dens interval, individually, is less than 12 mm. Fracture of the occipital condyle may be either impacted or avulsion of the condyle or basilar skull fracture extending into occipital condyle. Injury to the occipital condyle may result in an impacted fracture of the condyle, avulsion fracture of the condyle, or extension of fracture line from the base of the skull into the condyle. Fracture of the atlas may be in the posterior arch, lateral mass, or in both the anterior and posterior arch. Fracture of both the anterior and posterior arch or fracture of lateral mass with disruption of its ligaments may result in instability of the atlantooccipital joint. Overhanging of lateral mass more than 6.9 mm in open-mouth odontoid radiograph indicates disruption of transverse ligament. Injury to alar and transverse ligament leads to anterior/posterior displacement of the atlas resulting in atlantoaxial rotatory instability. Disruption of transverse ligament/alar ligament/tectorial membrane causes atlanto-dens instability. The anterior atlanto-dens interval of more than 3 mm indicates atlanto-dens instability. Fracture of odontoid may occur at the junction of the base and body or fracture line extending to the body of the C_2 vertebra (13).

The Spine Trauma Study Group (STSG) describes the severity of a sub-axial spinal injury based on injury morphology, disco-ligamentous complex, and neurological status (18,19). The spinal motion segment becomes unstable when it manifests abnormal mobility. Radiological evidence of anterior translation motion more than 3 mm and sagittal rotation more than 10° indicates segmental instability. A stress X-ray or kinetic MRI of neutral flexion, extension, and upright weight loading position is useful to ascertain segmental instability (20). The severity of thoracolumbar injury depends on injury morphology, disco-ligamentous complex, and neurological status (21). The defect in pars interarticularis is one of the causes of instability of the spine. Forward displacement of the slipped upper vertebra from its posterior cortex to the posterior cortex of the undisplaced lower vertebra defines the degree of spondylolisthesis (22).

Clinical and radiological examination ascertains evidence for instability of sacroiliac joint and symphysis pubis, if any. The spine derives a maximum impairment of 15%. Cervical spine and sub-axial cervical spine together derives an impairment of 7.5% (Table 7.10).

Table 7.10 Impairment evaluation of instability of spine

Stability of joint function	Clinical tools	Class 1	Class 2	Class 3	Maximum 15%
Cervical spine—7.5%					
Upper cervical spine					
Occipito-cervical dissociation	Harris Rule of 12's (Displacement of occiput)	Anterior subluxation 1.0%	Vertical distraction >2 mm of atlanto-occipital joint 2.5%	Posterior dislocation 5.0%	
Fracture of occipital condyle	Plain radiograph or CT radiograph	Impacted fracture (or) basilar skull fracture extending into occipital condyle with intact alar and tectorial membrane 0%	Avulsion of occipital condyle associated with disruption of alar ligament and tectorial membrane 2.5%		
Fracture of atlas	Open-mouth odontoid radiograph: overhanging of lateral mass >6.9 mm	Fracture of posterior arch 1.0%	Fracture of lateral mass associated with disruption of ligament 2.5%	Fracture of both anterior and posterior arch with disruption of transverse ligament (Jefferson's fracture) 5.0%	
Fracture of dens	Open-mouth odontoid radiograph	Fracture tip of odontoid associated with avulsion of alar ligament 1.0%	Fracture at the junction of base and body of odontoid 2.5%	Fracture of odontoid extending into body of C2 vertebra with displacement >5 mm or angulation >10 mm 5.0%	
Atlantoaxial rotatory instability	Dynamic CT: Disruption of alar and transverse ligament	Anterior displacement of Atlas >3–5 mm 1.0%	Anterior displacement of Atlas >5 mm 2.5%	Posterior displacement of atlas 5.0%	

(Continued)

Table 7.10 (*Continued*) Impairment evaluation of instability of spine

Stability of joint function	Clinical tools	Class 1	Class 2	Class 3	Maximum 15%
Atlanto-dens instability	Atlanto-dens interval >3 mm	Disruption of transverse ligament 1.0%	Disruption of transverse and alar ligaments 2.5%	Disruption of transverse, alar ligaments, and tectorial membrane 5.0%	
Sub-axial cervical spine					
Clinical and radiological evidence	Status of ligamentous complex	Only anterior longitudinal ligament disruption 0.5%	Only posterior ligamentous complex disruption 1.25%	Both anterior and posterior ligamentous complex disruption 2.5%	
	Status of osseous component	Compression fracture 0.5%	Compression fracture with teardrop or burst fracture 1.25%	Quadrangular fracture 2.5%	
	Status of facet joint	Unilateral subluxation 0.5%	Bilateral subluxation 1.25%	Dislocation 2.5%	
Dorsolumbar spine—5%					
Clinical and radiological evidence	Status of ligamentous complex	Only anterior longitudinal ligament disruption 0.5%	Only posterior ligamentous complex disruption 1.0%	Both anterior and posterior ligamentous complex disruption 1.5%	
	Status of osseous component or pars-interarticularis defect	Simple compression fracture 0.5%	Compression fracture with teardrop or burst fracture without canal compromise 1.0%	Compression fracture or burst fracture with loss of vertebral body height ≥50% and canal compromise ≥30% 1.5%	
		Grade 1 listhesis 0.5%	Grade 2 listhesis 1.0%	Grade 3 or 4 listhesis 1.5%	
	Status of facet joint	Unilateral subluxation 0.5%	Bilateral subluxation 1.0%	Dislocation 1.5% or spondyloptosis 2.0%	
Sacroiliac joint and symphysis pubis—2.5%					
Clinical and radiological evidence	Disruption with displacement of sacroiliac joint			2.5%	
	Disruption with horizontal displacement of symphysis pubis			0.5%	
	Disruption with vertical displacement of symphysis pubis			0.5%	
	Sum of whole spine impairment should not exceed 15%				

Note: Assigns impairment only if medical reason(s) defer surgery.

7.3 SENSORY FUNCTIONS

7.3.1 Exteroceptive sensations of peripheral nerves

Sensory functions comprise touch, pain, temperature, and vibration sensations. Maximum impairment of sensory function of one upper extremity obtains a score of 60%: 30% for the impairment of exteroceptive and proprioceptive sensation, 10% for sensory perversions, 10% for pain, and 10% for cortical sensation (applicable only in cortical lesions). Maximum impairment of sensory function of one lower extremity obtains a score of 40%: 20% for exteroceptive and proprioceptive sensation, 10% for sensory perversions, and 10% for pain. One-half of the neck and trunk receives an impairment score of 30%: 10% for impairment of exteroceptive and proprioceptive sensation, 10% for sensory perversions, and 10% for pain (Illustration 7.2).

The "Three-Point Scale" defines sensory impairment for each sensory modality of an individual nerve: normal sensory function (no impairment), partial loss (partial impairment), and total loss (complete impairment). Figures 7.2 and 7.3 depict the sensory distribution of peripheral nerves in upper and lower extremities respectively. Table 7.11 describes impairment for a total loss of sensory function in the upper extremity, and Table 7.12

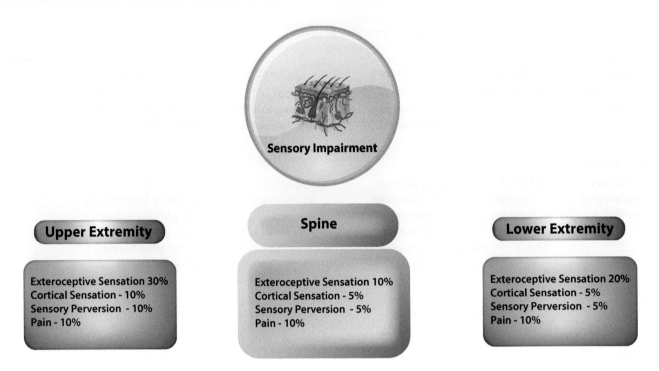

Illustration 7.2 Sensory impairment.

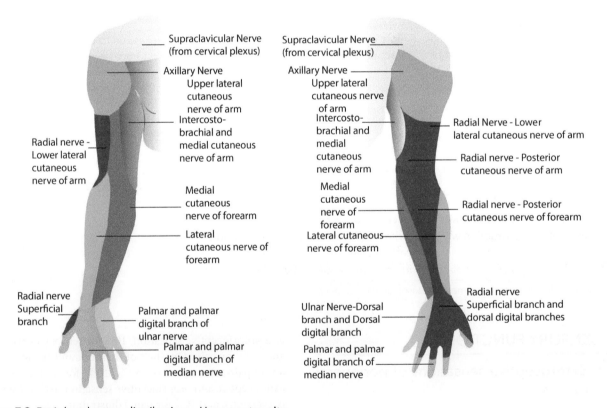

Figure 7.2 Peripheral nerve distribution—Upper extremity.

describes impairment for a total loss of sensation of peripheral nerves in the lower extremity.

The evaluators should make sure that there are definite correlating neurological findings before assigning impairment to the sensory deficit, since it is a subjective symptom.

7.3.2 Pain

The Visual Analogue Scale (VAS) assesses the severity of chronic pain and assigns 1% if VAS is 1, 2% if VAS is 2, 3% if VAS is 3, and a maximum of 10% impairment if VAS is 10 (Table 7.13). A person can apply the following guidelines, if

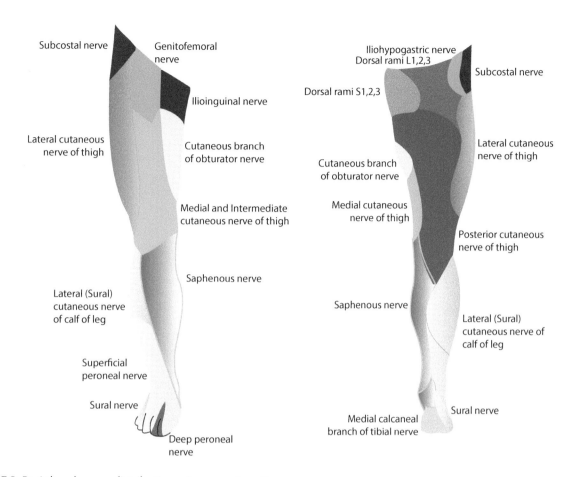

Figure 7.3 Peripheral nerve distribution—Lower extremity.

Table 7.11 Impairment of peripheral nerves—Upper extremity

Segment	Peripheral nerves	Impairment
Arm: 3%	Axillary nerve—upper lateral cutaneous nerve of arm	0.5%
	Radial nerve—lower lateral cutaneous nerve of arm	0.5%
	Intercostobrachial nerve	0.5%
	Medial cutaneous nerve of arm	0.5%
	Radial nerve—posterior cutaneous nerve of arm	1.0%
Forearm: 6%	Musculocutaneous nerve—lateral cutaneous nerve of forearm	2.0%
	Medial cutaneous nerve of forearm	2.0%
	Radial nerve—posterior cutaneous nerve of forearm	2.0%
Wrist: 1%	Lateral cutaneous nerve of forearm, medial cutaneous nerve of forearm and posterior cutaneous nerve of forearm, dorsal branch of ulnar nerve and superficial branch of radial nerve	1%
Hand: 5%	Palmar branch of median nerve	2.0%
	Palmar cutaneous branch of ulnar nerve and superficial terminal branch of ulnar nerve	1.0%
	Superficial branch of radial nerve	1.5%
	Dorsal branch of ulnar nerve	0.5%
Thumb: 6%	Palmar digital branch of median nerve: anterior surface of thumb	4.0%
	Superficial radial nerve: (1) Lateral branch: Posterior surface of radial side of thumb (2) Medial branch—digital nerve: Posterior surface of ulnar side of thumb	2.0%
Index finger: 3%	Median nerve—palmar digital branch: anterior surface of index finger	2.0%
	Dorsal digital branch of superficial radial nerve: posterior surface of index	1.0%

(Continued)

Table 7.11 (*Continued*) Impairment of peripheral nerves—Upper extremity

Segment	Peripheral nerves	Impairment
Middle finger: 3%	Median nerve—palmar digital branch: anterior surface of middle finger	2.0%
	Dorsal digital branch of superficial radial nerve: posterior surface of middle finger	1.0%
Ring finger: 1.5%	Median nerve—palmar digital branch: anterior surface of ring finger on the radial side	0.5%
	Ulnar nerve—palmar digital branch: anterior surface of ring finger on the ulnar side	0.5%
	Dorsal digital branch of superficial radial nerve: posterior surface of ring finger on the radial side	0.25%
	Ulnar nerve—dorsal digital branch: posterior surface of ring finger on the ulnar side	0.25%
Little finger: 1.5%	Ulnar nerve—palmar digital branch: anterior surface of little finger	1.0%
	Ulnar nerve—dorsal digital branch: posterior surface of little finger	0.5%

Table 7.12 Impairment of peripheral nerves—Lower extremity

Segment	Peripheral nerves	Impairment
Thigh: 4%	Dorsal rami (L1,2,3)	0.250%
	Dorsal rami (S1,2,3)	0.125%
	Cutaneous branch of obturator nerve (L2,3,4)	0.250%
	Iliohypogastric nerve (L1)	0.125%
	Subcostal nerve: upper lateral surface of thigh (T12)	0.125%
	Ilioinguinal nerve: upper medial surface of the thigh etc. (L1)	0.125%
	Femoral branch of genitofemoral: upper part of the thigh on the anterior surface (L1,2)	0.250%
	Lateral cutaneous nerve of thigh: anterior, lateral, and posterior surface of the thigh (L2,3)	0.750%
	Medial and intermediate cutaneous nerve of thigh:anterior part of the thigh and knee (L2,3)	1.00%
	Posterior cutaneous nerve of thigh: posterior surface of the thigh and leg (S1,2,3)	1.00%
Leg: 4%	Common peroneal nerve: lateral sural cutaneous nerve (Lateral cutaneous nerve of calf of the leg): lateral and posterior surface of the leg (L5, S1,2)	1.50%
	Saphenous nerve: anterior and medial surface of the leg and skin over the patella (L3,4)	1.50%
	Superficial peroneal nerve: lower lateral surface in the distal third of leg (L4,5 S1)	0.50%
	Sural nerve: Supply the posterior and lateral surface of distal third of leg (L5, S1,2)	0.50%
Ankle and foot: 12%	Medial calcaneal branch of tibial nerve (S1,2): heel and medial aspect of the sole	1.50%
	Saphenous Nerve (L3,4): inner side of the foot	0.75%
	Superficial peroneal nerve: dorsum of the foot and ankle, and all toes except lateral side of little toe, and adjacent sides of big toe and second toe (L4,5 S1)	3.50%
	Deep peroneal nerve (L4,5): first dorsal web space	0.50%
	Medial plantar nerve: cutaneous branches: medial three and a half area in the sole, medial side of the big toe and adjoining sides of the big toe and second toe, second and third toes, and third and fourth toes (L4,5)	3.50%
	Lateral plantar nerve: cutaneous branches: lateral one and half area in the sole and lateral half of the fourth toe and little toe (S1,2)	1.50%
	Sural nerve (S1,2): lateral side of foot and little toe	0.75%

Table 7.13 Impairment of sensory functions—Pain

Pain	VAS 1	VAS 2	VAS 3	VAS 4	VAS 5	VAS 6	VAS 7	VAS 8	VAS 9	VAS 10	Max 10

Table 7.14 Impairment of sensory perversion upper/lower extremity or spine

Sensory perversions	Normal sensation	Intermittent manifestation	Persistent whole day	Maximum impairment 10%
Paresthesia: Paresthesia are abnormal sensation evoked without any stimulus. It may be tactile, thermal, and burning.	0%	2.5%	5%	
Dysesthesia: Dysesthesia is painful stimulation evoked by a light touch over the affected area.	0%	2.5%	5%	

he/she finds difficult to grade pain by VAS. This guideline assigns a 0 to no pain, 1 to rarely experience pain, 2 to annoying minimal pain, and 4 to uncomfortable resting pain eased away by activity. The guideline further refers 6 as dreadful pain and performs an activity with discomfort, 8 as persistent severe pain and cannot perform any activity, and 10 as maximum unbearable pain. Congenital absence of pain or congenital indifference to pain derives maximum impairment of 10% and additional impairment if associated with amputation.

7.3.3 Sensory perversions

Sensory perversions comprise paresthesia and dysesthesia. Paresthesia is abnormal sensations evoked without any stimulus. It may be a tactile, thermal or burning sensation.

Dysesthesia is painful sensations evoked by a light touch over the affected area. Table 7.14 describes impairment related to sensory perversions.

7.4 COMBINING MOTOR AND SENSORY IMPAIRMENTS

In lower motor neuron lesions, evaluation covers only muscle power and muscle tone functions, mobility and stability of joint functions, movement functions and sensory functions. However, the evaluation does not include endurance functions.

Formula $A + B\left[\frac{100-A}{100}\right]$ combines motor and sensory impairments of extremities to arrive at a whole person impairment score (Illustration 7.3).

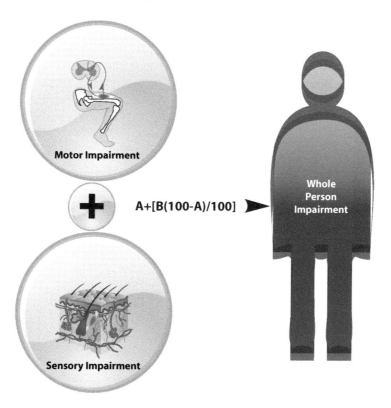

Illustration 7.3 Combining motor and sensory impairment.

REFERENCES

1. Griffin M, Hindocha S, Jordan D, Saleh M, Khan W. An overview of the management of flexor tendon injuries. *Open Orthop J.* 2012;6:28–35.
2. Kirkendall DT, Garrett WE. Function and biomechanics of tendons. *Scand J Med Sci Sports.* 1997;7(2):62–66.
3. Niebulski HZ, Richardson ML. High-grade pronator teres tear in a cricket batsman. *Radiol Case Rep.* 2011;6(3):540.
4. Chen CC, Chiou H-J, Kao C-L, Chan R-C. Sonographic appearance of a partial rupture of the supinator muscle. *J Clin Ultrasound.* 2008;36(4):247–250.
5. Lee SG, Kim JH, Lee SY, Choi IS, Moon ES. Winged scapula caused by rhomboideus and trapezius muscles rupture associated with repetitive minor trauma: A case report. *J Korean Med Sci.* 2006;21(3):581–584.
6. Burdett-Smith P, Davies MJ. A rupture of the serratus anterior. *Arch Emerg Med.* 1988; 5(3):191.
7. Bhatia DN, de Beer JF, van Rooyen KS, Lam F, du Toit DF. The "bench-presser's shoulder": An overuse insertional tendinopathy of the pectoralis minor muscle. *Br J Sports Med.* 2007;41(8):e11.
8. Decostre V, Canal A, Ollivier G, Ledoux I, Moraux A, Doppler V et al. Wrist flexion and extension torques measured by highly sensitive dynamometer in healthy subjects from 5 to 80 years. *BMC Musculoskelet Disord.* 2015;16:4.
9. Jaiswal A, Kacchap ND, Tanwar YS, Kumar D, Kumar B. Rupture of the triceps tendon - A case series. *Chin J Traumatol.* 2016;19(4):235–238.
10. Swanson AB, Hagert CG, Swanson GD. Evaluation of impairment of hand function. *J Hand Surg Am.* 1983;8(5 Pt 2):709–722.
11. Reeves NP, Narendra KS, Cholewicki J. Spine stability: The six blind men and the elephant. *Clin Biomech.* 2007;22(3):266–274.
12. Chapter 3: Stability and instability of the spine. In: Benzel EC, editor. *Biomechanics of Spine Stabilization.* Rolling Meadows, IL: American Association of Neurological Surgeons; 2001.
13. Torretti JA, Sengupta DK. Cervical spine trauma. *Indian J Orthop.* 2007;41(4):255–267.
14. Patel S, Potty A, Taylor EJ, Sorene ED. Collateral ligament injuries of the metacarpophalangeal joint of the thumb: a treatment algorithm. *Strategies Trauma Limb Reconstr.* 2010;5(1):1–10.
15. Kakarlapudi TK, Bickerstaff DR. Knee instability: Isolated and complex. *West J Med.* 2001;174(4):266–272.
16. Freeman MA. Instability of the foot after injuries to the lateral ligament of the ankle. *J Bone Joint Surg Br.* 1965;47(4):669–677.
17. Karlsson J, Eriksson BI, Renstrom PA. Subtalar ankle instability. A review. *Sports Med.* 1997;24(5):337–346.
18. Vaccaro AR, Hulbert RJ, Patel AA, Fisher C, Dvorak M, Lehman RA Jr. et al. The subaxial cervical spine injury classification system: A novel approach to recognize the importance of morphology, neurology, and integrity of the disco-ligamentous complex. *Spine.* 2007;32(21):2365–2374.
19. Whang PG, Patel AA, Vaccaro AR. The development and evaluation of the subaxial injury classification scoring system for cervical spine trauma. *Clin Orthop Relat Res.* 2011;469(3):723–731.
20. Jang SY, Kong MH, Hymanson HJ, Jin TK, Song KY, Wang JC. Radiographic parameters of segmental instability in lumbar spine using kinetic MRI. *J Korean Neurosurg Soc.* 2009;45(1):24–31.
21. Koh YD, Kim DJ, Koh YW. Reliability and validity of thoracolumbar injury classification and severity score (TLICS). *Asian Spine J.* 2010;4(2):109–117.
22. Wiltse L. Classification, terminology and measurements in spondylolisthesis. *Iowa Orthop J.* 1981;1:52–57.

Impairment of urogenital functions

8.1 EXCRETORY FUNCTION OF KIDNEY

Excretory function refers to the filtering function of the kidneys. The kidneys retain the materials needed and expel the toxic metabolic by-products in the urine, which is stored in the bladder for discharge. The glomerular filtration rate (GFR) assesses the severity of renal function. The Cockcroft–Gault formula (Equation 8.1) is a measurement for estimating the GFR (1).

$$\text{Creatinine clearance}\left(\text{mL/min}\right)$$
$$= \frac{\left(140 - \text{age in year}\right) \times \text{lean body weight}\left(\text{kg}\right)}{\text{plasma creatinine}\left(\dfrac{\text{mg}}{\text{dL}}\right) \times 72}\left(\times 0.85 \text{ in women}\right) \tag{8.1}$$

The normal GFR is equal to or more than 90 mL/min/1.73 m^2. GFR defines and classifies chronic renal failure into five stages (2). Persons with chronic kidney disease with a GFR of <30 mL/min/1.73 m^2 need maintenance with dialysis and require kidney transplantation (3). Congenital absence of kidney, the functioning of only one kidney, the glomerular filtration rate, dependency on dialysis, and kidney transplantation serve as parameters to define impairment class. Illustration 8.1 describes impairment of chronic renal failure.

8.2 MICTURITION FUNCTION

Micturition function refers to the evacuation of the bladder to expel urine (4). It also includes a sensation of bladder fullness, the sensation of desire, and sensation of voiding.

Impairment of micturition function includes the inability to hold urine resulting in incontinence, inability to initiate micturition resulting in hesitancy of micturition or retention requiring catheterization/diapers, loss of sensation of desire/fullness/voiding. Urodynamic study aids to assess an impairment of micturition function. Valsalva leak point pressure measures sphincter weakness. Sphincter electromyography ascertains suspected neuropathy. Tables 8.1 and 8.2 describe the impairment class for micturition function.

8.3 GENITAL FUNCTIONS

8.3.1 Sexual function

Sexual functions refer to mental and physical aspects of sexual arousal, sexual act, orgasm, ejaculation, and resolution (4). The International Index of Erectile Function questionnaire and Nocturnal penile tumescence test (NPT) elicits the occurrence of the spontaneous erection of the penis (normal—3–5 per night), color Doppler ultrasonography (CDU), and serum testosterone and prolactin measurements determine erectile dysfunction (5). *Integrated Evaluation of Disability* assigns an impairment of 15% for erectile dysfunction or anatomical loss of penis after maximum medical improvement (Table 8.3).

8.3.2 Menstrual function

Menstrual function refers to the regular cyclic discharge of menstrual fluid (4). Primary amenorrhea derives an impairment of 15% (Table 8.3).

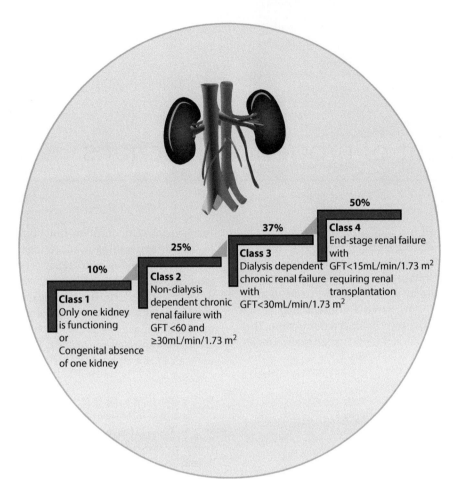

Illustration 8.1 Impairment class in chronic renal failure.

Table 8.1 Impairment class—Micturition function: Non-neurogenic lesion

Impairment class	Clinical status of micturition function	Impairment	Maximum impairment 15%
Class 1	**Urgency** of micturition without incontinence	5%	
Class 1	**Hesitancy** of micturition	5%	
Class 2	**Urgency** of micturition with incontinence	15%	
Class 2	**Stress incontinence** (1) Valsalva leak point pressure measures sphincter weakness (2) The urodynamic study assesses sphincter dysfunction (3) Sphincter electromyography ascertains suspected neuropathy	15%	

8.3.3 Procreation function

Procreation function relates to potency for fertility, pregnancy, childbirth, and lactation (4).

Impairment of procreation function in men includes azoospermia. It requires confirmation by hormone (or) semen analysis and (or) vasography (Table 8.3). Impairment of procreation in women of reproductive age may be due to primary amenorrhea and cervical, uterine, ovarian, tubal, or peritoneal factors, which may fail to initiate/continue the pregnancy. It requires confirmation by lab or imaging studies for cervical, uterine, ovarian, tubal, or peritoneal factors. Natural fertility and outcome after assisted reproductive technology in persons with low ovarian reserve declines between 30 and 50 years of age. There is a limitation of normal procreative function with advanced paternal age due to the associated risk of spontaneous abortion, autosomal dominant disorders, autism, and schizophrenia (6). Hence, *Integrated Evaluation of Disability* assigns an impairment of 15% for procreation function before the age of 50 years if the dysfunction persists even after maximum medical treatment (Table 8.3). Illustration 8.2 describes the impairment class for genital functions.

Table 8.2 Impairment class—Micturition function: Neurogenic lesion

Impairment class	Clinical status of micturition function	Impairment	Maximum impairment 50%
Class 1	**Urgency** of micturition without incontinence	5%	
Class 2	**Urgency** of micturition with incontinence	15%	
Class 2	Voiding by abdominal straining (Valsalva Maneuver)/Credé maneuver with no post-void residual urine	15%	
Class 3	Uninhibited neurogenic bladder	25%	
Class 3	(1) Reflex voiding (2) No detrusor sphincter dyssynergia (3) No sensation of desire/fullness/voiding	25%	
Class 4	(1) Reflex voiding (2) Detrusor-sphincter dyssynergia (3) No sensation of desire/ fullness/voiding associated with detrusor dysfunction (4) Requires alpha blockers or Botulinum toxin injection or transurethral sphincterotomy or endo-urethral stents to eliminate post-void residual urine	37%	
Class 5	(1) Inability in initiating micturition resulting in retention/inability to hold urine resulting in incontinence (or) Persistent post-void residual urine even after abdominal straining/Credé maneuver or sphincter management (2) No sensation of desire/fullness/voiding (3) Voiding by catheter/ requiring diapers (4) Neurogenic status confirmed by Urodynamic study	50%	

Table 8.3 Impairment class—Genital functions

Genital functions	Clinical tools	Reference impairment score
Sexual functions	Erectile dysfunction assessed by International Index of Erectile Function questionnaire, nocturnal penile tumescence test, Color Doppler Ultrasonography; anatomical loss of testes or anatomical loss of penis	15%
Menstrual functions	Primary amenorrhea in reproductive age after maximum medical management	15%
Procreation functions	(1) Azoospermia confirmed by hormone or semen analysis and/or vasography before 50 years of age or	15%
	(2) Structural and/or functional impairment failing to initiate/continue pregnancy due to cervical/uterine/ovarian/tubal or peritoneal factors before 50 years of age after maximum medical management	15%

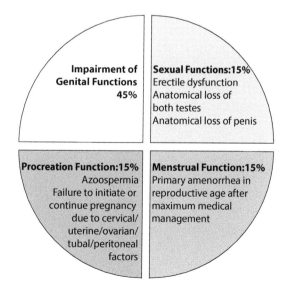

Illustration 8.2 Impairment class genital functions.

REFERENCES

1. Botev R, Mallie JP, Couchoud C, Schuck O, Fauvel JP, Wetzels JF et al. Estimating glomerular filtration rate: Cockcroft-Gault and modification of diet in renal disease formulas compared to renal inulin clearance. *Clin J Am Soc Nephrol.* 2009;4(5):899–906.
2. *Clinical Practice Guidelines for Chronic Kidney Disease: Evaluation, Classification and Stratification* [Internet]. New York: National Kidney Foundation Kidney Disease Outcomes Quality Initiative; 2002.
3. National Kidney Foundation. KDOQI clinical practice guideline for hemodialysis adequacy: 2015 update. *Am J Kidney Dis.* 2015;66(5):884–930.
4. *International Classification of Functioning, Disability and Health.* Geneva, Switzerland: World Health Organization; 2001.
5. Miller TA. Diagnostic evaluation of erectile dysfunction. *Am Fam Physician.* 2000;61(1):95–104.
6. Liu K, Case A. Advanced reproductive age and fertility. *J Obstet Gynaecol Can.* 2011;33(11):1165–1175.

9

Impairment of cardiovascular functions

9.1 CARDIOVASCULAR FUNCTIONS

The heart pumps the blood to move continuously with essential pressure throughout the whole body. The functions of the heart include sustaining the contractile force of cardiac muscle, maintaining optimum heart rate, rhythm, and cardiac output; valvular functions; pumping sufficient blood to the pulmonary circulation for the exchange of oxygen and carbon dioxide, and providing a continuous supply of blood to the heart. The overall function of the heart is to deliver oxygen and nutrients to all organs and tissues, and transport carbon dioxide and waste products through the venous circulation to the appropriate organs for excretion.

9.1.1 Heart rate

Heart rate refers to the number of heart beats per minute. Tachycardia (>100 bpm) manifests as palpitation and bradycardia manifests (<60 bpm) as fatigue and weakness. Electrocardiogram (ECG) assesses the heart rate.

9.1.2 Rhythmic functions of the heart

The rhythm of heart refers to regular beating of the heart. Dysrhythmia refers to impairment of rhythm of the heartbeat. Dysrhythmia clinically manifests as palpitation, syncope, dizziness, chest heaviness, and dyspnea. Examination of the pulse, auscultation of the chest, ECG and/or Holter monitoring, and echocardiography aid in the evaluation of dysrhythmia. Dysrhythmia may occur in persons with structural abnormalities namely congenital heart disease, valvular heart disease, hypertensive heart disease, ischemic heart disease, and cardiomyopathy. Dysrhythmia can arise in the structurally normal heart also.

9.1.3 Functions of the ventricular muscles

The contractile force of the ventricular muscle ejects the blood during every heartbeat. The impairment of the contraction of cardiac muscle results in diminished cardiac output manifesting as exertional angina/breathlessness. Echocardiography assesses systolic and diastolic functions of the heart.

9.2 EVALUATION OF FUNCTIONS OF THE HEART

Guidelines for the Diagnosis and Management of Heart Failure in Adults classify heart failure into four stages based on structural, functional impairment, and response to medical management (1).

The New York Heart Association (NYHA) functional classification is based on limitations of activities describes the stages of functional capacity of the heart in persons with heart failure (2).

VO_2 max refers to maximum oxygen uptake or consumption during maximum high-intensity exercise. It is an index of cardiopulmonary capacity to deliver oxygen to the tissues with existing physical conditioning and oxygen resource (3). Metabolic equivalents (METs) is an expression of functional capacity. A MET is the ratio of a person's metabolic rate during physical activity to their resting metabolic rate. One MET refers to the energy cost required to sit quietly without performing any work, and measures 1 kcal/kg/hour or 3.5 mL of oxygen/minute/

kg body weight (4,5). An exercise test with or without respiratory gas analysis using the motorized treadmill or stationary cycle ergometer (5) measure functional capacity. The intensity of physical activity indirectly measures functional capacity. A physician chooses a maximal or submaximal exercise test depending on the clinical situation. The Specific Activity Scale (SAS) describes a METs scale based on specific physical activity (6). Moderate and vigorous physical activity intensity indirectly indicates METs. There is an increase in heart rate during moderately intense physical activity, and an increase in heart rate and respiratory rate during vigorously intense physical activity with a corresponding increase in energy expenditure. Moderate-intensity activities include brisk walking, dancing, gardening, housework and domestic chores, active participation in games, and carrying/moving loads less than 20 kg and require energy equal to 3–6 METs. Vigorous-intensity activities include running, walking/climbing briskly up a hill, fast cycling, fast swimming, digging ditches, competitive sports/games, and carrying/moving loads more than 20 kg and require energy more than 6 METs (4). According to WHO-International Classification of Functioning, Disability and Health (ICF), function and activity are two different entities, and, hence, evaluation of impairment of function should not mix with the assessment of limitation of physical activity. *Integrated Evaluation of Disability* applies the intensity of physical activity to derive METs indirectly for impairment evaluation, only if there is medical contraindication to perform an exercise test.

Ejection fraction refers to the amount of blood pumped by the ventricle during each heartbeat. Ejection fraction of 55%–70% is normal, and less than 55% indicates left ventricular dysfunction (7). Abnormal ejection fraction refers to the subnormal volume of blood ejected by the ventricle namely mild: ≥45% to <55%, moderate: ≥30% to <45%, and severe: <30%. In echocardiography, "E" velocity refers to peak early filling velocity, and "A" velocity relates to the velocity during atrial contraction. Normally, "E" velocity is slightly greater than "A" velocity in middle-aged persons. "E" velocity is low if the rate of ventricular relaxation is slow (8). The measurement of "E" and "A" velocity is useful in evaluating diastolic dysfunction.

9.2.1 Coronary artery disease and hypertensive cardiovascular disease

Integrated Evaluation of Disability defines the parameters of severity of cardiovascular symptoms, METs aerobic functional capacity by exercise test with treadmill, and echocardiographic evidence of systolic and diastolic dysfunction in order to classify impairment class in coronary artery disease or hypertensive cardiovascular disease (Illustration 9.1 and Table 9.1).

Integrated Evaluation of Disability obtains METs from the intensity of physical activity only if there is a medical contraindication for performing exercise test.

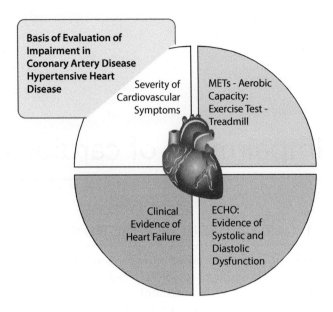

Illustration 9.1 Basis of evaluation of impairment in coronary artery disease (CAD), hypertensive heart disease.

Moderate-intensity physical activities, such as brisk walking, dancing, gardening, domestic chores, active participation in games, and carrying/moving loads less than 20 kg denotes 3–6 METs. Vigorous-intensity physical activities refers to running, walking, climbing a hill fast, fast cycling, fast swimming, digging ditches, competitive sports/games, and carrying/moving loads more than 20 kg and it indicates more than 6 METs.

9.2.2 Cardiomyopathy

Cardiomyopathy denotes a disease of the heart with enlargement and weakness of the cardiac muscle. It may be dilated cardiomyopathy, restrictive cardiomyopathy, hypertrophic cardiomyopathy, arrhythmogenic right ventricular dysplasia, and so on. Cardiomyopathy may manifest as arrhythmias and cardiac failure. Table 9.2 describes impairment class for cardiomyopathy.

9.2.3 Dysrhythmia

Dysrhythmia refers to the impairment of function relating to the regular beating of the heart. It may be either bradycardia or tachyarrhythmia. Diseases of the sinus node and atrioventricular node lead to bradycardia. Pacing corrects bradycardia due to sick sinus syndrome. Asystole of more than three seconds in carotid sinus syndrome needs permanent dual-chamber pacing. Atrial fibrillation with symptomatic bradycardia due to sick sinus syndrome benefits from atrial or dual chamber pacemaker (9). Heart failure can increase the risk of atrial fibrillation (10). A first-degree atrioventricular (AV) block does not require any specific treatment. Symptomatic second-degree AV block may

Table 9.1 Impairment class—CAD and hypertensive heart disease

Impairment class and severity of cardiovascular symptoms	Echocardiographic evidence of systolic and/or diastolic function	METs aerobic capacity	Maximum impairment 75%
Class 1: Person experiences fatigue, angina, and dyspnea during moderate-vigorous-physical exertion	Minimal left ventricular systolic dysfunction or diastolic dysfunction (EF ≥45% to <55% or E = A)	≥3 METs to ≤6 METs	15%
Class 2: Person experiences fatigue, angina, and dyspnea during moderate-vigorous-physical exertion	Minimal left ventricular systolic dysfunction and diastolic dysfunction (EF ≥45% to <55% and E = A)	≥3 METs to ≤6 METs	25%
Class 3: Person experiences fatigue, angina, and dyspnea during moderate physical exertion	Moderate left ventricular systolic dysfunction or diastolic dysfunction (EF ≥30% to <45% or E = A)	<3 METs to ≥1.5 METs	37%
Class 4: Person experiences fatigue, angina, and dyspnea during moderate physical exertion	Moderate systolic and diastolic left ventricular dysfunction (EF ≥30% to <45% and E = A)	<3 METs to ≥1.5 METs	50%
Class 5: Person experiences fatigue, angina, and dyspnea during minimal physical exertion and/or at rest	Severe systolic and diastolic left ventricular dysfunction (EF <30% and E < A)	<1.5 METs	75%

Table 9.2 Impairment class—Cardiomyopathy

Impairment class and severity of cardiovascular symptoms	Nature of intervention	Echocardiographic evidence of systolic and/or diastolic function	Maximum impairment 75%
Class 1: Asymptomatic	Isolated dysrhythmia controlled under Guideline-Directed Medical Therapy (GDMT)	Normal left ventricular function and diastolic function LVEF ≥55% to <70% or E > A	5%
Class 2: Palpitation	Isolated dysrhythmia requiring or underwent implantation of pacemaker and/or AICD	Normal left ventricular function and diastolic function LVEF ≥55% to <70% or E > A	10%
Class 3: Person experiences fatigue, angina, and dyspnea during moderate-vigorous-physical exertion, palpitation, missing of heartbeat, dizziness, sweating, anxiety	Dysrhythmia requiring or underwent implantation of pacemaker and/or AICD	Minimal left ventricular systolic dysfunction or diastolic dysfunction LVEF ≥45% to <55% or E = A	15%
Class 4: Person experiences fatigue, angina, and dyspnea during moderate-vigorous-physical exertion, palpitation, missing of heartbeat, dizziness, sweating, and anxiety	Dysrhythmia requiring or underwent implantation of pacemaker and/or AICD	Minimal left ventricular systolic dysfunction and diastolic dysfunction LVEF ≥45% to <55% and E = A	25%
Class 5: Person experiences fatigue, angina, and dyspnea during moderate physical exertion, palpitation, missing of heartbeat, dizziness, sweating, anxiety, dyspnea, chest pain, and syncope	Dysrhythmia requiring or underwent implantation of pacemaker and/or AICD	Moderate left ventricular systolic dysfunction or diastolic dysfunction (LVEF ≥30% to <45% or E = A)	37%
Class 6: Person experiences fatigue, angina, and dyspnea during moderate physical exertion, palpitation, missing of heartbeat, dizziness, sweating, anxiety, dyspnea, chest pain, and syncope	Dysrhythmia requiring or underwent implantation of pacemaker and/or AICD	Moderate systolic and diastolic left ventricular dysfunction (LVEF ≥30% to <45% and E = A)	50%
Class 7: Person experiences fatigue, angina, and dyspnea during minimal physical exertion and/or at rest, palpitation, missing of heartbeat, dizziness, sweating, anxiety, dyspnea, chest pain, and syncope	Dysrhythmia requiring or underwent implantation of pacemaker and/or AICD	Severe systolic and diastolic left ventricular dysfunction (LVEF <30% and E < A)	75%

benefit from permanent pacing because of the frequent association of the complete AV block resulting in Stokes-Adam attacks. A third-degree AV block (complete heart block) has a greater risk of asystole and requires permanent pacing. Persons with NYHA Class II symptoms and Left bundle branch block (LBBB) with QRS (a complex of wave forms recorded in ECG comprising of 'Q' wave, 'R' wave, 'S' wave) duration ≥150 milliseconds, or LBBB with QRS duration ≥150 milliseconds and Left ventricular ejection fraction (LVEF) ≤30%, or NYHA Class I symptoms and LBBB with QRS duration ≥150 milliseconds secondary to ischemia benefit from cardiac resynchronization therapy with greater reduction of ventricular fibrillation, ventricular tachycardia, and death (11). Atrial tachycardia refractory to medication needs radiofrequency ablation with a permanent dual-chamber pacemaker. Symptomatic atrioventricular re-entrant nodal supraventricular tachycardia with frequent recurrence requires radiofrequency ablation of the slower pathway. Wolff–Parkinson–White syndrome also benefits from radiofrequency ablation of the accessory pathway. Sustained ventricular tachycardia with hemodynamic compromise may benefit from ablation of the right ventricular outflow tract or automatic implantable cardiac defibrillator (AICD) (Illustration 9.2).

Integrated Evaluation of Disability assigns impairment based on the severity cardiovascular symptoms, the burden

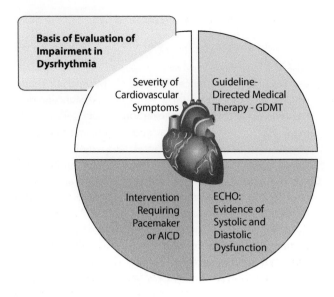

Illustration 9.2 Basis of evaluation of impairment in dysrhythmia.

of treatment including the failure of pacemaker, AICD devices, replacement of devices, and coexisting left ventricular dysfunction. Table 9.3 describes impairment class for dysrhythmia.

Table 9.3 Impairment class—Dysrhythmias

Impairment class and severity of cardiovascular symptoms	Nature of intervention	Echocardiographic evidence of systolic and/or diastolic function	Maximum impairment 75%
Class 1: Asymptomatic	Isolated dysrhythmia controlled under Guideline-Directed Medical Therapy (GDMT)	Normal left ventricular function and diastolic function LVEF ≥55% to <70% or E > A	5%
Class 2: Palpitation	Isolated dysrhythmia requiring or underwent implantation of pacemaker and/or AICD	Normal left ventricular function and diastolic function LVEF ≥55% to <70% or E > A	10%
Class 3: Palpitation, missing of heartbeat, dizziness, sweating, and anxiety	Dysrhythmia requiring or underwent implantation of pacemaker and/or AICD	Minimal left ventricular systolic dysfunction or diastolic dysfunction LVEF ≥45% to <55% or E = A	15%
Class 4: Palpitation, missing of heartbeat, dizziness, sweating, and anxiety	Dysrhythmia requiring or underwent implantation of pacemaker and/or AICD	Minimal left ventricular systolic dysfunction and diastolic dysfunction LVEF ≥45% to <55% and E = A	25%
Class 5: Palpitation, missing of heartbeat, dizziness, sweating, anxiety, dyspnea, chest pain, and syncope	Dysrhythmia requiring or underwent implantation of pacemaker and/or AICD	Moderate left ventricular systolic dysfunction or diastolic dysfunction (EF ≥30% to <45% or E = A)	37%
Class 6: Palpitation, missing of heartbeat, dizziness, sweating, anxiety, dyspnea, chest pain, and syncope	Dysrhythmia requiring or underwent implantation of pacemaker and/or AICD	Moderate systolic and diastolic left ventricular dysfunction (EF ≥30% to <45% and E = A)	50%
Class 7: Palpitation, missing of heartbeat, dizziness, sweating, anxiety, dyspnea, chest pain, and syncope	Dysrhythmia requiring or underwent implantation of pacemaker and/or AICD	Severe systolic and diastolic left ventricular dysfunction (EF <30% and E < A)	75%

9.2.4 Valvular heart disease

Evaluation of impairment in a person with valvular heart disease entails clinical examination and imaging studies. Echocardiogram assesses the impact of the valvular lesions on the size of the atrium and ventricle and its functions besides the severity of valvular lesions.

Guidelines for the management of persons with valvular heart disease provides definitions of the severity of valvular disease based on valve anatomy, hemodynamics, hemodynamic consequences, and symptoms (12).

Aortic stenosis leads to an increase in left ventricular pressure and results in left ventricular hypertrophy. Initially left ventricular function remains normal due to compensatory left ventricular hypertrophy. Left ventricular systolic dysfunction develops toward the end stage of the disease, though diastolic dysfunction occurs early. A person with aortic stenosis may develop breathlessness in spite of normal systolic function due to increase in diastolic filling pressure in progressive severe aortic stenosis (13,14).

In aortic regurgitation, the increase in preload and afterload imposed on the left ventricle produces progressive dilatation of the left ventricle, left ventricular dysfunction and heart failure (14).

In mitral stenosis, atrioventricular compliance represents hemodynamic consequences. It serves as a powerful predictor of pulmonary hypertension, an important determinant of functional capacity and prognosis independent of severity of stenosis. In mitral stenosis, compensatory mechanisms namely alteration of heart rate, cardiac output, and pulmonary vasoreactivity may delay the onset of symptoms. Atrioventricular compliance predicts progressive loss of functional capacity even in asymptomatic persons with mitral stenosis (15).

Mitral regurgitation places the left ventricle with an additional volume load resulting in a compensatory adaptation by enlargement of the left ventricle. Ejection fraction may remain normal or may increase. Reduced myocardial contraction or increase in afterload may decrease ejection fraction. In advanced disease, the person with mitral valve disease regurgitation develops signs and symptoms of pulmonary hypertension (14,16).

In tricuspid regurgitation, there is an increase in right atrial pressure resulting in hepatic congestion and peripheral edema. In severe tricuspid regurgitation, there is progressive volume overload of right ventricle and atrium resulting in enlargement of right atrium and ventricle. In the chronic condition, it leads to right heart failure, ascites, and anasarca (17).

In tricuspid stenosis, right atrial pressure increases with resultant enlargement of the right atrium, elevated jugular venous pressure, and enlargement of the liver. Persons with severe stenosis develop symptoms such as fatigue, discomfort in the right hypochondrium due to venous congestion and enlargement of the liver, discomfort in the neck due to jugular distension, and cold extremities due to decreased cardiac output (Illustration 9.3).

Integrated Evaluation of Disability assigns impairment based on symptomatic/asymptomatic valvular disease,

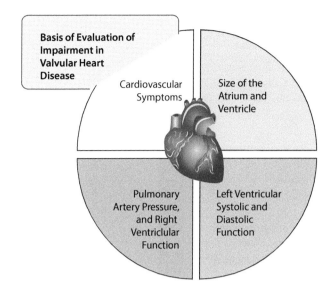

Illustration 9.3 Basis of evaluation of impairment in valvular heart disease.

left ventricular systolic and diastolic function, pulmonary artery pressure, and right ventricular function in persons with valvular heart disease. Table 9.4 describes the impairment class in valvular heart disease.

9.3 FUNCTIONS OF THE VESSELS

9.3.1 Functions of the arteries

The functions of the arteries refer to the carrying of oxygenated blood from the heart to the tissues throughout the body. It can produce vasodilation or vasoconstriction. Peripheral vascular disease displays atherosclerosis or narrowing of blood vessels. It has an increased risk of infection and amputation resulting in severe disability (18). The peripheral vascular disease is asymptomatic during its initial stage. As the disease progresses, it may present with claudication pain, resting pain and ulcer and gangrene of the extremities. The difference in blood pressure of >20 mm of Hg in upper extremities signifies the progression of the peripheral vascular disease. Doppler ultrasound calculates the Ankle-Brachial Index (ABI), which refers to the ratio of the blood pressure at the ankle (either dorsalis pedis or posterior tibial artery) to the blood pressure at the (brachial artery) upper arm. It indicates the blockage of blood flow, if any, to the lower extremity. Normal ABI is 0.9–1.4. It may represent the reduced blood flow as mild 0.71 to ≤0.90, moderate 0.41 to ≤0.70, and severe as ≤0.40 (19,20). Doppler ultrasound, magnetic resonance angiogram, computed tomographic angiography, and digital subtraction angiography may assist the physicians to assess the severity of the peripheral vascular disease. Pulse volume recording Doppler ultrasound qualitatively measures the perfusion of the affected segment. *Integrated Evaluation of Disability* applies the parameters namely, atypical leg pain,

Table 9.4 Impairment class—Valvular heart diseases

Impairment class symptoms	Size of atrium/ventricle	Systolic and diastolic ventricular function	Impairment score
Class 1: Asymptomatic valvular heart disease	Normal size of atrium/ventricle	(1) Left ventricular systolic and diastolic function—Normal: EF: 55%–70% and E > A (2) Normal pulmonary artery pressure: 8–20 mm of Hg at rest, and normal right ventricular function	5%
Class 2: Symptomatic valvular heart disease—syncope	Mild enlargement of atrium/ventricle	(1) Minimal left ventricular systolic dysfunction EF: ≥45 to <55% or minimal diastolic dysfunction: E = A **and/or** (2) Increased pulmonary artery pressure: >20 to ≤30 mm of Hg with normal right ventricular function	15%
Class 3: Symptomatic valvular heart disease—syncope	Mild enlargement of atrium/ventricle	(1) Minimal left ventricular systolic dysfunction EF: ≥45 to <55% and minimal diastolic dysfunction: E = A **and/or** (2) Pulmonary hypertension: >30 to ≤50 mm of Hg with normal right ventricular function	25%
Class 4: Symptomatic valvular heart disease—syncope, angina, dyspnea	Moderate enlargement of atrium/ventricle	(1) Moderate left ventricular systolic dysfunction EF: ≥30% to <45% or diastolic dysfunction: E = A **and/or** (2) Pulmonary hypertension: >30 to ≤50 mm of Hg with minimal right ventricular dysfunction	37%
Class 5: Symptomatic valvular heart disease—syncope, angina, dyspnea	Moderate enlargement of atrium/ventricle	(1) Moderate left ventricular systolic dysfunction EF: ≥30% to <45% and diastolic dysfunction: E = A **and/or** (2) Pulmonary hypertension: >30 to ≤50 mm of Hg with moderate right ventricular dysfunction	50%
Class 6: Symptomatic valvular heart disease—syncope, angina, dyspnea, decreased exercise tolerance	Severe enlargement of atrium/ventricle	(1) Severe left ventricular systolic dysfunction EF: <30% and diastolic dysfunction: E < A **and/or** (2) Pulmonary hypertension: >50 mm of Hg with severe right ventricular dysfunction	75%

claudication pain, resting pain, and severity of the ABI to define impairment class. Table 9.5 describes the impairment class. Illustration 9.4 depicts the basis of assigning impairment in peripheral vascular disease.

In Raynaud's disease, there is dysfunction of microvascular circulation in the fingers, toes, ear, nose, and nipple resulting in dysregulated vasoconstriction of arterioles at the pre-capillary level. Cold exposure, emotional stress, beta blockers, vibration, overuse of fingers, and smoking triggers ischemia of the digits. The manifestation of triphasic color changes, namely pallor due to vasoconstriction, cyanosis due to hypoxia of the tissues, and redness due

Table 9.5 Impairment class—Peripheral arterial disease upper/lower extremities

Impairment class	Clinical symptoms and/or signs	Clinical tools	Maximum impairment 10%
Class 1	Raynaud's phenomena: Triphasic color changes, triggered by exposure to cold, and so on	—	5%
Class 1	Elicits claudication pain on 6-minute walk test, and refractory to medical management	Ankle-Brachial Index: 0.71 to ≤0.90	5%
Class 2	Resting pain due to acute limb ischemia Contraindication for endovascular interventions and revascularization surgery due to medical reasons	Ankle-Brachial Index: 0.41 to ≤0.70	10%
Class 3	Gangrene and amputation	Ankle-Brachial Index: ≤0.40	According to level of amputation

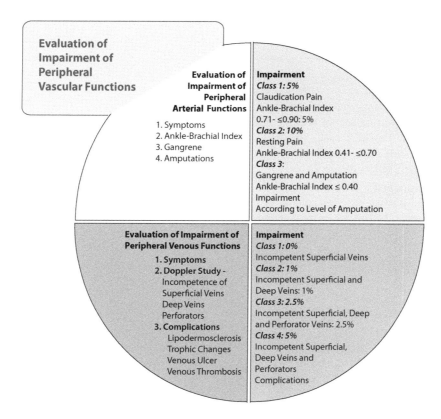

Illustration 9.4 Basis of evaluation of impairment of peripheral vascular functions.

to reperfusion of the tissue; swelling and numbness point toward the diagnosis of Raynaud's disease (21).

9.3.2 Functions of the veins

The functions of the vein refer to returning deoxygenated blood from the tissues to the heart. It can produce venous constriction, venous dilatation, and incompetence of the valves of the vein resulting in varicose veins.

A varicose vein is a common clinical condition due to chronic degenerative changes in the vessel and valves. The resultant chronic venous insufficiency may lead to venous ulceration and venous thrombosis if untreated. It may affect superficial veins, deep veins, and perforators. It can manifest as spider veins, reticular veins, edema, pigmentation, lipoderma-tosclerosis, trophic changes, and venous ulcer (22). *Integrated Evaluation of Disability* assigns impairment based on clinical symptoms, incompetence of superficial, deep veins and perforators, and complications of venous insufficiency (Table 9.6).

Table 9.6 Impairment class—Varicose veins: Upper/lower extremities

Impairment class	Clinical symptoms and/or signs	Clinical tools	Maximum impairment 10%
Class 1	Asymptomatic varicose veins	Doppler ultrasound—Incompetent superficial veins	0%
Class 2	Varicose veins with pain, heaviness in the leg, muscle cramps, and edema	Doppler ultrasound—Incompetent superficial and deep veins	1%
Class 3	Varicose veins with pain, heaviness in the leg, muscle cramps, edema, and pigmentation with irritation of the skin	Doppler ultrasound—Incompetent superficial, deep and perforator veins	2.5%
Class 4	Varicose veins with chronic venous insufficiency and pain, heaviness of the leg, muscle cramps, edema, pigmentation with irritation of the skin, lipodermatosclerosis, trophic changes, venous ulcer, and venous thrombosis	Doppler ultrasound—Incompetent superficial, deep, and perforator veins	5%

9.4 FUNCTIONS OF THE LYMPHATIC SYSTEM

The lymphatic system transmits lymphatic fluid (23). The function of the lymphatic system is to return the fluid, proteins, and immune cells from the interstitial space into intravascular space. Dysfunction of the lymphatic vessels results in accumulation of protein-rich fluid in the interstitial space. The collection of protein-rich fluid in the interstitial space, that is, lymphedema, may be due to congenital or acquired causes. Primary lymphedema is due to congenital absence or anomaly of the lymph node or vessels, for example, Milroy's disease. Secondary lymphedema is due to infections, such as filarial infection, malignancy per se, removal of lymph glands for the treatment of cancer, and radiotherapy. Secondary lymphedema may be attributable to the sequel of treatment for cancer, such as breast cancer, soft tissue sarcoma, gynecologic malignancy, and melanoma (24,25). Lymphedema may result in disfigurement, impairment of mobility of a joint, limitation of activities, and restriction of participation. *Integrated Evaluation of Disability* defines impairment based on parameters, namely lymphedema, disfigurement, limitation of ROM joint, and sequels such as infections, sarcoidosis, lymphangiosarcoma, and amputations (Illustration 9.5 and Table 9.7).

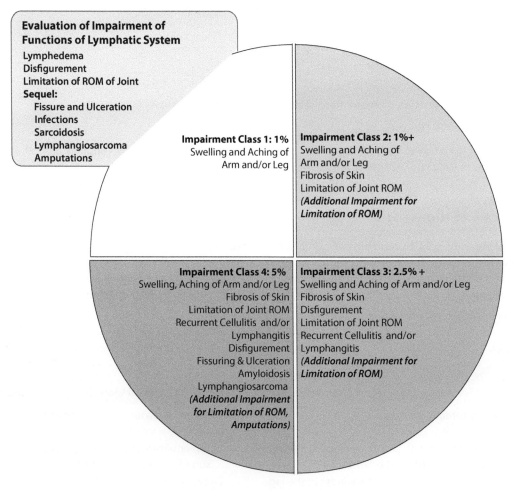

Illustration 9.5 Basis of evaluation of impairment of functions of lymphatic system.

Table 9.7 Impairment class—Lymphedema: Upper/lower extremities

Impairment class	Clinical symptoms and/or signs	Maximum impairment
Class 1	Swelling of arm and/or leg Aching of swollen arm and/or leg	1%
Class 2	Swelling of arm and/or leg with disfigurement Aching of swollen arm and/or leg Fibrosis of skin Limitation of ROM of joint	1% + Impairment score according to limitation of ROM of affected joint
Class 3	Swelling of arm and/or leg with disfigurement Aching of swollen arm and/or leg Fibrosis of skin Limitation of ROM of joint Recurrent cellulitis/lymphangitis	2.5% + Impairment score according to limitation of ROM of affected joint
Class 4	Swelling of arm and/or leg with disfigurement Aching of swollen arm and/or leg Fibrosis of skin Limitation of ROM of joint Recurrent cellulitis/lymphangitis Chronic fissuring and ulceration Amyloidosis Lymphangiosarcoma	5% + Impairment score according to limitation of ROM of affected joint + Impairment score according to level of amputation if deemed necessary

REFERENCES

1. Hunt SA, Abraham WT, Chin MH, Feldman AM, Francis GS, Ganiats TG et al. 2009 Focused update incorporated into the ACC/AHA 2005 guidelines for the diagnosis and management of heart failure in adults a report of the American College of Cardiology Foundation/American Heart Association task force on practice guidelines developed in collaboration with the International Society for Heart and Lung Transplantation. *J Am Coll Cardiol.* 2009;53(15):e1–e90.

2. The Criteria Committee of the New York Heart Association. *Nomenclature and Criteria for Diagnosis of Diseases of the Heart and Great Vessels: Functional Capacity and Objective Assessment of Patients with Diseases of the Heart.* Boston, MA: Little, Brown; 1994. pp. 253–256.

3. Hawkins MN, Raven PB, Snell PG, Stray-Gundersen J, Levine BD. Maximal oxygen uptake as a parametric measure of cardiorespiratory capacity. *Med Sci Sports Exerc.* 2007;39(1):103–107.

4. *Global Strategy on Diet, Physical Activity and Health: What is Moderate-Intensity and Vigorous-Intensity Physical Activity?* Geneva, Switzerland: World Health Organization; 2014.

5. Fleg JL, Pina IL, Balady GJ, Chaitman BR, Fletcher B, Lavie C et al. Assessment of functional capacity in clinical and research applications: An advisory from the Committee on Exercise, Rehabilitation, and Prevention, Council on Clinical Cardiology, American Heart Association. *Circulation.* 2000;102(13):1591–1597.

6. Goldman L, Hashimoto B, Cook EF, Loscalzo A. Comparative reproducibility and validity of systems for assessing cardiovascular functional class: Advantages of a new specific activity scale. *Circulation.* 1981;64(6):1227–1234.

7. Ejection fraction heart failure measurement. The American Heart Association; 2014. Available from: www.heart.org/.

8. Nishimura RA, Tajik AJ. Evaluation of diastolic filling of left ventricle in health and disease: Doppler echocardiography is the clinician's Rosetta Stone. *J Am Coll Cardiol.* 1997;30(1):8–18.

9. January CT, Wann LS, Alpert JS, Calkins H, Cigarroa JE, Cleveland JC Jr. et al. 2014 AHA/ACC/HRS guideline for the management of patients with atrial fibrillation: A report of the American College of Cardiology/American Heart Association task force on practice guidelines and the Heart Rhythm Society. *Circulation.* 2014;130(23):e199–e267.

10. Anter E, Jessup M, Callans DJ. Atrial fibrillation and heart failure: Treatment considerations for a dual epidemic. *Circulation.* 2009;119(18):2516–2525.

11. Tracy CM, Epstein AE, Darbar D, DiMarco JP, Dunbar SB, Mark Estes NA et al. 2012 ACCF/AHA/HRS focused update of the 2008 guidelines for device-based therapy of cardiac rhythm abnormalities: A report of the American College of Cardiology Foundation/American Heart Association Task Force on Practice Guidelines. *J Thorac Cardiovasc Surg.* 2012;144(6):e127–e145.

12. Nishimura RA, Otta CM, Bonow RO, Carabello BA, Erwin JP III, Guyton RA et al. 2014 AHA/ACC guideline for the management of patients with valvular heart disease. *J Am Coll Cardiol.* 2014:63:2438–2488.

13. Lindman BR, Bonow RO, Otto CM. Current management of calcific aortic stenosis. *Circ Res.* 2013;113(2):223–237.

14. Maganti K, Rigolin VH, Sarano ME, Bonow RO. Valvular heart disease: Diagnosis and management. *Mayo Clinic Proc.* 2010;85(5):483–500.

15. Nunes MC, Hung J, Barbosa MM, Esteves WA, Carvalho VT, Lodi-Junqueira L et al. Impact of net atrioventricular compliance on clinical outcome in mitral stenosis. *Circ Cardiovasc Imaging.* 2013;6(6):1001–1008.

16. Gaasch WH, Meyer TE. Left ventricular response to mitral regurgitation: Implications for management. *Circulation.* 2008;118(22):2298–2303.

17. Bruce CJ, Connolly HM. Right-sided valve disease deserves a little more respect. *Circulation.* 2009;119(20):2726–2734.

18. *Peripheral Vascular Disease.* Geneva, Switzerland: World Health Organization; 2015.

19. American College of Cardiology Foundation, American College of Radiology, American Institute of Ultrasound in Medicine, American Society of Echocardiography, American Society of Nephrology, Intersocietal Commission for the Accreditation of Vascular Laboratories, Society for Cardiovascular Angiography and Interventions et al. ACCF/ACR/AIUM/ASE/ASN/ICAVL/SCAI/SCCT/SIR/SVM/SVS/SVU [corrected] 2012 appropriate use criteria for peripheral vascular ultrasound and physiological testing part I: Arterial ultrasound and physiological testing: A report of the American College of Cardiology Foundation appropriate use criteria task force, American College of Radiology, American Institute of Ultrasound in Medicine, American Society of Echocardiography, American Society of Nephrology, Intersocietal Commission for the Accreditation of Vascular Laboratories, Society for Cardiovascular Angiography and Interventions, Society of Cardiovascular Computed Tomography, Society for Interventional Radiology, Society for Vascular Medicine, Society for Vascular Surgery, [corrected] and Society for Vascular Ultrasound. [corrected]. *J Am Coll Cardiol.* 2012;60(3):242–276.

20. Olin JW, Sealove BA. Peripheral artery disease: Current insight into the disease and its diagnosis and management. *Mayo Clinic Proc.* 2010;85(7):678–692.

21. Maverakis E, Patel F, Kronenberg DG, Chung L, Fiorentino D, Allanore Y et al. International consensus criteria for the diagnosis of Raynaud's phenomenon. *J Autoimmun.* 2014;48–49:60–65.

22. Chwala M, Szczeklik W, Szczeklik M, Aleksiejew-Kleszczynski T, Jagielska-Chwala M. Varicose veins of lower extremities, hemodynamics and treatment methods. *Adv Clin Exp Med.* 2015;24(1):5–14.

23. *International Classification of Functioning, Disability and Health.* Geneva, Switzerland: World Health Organization; 2001. p. 78.

24. Mendola A, Schlogel MJ, Ghalamkarpour A, Irrthum A, Nguyen HL, Fastre E et al. Mutations in the VEGFR3 signaling pathway explain 36% of familial lymphedema. *Mol Syndromol.* 2013;4(6):257–266.

25. Hodgson P, Towers A, Keast DH, Kennedy A, Pritzker R, Allen J. Lymphedema in Canada: A qualitative study to help develop a clinical, research, and education strategy. *Curr Oncol.* 2011;18(6):e260–e264.

10

Impairment of pulmonary functions

10.1 PULMONARY FUNCTION

Pulmonary function is a conglomerate of ventilation, diffusion, and gas exchange. Plethysmography, spirometry, and blood gas analysis are useful tools in the evaluation of pulmonary function. Tidal volume (TV) is the volume of air inhaled or exhaled during normal respiration without effort. Inspiratory reserve volume (IRV) is the maximum volume of air inhaled after the end-tidal inspiration. Expiratory reserve volume (ERV) is the maximum volume of air exhaled after the end-tidal expiration. Functional residual capacity (FRC) is the volume air remaining at the end-tidal expiration. Inspiratory capacity (IC) is the volume of air inhaled from the beginning of tidal inspiration, that is, from FRC. Forced vital capacity (FVC) is the volume of air exhaled during forced expiration from forced inspiration to the end of expiration. Total lung capacity is the volume of air present in the lung after maximum inspiration (Illustration 10.1) (1).

Pulmonary function tests namely forced expiratory volume in one second (FEV_1), FVC, FEV_1/FVC ratio, and Total Lung Capacity (TLC) interpret impairment of lung function. FEV_1/FVC ratio ≥ 0.7 and FVC >80% of predicted are normal spirometry values. FEV_1/FVC ratio <0.7 indicate airway obstruction. FEV_1/FVC ratio ≥ 0.7 and FVC <80% of predicted refer to the restrictive pattern. FEV_1/FVC ratio <0.7 and FVC <80% of predicted indicate mixed pattern (2). In general, FEV_1 grades the degree of impairment of pulmonary function (3). Post-bronchodilator FEV_1 assesses airway responsiveness, and a FEV_1 less than 80% of predicted indicates a limitation of airflow (4). The ratio of post-bronchodilator FEV_1/FVC to forced vital capacity less than 0.70 indicates airflow limitation in obstructive pulmonary diseases. A decrease in TLC below the fifth percentile and normal FEV_1/VC ratio represent restrictive lung diseases.

An increase in arterial partial pressure of carbon dioxide ($PaCO_2$), end-tidal PCO_2 or an elevation of transcutaneous PCO_2 more than 55 mm of Hg for ≥ 10 minutes; or an elevation of $PaCO_2$ or end-tidal PCO_2 or transcutaneous PCO_2 by 10 mm above 50 mm of Hg for ≥ 10 minutes during sleep refers to hypercapnic failure.

Impulse oscillometry (IOS) is a noninvasive method to measure airway impedance comprising of resistance and reactance (5). IOS generates pressure oscillation. The pressure oscillation travels along with air in the air passage. It produces distension and elastic recoil of the lung tissues and creates back pressure. The person breaths normally (tidal breathing). IOS measures the resistance in Hertz (Hz) (proximal R5, total resistance R20), and reactance—X at 5 Hz. Resistance and reactance increases in inflammation of airways—asthma, chronic obstructive pulmonary diseases (COPD), and reverses with bronchodilators and increases with methacholine. IOS can quantify the severity of asthma/COPD. As it is not effort dependent, it is preferable to use IOS in elderly persons, children, a person with respiratory muscle weakness, and during pregnancy and postoperative period.

10.2 CHRONIC OBSTRUCTIVE PULMONARY DISEASES

Indoor and outdoor air pollutants, tobacco smoke, and occupational dust and chemicals predispose people to the risk of developing COPD. Chronic irritants trigger inflammation of airways, parenchyma, and pulmonary vessels. It may lead to a chronic cough, expectoration of sputum, and breathlessness. The modified Medical Research Council's (mMRC) dyspnea scale assesses dyspnea (6,7). Furthermore, a person with COPD may develop pulmonary hypertension, respiratory failure, and/or right heart failure. The number of exacerbations the person has

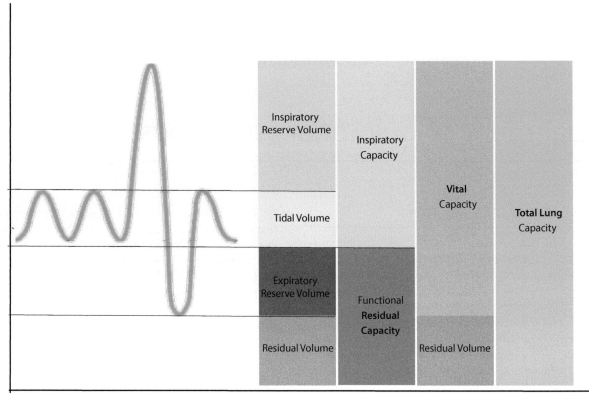

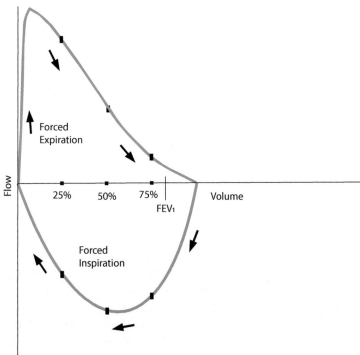

Illustration 10.1 Lung volumes.

had within the previous 12 months may signify the risk associated with COPD. Persistent non-reversible airflow obstruction evinced by the FEV_1-to-FVC ratio of less than 0.7 confirms the diagnosis of COPD if clinical signs and symptoms exist (4). *Integrated Evaluation of Disability* defines impairment in COPD based on clinical symptoms, such as a chronic cough, chronic productive cough, dyspnea; frequency of exacerbations, and post-bronchodilator airflow limitation, respiratory failure, and right heart failure. Illustration 10.2 describes Class 1 impairment of 5%, Class 2 impairment of 25%, and Class 3 impairment of 50% in COPD.

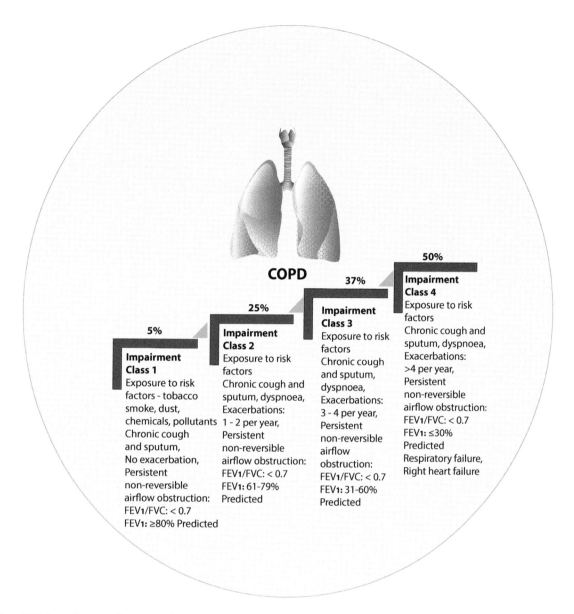

Illustration 10.2 Impairment classes in COPD.

10.3 ASTHMA

Asthma is a common cause of pulmonary disability. In asthma, there is hyperresponsiveness of the airways and obstruction due to chronic inflammation of the airways (8). Chronic obstruction may lead to occlusion of the small airway with uneven ventilation. It manifests as a cough, expectoration, breathlessness, tightness in chest, wheezing, and expiratory airflow limitation. In asthma, both symptoms and expiratory airflow limitation may vary in intensity over a period (9). FEV_1 and FEV_1-to-FVC ratio measures airflow limitation. The normal value of FEV_1-to-FVC ratio is 0.75–0.80. A value less than this indicates airflow limitation. Post-bronchodilator FEV_1 determines the level of airflow limitation. The degree of reversibility, that is, post-bronchodilator increase in FEV_1 of 12% and more than 200 mL confirms reversible airflow obstruction

and thus favors the diagnosis of asthma (10). Persistent non-reversible airflow obstruction indicates the diagnosis of COPD. Elevated exhaled nitric oxide reveals the degree of airway mucosal inflammation, that is, airway reactivity in asthma (11). Exhaled nitric oxide aids to distinguish asthma from COPD. Peak expiratory flow (PEF) rate refers to the maximum flow rate of exhaled air during forced expiration after maximum inspiration. It assesses the severity of asthma and monitors asthma control. As PEF is effort dependent on the person, it is necessary to select the best measurement during the asymptomatic period for comparison (12). Asthma control is good when the PEF rate is more than ≥95% predicted of the individual's best measurement. The asthma control is fair when PEF rate is ≥80% predicted, asthma control is inadequate when PEF rate is 70%–79% predicted, asthma control is poor when PEF rate is 60%–69% predicted, and asthma control is at

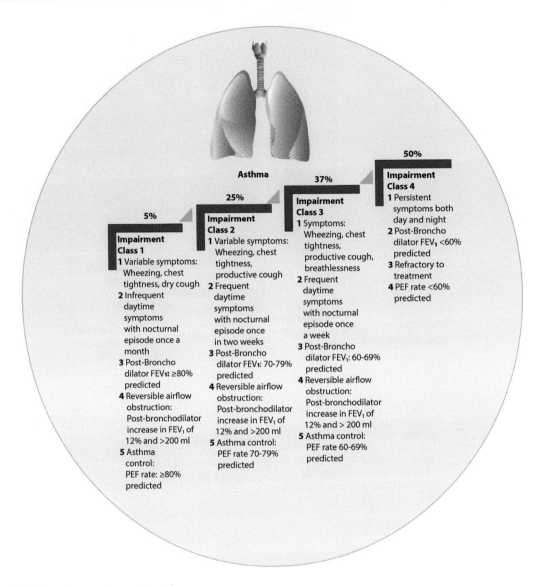

Illustration 10.3 Impairment classes in asthma.

a low ebb when PEF rate <60% predicted. Clinical symptoms, post-bronchodilator FEV_1, reversibility of airflow obstruction, and asthma control serve as parameters to define the impairment of asthma in *Integrated Evaluation of Disability*. Illustration 10.3 describes the impairment scores for asthma.

10.4 RESTRICTIVE LUNG DISEASES

Diseases of the lung parenchyma, pleura, chest wall, and neuromuscular apparatus produce restrictive lung diseases. Reduced lung volume suggests restrictive lung disease. In restrictive lung disease, there is decreased total lung capacity below the fifth percentile of the predicted value, and reduced FEV_1 and FVC but preserved or increased FEV_1-to-FVC ratio. However, caution is necessary for interpretation as submaximal inspiratory or expiratory efforts and/or patchy peripheral airflow

obstruction may result in decreased vital capacity and normal or increased FEV_1/VC (3).

The diffusing capacity of the lung for carbon monoxide (D_Lco)/transfer factor decreases in intrinsic lung disease, whereas it remains normal in extrinsic lung diseases. It is necessary to interpret D_Lco along with spirometry and lung volumes (body plethysmography). The degree of diffusing capacity for carbon monoxide grades the impairment as mild, moderate and severe (3). *Integrated Evaluation of Disability* defines impairment in extrinsic lung diseases based on FEV_1 % in the presence of decreased total lung capacity below the fifth percentile of the predicted value. In intrinsic lung disease, impairment is based on the degree of reduction of D_Lco percentage predicted. Illustration 10.4 describes the impairment classes for intrinsic and extrinsic restrictive lung diseases Illustration 10.5 describes the spirometry findings in persons with normal lung function, COPD, asthma, and restrictive lung disease.

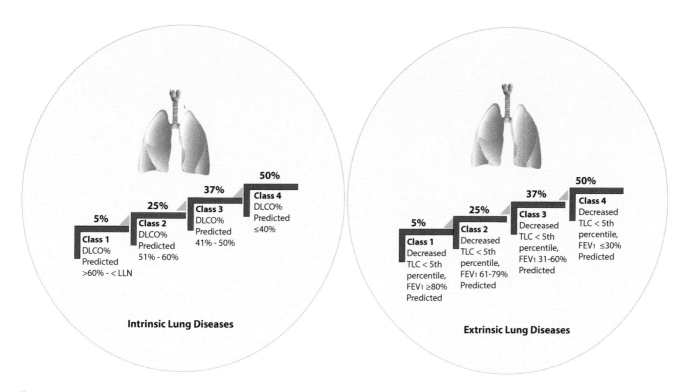

Illustration 10.4   Impairment classes in restrictive lung diseases.

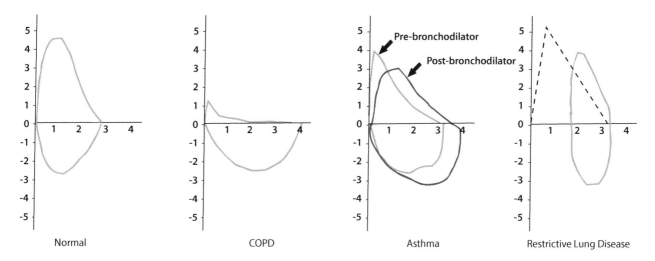

Illustration 10.5   Spirometry—Diseases of the lung.

10.5 CHRONIC RESPIRATORY FAILURE

Respiratory failure is a derangement in gas exchange function, that is, oxygenation and CO_2 elimination. It may be either hypoxemic or hypercapnic respiratory failure. In hypoxemic respiratory failure (type I respiratory failure), PaO_2 is less than 60 mm of Hg and $PaCO_2$ is normal or less than 50 mm of Hg. In hypercapnic respiratory failure (type II respiratory failure), $PaCO_2$ is more than 50 mm of

Hg, and arterial pH 7.45 (12). Chronic hypercapnic respiratory failure may be due to central hypoventilation, asthma, restrictive pulmonary diseases, obstructive pulmonary diseases, and obesity hypoventilation syndrome. Chronic hypercapnic respiratory failure may lead to pulmonary hypertension, right ventricular failure, and cor pulmonale. Illustration 10.6 describes the basis of impairment evaluation. *Integrated Evaluation of Disability* assigns an impairment of 50% for type II respiratory failure.

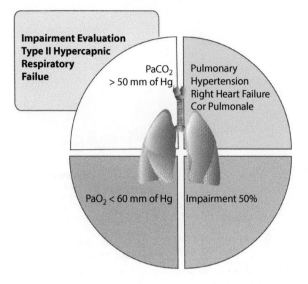

Illustration 10.6 Impairment evaluation in type II chronic respiratory failure.

10.6 RESPIRATORY MUSCLE PARALYSIS

An evaluation of respiratory muscles—diaphragm, intercostal muscles, and accessory muscles namely, scalenus, sternocleidomastoid, pectoralis major, serratus anterior, and lattissmusdorsi aids to define the impairment of respiratory muscle functions. The vital capacity of a normal person is about 3000–5000 cc. In inherited muscle disorders the vital capacity remains normal until it manifests respiratory muscle weakness of more than 50% (13). In a spinal cord injury with complete diaphragmatic paralysis, the vital capacity is very low (C3: 100 ccs, C4: 670 ccs). In unilateral diaphragmatic paralysis, vital capacity is less than 1000–1100 ccs. These persons may require assisted ventilation to restore and maintain alveolar ventilation to meet the metabolic demands as well as to correct arterial hypoxia. The vital capacity of individuals with intercostal and abdominal muscle paralysis but with intact diaphragm and accessory muscles of respiration varies from 1250 to 2500 cc (14).

Assisted ventilation is a vital requirement for persons with a vital capacity less than 500 ccs, and when higher vital capacity is rapidly declining (15).

The person with bilateral diaphragmatic paralysis remains ventilator dependent during his/her lifetime.

Integrated Evaluation of Disability relates the level of spinal cord injury, vital capacity, cough reflex and need for assisted ventilation to define impairment. It assigns Class 1 impairment of 15%, Class 2 impairment of 25%, Class 3 impairment of 50%, and Class 4 impairment of 75% as described in Illustration 10.7.

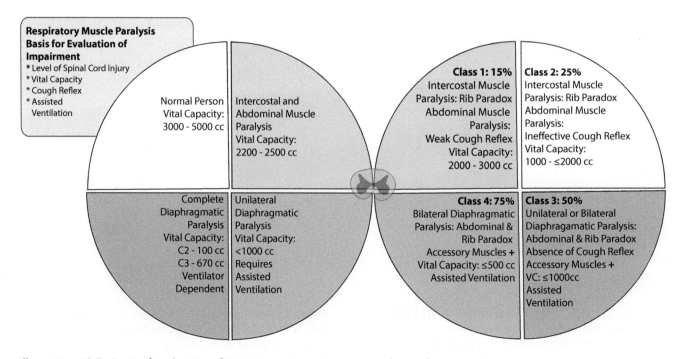

Illustration 10.7 Basis of evaluation of impairment in respiratory muscle paralysis.

10.7 SLEEP APNEA/HYPOPNEA SYNDROME

Sleep apnea results in disturbed sleep during the night and excessive daytime sleepiness. There are multiple events of apnea or hypopnea throughout sleep. It may last longer than 3 months (16). The sleep apnea may be either central apnea or obstructive sleep apnea. Obstructive sleep apnea is due to occlusion of the upper airway. There is a reduction in airflow due to the resistance of the upper airway passage in obstructive sleep apnea. Respiratory effort accompanies respiratory event in obstructive sleep apnea. In central apnea, there is a reduction in airflow due to decreased ventilatory drive. There is lack of respiratory effort in central apnea (17). The criteria for obstructive sleep hypopneas are snoring, drop in positive-airway-pressure device flow signal, or flattening of the nasal pressure from the pre-hypopnea reference level, and thoracoabdominal paradox during hypopnea. Snoring, drop in positive-airway-pressure device flow signal or flattening of nasal pressure, and thoracoabdominal paradox is absent in central apnea (18).

Persons with obstructive sleep apnea have a greater risk of developing hypertension, and about 50% of individuals with severe obstructive sleep apnea develop arrhythmias, such as bradyarrhythmias, premature ventricular contractions, and atrial fibrillation or flutter. Persons with severe obstructive sleep apnea have a greater risk of developing coronary artery disease, congestive failure, and stroke. There is an independent association between coronary artery disease and hypopneas with oxygen desaturation of more than 4%. There was a correlation between treatment of sleep apnea with Continuous positive airway pressure (CPAP) and decrease in systolic blood pressure, increase in

left ventricular function, and decrease in platelet activation (19,20). Furthermore being an independent risk factor, persons with obstructive sleep apnea may also develop pulmonary hypertension and subsequently cor pulmonale (21).

The oronasal thermal sensor detects the variation in airflow through the nose or mouth by changes in temperature in inhaled and exhaled air in apnea. Nasal pressure transducers are sensors that detect changes in airflow in hypopneas (18). It is preferable to use the alternative sensor signal when the oronasal thermal sensor is deferred (22). It is preferred to perform overnight pulse oximetry before planning polysomnography.

In "apnea," there is a reduction in airflow by 90% or more of the pre-apnea reference level detected by an oronasal thermal sensor or other recommended sensors, and the decrease in airflow extends for 10 seconds or longer. In "hypopnea," there is a decline in airflow by 30% or more of the pre-hypopnea reference level detected by nasal pressure sensors or other specified sensors, and the decrease in airflow remains for 10 seconds or longer, and oxygen desaturation also remains 3% or more from the pre-hypopnea reference level. Respiratory effort related arousal (RERA) may accompany hypopnea (18). Alpha and theta activity, or waveforms, greater than 16 cycles/second in EEG detect respiratory effort related arousal RERA (17). Respiratory disturbance index (RDI) refers to the combined number of respiratory events, namely hypopnea, apnea, and RERA per hour of sleep. RDI is 5-15 events per hour of sleep in mild apnea, 15-30 per hour of sleep in moderate apnea, and over 30 per hour of sleep in severe apnea (17).

Illustration 10.8 describes the impairment class for central/obstructive sleep apneas defined by *Integrated Evaluation of Disability*. It computes the additional percentage of impairment for the associated cognitive deficit if any.

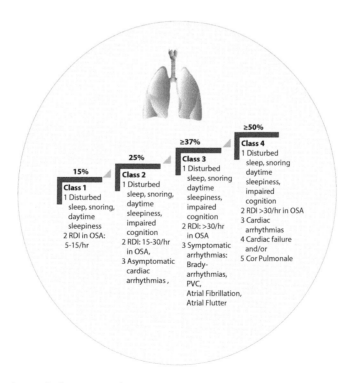

Illustration 10.8 Impairment classes in hypopneas/apneas.

REFERENCES

1. Wanger J, Clausen JL, Coates A, Pedersen OF, Brusasco V, Burgos F et al. Standardisation of the measurement of lung volumes. *Eur Respir J.* 2005;26:511–522.

2. Lusuardi M, De Benedetto F, Paggiaro P, Sanguinetti CM, Brazzola G, Ferri P, Donner CF. A randomized controlled trial on office spirometry in asthma and COPD in standard general practice data from spirometry in asthma and COPD: A comparative evaluation Italian study. *Chest.* 2006;129(4):844–852.

3. Pellegrino R, Viegi G, Brusasco V, Crapo RO, Burgos F, Casaburi R et al. Interpretative strategies for lung function tests. *Eur Respir J.* 2005;26(5):948–968.

4. Global Initiative for Chronic Obstructive Lung Disease. Global strategy for the diagnosis, management, and prevention of chronic obstructive pulmonary disease (Updated 2013) [Internet]. Global Initiative for Chronic Obstructive Lung Disease; 2013.

5. Komarow HD, Myles IA, Uzzaman A, Metcalfe DD. Impulse oscillometry in the evaluation of diseases of the airways in children. *Ann Allergy Asthma Immunol.* 2011;106(3):191–199.

6. Kim S, Oh J, Kim Y-I, Ban H-J, Kwon Y-S, Oh I-J, Kim K-S, Kim Y-C, Lim S-C. Differences in classification of COPD group using COPD assessment test (CAT) or modified Medical Research Council (mMRC) dyspnea scores: A cross-sectional analyses. *BMC Pulm Med.* 2013(13):35.

7. Hsu KY, Lin JR, Lin MS, Chen W, Chen YJ, Yan YH. The modified Medical Research Council dyspnoea scale is a good indicator of health-related quality of life in patients with chronic obstructive pulmonary disease. *Singapore Med J.* 2013;54(6):321–327.

8. National Asthma Education and Prevention Program. Expert panel report 3 (EPR-3): Guidelines for the diagnosis and management of asthma-summary report 2007. *J Allergy Clin Immunol.* 2007;120(5 Suppl):S94–S138.

9. Reddel HK, Bateman ED, Becker A, Boulet LP, Cruz AA, Drazen JM et al. A summary of the new GINA strategy: A roadmap to asthma control. *Eur Respir J.* 2015;46(3):622–639.

10. Bateman ED, Hurd SS, Barnes PJ, Bousquet J, Drazen JM, FitzGeralde JM et al. GLOBAL GUIDELINES Global strategy for asthma management and prevention: GINA executive summary. *Eur Respir J.* 2008;31(1):143–178.

11. Skloot GS, Busse PJ, Braman SS, Kovacs EJ, Dixon AE, Vaz Fragoso CA et al. An official American Thoracic Society workshop report: Evaluation and management of asthma in the elderly. *Ann Am Thorac Soc.* 2016;13(11):2064–2077.

12. Mokhlesi B, Tulaimat A, Evans AT, Wang Y, Itani AA, Hassaballa HA et al. Impact of adherence with positive airway pressure therapy on hypercapnia in obstructive sleep apnea. *J Clin Sleep Med.* 2006;2(1):57–62.

13. Australian Bureau of Statistics. 4430.0 - Disability, ageing and carers, Australia: Summary of findings, 2003 [Internet]. Available from: http://www.abs.gov.au/AUSSTATS/abs@.nsf/Lookup/4430.0Main+Features12003?

14. Carter RE. Respiratory aspects of spinal cord injury management. *Paraplegia.* 1987;25(3):262–266.

15. Gardner BP, Watt JW, Krishnan KR. The artificial ventilation of acute spinal cord damaged patients: A retrospective study of forty-four patients. *Paraplegia.* 1986;24(4):208–220.

16. *The International Classification of Sleep Disorders, Revised: Diagnostic and Coding Manual* [Internet]. American Academy of Sleep Medicine; 2001.

17. Tsara V, Amfilochiou A, Papagrigorakis MJ, Georgopoulos D, Liolios E. Guidelines for diagnosis and treatment of sleep-related breathing disorders in adults and children. Definition and classification of sleep related breathing disorders in adults: different types and indications for sleep studies (Part 1). *Hippokratia.* 2009;13(3):187–191.

18. Berry RB, Budhiraja R, Gottlieb DJ, Gozal D, Iber C, Kapur VK et al. Rules for scoring respiratory events in sleep: update of the 2007 AASM Manual for the Scoring of Sleep and Associated Events. Deliberations of the Sleep Apnea Definitions Task Force of the American Academy of Sleep Medicine. *J Clin Sleep Med.* 2012;8(5):597–619.

19. Dempsey JA, Veasey SC, Morgan BJ, O'Donnell CP. Pathophysiology of sleep apnea. *Physiol Rev.* 2010;90(1):47–112.

20. Jean-Louis G, Zizi F, Clark LT, Brown CD, McFarlane SI. Obstructive sleep apnea and cardiovascular disease: role of the metabolic syndrome and its components. *J Clin Sleep Med.* 2008;4(3):261–272.

21. Adegunsoye A, Ramachandran S. Etiopathogenetic mechanisms of pulmonary hypertension in sleep-related breathing disorders. *Pulm Med.* 2012;2012:273591.

22. Berry RB, Wagner MH. Fundamentals 13 - Respiratory event definitions in adults. In: *Sleep Medicine Pearls,* 3rd ed. Philadelphia, PA: Elsevier; 2015.

Impairment of functions in hematological and immunological systems

11.1 HEMATOLOGICAL SYSTEM

11.1.1 Anemia

In anemia, there is the insufficient oxygen-carrying capacity to meet the physiological needs of the body. Decreased red cell production results in anemia. Nutritional deficiencies, such as iron, folic acid, vitamin B12, inherited or acquired disorders affecting hemoglobin synthesis, decreases the production of the red cell. An inflammatory block due to acute and chronic inflammations or increased destruction due to autoantibodies causes a reduction in red blood cell count. Hemoglobin (Hgb) level in the blood defines the severity of anemia. Hemoglobin level of 110–129 g/L refers to mild anemia, 80–109 g/L to moderate anemia, and lower than 80 g/L to severe anemia in men 15 years of age and above. A hemoglobin level of 110–119 g/L refers to mild anemia, 80–109 g/L to moderate anemia, and lower than 80 g/L to severe anemia in non-pregnant women 15 years of age and above (1). A hemoglobin level of 70 g/L serves as a threshold for transfusion of red blood cell (2).

Persons with anemia develop palpitations, dyspnea, tachycardia, angina pectoris, dizziness, and syncope. ECG reveals de novo ST depression, or elevation on the electrocardiogram and new arrhythmia. Symptomatic anemia with hemoglobin less than 80 g/L requires transfusion of red blood cells. *Integrated Evaluation of Disability* describes asymptomatic chronic anemia with Hgb 110–129 g/L as Class 1 impairment of 0%. It assigns Class 2 impairment of 15% for symptomatic chronic anemia without cardiopulmonary limitations and Hgb >70–109 g/L requiring an occasional blood transfusion. It allocates Class 3 impairment of 37% for symptomatic chronic anemia with cardiopulmonary limitations,

Hgb ≤70 g/L requiring monthly blood transfusion and becoming transfusion-dependent for survival. It assigns impairment for chronic anemia only after having reached maximum medical improvement with maximum medical treatment (Illustration 11.1).

11.1.2 Leukemia

11.1.2.1 CHRONIC MYELOID LEUKAEMIA

Discovery of the Philadelphia chromosome and abnormal gene *BCR-ABL* in the blood and bone marrow of persons with chronic myeloid leukemia led to the development of newer drugs, such as Imatinib and later Dasatinib and Nilotinib. It has improved the management of chronic myeloid leukemia with a prospect of a good prognosis (3). The advent of tyrosine kinase inhibitors has completely changed the prognosis, and now chronic myeloid leukemia is a curable disease in many persons (4). Hence, persons with chronic myeloid leukemia do not develop any impairment of function. However, *Integrated Evaluation of Disability* recommends an impairment of 10% for the burden of treatment compliance if chronic myeloid leukemia remains uncured and under medication for more than the stipulated period.

11.1.2.2 CHRONIC LYMPHOID LEUKAEMIA

In typical B cell chronic lymphoid leukemia, the circulating lymphocytes are more than 4×10^9/L. *Integrated Evaluation of Disability* defines impairment in chronic lymphoid leukemia based on parameters namely lymphocytosis in the blood and bone marrow, lymphadenopathy, hepatomegaly, splenomegaly, anemia, and thrombocytopenia (Illustration 11.2).

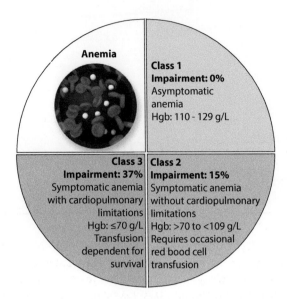

Illustration 11.1 Impairment classes in anemia.

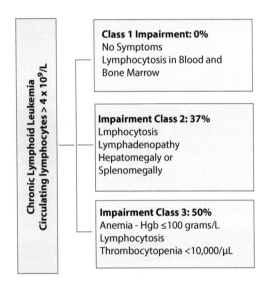

Illustration 11.2 Impairment classes in chronic lymphoid leukemia.

11.1.3 Clotting functions

11.1.3.1 THROMBOCYTOPENIA

Thrombocytopenia refers to a platelet count below $150 \times 10^9/L$, and $120 \times 10^9/L$ in late pregnancy (5). A person with thrombocytopenia manifests skin bruising, petechiae, bleeding gum and nasal bleeding, bleeding in gastrointestinal, urinary tracts, and menorrhagia. Platelet count defines the severity of thrombocytopenia. Persons with a platelet count over 50,000/μL do not have any significant bleeding diathesis. A platelet count between 20,000 and 50,000/μL denotes mild thrombocytopenia. These persons will bleed only as a result of major trauma or surgery. A platelet count between 10,000 and 20,000/μL denotes moderate thrombocytopenia.

In general, there is no serious spontaneous bleeding with a platelet count of above 10,000/μL. A platelet count below 10,000/μL indicates severe thrombocytopenia, and it triggers spontaneous bleeding (6). The modified WHO scale describes four grades of bleeding severity. Epistaxis, or oropharyngeal, bleeding for a less than 1 hour on a previous day, occult blood in the motion, petechiae, hematuria on a microscope, or vaginal bleeding refers to grade 1 bleeding. Epistaxis for about 1 hour or more on the previous day, hematoma, hemoptysis, melena, and purpura of more than one inch denote grade 2 bleeding. Bleeding in the central nervous system without symptoms requiring transfusion of red blood cells refers to grade 3 bleeding. Hemarthrosis, retinal hemorrhage with visual impairment, and bleeding in the central nervous system with severe hemodynamic instability often with fatal bleeding refers to grade 4 bleeding (7). *Integrated Evaluation of Disability* assigns Class 1 impairment of 5% for thrombocytopenia with platelet count of 20,000–50,000/μL, Class 2 impairment of 25% for thrombocytopenia with platelet count of 10,000–20,000/μL, and 50% for thrombocytopenia with platelet count of less than 10,000/μL refractory to treatment. It does not assign impairment to thrombocytopenia of temporary nature following infection or following drug therapy (Illustration 11.3).

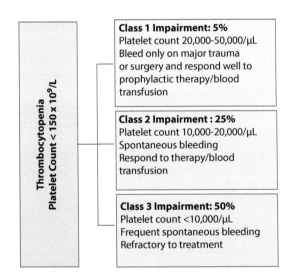

Illustration 11.3 Impairment classes in thrombocytopenia.

11.1.3.2 HEMOPHILIA

Hemophilia is a bleeding disorder due to a deficiency of a specific protein necessary for clotting of blood namely factor VIII and factor IX. A deficiency of factor VIII produces hemophilia "A" and a deficiency of factor IX produces hemophilia "B." Hemophilia "A" and "B" are inherited X-linked recessive disorders. Persons with severe hemophilia synthesize less than 1% of normal amount of these factors. Hence, they depend on the replacement of factors to prevent bleeding diathesis. A 30%–35% of persons with hemophilia "A" and 1%–3% of persons with hemophilia "B" develop inhibitory antibodies, which interfere with the functions of these factors VIII and IX (8). Hemophilia "C" is an autosomal recessive disorder due to deficiency factor XI. The bleeding tendency in "A" and "B" mainly relates to a factor level, whereas in "C" the bleeding does not correlate well with factor levels.

Bleeding and hemorrhage manifests spontaneously, during minor trauma, moderate/severe trauma, and during surgery. The bleeding in hemophilia may be intracranial, hemarthrosis, hematoma in muscles commonly gastrocnemius/iliopsoas/flexor muscles of the arm, and hematuria. If an adequate factor replacement is not controlling bleeding, it is necessary to confirm the presence of factor VIII or IX antibodies in the blood.

The level of coagulation factor serves to grade the severity of hemophilia. Class 1 impairment indicates coagulation factor level of more than 5% and less than 40%, that is, more than 0.05 and less than 0.40 IU/mL and hemorrhage occurs only during major trauma and surgery. Class 2 impairment denotes 1%–5% of normal factor level, that is, 0.01–0.05 IU/mL and triggers hemorrhage even with mild to moderate trauma. Class 3 impairment defines less than 1% of normal factor level, that is, less than 0.01 IU/mL and manifests spontaneous hemorrhage and hemarthrosis (6,9).

Illustration 11.4 describes the impairment class of hemophilia. Arthropathy, due to repeated bleeding, often results in a severe limitation of mobility and pain. Furthermore, there is coexisting hemophilia related nerve lesions, compartment syndrome, sequel due to intracranial bleeding, and so on, which can derive additional impairment.

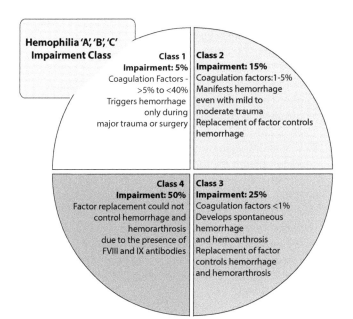

Illustration 11.4 Impairment classes in hemophilia.

11.2 IMMUNE FUNCTIONS

11.2.1 HIV

HIV refers to a human immunodeficiency virus infection. HIV depletes helper T lymphocytes "CD4+ cells" and produces a cellular immune deficiency. The clinical status of the disease namely activity of illness, advanced stage of disease, and CD4+ T- lymphocyte counts serve to classify the AIDS disease into three categories (10).

AIDS begins with a primary infection with HIV, stays as an asymptomatic chronic disease, and finally emerges as a progressive disease with severe immune deficiency, opportunistic infections, and neoplasms (11).

Category "A" comprises of asymptomatic infection, persistent generalized lymphadenopathy, acute primary infection, or a history of acute primary infection. Category "B" includes symptomatic infection due to HIV or due to impairment of cell-mediated immunity. Category "C" comprises of clinical conditions included in the 1993 AIDS surveillance definition. "CD4+ T cells" count subdivides category "A" into A1—≥500/μL, A2—200–499 cell/μL and A3—<200 cell/μL. "CD4+ T cells" count subdivides category "B" into B1—≥500/μL, B2—200–499 cell/μL and B3—<200 cell/μL, and category "C" into C1—≥500/μL, C2—200–499 cell/μL and C3—<200 cell/μL (10).

In advanced AIDS, there is the persistence of low CD4 less than 50 cells/cc, viral burden with 100,000 copies/mL despite combination therapy, and failure of optimized treatment due to multidrug resistance. Further, progressive hepatitis C with hepatic failure, progressive leukoencephalopathy with dementia, unresponsive Kaposi's sarcoma, end-stage renal and cardiac failure, and unresponsive lymphoma/other malignancy accompanies advanced disease (12).

Antiretroviral therapy (ART) decreases the risk of the progression of the HIV infection (13). ART is necessary for individuals with the severe and advanced disease, in people with CD4 count ≤500 cells/mm³, combined HIV and tuberculosis, combined HIV and Hepatitis B Virus (HBV), and in partners without HIV infection (14). *Integrated Evaluation of Disability* assigns Class 1 impairment of 15% for persons with HIV infection (category "A" on ART) for the burden of treatment compliance and stigma associated with HIV infection. It allocates Class 2 impairment of 25% for persons with AIDS disease (category "B") for the burden of disease due to poor response to treatment or failure of treatment, burden treatment compliance, and stigma associated with HIV infection. It assigns Class 3 impairment of 25% + for individuals with advanced AIDS disease (category "C"). Dementia, renal failure, cardiac failure, liver failure, neoplasms, and so on, add an additional impairment score for category "C" (Illustration 11.5).

11.2.2 Splenectomy

The spleen plays a significant role in immune functions and removes encapsulated bacteria and foreign matter. Traumatic injuries (such as a blunt injury to the spleen),

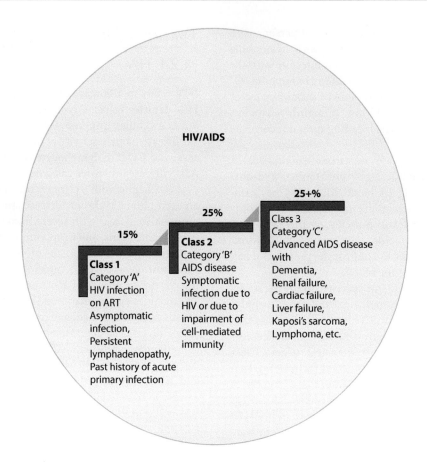

Illustration 11.5 Impairment classes in HIV/AIDS.

idiopathic thrombocytopenic purpura, hereditary spherocytosis, autoimmune hemolytic anemia, thrombocytopenic purpura, Hodgkin and non-Hodgkin lymphoma, chronic lymphocytic leukemia, hemangiomas, idiopathic myelofibrosis, myelodysplastic syndrome, hairy cell leukemia, splenic abscess or cyst, and tuberculosis require splenectomy (15).

A splenectomy removes 25% of lymphoid tissue and most of the macrophages. Persons who undergo a splenectomy are liable for infection with encapsulated bacteria. Vaccines are available to protect them against pneumococcal and Haemophilus Influenza infections. Hence, *Integrated Evaluation of Disability* does not assign any impairment for splenectomy.

REFERENCES

1. *Haemoglobin Concentrations for the Diagnosis of Anaemia and Assessment of Severity*. Vitamin and Mineral Nutrition Information System (VMNIS). Geneva, Switzerland: World Health Organization; 2011.
2. Tobian AA, Heddle NM, Wiegmann TL, Carson JL. Red blood cell transfusion: 2016 clinical practice guidelines from AABB. *Transfusion.* 2016;56(10):2627–2630.
3. Druker B. *Targeted Therapy for Chronic Myeloid Leukemia.* Washington, DC: American Society of Hematology; 2008.
4. Thompson PA, Kantarjian HM, Cortes JE. Diagnosis and treatment of chronic myeloid leukemia in 2015. *Mayo Clin Proc.* 2015;90(10):1440–1454.
5. Duodecim FMS. Thrombocytopenia. In: *EBM Guidelines. Evidence-Based Medicine* [Internet]. Helsinki, Finland: Wiley Interscience; 2007.
6. Thiagarajan P. *Expert Opinion on 'Integrated Evaluation of Disability: Thrombocytopenia'.* Houston, TX: Department of Hematopathology, Bayer College of Medicine; 2011.
7. Bercovitz RS, O'Brien SH. Measuring bleeding as an outcome in clinical trials of prophylactic platelet transfusions. *Hematology.* 2012;2012:157–160.
8. Lusher JM. *Hemophilia: From Plasma to Recombinant Factors.* Washington, DC: American Society of Hematology; 2008.
9. White GC 2nd, Rosendaal F, Aledort LM, Lusher JM, Rothschild C, Ingerslev J et al. Definitions in hemophilia. Recommendation of the scientific subcommittee on factor VIII and factor IX of the scientific and standardization committee of the International Society on Thrombosis and Haemostasis. *Thromb Haemost.* 2001;85:560.
10. *1993 Revised Classification System for HIV Infection and Expanded Surveillance Case Definition for AIDS Among Adolescents and Adults.* Atlanta, GA:

Morbidity and Mortality Weekly Report, Centers for Disease Control and Prevention, Department of Health and Human Services; 1992.

11. *The Relationship Between the Human Immunodeficiency Virus and the Acquired Immunodeficiency Syndrome.* In: National Institute of Allergy and Infectious Disease - National Institute of Health UDoHaHS, editor. Rockville, MD: US Department of Health and Human Services; 2010.

12. Anderson JR. *A Guide to the Clinical Care of Women with HIV, 2005 Edition.* Rockville, MD: Department of Health and Human Services, Health Resources and Services Administration, HIV/AIDS Bureau; 2005.

13. Adolescent PoAGfAa. *Guidelines for the Use of Antiretroviral Agents in HIV-1-Infected Adults and Adolescents.* In: Department of Health and Human Services, editor. 2013.

14. *Consolidated Guidelines on the Use of Antiretroviral Drugs for Treating and Preventing HIV Infection - Recommendations for a Public Health Approach.* Geneva, Switzerland: World Health Organization; 2013. p. 28.

15. Gamme G, Birch DW, Karmali S. Minimally invasive splenectomy: An update and review. *Can J Surg.* 2013;56(4):280–285.

12

Impairment of swallowing, liver, and defecation functions

12.1 SWALLOWING FUNCTIONS

Dysphagia refers to a subjective feeling of difficulty in swallowing when the food, either solid or liquid, traverses from mouth to stomach (1).

12.1.1 Oral swallowing

Oral swallowing refers to the transfer of solid or liquid food through the mouth at optimum speed (2).

There is impairment in the control of tongue during preparatory and propulsive phases of swallowing in conditions such as in paralysis of the tongue resulting in dysphagia. In oral dysphagia, there is difficulty in chewing solid food, difficulty in initiating swallowing or containing liquid food in the oral cavity before swallowing, and dribbling of food from the mouth.

12.1.2 Pharyngeal swallowing

Pharyngeal swallowing refers to the transfer of either solid or liquid food through the pharynx at optimum speed (2). In the pharyngeal dysphagia, there is the aspiration of food, nasal penetration of food, nasal quality of voice, the unilateral and bilateral absence of pharyngeal and palatal reflex, and lack of upward migration of larynx during attempted swallowing.

12.1.3 Esophageal swallowing

Esophageal swallowing refers to the transfer of either solid or liquid food through the esophagus at optimum speed (2).

A person with an impairment of esophageal swallowing retains food or liquid in the esophagus after swallowing and develops a localized sensation of blockage or discomfort in the retrosternal region, oral and pharyngeal regurgitation, and recurrent pneumonia. Impairment of esophageal swallowing also includes esophageal vomiting, that is, passive vomiting with undigested food, and associated loss of weight.

Video-fluoroscopic imaging can identify stricture esophagus due to corrosive intake, space occupying lesion, and esophageal paresis/paralysis. Esophagoscopy and biopsy may confirm space-occupying lesions. Esophageal motility studies may contribute to improving the diagnosis when fluoroscopy and esophagoscopy are unremarkable and noncontributory.

Postural techniques for minimizing the risk of aspiration include chin tug, head rotation to the weaker side, side lying position, and compensatory maneuvers, for example, Mendelsohn, effortful swallow, supraglottic swallow, and super-supraglottic swallow. In the Mendelson maneuver, the person maintains hyolaryngeal elevation for about two seconds to prolong the upper esophageal sphincter opening during swallowing (3). Individuals with severe dysphagia require feeding by nasogastric tube or gastrostomy (Percutaneous Endoscopic Gastrostomy) to maintain nutrition.

Integrated Evaluation of Disability defines impairment based on the variables namely drooling, the risk of aspiration, postural techniques, and compensatory maneuvers adopted to minimize the possibility of aspiration during swallowing and alternate feeding methods, namely nasogastric feeding and feeding through gastrostomy (percutaneous endoscopic gastrostomy) (Table 12.1).

Table 12.1 Impairment class—Oral, pharyngeal, and esophageal swallowing functions

Impairment class	Criteria	Reference impairment score
Class 1	Difficulty in swallowing with drooling of saliva or drooling during drinking liquids or accumulation of solid food in the alveoli of mouth	2.5%
Class 2	Prolonged duration of meal with sensation of holding of food in the throat Difficulty in swallowing with nasal regurgitation and/or occasional choking	5.0%
Class 3	Difficulty in swallowing with nasal regurgitation and on-and-off choking or Limited swallowing ability by modifying food consistency	15%
Class 4	Difficulty in swallowing with frequent nasal regurgitation and choking or Limited swallowing ability by modifying food consistency, and postural techniques and compensatory maneuvers to minimize the risk of aspiration	25%
Class 5	Inability to swallow, develop significant aspiration on attempted swallowing and require feeding by nasogastric tube or PEG (Percutaneous Endoscopic Gastrostomy)	50%

12.2 LIVER FUNCTION

The liver performs principal functions namely synthesis of albumin, carrier proteins, coagulation factors, growth and hormonal factors, bile acid, cholesterol, lecithin, phospholipids; regulation of nutritive products such as glucose, glycogen, amino acids, lipids, cholesterol; metabolism of drugs; and so on.

Hepatitis B and C, autoimmune hepatitis, alcoholic liver disease, non-alcoholic fatty liver disease, non-alcoholic steatohepatitis, primary biliary cirrhosis, primary sclerosing cholangitis, alpha-1-antitrypsin deficiency, Wilson disease, and hemochromatosis are all common causes of liver failure (4).

Hepatic encephalopathy is the major complication of chronic hepatic insufficiency. Elevated serum level of ammonia and manganese, swelling of astrocyte, intra-astrocytic glutamine, and upregulation of translocator protein 18-kDa (TPSO) may precipitate encephalopathy in hepatic insufficiency. Hyponatremia in liver failure may increase the risk of developing raised intracranial pressure and in turn brain edema (5). Hepatic encephalopathy manifests as impairments of consciousness, sleep, cognition, sensory and motor functions, and personality changes (6).

Hyponatremia is an important predictor of prognosis in persons with the end-stage liver disease. Further, ascites and renal impairment accompany hepatic encephalopathy. There was a linear increase in mortality for every mmol/L (millimole per liter) reduction of serum sodium in the blood with significant correlation (7).

Serum level of bilirubin indicates the ability of the liver to excrete bile; International Normalized Ratio (INR) measures coagulopathy, that is, the ability of the liver to produce blood clotting factors (7) and is a useful prognostic tool rather than an indicator of bleeding risk in patients with the chronic liver disease.

There is associated impairment of renal function in persons with end-stage liver failure, and is a significant predictor of mortality in liver failure (7). Chapter 8 describes the evaluation of the excretory function of the kidney.

Serum levels of bilirubin, albumin, sodium, INR, and hepatic encephalopathy define the impairment class in chronic liver failure (Table 12.2 and Illustration 12.1).

Table 12.2 Impairment class—Chronic liver failure

Impairment class	Encephalopathy	Serum level of bilirubin	INR	Serum level of albumin	Serum level of sodium	Impairment score
Class 1	Anxiety or euphoria	1–2 mg/dL	1.1–2.0	>3.5 gm/dL	136–140 mmol/L	25%
Class 2	(1) Lethargy and minor impairment of awareness; (2) Impairment of cognition: poor attention span, difficulty in orientation for time and place, difficulty in calculation for addition, subtraction; (3) Asterixis (flapping tremor) (4) Inappropriate; behavior	2.1–3 mg/dL	2.1–3.0	3.1–3.5 gm/dL	131–135 mmol/L	50%
Class 3	(1) Somnolent but arousable; (2) Impairment of cognition: lack of orientation for place/time/ person; (3) Asterixis (flapping tremor), hyperreflexia, and plantar extensor response; (4) Bizarre behavior	3.1–4 mg/dL	3.1–4	2.6–3.0 gm/dL	126–130 mmol/L	75%
Class 4	Coma not responding to verbal or painful stimuli	>4 mg/dL	>4	≤2.5 gm/dL	≤125 mmol/L	95%
Class 1	*Integrated Evaluation of Disability* assigns Class 1 impairment to persons who underwent liver transplantation because of burden of treatment compliance					25%

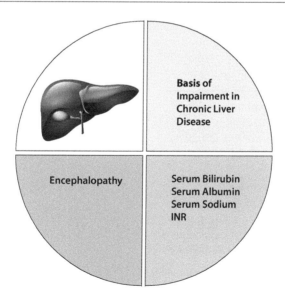

Illustration 12.1 Basis for defining impairment in chronic liver failure.

12.3 DEFECATION FUNCTION

Defecation refers to expulsion of waste and undigested food as fecal matter (8). Inability to control bowel movement results in incontinence. Inability to initiate bowel movement results in constipation. In neurogenic bowel dysfunction, there is also loss of sensation of bowel fullness and loss of sensation of bowel movement. Neurological cause, frequency of bowel movement, response to fiber supplements and suppositories, need for prokinetic agents, and mandate for colostomy are essential variables to define impairment class in constipation. *Integrated Evaluation of Disability* assigns an impairment of 37% for incontinence, that is, inability to control bowel movement associated with lack of sensation of bowel fullness and movement. Table 12.3 describes various impairments of defecation function.

Table 12.3 Impairment class—Defecation function

Impairment class	Nature of impairment	Impairment
Class 1	**Constipation:** Difficulty in initiating bowel movement and evacuating bowel less than three times per week due to neurological cause and requiring fiber supplements, and suppositories for evacuation of bowel	5%
Class 2	**Constipation:** Difficulty in initiating bowel movement and evacuating bowel less than three times per week due to a neurological cause; Refractory to fiber supplements and suppositories Requires prokinetic agents	10%
Class 3	**Constipation:** Difficulty in initiating bowel movement and evacuating bowel one time per week due to neurological cause and requiring enema for evacuation	15%
	Constipation: Anismus, dyssynergia, descending perineal syndrome	15%
	Constipation: Mechanical obstruction due to partial occlusion of anus, e.g., following burns	15%
Class 4	**Constipation:** Mechanical obstruction due to complete occlusion of anus, for instance, following burns	25%
Class 5	**Incontinence:** Inability in controlling bowel movement resulting in incontinence and lack of sensation of bowel fullness and movement due to neurological cause and requiring diapers	37%
Class 6	**Permanent colostomy**	50%

REFERENCES

1. ACR Appropriateness Criteria® dysphagia [Internet]. American College of Radiology. 2010.
2. *International Classification of Functioning, Disability and Health*. Geneva, Switzerland: World Health Organization; 2001. p. 82.
3. Wheeler-Hegland K, Ashford J, Frymark T, McCabe D, Mullen R, Musson N et al. Evidence-based systematic review: Oropharyngeal dysphagia behavioral treatments. Part II–impact of dysphagia treatment on normal swallow function. *J Rehabil Res Dev.* 2009;46(2):185–194.
4. Murray KF, Carithers RL Jr. AASLD practice guidelines: Evaluation of the patient for liver transplantation. *Hepatology.* 2005;41(6):1407–1432.
5. Manka P, Bechmann LP, Tacke F, Sowa JP, Schlattjan M, Kalsch J et al. Serum sodium-based modification of the MELD does not improve prediction of outcome in acute liver failure. *BMC Gastroenterol.* 2013;13:58.
6. Poh Z, Chang PE. A current review of the diagnostic and treatment strategies of hepatic encephalopathy. *Int J Hepatol.* 2012;2012:480309.
7. Asrani SK, Kim WR. Model for end-stage liver disease: End of the first decade. *Clin Liver Dis.* 2011;15(4):685–698.
8. *International Classification of Functioning, Disability and Health*. Geneva, Switzerland: World Health Organization; 2001. p. 83.

13

Impairment of visual functions

13.1 VISUAL FUNCTIONS

Visual functions refer to a multitude of functions comprising of acuity of vision, color vision, acuity of alignment, the perception of movement and perception of changing luminous intensity or differentiating luminous intensity, that is, contrast (1). Visual impairments include myopia, hypermetropia, astigmatism, hemianopia, color blindness, tunnel vision, central and peripheral scotoma, diplopia, night blindness, and impaired adaptability to light (2). The World Health Organization estimates that 285 million people in the world have a visual impairment. The primary causes of visual impairment are refractive error, cataract, and glaucoma (3).

Eighty percent of sensory information processed by the brain is from the eye (4). Eye processes 80%–85% of sensory information for visual perception, performing a cognitive function, and participating major life activities including learning (5). Hence, *Integrated Evaluation of Disability* assigns maximum impairment of 85% for the total blindness of both eyes. A person with complete blindness of one eye can function independently with the normal functioning another eye, though there is impairment of depth perception. Hence, *Integrated Evaluation of Disability* assigns maximum impairment of only 15% in persons with total blindness of one eye for lack of depth perception and low level of safety for the normal eye.

13.2 ACUITY OF VISION

Acuity of vision refers to the clarity of vision with details of perception such as form and contour of visual stimuli for both distant and near vision.

13.2.1 Distance vision

The Snellen chart assesses the acuity of vision within 6 meters (20 feet). The evaluator assesses each eye separately with a pinhole occluder and current spectacles. The person reads the multi-letter, or "E," or "C" Snellen chart with proper illumination. The line with the smallest letters that the person could read refers to a fraction, for example, 6/60 where numerator 6 denotes the test distance in meters at which the person could recognize the symbol and denominator 60 indicates the distance in meters at which the person with normal vision could recognize the symbol. The evaluator ascertains if the person could not read the largest letter on the Snellen chart at 6 m whether he/she could read at 5 m from the chart (5/60). If the person could not read the letters at 5 m, the evaluator assess whether he/she could read at 4 m (4/60), 3 m (3/60), 2 m (2/60). If the person could not read even at a 1-meter distance (1/60), the evaluator further ascertains whether he/she could count the fingers at less than one-meter distance, and, if it is not possible, whether he/she could recognize hand movement. Finally, the evaluator examines whether he/she could perceive the light splashed on his/her eye (6).

In clinical conditions, such as multiple sclerosis, low-contrast grayscale rather than a black and white letter chart (or Sloan letter chart) can detect visual impairment early. Multiple sclerosis also manifests as photophobia, excessive glare, visual fading, diplopia, and photopsia. The King-Devick test evaluates impairment of saccades related to fatigue associated with multiple sclerosis (7).

The International Statistical Classification of Diseases and Related Health Problems 10th Revision (ICD-10 Version: 2015) classifies visual impairment as (1) no or mild visual impairment, (2) moderate visual impairment, (3) severe visual impairment, and (4) blindness. It has classified visual impairment into five categories (8) (Tables 13.1 and 13.2).

13.2.2 Near acuity of vision

The evaluator uses either reduced Snellen acuity card to evaluate near vision at distance of 16″ (40 cm) or Jaeger acuity card—20 letter sizes from J1 to J20 or "M" notation

Table 13.1 Impairment class—Distance acuity of monocular vision: Both eyes

Impairment class	ICD-10 version: 2015 categories (8)	Presenting distance visual acuity			Reference impairment score acuity of vision	Select impairment score Right eye	Select impairment score Left eye	Impairment score of both eyes
		Snellen notation	US notation	Decimal notation				
Class 0	Category 0—Mild or "no" visual impairment	Equal to or better than 6/18	Equal to or better than 20/70	Equal to or better than 3/10 (0.3)	0%			
Class 1	Category 1—Moderate impairment	Equal to or better than 6/60 Worse than 6/18	Equal to or better than 20/200 Worse than 20/70	Equal to or better than 1/10 (0.1) Worse than 3/10 (0.3)	5%			
Class 2	Category 2—Severe impairment	Equal to or better than 3/60 Worse than 6/60	Equal to or better than 20/400 Worse than 20/200	Equal to or better than 1/20 (0.05) Worse than 1/10 (0.1)	15%			
Class 3	Category 3—Blindness	Equal to or better than 1/60 Worse than 3/60	Equal to or better than 20/1200 Worse than 20/400	Equal to or better than 1/50 (0.02) Worse than 1/20 (0.05)	25%			
Class 4	Category 4—Blindness	Equal to or better than Light Perception Worse than 1/60	Equal to or better than Light Perception Worse than 20/1200	Equal to or better than Light Perception Worse than 1/50 (0.02)	37%			
Class 5	Category 5—Blindness	No light perception			42.5%			

Total impairment of right and left eye

Table 13.2 Impairment class—Distance acuity of vision with normal vision in another eye

Impairment class	ICD–10 version: 2015 categories (8)	Presenting distance visual acuity			Reference impairment score acuity of vision	Select impairment score of affected eye
		Snellen notation	US notation	Decimal notation		
Class 0	Category 0—Mild or "no" visual impairment	Equal to or better than 6/18	Equal to or better than 20/70	Equal to or better than 3/10 (0.3)	0%	
Class 1	Category 1—Moderate impairment	Equal to or better than 6/60 Worse than 6/18	Equal to or better than 20/200 Worse than 20/70	Equal to or better than 1/10 (0.1) Worse than 3/10 (0.3)	1%	
Class 2	Category 2—Severe impairment	Equal to or better than 3/60 Worse than 6/60	Equal to or better than 20/400 Worse than 20/200	Equal to or better than 1/20 (0.05) Worse than 1/10 (0.1)	2.5%	
Class 3	Category 3—Blindness	Equal to or better than 1/60 Worse than 3/60	Equal to or better than 20/1200 Worse than 20/400	Equal to or better than 1/50 (0.02) Worse than 1/20 (0.05)	5%	
Class 4	Category 4—Blindness	Equal to or better than Light Perception Worse than 1/60	Equal to or better than Light Perception Worse than 20/1200	Equal to or better than Light Perception Worse than 1/50 (0.02)	10%	
Class 5	Category 5—Blindness	No light perception			15%	

Table 13.3 Impairment class—Near acuity of vision

Impairment class	Distance for letter recognition of 1M print	Reference impairment score binocular vision	Select the impairment score
Class 0	160 cm	0%	
	125 cm		
	100 cm		
	80 cm		
Class 1	63 cm	5%	
	50 cm		
	40 cm		
	32 cm		
Class 2	25 cm	25%	
	20 cm		
	16 cm		
	12 cm		
Class 3	10 cm	50%	
	8 cm		
	6 cm		
	5 cm		
Class 4	4 cm	75%	
	3 cm		
	2.5 cm		
	2 cm		
Class 5		85%	

(1 "M" unit = 1.454 mm or 1/16″) or point system with each point measuring 0.35 mm. Continuous text reading chart with various print sizes at different distances aids to measure the impairment of functional near vision. It is necessary to evaluate near vision, if near vision impairment is severe than distant vision (Table 13.3).

Integrated Evaluation of Disability combines both near and distance acuity of vision to arrive an average impairment of acuity of vision.

13.3 FIELD OF VISION

Field of vision refers to the perception of the whole visual field during fixation of gaze (2). Accurate evaluation and interpretation of field defect are necessary to classify visual impairment. The confrontation test evaluates visual field at the bedside. Equipment, such as Tangent screen, Goldmann perimetry, and standard automated perimetry (SAP) also serve to assess the field of vision (9). The confrontation test identifies only larger defects in the field in four locations in the visual field. Tangent screen estimates only the central 30° of the visual field. Goldmann perimetry is a kinetic perimetry in which the stimulus starts from outside the visual field and moves into the visual field. Automated perimetry evaluates the visual field using a computer either by a stationary stimulus or by a kinetic stimulus remaining for about 200 millisecond. Depending on the visual impairment, the size (0.5°–2° diameter) and intensity of the stimulus (brightest stimulus 0 dB to the dimmest stimulus 51 dB) increases or decreases to the level the person could recognize (1). Goldmann perimetry applies stimulus size I (0.25 mm²) to V (64 mm²), and Humphrey perimetry uses 4 mm² stimuli (equivalent to Goldmann size III stimulus) (10). The stimulus tests the points in one meridian in a radial or a circular pattern. The visibility of a white target in the perimetry depends on the size and the luminous intensity of the spot as well as background illumination. It identifies peripheral limits or boundaries of the visual field and relative visual acuity. Isopters refers to boundaries or contour lines.

In binocular vision, the two images fuse to form a single image (Figure 13.1). The binocular fusion also provides depth perception (11). The evaluation of impairment of binocular visual field requires the Esterman test in Humphrey Field Analyzer, or integrating visual fields by combining right and left visual fields (10).

The central field refers to inner 30° of the visual field (12). The visual field extends laterally (temporally) for 100°, medially (nasally) 60°, superiorly 60° and inferiorly 70° from central fixation (Illustration 13.1) (10). The absence of vision anywhere in the visual field excepting the blind spot is abnormal. The blind spot lies in the temporal field approximately 12° to 17° from the central fixation and 1.5° below the horizontal meridian (12) (Illustration 13.2).

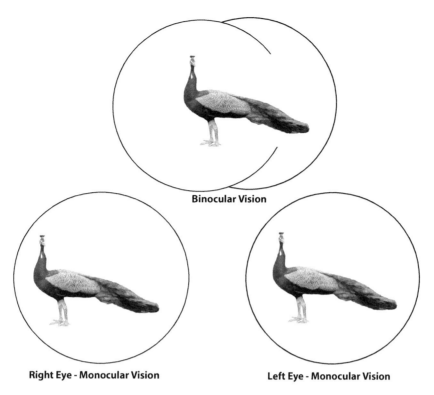

Figure 13.1 Binocular vision.

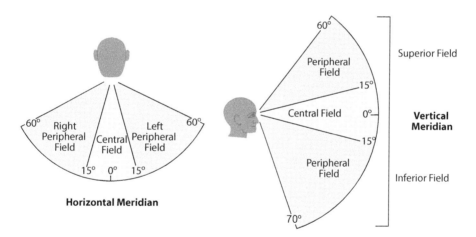

Illustration 13.1 Field of vision—Vertical and horizontal meridians.

The visual field in the center is light adaptive. It has a high acuity of vision with excellent color sensitivity and works efficiently with high illumination (photopic system). The visual field in the periphery is dark adapted and has reduced acuity and poor color sensitivity. It works effectively with minimum illumination (scotopic system) (11). Thus, the central field is essential for reading, working on the computer, and manipulative tasks involved in domestic, educational, vocational, and avocational activities. The peripheral field is vital for activities in the dark as well as during mobility. A defect in the central and inferior field is more disabling than that of the superior field and, hence, derives more weight for a

defect in the central and inferior field. The nasal field obtains lesser impairment than that of the temporal field because of the smaller field area.

Integrated Evaluation of Disability assigns an impairment of 42.5% for loss of field of monocular vision. The visual field comprises of central (inner 30°) and peripheral field. The central field receives an impairment of 24% and peripheral field an impairment of 18.50%. The central field consists of four quadrants namely central superior temporal, central superior nasal, central inferior temporal, and central inferior nasal fields. Each central field gets an impairment of 6%. *Integrated Evaluation of Disability* divides peripheral

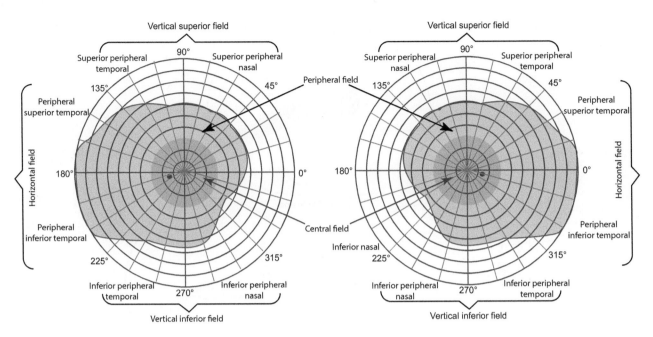

Illustration 13.2 Perimetry—Fields of vision.

field based on vertical and horizontal meridians into vertical superior temporal, vertical superior nasal, horizontal superior temporal, horizontal superior nasal, horizontal inferior temporal, horizontal inferior nasal, vertical inferior temporal, and vertical inferior nasal fields. It assigns an impairment of 2% for vertical superior temporal, 2% for vertical superior nasal, 3% for vertical inferior temporal, 3% for vertical inferior nasal, 2.75% for horizontal superior temporal, 2.75%

for horizontal inferior temporal, 1.50% for horizontal superior nasal, and 1.50% for horizontal inferior nasal field. If the visual field defect is partial and/or incongruous, it assigns an impairment for the field based on the percentage of the size of the defect, for example, if the size of the vertical superior nasal peripheral is 50%, the impairment is only 1.00% for the field defect. The maximum impairment for visual field defect in both eyes should not exceed 85% (Illustration 13.3).

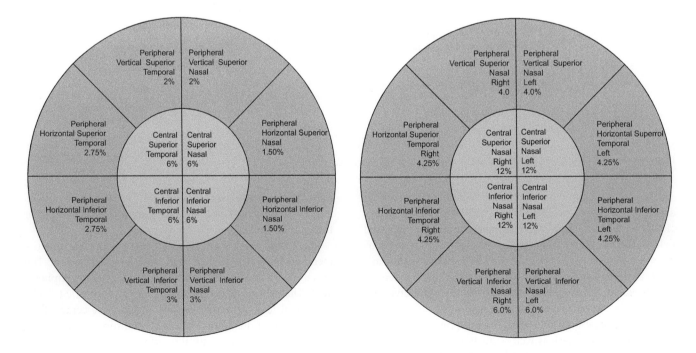

Illustration 13.3 Impairment monocular and binocular fields of vision.

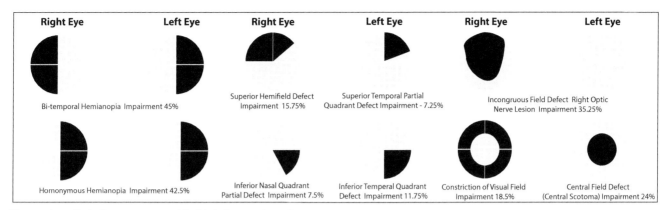

Illustration 13.4 Common visual field defects—Impairment.

ICD-10 Version 2015 (8) classifies visual field defects. It comprises of the enlarged blind spot, generalized contraction of the visual field, hemianopsia (heteronymous) (homonymous), quadrant anopsia, and scotoma: Arcuate, Bjerrum, Central, and Ring (Illustration 13.4).

13.4 CONTRAST SENSITIVITY

Contrast sensitivity refers to the function of discriminating figures from the ground with minimum luminance. It may not impair acuity of vision. The tendency to perceive larger objects with minimum contrast may interfere with activities of daily living (13). The Pelli-Robson Contrast Sensitivity Chart measures contrast sensitivity in which the contrast of the capital letters in the successive lines are decreasing without decreasing the size of the letters on white background. Low/poor contrast sensitivity triggers risk of accidents during driving in the night. *Integrated Evaluation of Disability* assigns an impairment of 5% for low contrast sensitivity and 10% for poor contrast sensitivity (Table 13.4).

13.5 LIGHT SENSITIVITY

Light sensitivity refers to visual functions of detecting minimum amount of light, and discriminate the minimum difference in intensity. It includes functions of dark adaptation, night blindness, and photophobia.

13.5.1 Night blindness

Retinitis pigmentosa, vitamin A deficiency, glaucoma, X-linked congenital stationary night blindness, gyrate atrophy, Laurence-Moon syndrome, Oguchi disease, optic atrophy, peripheral chorioretinitis, siderosis retinae, cancer-associated retinopathy or hypoxia, and uncorrected myopia causes night blindness (nyctalopia). If night blindness is irreversible even after maximum medical management, *Integrated Evaluation of Disability* assigns an impairment of 25%.

13.5.2 Photophobia

The causes for photophobia include iritis, uveitis, and corneal disease. The photogenic stimulus of 2–8 cycles/second causes photophobia in persons with migraine. There are evidences that FL-41 pinkish tinted sunglasses have a mixture of colors, which block the blue-green wavelengths, and, hence, reduce the blepharospasm (14). *Integrated Evaluation of Disability* assigns an impairment of 10% if photophobia persists, and 25% for irreversible night blindness even after maximum medical management (Table 13.5).

Table 13.4 Impairment class—Contrast sensitivity

Clinical tool—Pelli Robson contrast sensitivity chart	Reference impairment score	Impairment score
Normal contrast sensitivity: Can read all the eight lines without difficulty	0%	
Low contrast sensitivity: Difficulty in reading last three lines	5%	
Poor contrast sensitivity: Cannot read the last three lines	10%	

Table 13.5 Impairment class—Light sensitivity

Light sensitivity	Reference impairment score	Maximum impairment 25%
Persistent photophobia even after maximum medical treatment	10%	
Irreversible night blindness even after maximum medical treatment	25%	

13.6 COLOR VISION

Color vision refers to the visual functions of perception, and distinguishing and matching colors (2). The causes for color blindness include congenital, optic neuropathies, macular diseases, media opacities, and amblyopia. Congenital color blindness is mostly for red and green. Glaucoma and diseases of the optic nerve produces color blindness for blue and yellow (15).

Photoreceptors, or "cones," concentrated in the center of the retina (mainly fovea) perceive the color of an object. The photoreceptors, which are the long, medium and short wavelength sensitive cones, recognize primary colors respectively, namely red, green, and blue. Color blindness due to deficiencies of photoreceptors, namely the long and medium cones, are gender-linked deficiencies. The color blindness, due to deficiency of small cones, is autosomal inheritance. Protanopia refers to color blindness for red light due to the absence of large cones. Deuteranopia refers to color blindness for green light due to lack of medium cones. Tritanopia refers to color blindness for blue light due to lack of small cones. The person with anomalous photoreceptors can recognize all colors but with reduced discrimination. Protanomaly refers to reduced sensitivity to red light due to the anomaly of large cones, deuteranomaly to reduced sensitivity to green light due to the anomaly of medium cones, and tritanomaly to reduced sensitivity to blue light due to the anomaly of small cones.

Normal persons (trichromats) are sensitive to red, green, and blue light. Dichromats, with two photoreceptors, can recognize two colors. Most of the dichromats are red and green color deficient. Yellow and blue color deficient persons are rare. Monochromats with a single photoreceptor are color blind as they cannot recognize any color signal. They perceive only grayscale between black and white. Persons with achromatopsia (13) (monochromats) are deprived of the full experience of color perception in their environment, and this may interfere with activities of daily living. They also find it difficult to identify the color signal in a traffic light, and can drive only by locating the illumination of upper, middle, or lower lights. Thus, they have the risk of being involved in an accident. Furthermore, color discrimination is significantly important in certain occupations requiring critical safety tasks, such as in air, marine, road, and train transport systems as well as in certain trades. Hence, they may not be eligible for occupations such as a pilot, train engineer, railroad worker, firefighter, and signalman on railways. In dichromatopsia and those with anomalous color vision, there is an inaccurate recognition of the actual color and the perception of the reduced intensity of color may further augment the difficulty in identifying standard colors at a regular distance or in the presence of mist, smoke, or during rain. Thus, the quality of life is at a low ebb in persons with impairment of color vision.

Ishihara, Holmes-Wright lantern tests, FM test (Farnsworth Munsell 100 hue test), and the wire test evaluate color vision (15,16). *Integrated Evaluation of Disability* assigns maximum impairment of 25% for loss of color perception (Table 13.6).

13.7 DOUBLE VISION

Monocular diplopia occurs when there is defective transmission of light through the eyes to the retina. One of the images is normal quality and the other poor quality in respect to brightness, contrast and clarity. Early cataract, corneal opacity, dislocation of the lens and severe astigmatism may result in monocular diplopia (17).

The normally functioning fovea and synergistic and balanced action of yoked extraocular muscles facilitate the coordinated action of both eyes in creating a single binocular vision. Double vision occurs when there is an imbalance of muscle power in the yoked extraocular muscles. Double vision is due to the non-fusion of the images resulting in malprojection of the images to the corresponding points on the retina. Double vision becomes severe in the visual field of affected muscles. Horizontal diplopia becomes severe in tasks involving near vision such as reading. Adjustment of the posture may mask the diplopia by movement of the head to the right or left in horizontal diplopia, upward or downward rotation of the head in vertical diplopia, and tilting of the head in diplopia with the torsional element.

Table 13.6 Impairment class—Color vision

Impairment class	Clinical tools	Severity of impairment	Impairment score
Class 1	1. Ishihara test	Anomalous dichromacy—Yellow and blue deficiency	5%
Class 2	2. Holmes-Wright lantern test 3. FM test (Farnsworth Munsell 100 hue test)	Anomalous dichromacy with red and green deficiency due to protanomaly and deuteranomaly	10%
		Anomalous trichromacy	15%
Class 3	4. Wire test	Dichromacy	20%
Class 4		Monochromacy	25%

The Cervical Range of Motion (CROM) and Goldmann Perimetry methods quantify diplopia. The CROM method is a simpler method than Goldmann perimetry. The CROM method uses a 20/200 "E" target with a head-mounted device. It uses an "E" target in 10 gaze positions. The gaze positions include primary position, reading position, 10° upward, 30° upward, 10° downward, 30° downward, 10° rotation to the right, 30° rotation to the right, 10° rotation to the left, 30° rotation to the left, and any position at a distance 20/200. The CROM method has a constraint in evaluating persons with a restriction of cervical range of motion and people with pacemaker because of the built-in magnet in the CROM device. These individuals require the application of Goldmann perimetry (18). The diplopia score evaluated by the CROM method serves as a basis for assigning the percentage of impairment (Table 13.7). It assigns maximum impairment of 25% if the diplopia score is between 16 and 25.

1. Diplopia is present in primary position: Diplopia score 6
2. Diplopia is present during reading: Diplopia score 4
3. Diplopia is present during downward movement at 10°: Diplopia score 2
4. Diplopia is present during downward movement at 30°: Diplopia score 2
5. Diplopia is present during rotation to right at 30°: Diplopia score 2
6. Diplopia is present during rotation to left at 10°: Diplopia score 2
7. Diplopia is present during rotation to left at 30°: Diplopia score 2
8. Diplopia is present during rotation to left at 10°: Diplopia score 1
9. Diplopia is present during upward movement at 10°: Diplopia score 1
10. Diplopia is present during upward movement at 30°: Diplopia score 1
11. Any position: Diplopia score 1

The International Council of Ophthalmology recommends visual standards covering the requirements for driving safety, namely visual acuity of 20/40 (0.5, 6/12) and binocular visual field of at least 120° horizontal and 40° vertical. The other visual function evaluation includes glare sensitivity, Useful Field of View (UFOV), diplopia, color vision, and night vision. Persons with monocular vision adapt well within about six months for depth perception (19).

The formula $A + B(100 - A)/100$ combines the impairment of acuity of vision, the field of vision, double vision, color vision, night blindness, and photophobia to arrive at global impairment of vision (Illustration 13.5).

Table 13.7 Impairment class—Diplopia

Impairment class	Diplopia score	Reference impairment score	Impairment score
Class 1	Diplopia score 1–5	5%	
Class 2	Diplopia score 6–10	10%	
Class 3	Diplopia score 11–15	15%	
Class 4	Diplopia score 16–25	25%	

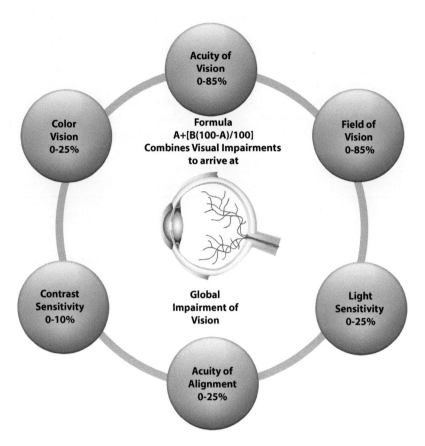

Illustration 13.5 Global impairments of vision.

REFERENCES

1. Visual field testing: From one medical student to another [Internet]. 2013. Available from: EYE ROUNDS.ORG.
2. International Classification of Functioning, Disability and Health. Geneva, Switzerland: World Health Organization; 2001. pp. 62–64.
3. Visual Impairment and Blindness. Geneva, Switzerland: World Health Organization; 2014.
4. Module 4 sensation & perception [Internet]. 2017 [cited August 24, 2017]. Available from: https://www.smore.com/wmp4q-module-4-sensation-perception.
5. Vision is our dominant sense [Internet]. Brainline.org, and NORA Neuro-Optometric Rehabilitation Association [cited August 24, 2017].
6. Sue S. Test distance vision using a Snellen chart. Community Eye Health. 2007;20(63):52.
7. Balcer LJ, Miller DH, Reingold SC, Cohen JA. Vision and vision-related outcome measures in multiple sclerosis. Brain. 2015;138(Pt 1):11–27.
8. ICD-10 Version: 2015 (International Statistical Classification of Diseases and Related Health Problems 10th Revision). Geneva, Switzerland: World Health Organization.
9. Kedar S, Ghate D, Corbett JJ. Visual fields in neuro-ophthalmology. Indian J Ophthalmol. 2011;59(2):103–109.
10. Standard automated perimetry [Internet]. EyeWiki, 2014. Available from: http://eyewiki.aao.org.
11. Dragoi V. Section 2: Sensory systems - Chapter 14: Visual processing: Eye and retina. In: Neuroscience online [Internet]. Houston, TX: Department of Neurobiology and Anatomy, University of Texas Medical School; 1997.
12. Spector RH. Chapter 116: Visual fields. In: Walker HK, Hall WD, Hurst JW, editor. Clinical Methods: The History, Physical, and Laboratory Examinations, 3rd ed. Boston, MA: Butterworths; 1990.
13. Rehabilitation ISfLvRa, editor. GUIDE for the evaluation of VISUAL impairment. International Low Vision Conference VISION-99. San Francisco, CA: Pacific Vision Foundation; 1999.
14. Clinical update: Neuro-ophthalmology photophobia: Looking for causes and solutions [Internet]. American Academy of Ophthalmology, 2005. Available from: http://www.aao.org/.
15. Almog Y, Nemet A. The correlation between visual acuity and color vision as an indicator of the cause of visual loss. Am J Ophthalmol. 2010;149(6):1000–1004.

16. Colour vision deficiency part 3 – occupational standards [Internet]. *OT CET Continuing Education and Training*, 2014. Available from: http://www.optometry.co.uk/.

17. Spector RH. Chapter 113: Diplopia. In: Walker HK, Hall WD, Hurst JW, editor. *Clinical Methods: The History, Physical, and Laboratory Examinations*, 3rd ed. Boston, MA: Butterworths; 1990.

18. Hatt SR, Leske DA, Holmes JM. Comparing methods of quantifying diplopia. *Ophthalmology*. 2007;114(12):2316–2322.

19. (ICO) ICoO, editor. Vision requirements for driving safety – International Council of Ophthalmology – December 2005. *30th World Ophthalmology Congress*. Sao Paulo, Brazil: International Council of Ophthalmology (ICO); 2006.

14

Impairment of hearing functions

14.1 HEARING FUNCTIONS

Hearing function comprises the transformation of sound waves into vibration, and transduction into the electrical impulse for transmission into the brain for interpretation of its location, pitch, loudness, and quality.

Hereditary sensorineural hearing disorder, craniofacial anomalies, inborn error metabolism (such as mucopolysaccharidosis), mucolipidosis, Refsum disease, and autism all produce hearing impairment. Maternal rubella, perinatal complications, meningitis, cytomegalovirus, syphilis, toxoplasmosis, and herpes may also lead to hearing impairment. Ototoxic drugs, chronic otitis media, otosclerosis, head injury with a skull fracture, exposure to excessive noise, and aging also produce hearing impairment.

Genetic disorders, maternal rubella, perinatal complications, meningitis, ototoxic drugs, excessive noise, and aging constitute major causes of hearing impairment (1). Hearing impairment may be sensory neural, conductive, central, and mixed. Sensory neural hearing impairment is due to lesions in the cochlea, and/or injury to the eighth nerve and/or brainstem. Conductive hearing impairment is due to lesions in the external and/or middle ear; and central hearing impairment is due to lesions in the cortex.

Hearing impairment leads to the difficulty or inability to interpret speech sounds, delay in acquisition of language skills, limitation of activities in communication, and participation restriction in education, work and employment, economic life, community, and social and civic life. Further, it adds stigma to the person with deafness.

14.2 SOUND

Sound displays a series of pressure changes in the air. The frequency and intensity of sound vary according to the nature of speech. A normal person can hear sounds between 20 and 20,000 Hz. The frequency of sound relates to the pitch of the sound. The best hearing exists between the frequency of 3000 and 4000 Hz. The decibel (dB) measures the intensity of sound and pressure. The decibel is a logarithmic unit that describes the ratio of a measured value of sound intensity and pressure to a reference value. There is a doubling in the intensity of sound for every 6 dB increase in sound pressure level (2). The sound of dropping a pin corresponds to 10 dB, ticking of a watch 20 dB, a whisper 30 dB, and a quiet library 40 dB. The sound of a refrigerator is 50 dB, normal conversation or sewing machine is 60 dB, a toilet flushing is 70 dB, the vacuum cleaner is 80 dB, truck traffic or MRI machine is 90 dB, the pneumatic drill is 100 dB, and a jet engine at takeoff measures 140 dB.

14.3 AUDIOMETRY

Pure tone audiometry evaluates hearing impairment. An audiometer delivers sounds of specific frequencies at 125, 250, 500, 1000, 2000, 3000, 4000, 6000, and 8000 Hz and different intensities with earphones for air conduction. It also delivers sounds at 125, 250, 500, 1000, 2000, 3000, and 4000 Hz with an oscillator held at mastoid or on the forehead for bone conduction to measure hearing thresholds. The threshold for normal hearing is 0 ± 10 dB.

14.4 HEARING IMPAIRMENT

The World Health Organization (WHO) defines hearing impairment as the permanent unaided hearing threshold level for the better ear of 41 dB or higher. WHO recommends average audiometric ISO value for four frequencies, that is, 500, 1000, 2000, and 4000 Hz to grade hearing impairment (3). *Integrated Evaluation of Disability* applies the WHO grading of Hearing Impairment (4). Persons with monaural hearing impairment can perform most of his/her life activities, whereas individuals with binaural

Table 14.1 Monaural hearing impairment with normal hearing function in another ear

Impairment class	WHO's grading of hearing impairment	ISO value—Pure tone average of the threshold at 500, 1000, 2000, and 4000 Hz	Impairment reference value	% of impairment
Class 0	No impairment	25 dB or better	0%	
Class 1	Slight impairment	25–40 dB	1%	
Class 2	Moderate impairment	41–60 dB	5%	
Class 3	Severe impairment	61–80 dB	10%	
Class 4	Profound impairment including deafness	>80 dB	15%	

Table 14.2 Impairment class—Binaural hearing impairment

Impairment class	WHO's grading of hearing impairment	ISO value—pure tone average of the threshold at 500, 1000, 2000, and 4000 Hz	Impairment reference value	% of impairment right ear	% of impairment left ear
Class 0	No impairment	25 dB or better	0%		
Class 1	Slight impairment	25–40 dB	1%		
Class 2	Moderate impairment	41–60 dB	5%		
Class 3	Severe impairment	61–80 dB	15%		
Class 4	Profound impairment including deafness	>80 dB	25%		

Total whole person impairment for right and left ear.

hearing impairment cannot perform activities requiring communication. Hence, *Integrated Evaluation of Disability* assigns maximum impairment of 15% for monaural hearing impairment and 50% for binaural hearing impairment (Tables 14.1 and 14.2).

A person with deafness would have a severe impairment, limitation of activity, and restriction of participation. A cochlear implant provides the perception of sounds by activation of the auditory nerve through an electronic device comprising a microphone, speech processor, transmitter, receiver/stimulator, and an array of electrodes. However, a cochlear implant does not replace normal hearing but provides the perception of sounds in the environment (5). *Integrated Evaluation of Disability* assigns an impairment of 50% for the person with deafness. The cochlear implant grossly decreases the impairment of hearing, limitation of activities, and participation restriction.

14.5 ILLUSTRATIONS: AUDIOGRAMS

Illustrations 14.1–14.5 present normal hearing function, conductive hearing loss, sensorineural hearing loss, and mixed hearing loss in an audiogram.

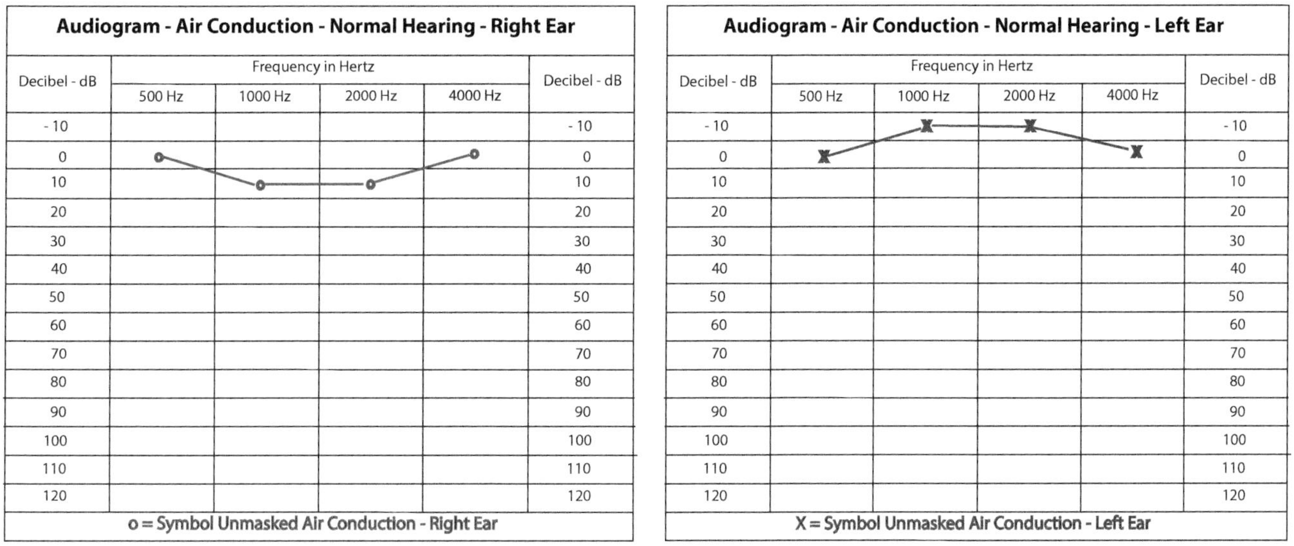

Audiogram - Air Conduction - Normal Hearing - Right Ear					
Decibel - dB	Frequency in Hertz				Decibel - dB
	500 Hz	1000 Hz	2000 Hz	4000 Hz	
- 10					- 10
0					0
10					10
20					20
30					30
40					40
50					50
60					60
70					70
80					80
90					90
100					100
110					110
120					120
o = Symbol Unmasked Air Conduction - Right Ear					

Audiogram - Air Conduction - Normal Hearing - Left Ear					
Decibel - dB	Frequency in Hertz				Decibel - dB
	500 Hz	1000 Hz	2000 Hz	4000 Hz	
- 10					- 10
0					0
10					10
20					20
30					30
40					40
50					50
60					60
70					70
80					80
90					90
100					100
110					110
120					120
X = Symbol Unmasked Air Conduction - Left Ear					

Illustration 14.1 Audiogram—Air conduction: Normal hearing function.

Audiogram - Bone Conduction - Normal Hearing - Right Ear					
Decibel - dB	Frequency in Hertz				Decibel - dB
	500 Hz	1000 Hz	2000 Hz	4000 Hz	
- 10					- 10
0					0
10					10
20					20
30					30
40					40
50					50
60					60
70					70
80					80
90					90
100					100
110					110
120					120
< = Symbol Unmasked Bone Conduction - Right Ear					

Audiogram - Bone Conduction - Normal Hearing - Left Ear					
Decibel - dB	Frequency in Hertz				Decibel - dB
	500 Hz	1000 Hz	2000 Hz	4000 Hz	
- 10					- 10
0					0
10					10
20					20
30					30
40					40
50					50
60					60
70					70
80					80
90					90
100					100
110					110
120					120
➤ = Symbol Unmasked Air Conduction - Left Ear					

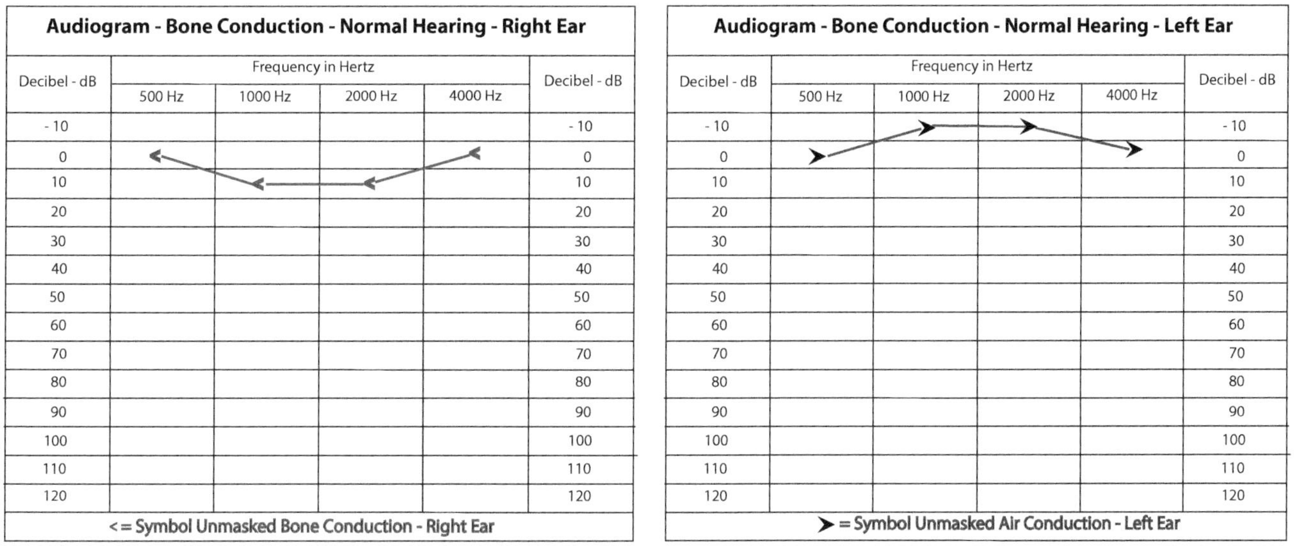

Illustration 14.2 Audiogram—Bone conduction: Normal hearing function.

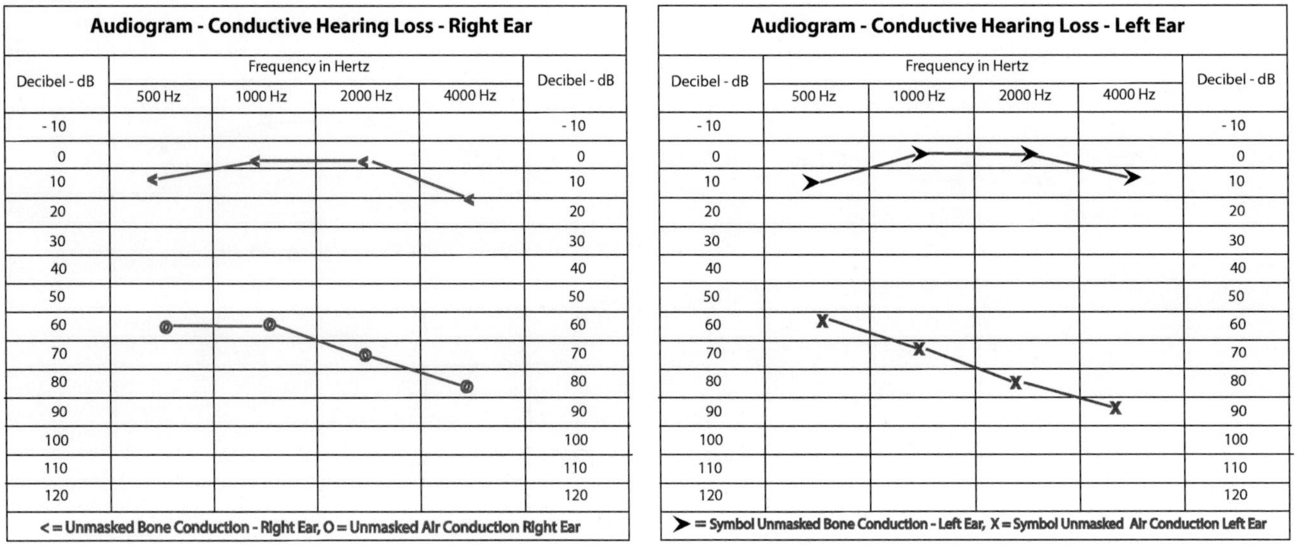

Audiogram - Conductive Hearing Loss - Right Ear

Decibel - dB	Frequency in Hertz				Decibel - dB
	500 Hz	1000 Hz	2000 Hz	4000 Hz	
- 10					- 10
0					0
10					10
20					20
30					30
40					40
50					50
60					60
70					70
80					80
90					90
100					100
110					110
120					120

< = Unmasked Bone Conduction - Right Ear, O = Unmasked Air Conduction Right Ear

Audiogram - Conductive Hearing Loss - Left Ear

Decibel - dB	Frequency in Hertz				Decibel - dB
	500 Hz	1000 Hz	2000 Hz	4000 Hz	
- 10					- 10
0					0
10					10
20					20
30					30
40					40
50					50
60					60
70					70
80					80
90					90
100					100
110					110
120					120

➤ = Symbol Unmasked Bone Conduction - Left Ear, X = Symbol Unmasked Air Conduction Left Ear

Illustration 14.3 Audiogram—Conductive hearing loss.

Audiogram - Sensory Neural Hearing Loss - Right Ear

Decibel - dB	Frequency in Hertz				Decibel - dB
	500 Hz	1000 Hz	2000 Hz	4000 Hz	
- 10					- 10
0					0
10					10
20					20
30					30
40					40
50					50
60					60
70					70
80					80
90					90
100					100
110					110
120					120

< = Unmasked Bone Conduction - Right Ear, O = Unmasked Air Conduction Right Ear

Audiogram - Sensory Neural Hearing Loss - Left Ear

Decibel - dB	Frequency in Hertz				Decibel - dB
	500 Hz	1000 Hz	2000 Hz	4000 Hz	
- 10					- 10
0					0
10					10
20					20
30					30
40					40
50					50
60					60
70					70
80					80
90					90
100					100
110					110
120					120

➤ = Symbol Unmasked Bone Conduction - Left Ear, X = Symbol Unmasked Air Conduction Left Ear

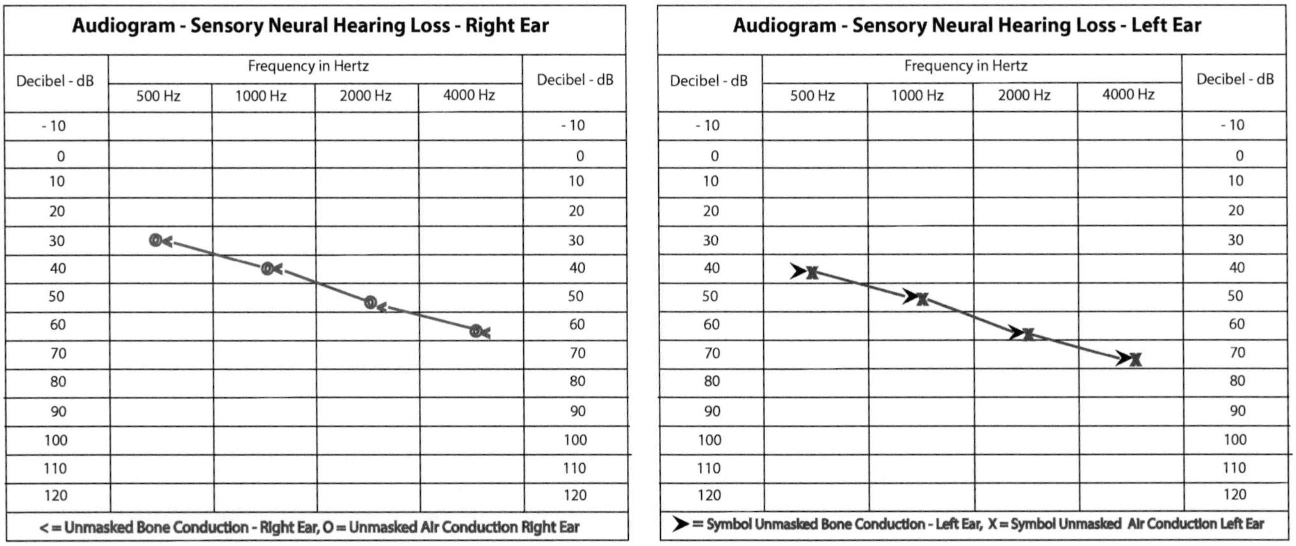

Illustration 14.4 Audiogram—Sensorineural hearing loss.

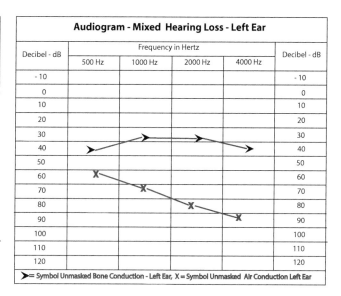

Audiogram - Mixed Hearing Loss - Right Ear					
Decibel - dB	Frequency in Hertz				Decibel - dB
	500 Hz	1000 Hz	2000 Hz	4000 Hz	
- 10					- 10
0					0
10					10
20					20
30					30
40					40
50					50
60					60
70					70
80					80
90					90
100					100
110					110
120					120
< = Unmasked Bone Conduction - Right Ear, O = Unmasked Air Conduction Right Ear					

Audiogram - Mixed Hearing Loss - Left Ear					
Decibel - dB	Frequency in Hertz				Decibel - dB
	500 Hz	1000 Hz	2000 Hz	4000 Hz	
- 10					- 10
0					0
10					10
20					20
30					30
40					40
50					50
60					60
70					70
80					80
90					90
100					100
110					110
120					120
>= Symbol Unmasked Bone Conduction - Left Ear, X = Symbol Unmasked Air Conduction Left Ear					

Illustration 14.5 Audiogram—Mixed hearing loss.

REFERENCES

1. *Deafness and Hearing Loss*. Geneva, Switzerland: World Health Organization; 2014.
2. Gray L. Section 2 - Sensory systems—Chapter 12: Auditory system: Structure and function. In: *Neurosciences Online*. Houston, TX: Department of Neurobiology and Anatomy, University of Texas Medical School; 1997.
3. *Report of the Informal Consultation on the Economic Analysis of Sensory Disabilities*. Geneva, Switzerland: World Health Organization; 2000.
4. *Prevention of Blindness and Deafness: Grades of Hearing Impairment*. Geneva, Switzerland: World Health Organization; 2014.
5. *Cochlear Implants*. In: (NIDCD) N-NIoDaOCD, editor. Washington, DC: U.S. Department of Health & Human Services; 2014.

Impairment of amputations

15.1 GUIDELINES FOR ASSIGNING IMPAIRMENT

Functional/structural loss of an upper extremity derives an impairment of 60% and lower extremity 40% by convention. A person with isolated flaccid motor paralysis involving one lower extremity can walk independently, with some gait deviation, after stabilization by surgery or by the appliance. A person with hip disarticulation/transfemoral amputation has loss of both structure and function. He/she cannot walk without an artificial limb. He/she can walk downhill, climb up the stairs, and run with a microprocessor-controlled prosthetic knee joint, though with some difficulty. But the person cannot feel sensations through the artificial limb.

A person with profound deafness or sever hard of hearing can understand speech by a cochlear implant. A series of electrodes in the cochlear implant in the base of the cochlea stimulate the auditory nerve for the perception of sounds by the brain (1,2). Similarly, a pacemaker corrects the abnormal heart rhythm and restores the function in a person with severe arrhythmias.

There is no mechanism to interpret the sensation in a person with an amputation fitted with an artificial limb. He/she cannot feel the touch sensation through his/her prosthesis. Thus, it is not logical to give the same impairment of motor loss for combined motor loss, sensory loss, vascular loss, and dermal loss. Hence, *Integrated Evaluation of Disability* combines impairment of motor loss, sensory loss, vascular loss, and dermal loss by formula (Box 15.1)

$$A + \frac{B(100 - A)}{100} \qquad (15.1)$$

to calculate a whole person impairment. Tables 15.1 through 15.11 illustrate the basis for assigning impairment in upper extremity amputations.

15.2 UPPER EXTREMITY AMPUTATIONS

Based on the concept of combined motor, sensory, vascular, and dermal loss, a forequarter amputation derives a whole person impairment of 80%, shoulder disarticulation 79%, elbow disarticulation 72%, and wrist disarticulation 65% (Figures 15.1 and 15.2).

The stiffness of the proximal joint and phantom pain/sensation also derive additional impairment. A person with

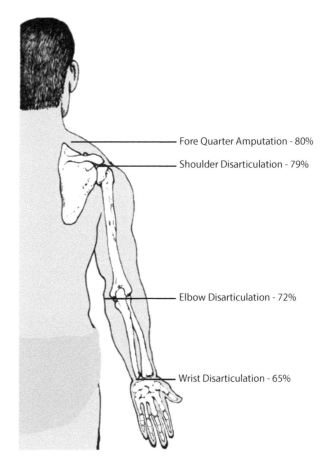

Figure 15.1 Impairment of upper extremity amputations.

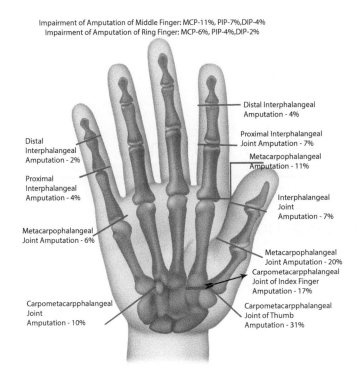

Impairment of Amputation of Middle Finger: MCP-11%, PIP-7%,DIP-4%
Impairment of Amputation of Ring Finger: MCP-6%, PIP-4%,DIP-2%

Distal Interphalangeal Amputation - 4%

Proximal Interphalangeal Joint Amputation - 7%

Metacarpophalangeal Amputation - 11%

Interphalangeal Joint Amputation - 7%

Metacarpophalangeal Joint Amputation - 20%

Carpometacarpphalangeal Joint of Index Finger Amputation - 17%

Carpometacarpphalangeal Joint of Thumb Amputation - 31%

Distal Interphalangeal Amputation - 2%

Proximal Interphalangeal Amputation - 4%

Metacarpophalangeal Joint Amputation - 6%

Carpometacarpphalangeal Joint Amputation - 10%

Figure 15.2 Impairment of finger amputations.

Table 15.1 Basis of assigning motor impairment—Upper extremity amputation

| Shoulder elbow and wrist: Hand = 1:3 | | | | | | | | | | | | | |
| 15% shoulder: elbow: wrist @ 2:2:1 | | | | 20% palm and dorsum 20% @ 4:2:2:1:1 | | | | | 25% fingers @ 4:2:2:1:1 | | | | | |
Shoulder girdle	Shoulder	Elbow	Wrist	1st ray	2nd ray	3rd ray	4th ray	5th ray	Thumb	Index	Middle	Ring	Little	Total
2.4%	3.6%	6%	3%	8%	4%	4%	2%	2%	10%	5%	5%	2.5%	2.5%	60%

Table 15.2 Basis of assigning sensory impairment—Upper extremity amputation

| Shoulder elbow and wrist: Hand = 1:2 | | | | | | | | | | | | | |
| Shoulder and arm, elbow and forearm, wrist—10% | | | Hand 5% @ 4:2:2:1:1 | | | | | Fingers 15% @ 4:2:2:1:1 | | | | | |
Shoulder and arm	Elbow and forearm	wrist	1st ray	2nd ray	3rd ray	4th ray	5th ray	Thumb	Index	Middle	Ring	Little	Total
3%	6%	1%	2%	1	1	0.5	0.5	6%	3%	3%	1.5%	1.5%	30%

Table 15.3 Basis of assigning vascular impairment—Upper extremity amputation 20%

| Arm and forearm—6.5% | | | | Palm and dorsum of hand—3.5% | | | | | Fingers 10% @ 4:2:2:1:1 | | | | | |
Shoulder	Arm	Elbow and forearm	Wrist	1st ray	2nd ray	3rd ray	4th ray	5th ray	Thumb	Index	Middle	Ring	Little	Total
2%		4%	0.5%	1%	0.75%	0.75%	0.5%	0.5%	4%	2%	2%	1%	1%	20%

Table 15.4 Basis of assigning dermal impairment—Upper extremity amputation

| Arm, forearm, wrist 3.25% | | | | Palm and dorsum of hand—1.75% | | | | | Fingers 5% @ 4:2:2:1:1 | | | | | |
Shoulder	Arm	Elbow and forearm	Wrist	1st ray	2nd ray	3rd ray	4th ray	5th ray	Thumb	Index	Middle	Ring	Little	Total
1%		2%	0.25%	0.5%	0.375%	0.375%	0.2 5%	0.25%	2%	1%	1%	0.5%	0.5%	5%

Table 15.5 Impairment of upper extremity amputations—Arm, forearm, and wrist

Level of amputation	Motor loss	Sensory loss	Combine ML + SL by $A + \dfrac{B(100-A)}{100}$	Vascular loss	Combine ML + SL by $A + \dfrac{B(100-A)}{100}$	Loss of skin	Combine ML + SL by $A + \dfrac{B(100-A)}{100}$	Impairment score	Select impairment score
Fore quarter	60%	30%	72%	20%	78%	10%	80%	80%	
Shoulder Disarticulation	57.6%	30%	71%	20%	77%	10%	79%	79%	
Transhumeral Upper third								78%	
Transhumeral Middle third								77%	
Transhumeral Lower third								76%	
Elbow Disarticulation	48%	27%	62%	18%	69%	9%	72%	72%	
Transradial Upper third								70%	
Transradial Middle third								68%	
Transradial Lower third								66%	
Wrist Disarticulation	45%	20%	56%	13.5%	62%	6.75%	65%	65%	

Table 15.6 Impairment of upper extremity amputations—Hand

Level of amputation	Motor loss	Sensory loss	Combine ML + SL by $A + \dfrac{B(100-A)}{100}$	Vascular loss	Combine ML + SL by $A + \dfrac{B(100-A)}{100}$	Loss of skin	Combine ML + SL by $A + \dfrac{B(100-A)}{100}$	Impairment score	Select impairment score
Hand									
Fingers transmetacarpal amputation all fingers								55%	
CMCP Amputation of four fingers except thumb at carpo-metacarpo-phalangeal (CMCP) joint	27%	12%	36%	8.5%	42%	4.25%	44%	44%	
Amputation of thumb at carpo-metacarpo-phalangeal joint	18%	8%	25%	5%	29%	2.5%	31%	31%	
Thumb Amputation of thumb at transmetacarpal level								26%	
Amputation of thumb at metacarpophalangeal joint	10%	6%	15%	4%	18%	2%	20%	20%	
Amputation of thumb at Interphalangeal joint	3.3%	2%	5%	1.33%	6%	0.66%	7%	7%	

Table 15.7 Impairment of upper extremity amputations—All fingers

Level of amputation	Motor loss	Sensory loss	Combine ML + SL by $A + \dfrac{B(100 - A)}{100}$	Vascular loss	Combine ML + SL by $A + \dfrac{B(100 - A)}{100}$	Loss of skin	Combine ML + SL by $A + \dfrac{B(100 - A)}{100}$	Impairment score	Select impairment score
All fingers Amputation of all fingers including thumb at metacarpophalangeal joint	25%	15%	36%	10%	42%	5%	44.9%	45%	
Amputation of four fingers except thumb at metacarpophalangeal joint	15%	9%	23%	6%	28%	3%	30%	30%	

Table 15.8 Impairment of upper extremity amputations—Index finger

Level of amputation	Motor loss	Sensory loss	Combine ML + SL by $A + \dfrac{B(100-A)}{100}$	Vascular loss	Combine ML + SL by $A + \dfrac{B(100-A)}{100}$	Loss of skin	Combine ML + SL by $A + \dfrac{B(100-A)}{100}$	Impairment score	Select impairment score
Index Amputation of index finger at carpo metacarpophalangeal joint	9%	4%	13%	2.75%	16%	1.375%	17%	17%	
Amputation of index finger at transmetacarpal level								14%	
Amputation of index finger at metacarpophalangeal joint	5%	3%	8%	2%	10%	1%	11%	11%	
Amputation of index finger at proximal interphalangeal joint	3.33%	2%	5%	1.33%	6.00%	0.66%	7%	7%	
Amputation of index finger at distal interphalangeal joint	1.66%	1%	2.66%	0.66%	4.00%	0.33%	4%	4%	

Table 15.9 Impairment of upper extremity amputations—Middle finger

Level of amputation	Motor loss	Sensory loss	Combine ML + SL by $A + \dfrac{B(100-A)}{100}$	Vascular loss	Combine ML + SL by $A + \dfrac{B(100-A)}{100}$	Loss of skin	Combine ML + SL by $A + \dfrac{B(100-A)}{100}$	Impairment score	Select impairment score
Middle finger Amputation of middle finger at carpo-metacarpophalangeal joint	9%	4%	13%	2.75%	16%	1.375%	17%	17%	17%
Amputation of middle finger at transmetacarpal level								14%	
Amputation of middle finger at metacarpophalangeal joint	5%	3%	8%	2%	10%	1%	11%	11%	
Amputation of middle finger at PIP joint	3.33%	2%	5%	1.33%	6%	0.66%	7%	7%	
Amputation of middle finger at DIP joint	1.66%	1%	2.66%	0.66%	4.00%	0.33%	4%	4%	

Table 15.10 Impairment of upper extremity amputations—Ring finger

Level of amputation	Motor loss	Sensory loss	Combine ML + SL by $A + \frac{B(100 - A)}{100}$	Vascular loss	Combine ML + SL by $A + \frac{B(100 - A)}{100}$	Loss of skin	Combine ML + SL by $A + \frac{B(100 - A)}{100}$	Impairment score	Select impairment score
Ring finger Amputation of ring finger at carpo-metacarpalphalangeal joint	4.5%	2%	7%	1.5%	9%	0.75%	10%	10%	
Amputation of ring finger at transmetacarpal level								8%	
Amputation of ring finger at metacarpophalangeal joint	2.5%	1.5%	4%	1%	5%	0.5%	6%	6%	
Amputation of ring finger at PIP Joint	1.66%	1%	3%	0.66%	4%	0.333%	4%	4%	
Amputation of ring finger at DIP Joint	0.83%	0.5%	2%	0.33%	2%	0.166%	2%	2%	

Table 15.11 Impairment of upper extremity amputations—Little finger

Level of amputation	Motor loss	Sensory loss	Combine ML + SL by $A + \dfrac{B(100-A)}{100}$	Vascular loss	Combine ML + SL by $A + \dfrac{B(100-A)}{100}$	Loss of skin	Combine ML + SL by $A + \dfrac{B(100-A)}{100}$	Impairment score	Select impairment score
Little finger Amputation of little finger at carpo-metacarpophalangeal joint	4.5%	2%	7%	1.5%	9%	0.75%	10%	10%	10%
Amputation of little finger at transmetacarpal level								8%	
Amputation of little finger at metacarpophalangeal joint	2.5%	1.5%	4%	1%	5%	0.5%	6%	6%	
Amputation of little finger at proximal interphalangeal joint	1.66%	1%	3%	0.66%	4%	0.333%	4%	4%	
Amputation of little finger at distal interphalangeal joint	0.83%	0.5%	2%	0.33%	2%	0.166%	2%	2%	

vascular amputation expends more energy for ambulation than in traumatic amputation with a consequent reduction in the endurance of walking. A person with congenital amputation adapts very well for most of the activities, whereas there is a limitation of activities in person with vascular or traumatic amputation. The "Activity Participation Skill Assessment Scale" evaluates limitation of activity to assign an appropriate weight for computing the additional percentage of disability.

15.3 LOWER EXTREMITY AMPUTATIONS

Similarly, based on the concept of combined motor, sensory, vascular, and dermal loss, hindquarter amputation derives a whole person impairment of 61%, hip disarticulation derives 60%, knee disarticulation 54%, and ankle disarticulation 45% in *Integrated Evaluation of Disability* (Figure 15.3). Tables 15.12 through 15.17 illustrate the basis for assigning impairment in lower extremity amputations.

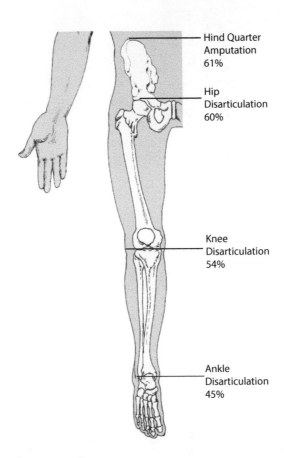

Figure 15.3 Impairment of lower extremity amputations.

Table 15.12 Basis of assigning motor impairment

Hip, knee, and ankle 28%			Foot 8%		Toes 4%					
Hip	Knee	Ankle	Hindfoot and midfoot	Forefoot	Bigtoe	2nd toe	3rd toe	4th toe	5th toe	Total
4%	8%	16%	6%	2%	1.5%	0.75%	0.75%	0.5%	0.5%	40%

Table 15.13 Basis of assigning sensory impairment

Thigh and leg 8%		Hindfoot 2.5%		Midfoot 2%	Forefoot 5%					Toes 2.5%					
Thigh	Leg	Ankle	Heel	Midfoot	Foot 1st ray	Foot 2nd ray	Foot 3rd ray	Foot 4th ray	Foot 5th ray	Big toe	2nd toe	3rd toe	4th toe	5th toe	Total
4%	4%	0.5%	2%	2%	2%	1%	1%	0.5%	0.5%	1%	0.5%	0.5%	0.25%	0.25%	20%

Table 15.14 Basis of assigning vascular impairment

Thigh and leg 6%		Hindfoot 1.5%		Midfoot 1.25%	Forefoot 3.75%					Toes 2.5%					
Thigh	Leg	Ankle	Heel	Midfoot	Foot 1st ray	Foot 2nd ray	Foot 3rd ray	Foot 4th ray	Foot 5th ray	Big toe	2nd toe	3rd toe	4th toe	5th toe	
3%	3%	0.5%	1%	1.25%	1.5%	0.75%	0.75%	0.375%	0.375%	1%	0.5%	0.5%	0.25%	0.25%	15%

Table 15.15 Basis of assigning dermal impairment

Thigh and leg 2%		Foot 0.5%		Midfoot 0.5%	Forefoot 1.25%					Toes 0.75%					
Thigh	Leg	Ankle	Heel	Midfoot	Foot 1st ray	Foot 2nd ray	Foot 3rd ray	Foot 4th ray	Foot 5th ray	Big toe	2nd toe	3rd toe	4th toe	5th toe	
1%	1%	0.25%	0.25%	0.5%	0.5%	0.25%	0.25%	0.125%	0.125%	0.25%	0.125%	0.125%	0.125%	0.125%	5%

Table 15.16 Impairment of lower extremity amputations—Hip and knee

Level of amputation	Motor loss	Sensory loss	Combine ML + SL by $A + \dfrac{B(100 - A)}{100}$	Vascular loss	Combine (ML + SL) and VL by $A + \dfrac{B(100 - A)}{100}$	Loss of skin	Combine (ML + SL + VL) and DL by $A + \dfrac{B(100 - A)}{100}$	Impairment score	Select impairment score
Hind quarter amputation	40%	20%	52%	15%	59%	5%	61%	61%	
Hip disarticulation	40%	19.5%	51.7%	14%	58%	4.5%	60%	60%	
Transfemoral—proximal third								59%	
Transfemoral—middle third								58%	
Transfemoral—distal third								55%	
Knee disarticulation	36%	16%	46%	12%	52%	4%	54%	54%	
Trans tibiofibular proximal third <3"								53%	
Trans tibiofibular proximal third ≥3"								51%	
Trans tibiofibular—middle third								49%	
Trans tibiofibular—lower third								47%	

Table 15.17 Impairment of lower extremity amputations—Ankle and foot

Level of amputation	Motor loss	Sensory loss	Combine ML + SL by $A + \dfrac{B(100-A)}{100}$	Vascular loss	Combine (ML + SL) and VL by $A + \dfrac{B(100-A)}{100}$	Loss of skin	Combine (ML + SL + VL) and DL by $A + \dfrac{B(100-A)}{100}$	Impairment score	Select impairment score
Ankle disarticulation	28%	12%	37%	9%	43%	3%	45%	45%	
Syme's amputation	20%	11.5%	30%	8%	36%	2.75%	38%	38%	
Chopart—midtarsal amputation	9%	9.5%	18%	7.5%	25%	2.5%	27%	27%	
Lisfranc tarsometatarsal	6%	7.5%	14%	6.25%	19%	2%	21%	21%	
Trans-metatarsal								16%	
All toes metatarsophalangeal	4%	2.5%	7%	2.5%	10%	0.75%	11%	11%	
All toes except big toe	2.5%	1.5%	4%	1.5%	6%	0.5%	7%	7%	
Big toe at MTP	1.5%	1%	3%	1%	4%	0.25%	4%	4%	
Big toe at IP								2%	
2nd toe at MTP	0.75%	0.5%	1.25%	0.50%	1.75%	0.125%	1.875%	2%	
2nd toe at PIP								1%	
2nd toe at DIP								0.50%	
3nd toe at MTP	0.75%	0.5%	1.25%	0.50%	1.75%	0.125%	1.875%	2%	
3rd toe at PIP								1%	
3rd toe at DIP								0.50%	
4nd toe at MTP	0.5%	0.5%	1.0%	0.25%	1.25%	0.125%	1.375%	1%	
4th toe at PIP								0.50%	
4th toe at DIP								0.25%	
5nd toe at MTP	0.5%	0.5%	1.0%	0.25%	1.25%	0.125%	1.375%	1%	
5th toe at PIP								0.50%	
5th toe at DIP								0.25%	

REFERENCES

1. Gray L. Section 2: Sensory systems - Chapter 12: Auditory system: Structure and function. In: *Neurosciences Online*. Houston, TX: Department of Neurobiology and Anatomy, University of Texas Medical School; 1997.

2. *Cochlear Implants*. In: (NIDCD) N-NIoDaOCD, editor. Washington, DC: U.S. Department of Health & Human Services; 2014.

16

Impairment of congenital skeletal limb deficiencies

16.1 FRANTZ AND O'RAHILLY CLASSIFICATION

In 1961, Frantz and O'Rahilly (1) proposed a classification for congenital skeletal limb deficiencies based on the embryologic and teratogenic manifestations. In this classification, the Latin words *amelia* refers to the total absence of a limb, *acheiria* to total absence of hand, *apodia* to total absence of foot, *adactylia* to total absence of a digit (including metacarpal/metatarsal), and *aphalangia* to total absence of one phalanx or more phalanges. Similarly, the Greek word *hemimelia* denotes half of the limb and *phocomelia* means part of the limb directly attached to the trunk.

Frantz and O'Rahilly classified skeletal limb deficiencies into terminal deficiencies and intercalary deficiencies.

16.1.1 Terminal transverse deficiencies

In terminal transverse deficiencies, *amelia* refers to the absence of a limb, *hemimelia* to the absence of forearm and hand or leg and foot, partial *hemimelia* to the absence of a portion of the forearm or leg. *Acheiria* refers to the absence of hand, *apodia* refers to the absence of a foot, complete *adactylia* to the absence of all five digits (including their metacarpals/metatarsals), and complete *aphalangia* to the absence of one or more phalanges in the five digits.

16.1.2 Terminal longitudinal deficiencies

In terminal longitudinal deficiencies, complete paraxial *hemimelia* denotes the complete absence of either radial or ulnar ray/tibial or fibular ray. Incomplete paraxial *hemimelia* represents the partial absence of either radial or ulnar ray/tibial or fibular ray, partial *adactylia* indicates the absence of either one or two or three or four digits (including metacarpals/metatarsals), and partial *aphalangia* refers to the absence of one or more phalanges from one to four digits.

16.1.3 Intercalary transverse deficiencies

In intercalary transverse deficiencies, complete *phocomelia* refers to either hand or foot directly attached to the trunk, proximal *phocomelia* to hand and forearm or foot and leg attached directly to trunk, distal *phocomelia* to hand or foot attached directly to arm or thigh with the absence of intermediate segments of the extremities.

16.1.4 Intercalary longitudinal deficiencies

Intercalary longitudinal deficiencies include complete paraxial *hemimelia*, incomplete paraxial *hemimelia*, partial *adactylia*, and partial *aphalangia* (1).

16.2 ISPO CLASSIFICATION

International Standard Organization (ISO)/International Society for Prosthetics and Orthotics (ISPO) classifies congenital skeletal limb deficiencies based on anatomical and radiological deficiencies resulting from the failure of formation of skeletal elements. International Standard Organization (ISO)/International Society for Prosthetics and Orthotics (ISPO) also describes the deficiencies into transverse and longitudinal deficiencies (1) (Illustration 16.1).

16.2.1 Transverse deficiencies

Transverse deficiencies are like amputations. In a transverse deficiency, no skeletal elements will exist beyond the normally developed residual limb. However, there may be digital buds. It labels the transverse deficiencies by indicating the part at which the extremity ends and further denotes the level within the part distal to which no skeletal structures exist (2).

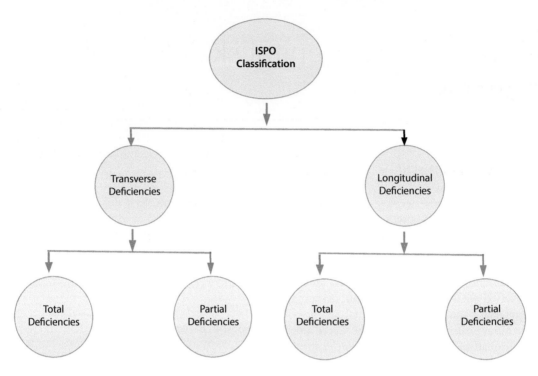

Illustration 16.1 ISPO—Classification: Congenital skeletal limb deficiencies.

16.2.1.1 UPPER EXTREMITY

1. Shoulder—total—transverse deficiency
2. Upper arm—total—transverse deficiency
3. Upper arm—upper third—transverse deficiency
4. Upper arm—middle third—transverse deficiency
5. Upper arm—lower third—transverse deficiency
6. Forearm—total—transverse deficiency
7. Forearm—upper third—transverse deficiency
8. Forearm—middle third—transverse deficiency
9. Forearm—lower third—transverse deficiency
10. Carpal—total—transverse deficiency
11. Carpal—partial—transverse deficiency
12. Metacarpal—total—transverse deficiency
13. Metacarpal—partial—transverse deficiency
14. Phalangeal—total—transverse deficiency
15. Phalangeal—partial—transverse deficiency (finger or thumb)

16.2.1.2 LOWER EXTREMITY

1. Pelvis—total—transverse deficiency
2. Thigh—total—transverse deficiency
3. Thigh—upper third—transverse deficiency
4. Thigh—middle third—transverse deficiency
5. Thigh—lower third—transverse deficiency
6. Leg—total—transverse deficiency
7. Leg—upper third—transverse deficiency
8. Leg—middle third—transverse deficiency
9. Leg—lower third—transverse deficiency
10. Tarsal—total—transverse deficiency
11. Tarsal—partial—transverse deficiency
12. Metatarsal—total—transverse deficiency
13. Metatarsal—partial—transverse deficiency
14. Phalangeal—total—transverse deficiency
15. Phalangeal—partial—transverse deficiency

16.2.2 Longitudinal deficiencies

In a longitudinal deficiency, there is the total or partial absence of bone in the long axis of the extremity with preserved normal distal skeletal elements. ISO/ISPO classification of congenital limb deficiency describes the longitudinal deficiencies by naming the affected bones in a proximal-distal sequence and any bones not labelled is present with intact structure (2).

16.2.2.1 UPPER EXTREMITY

1. Scapula—total—longitudinal deficiency
2. Scapula—partial—longitudinal deficiency
3. Clavicle—total—longitudinal deficiency
4. Clavicle—partial—longitudinal deficiency
5. Humerus—total—longitudinal deficiency
6. Humerus—partial—longitudinal deficiency

7. Radius—total—longitudinal deficiency
8. Radius—partial—longitudinal deficiency
9. Ulna—total—longitudinal deficiency
10. Ulna—partial—longitudinal deficiency
11. Carpal—total—longitudinal deficiency
12. Carpal—partial—longitudinal deficiency
13. Metacarpal (1) thumb—total—longitudinal deficiency
14. Metacarpal (1) thumb—partial—longitudinal deficiency
15. Metacarpal (2) index—total—longitudinal deficiency
16. Metacarpal (2) index—partial—longitudinal deficiency
17. Metacarpal (3) middle—total—longitudinal deficiency
18. Metacarpal (3) middle—partial—longitudinal deficiency
19. Metacarpal (4) ring—total—longitudinal deficiency
20. Metacarpal (4) ring—partial—longitudinal deficiency
21. Metacarpal (5) little—total—longitudinal deficiency
22. Metacarpal (5) little—partial—longitudinal deficiency
23. Phalangeal (1) thumb—total—longitudinal deficiency
24. Phalangeal (1) thumb—partial—longitudinal deficiency
25. Phalangeal (2) index—total—longitudinal deficiency
26. Phalangeal (2) index—partial—longitudinal deficiency
27. Phalangeal (3) middle—total—longitudinal deficiency
28. Phalangeal (3) middle—partial—longitudinal deficiency
29. Phalangeal (4) ring—total—longitudinal deficiency
30. Phalangeal (4) ring—partial—longitudinal deficiency
31. Phalangeal (5) little—total—longitudinal deficiency
32. Phalangeal (5) little—partial—longitudinal deficiency

16.2.2.2 LOWER EXTREMITY

1. Ilium—total—longitudinal deficiency
2. Ilium—partial—longitudinal deficiency
3. Ischium—total—longitudinal deficiency
4. Ischium—partial—longitudinal deficiency
5. Pubis—total—longitudinal deficiency
6. Pubis—partial—longitudinal deficiency
7. Femur—total—longitudinal deficiency
8. Femur—partial—longitudinal deficiency
9. Tibia—total—longitudinal deficiency
10. Tibia—partial—longitudinal deficiency
11. Fibula—total—longitudinal deficiency
12. Fibula -partial—longitudinal deficiency
13. Tarsal—total—longitudinal deficiency
14. Tarsal—partial—longitudinal deficiency
15. Metatarsal (1)—total longitudinal deficiency
16. Metatarsal (1)—partial—longitudinal deficiency
17. Metatarsal (2)—total longitudinal deficiency
18. Metatarsal (2)—partial—longitudinal deficiency
19. Metatarsal (3)—total longitudinal deficiency
20. Metatarsal (3)—partial—longitudinal deficiency
21. Metatarsal (4)—total longitudinal deficiency
22. Metatarsal (4)—partial—longitudinal deficiency
23. Metatarsal (5)—total longitudinal deficiency
24. Metatarsal (5)—partial—longitudinal deficiency
25. Phalangeal (1) Big toe—total longitudinal deficiency

26. Phalangeal (1) Big toe—partial—longitudinal deficiency
27. Phalangeal (2) Second toe—total longitudinal deficiency
28. Phalangeal (2) Second toe—partial—longitudinal deficiency
29. Phalangeal (3) Third toe—total longitudinal deficiency
30. Phalangeal (3) Third toe—partial—longitudinal deficiency
31. Phalangeal (4) Fourth toe—total longitudinal deficiency
32. Phalangeal (4) Fourth toe—partial—longitudinal deficiency
33. Phalangeal (5) Fifth toe—total longitudinal deficiency
34. Phalangeal (5) Fifth toe—partial—longitudinal deficiency

16.3 IMPAIRMENT

16.3.1 Impairment in transverse deficiencies

The transverse deficiency is like that of amputation and hence the whole person impairment is like that of amputation.

16.3.1.1 CONGENITAL SKELETAL LIMB TRANSVERSE DEFICIENCIES—UPPER EXTREMITY: IMPAIRMENT

Shoulder total transverse deficiency: 80%
Upper arm total transverse deficiency: 79%
Upper arm upper third transverse deficiency: 78%
Upper arm middle third transverse deficiency: 77%
Upper arm distal third transverse deficiency: 76%
Forearm total transverse deficiency: 72%
Forearm upper third transverse deficiency: 70%
Forearm middle third transverse deficiency: 68%
Forearm distal third transverse deficiency: 66%
Carpal total transverse deficiency: 65%
Metacarpal total transverse deficiency: 64%
Metacarpal partial transverse deficiency: 55%
Phalangeal all fingers total transverse deficiency: 45%
Phalangeal Thumb total transverse deficiency at CMCP: 31%
Phalangeal Thumb partial transverse deficiency at MCP: 20%
Phalangeal Thumb partial transverse deficiency at IP: 7%
Phalangeal Index total transverse deficiency at CMCP: 17%
Phalangeal Index partial transverse deficiency at MCP: 11%
Phalangeal Index partial transverse deficiency at PIP: 7%
Phalangeal Index partial transverse deficiency at DIP: 4%
Phalangeal middle finger total transverse deficiency at CMCP: 17%
Phalangeal middle finger partial transverse deficiency at MCP: 11%
Phalangeal middle finger partial transverse deficiency at PIP: 7%

Phalangeal middle finger partial transverse deficiency at DIP: 4%

Phalangeal ring finger total transverse deficiency at CMCP: 10%

Phalangeal ring finger partial transverse deficiency at MCP: 6%

Phalangeal ring finger partial transverse deficiency at PIP: 4%

Phalangeal ring finger partial transverse deficiency at MCP: 2%

Phalangeal little finger total transverse deficiency at CMCP: 10%

Phalangeal little finger partial transverse deficiency at MCP: 6%

Phalangeal little finger partial transverse deficiency at PIP: 4%

Phalangeal little finger partial transverse deficiency at MCP: 2%

(CMCP = Carpo-metacarpophalangeal joint, MCP = Metacarpophalangeal joint, PIP = Proximal interphalangeal joint, DIP = Distal interphalangeal joint)

16.3.1.2 CONGENITAL SKELETAL LIMB TRANSVERSE DEFICIENCIES—LOWER EXTREMITY: IMPAIRMENT

Pelvis total transverse deficiency: 61%
Thigh total transverse deficiency: 60%
Thigh upper third transverse deficiency: 59%
Thigh middle third transverse deficiency: 58%
Thigh lower third transverse deficiency: 55%
Leg total transverse deficiency: 54%
Leg upper third transverse deficiency <3″: 53%
Leg upper third transverse deficiency ≥3″: 51%
Leg middle third transverse deficiency: 49%
Leg lower third transverse deficiency: 47%
Tarsal total transverse deficiency: 45%
Tarsal partial transverse deficiency: 27%
Metatarsal total transverse deficiency: 21%
Metatarsal partial transverse deficiency: 16%

Phalangeal total transverse deficiency—all toes: 11%
Phalangeal total transverse deficiency—Big Toe: 4%
Phalangeal partial transverse deficiency—Big Toe: 2%
Phalangeal total transverse deficiency 2nd Toe: 2%
Phalangeal partial transverse deficiency 2nd Toe: 1%
Phalangeal total transverse deficiency 3rd Toe: 2%
Phalangeal partial transverse deficiency 3rd Toe: 1%
Phalangeal total transverse deficiency 4th Toe: 1%
Phalangeal partial transverse deficiency 4th Toe: 0.5%
Phalangeal total transverse deficiency 5th Toe: 1%
Phalangeal partial transverse deficiency 5th Toe: 0.5%

16.3.2 Impairment in longitudinal deficiencies

In a longitudinal deficiency, there may be the absence of joint, loss of muscle due to aplasia, or hypoplasia of the muscle in the corresponding missing skeletal element. There may be a loss of stability of the extremity due to the absence of the skeletal element. There may be a limitation of range of motion (ROM) in the knee/ankle joint due to the absence of tibia, loss of muscle power in the ankle due to aplasia or hypoplasia of the tibial muscles. There may be potential instability of the lower extremity due to the absence of tibia, for example, tibial total longitudinal deficiency. Hence, *Integrated Evaluation of Disability* computes impairment based on ROM of a joint, muscle power, stability, and shortening. *Integrated Evaluation of Disability* assigns impairment of 1% for each inch of shortening of the upper/lower extremity. Furthermore, the person also may obtain an additional percentage of disability according to their limitation of activity or participation.

REFERENCES

1. Frantz CH, O'Rahilly R. Congenital skeletal limb deficiencies. *J Bone Joint Surg.* 1961;43A(8):1202–1224.
2. Day HJB. The ISO/ISPO classification of congenital limb deficiency. *Prosthet Orthot Int.* 1991;15(2):67–69.

17

Impairment: Dwarfism, disfigurement, deformities, and shortening

17.1 DWARFISM/SHORT STATURE

17.1.1 History

The average height for a man varies from 5′2″ (Indonesia) to 5′11½″ (Germany), and the average female height varies from 4′8″ (Bolivia–Aymara) to 5′7½″ (Dinaric Alps) (1). Gul Mohammed of New Delhi, India was the shortest man until his death in October of 1997. Gul Mohammed was 0.57 meters (or 22.4 inches) tall on July 19, 1990 (2). An adult human with the shortest height on record is Chandra Bahadur Dangi of Nepal at 1′9½″ (1).

17.1.2 Definition

Idiopathic short stature refers to a height below -2 standard deviation score (SDS) based on the science of human growth and development with no evidence for any primary diseases (3). Little People of America defines dwarfism as a medical or genetic condition resulting in an adult height of 4′10″ or shorter (4). The height in dwarfism varies from 2′8″ to 4′8″ (5).

17.1.3 Classification

Dwarfism may be proportionate and disproportionate based on stem length and limb length. In proportionate dwarfism both the stem length, that is, crown to rump length and length of the extremity are equal. In disproportionate dwarfism, the stem length and length of the extremities are unequal. The proportionate short stature is due to endocrine, metabolic, chromosomal, and non-skeletal dysplasia abnormalities. The disproportionate short stature is due to skeletal dysplasia with the resultant abnormalities of bone and cartilage growth. It may produce abnormal shape and size of the skeleton and disproportion of long bones, spine,

and head. The most common skeletal dysplasias are achondroplasia, thanatophoric dysplasia, osteogenesis imperfecta, and achondrogenesis (6).

Dwarfism may be rhizomelic, mesomelic, and acromelic according to the distribution of anomaly. In rhizomelic dwarfism, shortening confines to the proximal segments namely the humerus and femur, for example, achondroplasia, hypochondroplasia, spondyloepiphyseal dysplasia congenita, congenital short femur, and so on. In mesomelic dwarfism, shortening confines to the middle segments, that is, radius, ulna, tibia, and fibula, for example, Robinow syndrome, Reinhardt syndrome, and so on. In acromelic shortening, the shortening confines to the distal segments namely metacarpals and phalanges, for example, acrodysostosis and peripheral dysostosis. In micromelia, shortening limits to the entire extremity, for example, achondrogenesis, fibrochondrogenesis, Roberts syndrome, and so on. Short stature with shortening of trunk occurs in Morquio syndrome, Kniest syndrome, spondyloepimetaphyseal dysplasia, and metatropic dysplasia.

17.1.4 Disability in persons with dwarfism

Persons with dwarfism have functional limitations in overhead activities due to short stature, increased cadence during walking, limitation of access to pedals for acceleration and brake, obstacles in vision during driving, using the ATM, gas/petrol pump, and so on.

Integrated Evaluation of Disability assigns an impairment of 1.72% for each inch of shortening from 4′10″ (Illustration 17.1). Furthermore, impairment of cognition, sensory-motor functions, bladder and bowel functions, heart function, pulmonary function, renal function, limitations of the joints due to skeletal deformities, and so on derive additional impairment score.

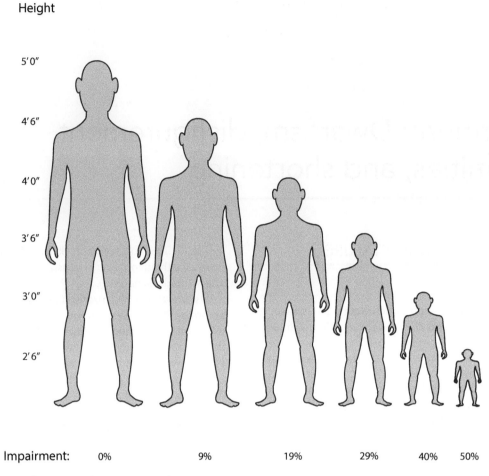

Illustration 17.1 Dwarfism—Height versus impairment.

17.2 DISFIGUREMENT AND DEFORMITIES

Disfigurement may be due to depigmentation of the skin, hypertrophic scar, keloid, amputation of pinna of the ear, saddle nose, amputation of the nose, cleft lip, facial scar, mastectomy, deformity, and so on (Tables 17.1 through 17.4).

17.3 SHORTENING OF EXTREMITY

Integrated Evaluation of Disability assigns impairment of one percent for each inch of shortening of the upper/lower extremity.

Table 17.1 Impairment class—Disfigurement and deformity: Head and neck

Region	Class 1 impairment	Class 2 impairment	Class 3 impairment	Class 4 impairment
Face	Depigmentation, such as leukoderma 1%	Hypertrophic scar involving less than 50% of the face 2.5%	Hypertrophic scar involving more than 50% of the face or keloid less than 50% of the face 5%	Keloid involving more than 50% of the face 10%
Ear	Depigmentation 0.25%	Hypertrophic scar 0.5%	Keloid 1.0%	Amputation of the pinna of the ear 2.5%
Eye	Scar and loss of hair in the eyebrow, for instance burns sequel 0.25%	Entropion/Ectropion 0.50%	Corneal opacity 0.75%	Enucleation of one eye 1%
Nose	Saddle nose 1.25%	Saddle nose with keloid 2.5%	Sub-total amputation 3.75%	Total nasal amputation 5%
Mouth	Depigmentation of lip—Leukoplakia 0.5%	Microstomia 1.0%	Cleft lip 2.5%	Cleft lip and palate 5%
Neck	Depigmentation 0.5%	Hypertrophic scar 1.00%	Keloid 2.0%	Torticollis 5.0%

Table 17.2 Impairment class—Disfigurement and deformity: Chest and trunk

Region	Class 1 impairment	Class 2 impairment	Class 3 impairment	Class 4 impairment
Chest	Depigmentation 0.25%	Hypertrophic scar 0.5%	Keloid 1.0%	Band like contracture 2.0%
Breast	Subcutaneous mastectomy 1.0%	Partial mastectomy 2.5%	Total unilateral mastectomy 5.0%	Bilateral total mastectomy 10.0%
Spine—scoliosis/ kyphosis cobb angle		Cobb: 10°–24° 2.5%	Cobb: 25°–50° 5.0%	Cobb: >50° 10.0%

Table 17.3 Impairment class—Disfigurement and deformity: Upper extremity

Region	Class 1 impairment	Class 2 impairment	Class 3 impairment	Class 4 impairment
Upper arm	Depigmentation 0.25%	Hypertrophic scar 0.5%	Keloid 0.75%	Contracture 1.0%
Forearm, wrist, and hand	Depigmentation 1.0%	Hypertrophic scar 2.0%	Keloid 3.0%	Contracture, e.g., club hand, claw hand deformity, or Resorption of fingers 4.0%

Table 17.4 Impairment class—Disfigurement and deformity: Lower extremity

Region	Class 1 impairment	Class 2 impairment	Class 3 impairment	Class 4 impairment
Hip and thigh			Keloid 0.25%	Deformity 0.5%
Knee and leg			Keloid 0.25%	Deformity 0.5%
Ankle	Depigmentation 0.25%	Hypertrophic scar 0.5%	Keloid 0.75%	Deformity, e.g., equinus deformity, calcaneal deformity 2.0%
Dorsum of the foot	Depigmentation 0.25%	Hypertrophic scar 0.5%	Keloid 1.0%	
Sole of the foot	Hypertrophic scar 1.0%	Keloid 2.0%	Pes cavus deformity 2.0%	Club foot 4.0%

REFERENCES

1. Wikipedia. Human height. Available from: http://en.wikipedia.org/wiki/Human_height.
2. Very big very short very small very tall [Internet]. Oracle Think Quest Educational Foundation [cited September 24, 2011]. Available from: http://library.thinkquest.org/4038/short.htm.
3. Cohen P, Rogol AD, Deal CL, Saenger P, Reiter EO, Ross JL et al. Consensus statement on the diagnosis and treatment of children with idiopathic short stature: a summary of the Growth Hormone Research Society, the Lawson Wilkins Pediatric Endocrine Society, and the European Society for Paediatric Endocrinology Workshop. *J Clin Endocrinol Metab.* 2008;93(11):4210–4217.
4. Dwarfism [Internet]. Little People of America. Available from: http://www.lpaonline.org/.
5. Frequently asked questions: Definition of dwarfism [Internet]. Little People of America; 2008–2011.
6. Chen H. *Skeletal Dysplasia.* New York: Medscape; 2013.

Burns: Impairment

18.1 FUNCTIONS OF THE SKIN

The skin shields the body from physical, chemical, and biological injury or threats (1), and regulates body temperature, secretes sebum, excretes sweat, synthesizes vitamin D from exposure to sunlight, and so on.

18.2 BURNS DEFINITION, CAUSES, CLASSIFICATION, AND SEQUEL

Burns, per se, refer to both total and partial absence of skin and sequel following repair functions of the skin. Heat, radiation, radioactivity, electricity, chemicals, and smoke inhalation can produce burn injury to the skin and respiratory tract. The World Health Organization (WHO) states that children under 5 years old and persons over 70 years have the highest incidence of mortality due to burns (2).

In first-degree burns, injury confines to the epidermis. In second-degree superficial partial-thickness burns, injury is limited to the epidermis and papillary dermis; and in second-degree deep partial-thickness burns injury is to the epidermis, papillary dermis, and deep reticular dermis. In third-degree burns, injury involves the epidermis and the full thickness of dermis. First-degree and second-degree superficial burns heal spontaneously by primary intention. Second-degree and third-degree burns heal by secondary intention involving epithelization and contraction. Third-degree burns heal only by surgical intervention, usually skin grafting. Hence, third-degree burns result in scars and deformities (3). Fourth-degree burns also involve the muscles and bones (4) (Figure 18.1).

Post-burn sequel includes loss of hair, loss of the nails, depigmentation of skin, hypertrophic scar, keloid formation, contracture, and deformities, for example, ectropion of the eyelid, and flexion contracture in the neck. It also includes loss of pinna of the ear, scar in the sclera, conjunctiva, cornea and loss of vision, deformity and scars on the face, microstomia, scarring or loss of a breast, and a scar or loss of genitals. It further includes axillary scars, contracture of the joints in the extremities, deformity or amputations, and disfigurement.

Burns may involve eyelid, conjunctiva, sclera, cornea, lens, and macula. Persons who have sustained high voltage burns involving the eyes may develop cataract and maculopathy (5,6). Ocular injury due to fireworks may result in open/globe injury with either partial or total loss of vision (7).

Burns to the external ear may lead to the baring of the cartilage of the external ear or amputation of the external ear (8). Burn injuries to the ear may also involve tympanic membrane and middle ear (9).

Burns to the nose may result in loss of alar lobule, subtotal amputation with complete loss of cartilaginous support, or total amputation of nose (10). Airway occlusion in the nose following burns may produce sleep apnea/hypopnea. Chapter 10: Impairment of pulmonary functions, Section 10.7 describes the evaluation of sleep apnea.

Burns to the perioral tissue may lead to microstomia, and it may produce pain during activities involving mouth. Microstomia may result in drooling, limited swallowing ability using only a straw, limitation of oral hygiene and dental care, inability to smile, and impairment of articulation of speech (11).

Burns to the perineum and genitals may present either with partial thickness injury or full thickness injury (12). Full thickness burns produce loss of sensation in the penis. Furthermore, there is discoloration and contracture of the penis (13). Post burns sequel of perineum and groin includes perineal obliteration, hidden genitalia, limitation of sexual function, restriction of hip movement, and limitation of perineal hygiene, megarectum, intestinal obstruction, and recurrent ulcerations in the contracture (14,15).

Acute renal injury is one of the major complications of burns. Among the survivors, the majority regain the normal renal function and few require long-term dialysis (16).

There is severe loss of plasma fluid due to increased capillary permeability. The resultant decreased cardiac

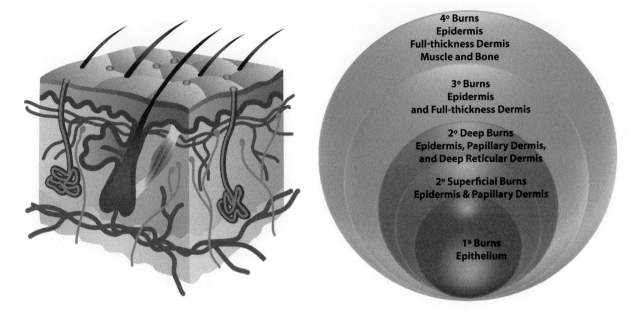

Figure 18.1 Degrees of burns.

output triggers a compensatory increase in heart rate, peripheral vascular resistance, and pulmonary resistance, which may lead to biventricular failure in persons with larger burns.

Loss of elasticity of scar tissue in third-degree burns may interfere with respiratory mechanics and ventilation. Smoke inhalation during burns may lead to increased pulmonary artery resistance, pulmonary hypertension, and increased right ventricular load (17). In a smoke inhalation injury, heat may result in occlusion of the upper respiratory tract. The toxins and particulate matter contained in the smoke may induce inflammation, infection and immunological changes in the lung, hypoxia due to interference with oxygen transport and utilization, and ventilation-perfusion mismatch (18,19).

18.3 IMPAIRMENT OF STRUCTURE AND FUNCTIONS FOLLOWING BURNS

Disfigurement and impairment of structure and function defines the impairment score. Tables 18.1 through 18.12 describe impairment class of post burns sequel. The formula

$$A + \left[\frac{B(100 - A)}{100} \right] \tag{18.1}$$

combines impairment of the scalp and face, eye, ear, nose, mouth, neck, chest and trunk, perineum and genitals, upper and lower extremities, and impairment of renal and

Table 18.1 Impairment class—Burns: Scalp and face

Impairment variables	Class 1	Class 2	Class 3	Class 4
Disfigurement	Depigmentation of the scar 1%	Hypertrophic scar less than 50% of the face 2.5%	Hypertrophic scar more than 50% or keloid less than 50% of the face 5%	Keloid involving more than 50% of the face 10%
Impairment of structure	Permanent hair Loss <25% of scalp 1.25%	Permanent hair loss 25%–50% of scalp 2.5%	Permanent hair loss 50%–75% of scalp 3.75%	Permanent hair loss >75% of scalp 5%
Impairment of function Trigeminal nerve – 3° burns	Loss of sensation of either maxillary or mandibular division 1.25%	Loss of sensation of both maxillary and mandibular divisions 2.5%	Loss of sensation of ophthalmic division 3.75%	Loss of sensation of all the three divisions 5%
C2 dermatome 3° burns	Loss of sensation of ≤25% of area behind vertico-mental-interaural line 0.25%	Loss of sensation of 26%–50% of area behind vertico-mental-interaural line 0.50%	Loss of sensation of 51%–75% of area behind vertico-mental-interaural line 0.75%	Loss of sensation of >75% of area behind vertico-mental-interaural line 1.00%

Table 18.2 Impairment class—Burns involving eye

Impairment variables	Class 1	Class 2	Class 3	Class 4
Disfigurement Right eye	Scar and loss of hair in the eyebrow 0.25%	Entropion/ectropion 0.5%	Corneal opacity 0.75%	
Left eye	Scar and loss of hair in the eyebrow 0.25%	Entropion/ectropion 0.5%	Corneal opacity 0.75%	
Impairment of structure			Enucleation of one eye 1%	Enucleation of two eyes 2%
Impairment of function	Refer to Chapter 13 "Impairment of Visual Functions"			

Table 18.3 Impairment class—Burns involving ear

Impairment variables	Class 1	Class 2	Class 3	Class 4
Disfigurement Right—ear	Depigmentation of the scar 0.25%	Hypertrophic scar 0.5%	Keloid 1%	
Left—ear	Depigmentation of the scar 0.25%	Hypertrophic scar 0.5%	Keloid 1%	
Impairment of structure Right ear	Loss of skin over pinna of the ear with intact bare cartilage 1.25%	Amputation of the pinna of the ear 2.5%	Amputation of pinna and injury to tympanic membrane 3.75%	Amputation of pinna, injury to tympanic membrane and middle ear 5%
Left ear	Loss of skin over pinna of the ear with intact bare cartilage 1.25%	Amputation of the pinna of the ear 2.5%	Amputation of pinna and injury to tympanic membrane 3.75%	Amputation of pinna, injury to tympanic membrane and middle ear 5%
Impairment of function ear (Refer to Chapter 14 "Impairment of Hearing Functions")	Monaural hearing impairment due to tympanic membrane	Binaural hearing impairment due to tympanic membrane	Monaural hearing impairment due to middle ear injury	Binaural hearing impairment due to middle ear injury

Table 18.4 Impairment class—Burns involving nose

Impairment variables	Class 1	Class 2	Class 3	Class 4
Disfigurement	Depigmentation 0.50%	Hypertrophic scar 1.00%	Keloid 2.00%	
Impairment of structure	Partial loss of alar lobule of nose 1.25%	Total loss of alar lobule of nose with intact cartilaginous support 2.5%	Sub-total amputation of nose with loss of cartilaginous support 3.75%	Total nasal amputation 5%
Impairment of function Occlusion of airway: Impairment of obstructive sleep apnea/hypopnea	Refer to Chapter 10 "Impairment of Pulmonary Functions"			
Nose—anosmia	Unilateral anosmia 2.5%	Bilateral anosmia 5%		

Table 18.5 Impairment class—Burns involving mouth

Impairment variables	Class 1	Class 2	Class 3	Class 4
Disfigurement	Depigmentation 0.50%	Hypertrophic scar 1.00%	Keloid 2.00%	
Impairment of structure	Microstomia with no impairment of function 1.00%			
Impairment of function Microstomia	Microstomia—Inability to smile or Intermittent drooling 2.50%	Microstomia with continuous drooling Or Dysarthria 5%	Microstomia with pain while opening the mouth for oral hygiene and drinking and eating (1% if VAS is 1, 2% if VAS is 2, 3% if VAS is 10% if VAS 10) 1%–10%	Microstomia with limited swallowing ability using only straw 15%

Table 18.6 Impairment class—Burns involving neck

Impairment variables	Class 1	Class 2	Class 3	Class 4
Disfigurement	Depigmentation of the scar 0.50%	Hypertrophic scar 1.00%	Keloid 2.00%	
Impairment of structure			Flexion contracture 2.50%	
Impairment of function	Partial loss of sensation 0.75%	Complete loss of sensation 1.50%		

Table 18.7 Impairment class—Burns: Chest and trunk

Impairment variables	Class 1	Class 2	Class 3	Class 4
Disfigurement Scar in the chest including breast	Depigmentation 0.25%	Hypertrophy 0.50%	Keloid 1.00%	Contracture (band like) 2.00%
Impairment of structure Breast	Unilateral loss of full-thickness skin 1.25%	Bilateral loss of full-thickness skin 2.50%	Unilateral total loss of breast 5.00%	Bilateral total loss of breast 10.00%
Impairment of function Lactation in childbearing age			Impairment of lactation in one breast 5%	Impairment of lactation in both breast 10%
Airway occlusion, smoke inhalation injury	Refer to Chapter 10 "Impairment of Pulmonary Functions"			

Table 18.8 Impairment class—Burns: Perineum and genitals

Impairment variables	Class 1	Class 2	Class 3	Class 4
Disfigurement	Discoloration 1.25%	Hypertrophic scar 2.5%	Keloid 3.75%	Contracture and/or recurrent ulceration of scar 5.0%
Impairment of structure Perineal obliteration		Occlusion of anus 2.5%	Occlusion of anus with megarectum 5%	Hidden genitals in male or occlusion of external genitalia in female 10%
Impairment of function Anus		Partial occlusion with difficulty in initiating bowel movement requiring suppositories 5%	Partial occlusion with constipation requiring enema 15%	Complete occlusion with obstipation 25%
Male genitals		Loss of sensation 2.5%	Painful erection 5%	Interfere with sexual intercourse 15%
Female genitals		Loss of sensation 2.5%		Interfere with sexual intercourse 15%

Table 18.9 Impairment class—Burns: Upper extremity

Impairment variables	Class 1	Class 2	Class 3	Class 4
Disfigurement	Depigmentation of the scar	Hypertrophic scar	Keloid	Contracture
Axillary scar	0.25%	0.5%	0.75%	1%
Upper arm scar	0.25%	0.5%	0.75%	1%
Forearm, wrist, and hand scar	1%	2%	3%	4%
Impairment of structure Amputations	Refer to Chapter 15 "Impairment of Amputations"			
Impairment of motor function Limitation of ROM of joints	Refer to Chapter 7 "Impairment of Functions in Neuromusculoskeletal System"			
Impairment of sensory function	Refer to Chapter 7 "Impairment of Functions in Neuromusculoskeletal System"			

Table 18.10 Impairment class—Burns: Lower extremity

Impairment variables	Class 1	Class 2	Class 3	Class 4
Disfigurement	Depigmentation of the scar	Hypertrophic scar	Keloid	Contracture
Thigh scar	—	—	0.25%	0.5%
Leg scar	—	—	0.25%	0.5%
Ankle scar	0.25%	0.50%	0.75%	2.0%
Foot scar including sole	0.5%	1%	2%	4% Keloid with contracture
Impairment of structure Amputations	Refer Chapter 15 "Impairment of Amputations"			
Impairment of function Limitation of ROM of joints	Refer to Chapter 7 "Impairment of Functions in Neuromusculoskeletal System"			
Impairment of sensory function	Refer to Chapter 7 "Impairment of Functions in Neuromusculoskeletal System"			

Table 18.11 Impairment class—Burns involving renal, and cardiopulmonary systems

Renal function	Refer to Chapter 8 "Impairment of Urogenital Functions"
Permanent dialysis	
Cardiac function	Refer to Chapter 9 "Impairment of Cardiovascular Functions"
Pulmonary function	Refer to Chapter 10 "Impairment of Pulmonary Functions"

Table 18.12 Burns—Whole person impairment 90%

Burns affecting region/systems/extremities	Reference value—Maximum impairment	Assigned whole person impairment combine by formula $A + [B(100 − A)/100]$
Head and neck	70%	
Eye	85%	
Ear	50%	
Chest	50%	
Perineum and genitals	35%	
Right upper extremity	80%	
Left upper extremity	80%	
Right lower extremity	61%	
Left lower extremity	61%	
Renal function	50%	
Cardiovascular function	75%	
Pulmonary function	75%	

cardiopulmonary functions due to burns. The maximum combined whole person impairment does not exceed 90%. Because of the impairment of functions and structure, there may be a limitation of activities, participation restriction and environmental barriers, fear of rejection by the society, and inadequate behavioral adaptation, sometimes with suicidal tendencies.

Furthermore, "Activity Participation Skill Assessment Scale," "Environmental Factors Measurement Scale," and "Personal Factors Measurement Scale" evaluate limitation of activities, participation restrictions, environmental factors, and adaptive behavior of the person for an additional percentage of disability.

REFERENCES

1. *International Classification of Functioning, Disability and Health.* Geneva, Switzerland: World Health Organization; 2001. p. 103, 4, 5, 22.

2. *Violence and Injury Prevention: Burns.* Geneva, Switzerland: World Health Organization; 2014.

3. Tiwari VK. Burn wound: How it differs from other wounds? *Indian J Plast Surg.* 2012;45(2):364–373.

4. Agbenorku P. Burns functional disabilities among burn survivors: A study in Komfo Anokye Teaching Hospital, Ghana. *Int J Burns Trauma.* 2013;3(2):78–86.

5. Faustino LD, Oliveira RA, Oliveira AF, Rodrigues EB, Moraes NS, Ferreira LM. Bilateral maculopathy following electrical burn: Case report. *Sao Paulo Med J.* 2014;132(6):372–376.

6. Reddy SC. Electric cataract: A case report and review of the literature. *Eur J Ophthalmol.* 1999;9(2):134–138.

7. Patel R, Mukherjee B. Crash & burn: Ocular injuries due to fireworks. *Semin Ophthalmol.* 2016;31:243–248.

8. Templer J, Renner GJ. Injuries of the external ear. *Otolaryngol Clin North Am.* 1990;23(5):1003–1018.

9. Lukan N. Burn injuries of the middle ear. *ORL J Otorhinolaryngol Relat Spec.* 1991;53(3):140–142.

10. Taylor HO, Carty M, Driscoll D, Lewis M, Donelan MB. Nasal reconstruction after severe facial burns using a local turndown flap. *Ann Plast Surg.* 2009;62(2):175–179.

11. Maragakis GM, Garcia-Tempone M. Microstomia following facial burns. *J Clin Pediatr Dent.* 1998;23(1):69–74.

12. Rutan RL. Management of perineal and genital burns. *J ET Nurs.* 1993;20(4):169–176.

13. Abdel-Razek SM. Isolated chemical burns to the genitalia. *Ann Burns Fire Disasters.* 2006;19(3):148–152.

14. Sajad W, Hamid R. Outcome of split thickness skin grafting and multiple z-plasties in postburn contractures of groin and perineum: A 15-year experience. *Plast Surg Int.* 2014;2014:358526.

15. Grishkevich VM. Postburn perineal obliteration: Elimination of perineal, inguinal, and perianal contractures with the groin flap. *J Burn Care Res.* 2010;31(5):786–790.

16. Ibrahim AE, Sarhane KA, Fagan SP, Goverman J. Renal dysfunction in burns: A review. *Ann Burns Fire Disasters.* 2013;26(1):16–25.

17. Abu-Sittah GS, Sarhane KA, Dibo SA, Ibrahim A. Cardiovascular dysfunction in burns: Review of the literature. *Ann Burns Fire Disasters.* 2012;25(1):26–37.

18. Jones SW, Zhou H, Ortiz-Pujols SM, Maile R, Herbst M, Joyner BL Jr. et al. Bronchoscopy-derived correlates of lung injury following inhalational injuries: A prospective observational study. *PloS one.* 2013;8(5):e64250.

19. Toon MH, Maybauer MO, Greenwood JE, Maybauer DM, Fraser JF. Management of acute smoke inhalation injury. *Crit Care Resusc.* 2010;12(1):53–61.

19

Intellectual disability or mental retardation

19.1 INTELLECTUAL FUNCTION

Intellectual function refers to the ability to comprehend and assimilate various mental actions, such as reasoning, thinking, planning, judging, problem-solving, and communicating to learn life skills. *Integrated Evaluation of Disability* prefers preliminary bedside clinical evaluation. The clinical evaluation comprises a questionnaire to assess intellectual functioning, such as awareness of the purpose of their visit to the doctor and reading and understanding the newspaper. It also presents calculations, such as the serial addition of 7 from 0 to 50 or subtracting 7 from 100. It further includes an abstract such as the use of proverbs and judgment; for example, what to do with a letter if you found one in front of the post box. If the preliminary evaluation reveals an impairment of IQ, the person may need an evaluation by a psychologist. The Wechsler Scale (1) and Raven's matrices (2) are widely used to evaluate IQ. A mean IQ of 100, one standard deviation above 100, which is 115, and one standard deviation below 100, which is 85, are all considered normal. An IQ score below two standard deviations from the mean, which is ≤70, represent a significant reduction in intellectual functioning (3). *Integrated Evaluation of Disability* assigns an impairment of 0% for an IQ of 85–115. It allocates negligible impairment of 4% for an IQ of 71–84, mild impairment of 14% (median score) for an IQ of 50–70, moderate impairment of 39% (median score) for an IQ score of 25–49, and severe impairment of 63% (median score) for an IQ score of <25. Table 19.1 describes the impairment class for deficiency of IQ.

Table 19.1 Impairment class—Intellectual functions

Impairment class	Clinical scales: Wechsler's scale/ Raven's matrices	Reference impairment median score
Class 1	IQ: 71–84	4%
Class 2	IQ: 50–70	14%
Class 3	IQ: 25–49	39%
Class 4	IQ: <25	63%

19.2 ADAPTIVE SKILLS

Diagnostic and Statistical Manual of Mental Disorders (DSM-5) (APA 2013) states that intellectual disability relates to cognitive functions—namely reasoning, problem-solving, abstract thinking, judgment; academic learning—both school learning and traditional learning; and experiential learning. It also requires an evaluation by culturally appropriate standard IQ tests.

Adaptive skills refer to the ability of a person, depending on their age and cultural requirements, to fulfill personal, common life, and social demands vital for performing life activities.

19.2.1 Social competence model and personal competence model

The social competence model and personal competence model include guidelines for the evaluation of adaptive behavior. The social competence model evaluates adaptive behavior: independent functioning, physical development, self-direction, personal responsibility, economic and vocational activity, and functional academic skills; and social skills: personal behavior, interpersonal behavior, academic-related behaviors, assertion, peer acceptance, and community skills. The personal competence model evaluates physical competence, affective competence, everyday competence, and academic competence. Vulnerability, gullibility (can be deceived without any difficulty) and credulity (believed without adequate evidence) are early markers of adaptive behavior evident in cognitive impairment (4).

19.2.2 Adaptive behavior

The American Association on Intellectual and Developmental Disability defines adaptive behavior as a conglomerate of conceptual skills, social skills, and practical skills learned and performed by people in their daily life (5).

Conceptual skills include the reception and expression of information using language, reading, writing, calculation, preparing notes, recognizing time, and measuring height, weight, distance. It also includes self-direction—namely, self-control/willpower—for independent living, understanding and accepting responsibility; planning, organizing, and executing a task independently or with assistance, time management, and prioritizing a work schedule.

Social skills comprise interpersonal relationships or attitudes toward extended family members, friends, neighbors, teachers, peer workers, superior officers, community members, and public servants. It also comprises of adhering to rules and following laws, as well as self-esteem, gullibility, carefulness.

Practical skills include self-care, namely washing oneself, toileting, dressing, eating and drinking; and health care such as preventing an injury, recognizing an illness, seeking medical advice, and following medical management.

Additionally, occupational skills include maintaining a good interpersonal relationship with peers, subordinates, superior officers, and completing the work within the schedule and with good productivity. It also includes planning, organizing, cooking, and serving food; cleaning the cooking area and utensils; washing, drying, and ironing clothes; and using the washing machine and dishwasher.

Further, it includes travel and transportation, following a daily schedule, participating in leisure activities, games and sports, conducting economic transactions, and using a device, like a telephone, to communicate. Some scales also consider motor skills, such as fine and gross motor skills for mobility, manipulating, and exploring the environment, when evaluating adaptive behavior (6).

19.3 INTELLECTUAL DISABILITY/MENTAL RETARDATION

Intellectual disability/mental retardation refers to subaverage intellectual functioning, which is an IQ score below two standard deviations from the mean, namely ≤70 accompanied by limited adaptive skills vital for personal and social activities, and educational and/or vocational and avocational pursuits depending on the age and culture in which he/she is living. Hence, evaluating IQ in conjunction with activity and participation skills is essential to reflect the true status of mental retardation/intellectual disability (Illustration 19.1). Chapter 20 describes in detail "Activities and Participation" and "Activity Participation Skill Assessment Scale." Table 19.2 describes the disability class and disability percentage for persons with intellectual disability/mental retardation.

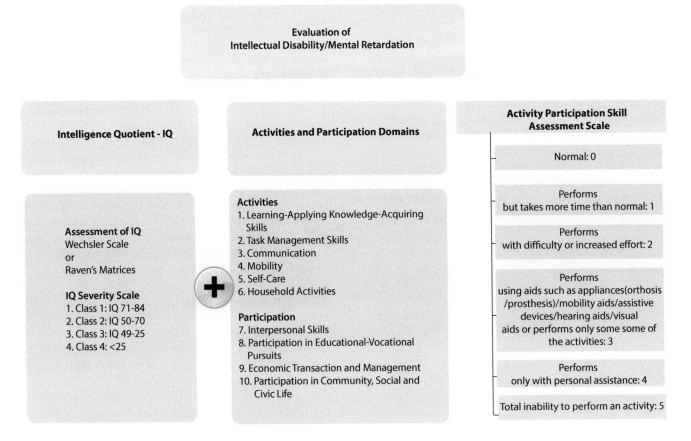

Illustration 19.1 Evaluation of intellectual disability.

Table 19.2 Disability class—Intellectual disability/mental retardation

Disability class	IQ	Impairment IQ	Activity Participation Skill Assessment score	Disability
Disability Class 1 (1%–4%)	70–84 (Median 60%)	4%	3.24%	3.62%
Disability Class 2 (5%–24%)	50–70 (Median 60%)	14%	17.30%	15.65%
Disability Class 3 (25%–49%)	25–49 (Median 37%)	39%	45.41%	42.20%
Disability Class 4 (≥50%)	<25 (Median 12.5%)	63%	62.16%	62.58%

REFERENCES

1. Wechsler DW. *Wechsler Adult Intelligence Scale-III (WAIS - III)*. San Antonio, TX: The Psychological Corporation; 1997.
2. Grossi D, Correra G, Calise C, Ruscitto MA, Vecchione V, Vigliardi MV et al. Evaluation of the influence of illiteracy on neuropsychological performances by elderly persons. *Percept Motor Skills*. 1993;77(3 Pt 1):859–866.
3. Trahan LH, Stuebing KK, Fletcher JM, Hiscock M. The Flynn effect: A meta-analysis. *Psychol Bull*. 2014;140(5):1332–1360.
4. National Research Council (US) Committee on Disability Determination for Mental Retardation. The role of adaptive behavior assessment. In: Reschly DJ, Myers TG, Hartel CR, editor. *Mental Retardation: Determining Eligibility for Social Security Benefits*. Washington, DC: National Academies Press (US); 2002.
5. Disabilities AAoIaD. *Definition of Intellectual Disability*. Washington, DC: American Association on Intellectual and Developmental Disabilities; 2013.
6. Jeffrey Ditterline TO. Relationships between adaptive behavior and impairment. In: Goldstein S, Naglieri JA, editors. *Assessing Impairment from Theory to Practice*. New York: Springer; 2009.

Activities and participation

20.1 ACTIVITY

Activity is an action performed by the person to execute essential personal demands of life. Thus, it denotes execution of a task with a personal perspective. Activity is a multidimensional construct comprising six domains of activity, namely, learning-applying knowledge-acquiring skills, task management, communication, mobility, self-care, and household activities. The WHO International Classification of Functioning, Disability and Health (ICF) states, *"Activity limitations are difficulties an individual may have in executing activities"* (1).

20.2 PARTICIPATION

Participation is a task of partaking in the society by the person in his/her life circumstances. Thus, it denotes execution of a task with a social perspective. It comprises of four domains, namely interpersonal skills, participation in educational-vocational pursuits, economic transaction and management, and participation in community, social, and civic life. ICF describes, *"Participation restrictions are problems an individual may experience in involvement in life situations"* (1).

20.3 "ACTIVITY PARTICIPATION SKILL ASSESSMENT SCALE"

Integrated Evaluation of Disability developed the "Activity Participation Skill Assessment Scale" and severity scale to assess impairment of bodily functions and structures, limitation of activities and participation restriction, environmental barriers, and behavior of the person toward their disability. It assigns a score after ascertaining his/her pre-morbid level of activities and participation (Illustration 20.1 and Tables 20.1 through 20.9).

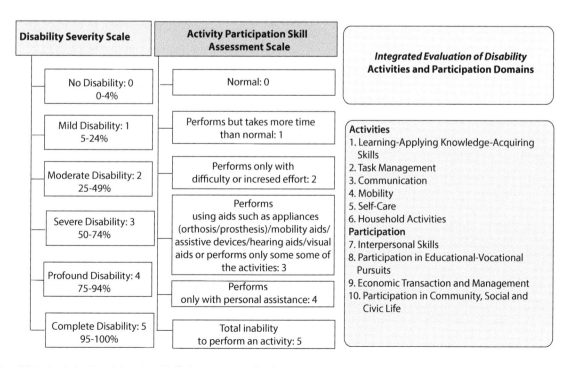

Illustration 20.1 Activity Participation Skill Assessment Scale.

Table 20.1 Activity Participation Skill Assessment Scale: Learning-applying knowledge-acquiring skills

1 Learning-applying knowledge-acquiring skills

Questions	Reference score	Assigned score
Can he/she copy an alphabet, learn a lesson, read, and write, calculate such as addition or subtraction or using Braille in persons with blindness?		
Can he/she rehearse a song?		
Can he/she acquire skills such as using a spoon and fork for eating food?		
Can he/she able to learn playing games such as football/soccer?		
Answers		
Cannot learn	5	
Can learn with maximum personal assistance	4	
Can learn only some of the items	3	
Can learn with difficulty/increased effort	2	
Can learn at slow pace	1	
Can learn normally	0	

Table 20.2 Activity Participation Skill Assessment Scale—Task management

2 Performing isolated single task

Questions	Reference score	Assigned score
Can he/she perform a single task such as identifying the books for his/her class or writing a letter?		
Answers		
Cannot perform the task	5	
Can perform the task with assistance	4	
Can perform only part of the task	3	
Can perform the task with difficulty/increased effort	2	
Can perform the task at slow pace	1	
Can perform the task normally	0	

3 Performing multiple tasks

Questions	Reference score	Assigned score
Can he/she plan, organize, and execute tasks at outstation independently? Can he/she locate the place of personal/official work, identifying time and date of travel, mode of travel—bus/train/air, purchasing a ticket, collecting travel kits, clothes, keeping the necessary money—cash or check or credit/debit card and work-related materials?		
Answers		
Cannot perform the task	5	
Can perform the task with assistance	4	
Can perform only part of the task	3	
Can perform the task with difficulty/increased effort	2	
Can perform the task at slow pace	1	
Can perform the task normally	0	

4 Performing daily activities

Questions	Reference score	Assigned score
Can he/she plan, manage, and complete daily activities namely getting up early from bed, toileting, washing his/her body/body parts, dressing, eating, and drinking, travelling and reaching the school/workplace? or Can he/she plan, organize, cook, serve food, clean cooking and dining area and clean utensils?		

(Continued)

Table 20.2 (*Continued*) Activity Participation Skill Assessment Scale—Task management

Answers

Cannot perform the task	5
Can perform the task with assistance	4
Can perform only part of the task	3
Can perform the task with difficulty/increased effort	2
Can perform the task at slow pace	1
Can perform the task normally	0

5 Managing responsibilities, stress, and emergency

Questions	Reference score	Assigned score
Can he/she coordinate, control psychological demands to accomplish the task namely driving to reach the airport during heavy road traffic? or Can he/she cope up with the stress while accompanying his wife/her husband with chest pain to come to an emergency service in the hospital?		

Answers

Cannot perform the task	5
Can perform the task with personal assistance	4
Can perform only part of the task	3
Can perform the task with difficulty	2
Can perform the task with moral support by accompanying person	1
Can cope up and perform the task normally	0

Table 20.3 Activity Participation Skill Assessment Scale—Communication

6 Communication—Reception

Questions	Reference score	Assigned score
Can he/she understand news in a TV?		
Can he/she read and understand a newspaper?		
Can he/she understand traffic signs?		
Can he/she visualize or interpret bus numbers?		
Can he/she visualize or interpret street numbers/name?		
Can he/she hear the safety alarm?		
or		
Can he/she understand messages by sign language?		
Can he/she read and understand a news by Braille?		
Can he/she follow safe lane by tactile surface?		

Answers

Cannot understand	5
Can understand only with maximum personal assistance	4
Can communicate or understand with hearing aids/visual aids/tactile surface	3
or	
Can understand the telephone voice with captioned telephone which displays every character in the conversation, or by TTY—device for communication by typing message forth and back	
or	
Can understand by hearing aid with amplifiers, or understand by speech recognition system	
or	
Can understand Braille language	
or	
Can use the joystick to open the computer and view the email or comprehend only some of the messages	

(*Continued*)

Table 20.3 (*Continued*) Activity Participation Skill Assessment Scale—Communication

Can understand with difficulty or increased effort	2
or	
Can understand traffic lights/signals with difficulty due to color blindness	
Can take longer time to understand	1
Can understand spoken, written, nonverbal messages	0
Persons with illiteracy	0

7 Communication—Expression

Questions	Reference score	Assigned score
Can he/she express a fact in a spoken message?		
Can he/she send a message by writing a letter to a friend?		
Can he/she express a message by gesture?		
Can he/she express a message by electronic devices?		
Answer		
Cannot express by verbal message or written message or gesture or email or by electronic devices	5	
Ability in any one modality rules out a score of 5		
Can express a message only with the assistance of a person or can write a letter only with the assistance of a person	4	
Can express a verbal message with voice amplifier	3	
Can use Braille writer to communicate		
Can use the computer with joystick to reply to an email		
Can express a message with difficulty or increased effort	2	
or		
Can write a letter with difficulty or increased effort		
Can write or express both verbal, nonverbal messages at slow pace	1	
or		
Can use only the left hand for writing if right hand is dominant		
Can use verbal, and non-verbal communication normally	0	
Persons with illiteracy (regarding written message)	0	

Table 20.4 Activity Participation Skill Assessment Scale—Mobility

8 Changing posture

Questions	Reference score	Assigned score
Can he/she lie down?		
Can he/she sit?		
Can he/she stand?		
Can he/she squat?		
Can he/she kneel?		
Can he/she bend down and pick up a coin from the floor?		
Can he/she change positions from lying down, from squatting, kneeling, from sitting or standing, bending?		
Answer		
Cannot change and maintain a posture	5	
Can change position only with personal help	4	
Can change position only with tools or equipment such as overhead sling, orthosis, or mobility aids and maintain position with restraints or perform only some of the activities	3	

(*Continued*)

Table 20.4 (*Continued*) Activity Participation Skill Assessment Scale—Mobility

	Reference score	Assigned score
Can change position with difficulty or increased effort	2	
Can change position but takes more than normal duration	1	
Can perform all activities normally	0	

9 Transfer

Question	Reference score	Assigned score
Can he/she transfer from a bed to a chair?		

Answer		
Cannot transfer	5	
Can transfer only with personal help	4	
Can transfer using equipment such as hoist or overhead sling, orthosis, or mobility aids	3	
Can transfer with difficulty or increased effort	2	
Can transfer but takes more than normal duration	1	
Can transfer normally	0	

10 Lifting and carrying objects

Questions	Reference score	Assigned score
Can he/she lift a suitcase weighing more than 20 kg (6 METs) and put the suitcase in a weighing machine or remove the suitcase from the conveyor belt and put it in the trolley?		
Can he/she carry a briefcase weighing 7 kg in the hands or carry an object in the arms or the shoulder or the hip or the back or the head or can he/she put down an object on the surface or place?		

Answer		
Cannot lift, carry, and put down an object weighing ≥23 kg and cannot carry an object weighing about 7 kg	5	
Cannot lift, carry, and put down an object weighing ≥23 kg including object weighing about 7 kg and requires personal help	4	
Can lift, use trolley to carry an object and can put down an object weighing ≥23 kg and carry an object weighing about 7 kg	3	
Can lift, carry, and put down an object weighing ≥23 kg with difficulty	2	
Can lift, carry with intermittent rest, and put down an object weighing ≥23 kg	1	
Can lift, carry, and put down an object weighing ≥23 kg without difficulty	0	

11 Fine actions of the hand

Questions	Reference score	Assigned score
Can he/she write?		
Can he/she turn the pages of a book?		
Can he/she pick up a coin from the purse and pay it to the cashier?		
Can he/she dial the telephone or press the key or swipe across a touchscreen on the cell phone?		
Can he/she turn the doorknob?		
Can he/she operate the computer keyboard/touchscreen/touchpad?		
Can he/she screw/unscrew a cap of a bottle?		

Answers		
Cannot perform any activity	5	
Can perform with personal help	4	

(*Continued*)

Table 20.4 (*Continued*) Activity Participation Skill Assessment Scale—Mobility

Can perform with assistive devices/remote control for opening doors or windows or operating electronic equipment or perform only some of the activities	3
Can perform with difficulty or increased effort	2
Can perform but takes longer time than normal	1
Can normally perform all the activities	0

12 Gross actions of the hand and arm

Questions	Reference score	Assigned score
Can he/she push the door/pull the door?		
Can he/she reach across the table for a book?		
Can he/she throw a ball/catch a ball?		

Answers	Reference score	Assigned score
Cannot perform any activity	5	
Can perform with personal help for opening doors or windows	4	
Can perform with remote control for opening doors or windows or perform only some of the activities	3	
Can perform with difficulty or increased effort	2	
Can perform but takes longer time than normal	1	
Can normally perform all the activities	0	

13 Walking

Questions	Reference score	Assigned score
Can he/she walk inside the house/office?		
Can he/she walk outside the house on different terrains or uneven surfaces?		
Can he/she walk long distance at his/her own pace continuously in open space/treadmill for about 30 minutes?		
Can he/she walk around the marketplace?		
Can he/she walk through traffic?		

Answers	Reference score	Assigned score
Cannot walk	5	
Can walk with personal assistance	4	
Can walk with cane/crutch	3	
Can walk with difficulty or increased effort or may fall	2	
Can walk long distance but takes longer time than normal	1	
Can walk long distance	0	

14 Mobility with wheelchair/walker

Questions	Reference score	Assigned score
Can he/she move inside the house in a wheelchair?		
Can he/she move on the street in a wheelchair?		
Can he/she move inside the house with walker?		
Can he/she move on the street with walker?		

Answers	Reference score	Assigned score
Cannot ambulate in a wheelchair and move only by stretcher	5	
Can ambulate in a wheelchair propelled by the caregiver	4	
Can ambulate in a motorized wheelchair	3	
Can propel the wheelchair/walker with difficulty or with increased effort for indoor mobility	2	

(Continued)

Table 20.4 (*Continued*) Activity Participation Skill Assessment Scale—Mobility

Can propel wheelchair/walk with walker indoor without difficulty but cannot move with walker/wheelchair in the street	1
Can ambulate in the street in a wheelchair/walker by himself/herself without difficulty	0

15 Mobility in and around

Questions	Reference score	Assigned score
Can he/she climb in a mountainous terrain/slope to reach his/her house or workplace?		
Can he/she climb the stairs?		
Can he/she run?		
Can he/she jog?		
Can he/she jump?		
Can he/she swim?		

Answers		
Cannot perform any activity	5	
or		
Can swim but restricted due to seizures		
Can perform with assistance from a person, e.g., climbing	4	
Can perform with mobility aids (e.g., crutches, walking cane)/equipment or perform only some of the activities	3	
Can perform with difficulty or increased effort	2	
Can perform independently but with deviation (e.g., run with abnormal pattern) or perform independently at a slow pace	1	
Can perform all activities normally	0	

16 Mobility using transportation

Questions	Reference score	Assigned score
Can he/she travel in a bus?		
Can he/she travel in a taxi?		
Can he/she travel on a train?		
Can he/she travel in a boat?		
Can he/she travel in an aircraft?		

Answers		
Cannot travel in any transport independently	5	
Can travel only with personal assistance	4	
Can travel in vehicles with the facility to lie and sleep, e.g., train/air	3	
Can travel with difficulty because of difficult to sit for a long time	2	
Can travel but takes longer time to get in and get out of the vehicle	1	
Can travel normally using a bus/taxi/train/boat/aircraft	0	

17 Driving

Questions	Reference score	Assigned score
Can he/she drive a car?		
Can he/she bicycle?		
Can he/she drive a motorbike?		
Can he/she row a boat?		
Can he/she drive a motorboat?		
Can he/she drive a horse-drawn cart/bullock cart?		

(*Continued*)

Table 20.4 (*Continued*) Activity Participation Skill Assessment Scale—Mobility

Answer

Cannot drive any vehicle	5
or	
Can drive but restriction due to seizures	
Can drive only in the presence of caregiver for want of moral support as well as to assist him/her to get in/out of the vehicle	4
Can drive a car after modification with hand control	3
Can drive a car only for less than 30 minutes because of difficulty in sitting	2
or	
Can drive with difficulty or increased effort to bicycle/row a boat	
Can bicycle or drive slowly	1
Can normally drive—bicycling fast/driving a car/driving a boat/driving a vehicle powered by animals such as horse-drawn cart or bullock cart	0
Not applicable	0
(*Applicable only to those who have already been trained to drive a vehicle and to use them*)	

Table 20.5 Activity Participation Skill Assessment Scale—Self-care

18 Washing

Questions	Reference score	Assigned score
Can he/she take a bath/shower using soap?		
Can he/she dry the body after bath/shower?		

Answer

	Reference score	
Cannot take a bath, and dry the body	5	
Cannot take a bath, and dry the body without personal assistance	4	
or		
Can take a bath independently but requires supervision due to seizures		
Can take a bath with supportive or safety devices such as raised shower, stool, and grab bar, and dry the body	3	
Can take a bath, and dry the body with difficulty or increased effort	2	
Can take a bath, and dry the body but takes more time than normal	1	
Can perform washing, and drying body normally	0	

19 Taking care of body parts

Questions	Reference score	Assigned score
Can he/she brush the teeth?		
Can he/she comb the hair?		
Can he/she trim the nail?		
Can he/she moisturize the skin?		

Answer

	Reference score	
Cannot brush the teeth, comb the hair, and trim the nail	5	
Cannot brush the teeth, comb the hair, and trim the nail without personal assistance	4	
Can brush the teeth, comb the hair, and trim the nail with self-help assistive devices or perform only some of the activities	3	
Can brush the teeth, comb the hair, and trim the nail with difficulty or increased effort or brush the teeth, comb the hair, and trim the nail with unaccustomed hand	2	

(*Continued*)

Table 20.5 (*Continued*) Activity Participation Skill Assessment Scale—Self-care

	Reference score	Assigned score
Can brush the teeth, comb the hair, and trim the nail but takes more time than normal	1	
Can caring for the body parts normally	0	

20 Toileting

Questions	Reference score	Assigned score
Can he/she adjust clothes and position before and after urination and cleaning after urination?		
Can he/she adjust clothes and position before and after defecation and cleaning after defecation?		
Can he/she adjust clothes and position, and clean to maintain hygiene during menstruation?		

Answer		
Cannot carry out toileting by himself/herself	5	
Cannot carry out toileting and needing personal assistance or nursing assistance to put an indwelling catheter or safely perform intermittent-catheterization or apply condom or clean and change diapers	4	
Can carry out toileting with raised toilet sheet, toilet frame and grab bar	3	
Can toilet with increased effort or with difficulty or adapt unaccustomed hand for cleaning	2	
Can carry out toileting but take more time than normal duration	1	
Can toilet normally	0	

21 Dressing

Questions	Reference score	Assigned score
Can he/she choose proper clothes as per the dress codes and climatic conditions?		
Can he/she put on/take off socks, stockings, and footwear?		

Answer		
Cannot dress	5	
Can carry out dressing with personal assistance	4	
Can dress with assistive devices/modified garments with Velcro tabs instead of buttons or perform only some of the activities, e.g., can dress but cannot put on or take of footwears or carry out either upper or lower body dressing	3	
Can carry out dressing with increased effort	2	
Can carry out dressing but take more time than normal duration	1	
Can carry out dressing normally	0	

22 Eating and drinking

Questions	Reference score	Assigned score
Can he/she perform the act of eating food and drinking?		

Answers		
Cannot perform the act of eating and drinking	5	
Can eat and drink only with personal help	4	
Can use only straw, e.g., microstomia following burns or adopt safe posture of the neck for safe drinking and eating or use assistive devices or perform only either drinking or eating	3	
Can eat and drink with difficulty or increased effort or adopt an unaccustomed hand	2	
Can eat/drink but take more time than normal duration	1	
Can eat/drink normally	0	

(*Continued*)

Table 20.5 (*Continued*) Activity Participation Skill Assessment Scale—Self-care

23 Looking after one's health

Questions	Reference score	Assigned score
Can he/she eat a nutritious diet, perform an appropriate physical activity, received immunizations, avoid drug, and abstain from unsafe sexual practice (AIDS)?		
Can he/she recognize an illness/injury, seek medical advice, and adhere to medical management?		

Answer		
Cannot understand to keep his/her body and mind in good health	5	
Can keep his/her body and mind in good health only with personal assistance	4	
Can take care of his/her health only during illness	3	
Can take intermittent care to keep his/her body and mind in good health after counseling	2	
Can take adequate care to maintain his/her body and mind in good health after counseling	1	
Can take proper care to maintain his/her body and mind in good health without counseling	0	

Table 20.6 Activity Participation Skill Assessment Scale—Household activities

24 Purchasing goods and services

Questions	Reference score	Assigned score
Can he/she perform shopping and gather daily needs such as cereals, crockery, vegetables, fruits, clothes, and cleaning material by verifying quality and price?		

Answers		
Cannot perform shopping and gather daily needs by himself/herself	5	
Can perform it with personal help	4	
Can perform only some of the activities	3	
Can perform with difficulty or increased effort	2	
Can perform at slow pace and taking more time than normal	1	
Can perform normally	0	

25 Preparing food

Question	Reference score	Assigned score
Can he/she select ingredients, arrange cooking utensils, cook, and serve food?		

Answers		
Cannot prepare food	5	
Can prepare food with personal assistance	4	
Can prepare food if provided with ingredients or perform only some of the activities	3	
Can plan, prepare, and serve with difficulty or increased effort	2	
Can plan, prepare, serve at slow pace, and taking more time than normal duration	1	
Can normally perform	0	
Not applicable	0	
(*Applicable only to those who have experience in cooking*)		

(*Continued*)

Table 20.6 (*Continued*) Activity Participation Skill Assessment Scale—Household activities

26 Cleaning the house and using household appliances

Questions	Reference score	Assigned score
Can he/she clean cooking and dining area and utensil?		
Can he/she clean living area?		
Can he/she wash, dry and iron clothes and garments?		
Can he/she polish footwear?		
Can he/she use household appliances such as washing machine, dryers, irons, vacuum cleaners, and dishwashers?		
Applicable only to those who have already experienced to do the above activities		

Answer		
Cannot perform any activity	5	
Can perform it with personal help	4	
Can perform only some of the activities	3	
Can perform with difficulty or increased effort	2	
Can perform at slow pace and take more time than normal duration	1	
Can perform it normally	0	

Table 20.7 Activity Participation Skill Assessment Scale—Interpersonal skill

27 Social interaction

Questions	Reference score	Assigned score
Can he/she create and maintain mutual esteem relationship with friends?		
Can he/she create an informal relationship with neighbors and acquaintances?		
Can he/she maintain an informal relationship with colleagues?		
(*In comparison to pre-morbid levels of interactions*)		

Answer		
Cannot create and maintain appropriate relationship with friends, neighbors, acquaintances, and peer because of the unsociable attitude following disability	5	
Cannot create and maintain appropriate relationship with friends, neighbors, acquaintances, and peer due to fear of neglect and inhibition	4	
Can sustain limited interaction with friends only after counseling	3	
Can interact with neighbors, acquaintances, and peer after initial hesitation	2	
Can sustain interaction with neighbors, acquaintances, and peer at a slow pace	1	
Can create and maintain always normal relationship with friends, neighbors, acquaintances, and peer	0	

28 Interaction with family

Questions	Reference score	Assigned score
Can he/she maintain a parent-child relationship and provides physical, intellectual, emotional nurture?		
Can he/she create and sustain child-parent relationship such as obeying his/her parents and taking care of his/her elderly parents?		
Can he/she maintain a brotherly or sisterly relationship with his or her siblings?		
Can he/she create and sustain an optimum relationship with members of the extended family such as cousins, aunts, uncles, and grandparents?		
(*In comparison to pre-morbid levels of interactions*)		

(*Continued*)

Table 20.7 (*Continued*) Activity Participation Skill Assessment Scale—Interpersonal skill

Answer	
Cannot create and maintain specified role	5
Cannot accomplish the role even after guidance by the caregiver	4
Can accept love and affection, and support from family members on guidance and cannot reciprocate	3
Can attempt to perform the role of parent/sibling/child, and exhibit limited interpersonal adjustment with on and off arguments	2
Can perform the role of parent/sibling/child at a slow pace, and maintain fair interpersonal adjustment with occasional tension	1
Can perform the role of parent/sibling/child normally and retain good interpersonal adjustment	0

29 Intimate interaction

Questions	**Reference score**	**Assigned score**
Can he/she maintain a sexual relationship with a spouse or another partner? *(In comparison to pre-morbid levels of intimacy)*		
Cannot participate in sexual life	5	
Can participate passively in sexual life	4	
Can participate in sexual life but clumsy or qualitatively inadequate and cannot satisfy his/her partner	3	
Can participate in sexual life with excessive effort and cannot completely satisfy his/her partner	2	
Can satisfy his/her partner in sexual life	1	
Can maintain normal sexual relationship (Happy as both a pleasure-receiver and pleasure-giver to the partner)	0	

Table 20.8 Activity Participation Skill Assessment Scale—Education and employment

30 Education

Questions	**Reference score**	**Assigned score**
Can he/she pursue school education or higher education?		

Answer	
Cannot pursue education	5
Can learn by peer support and mentoring	4
Can study only in school for special needs or learn only with Braille or learn sign language or learn by "Augmentative and Alternative Communication (AAC)"	3
Can learn with difficulty or increased effort	2
Can learn slowly	1
Can pursue education normally	0
Not applicable, e.g., not undergone education	0

31 Employment

Questions	**Reference score**	**Assigned score**
Can he/she perform sedentary work?		

1. The activity involves sitting most of the time, walking, and standing for the minimum period.
2. Activity is requiring a maximum force of 10 pounds to lift, carry, push, pull, or move objects, including the human body*.

(Continued)

Table 20.8 (*Continued*) Activity Participation Skill Assessment Scale—Education and employment

Can he/she perform light work?

1. Light work requires exerting a force of 10–20 pounds to move objects most of the time.
2. Sitting, standing, and walking most of the time
3. The activity involves pulling and pushing with hand/leg control*.

   Can he/she perform medium work?

   Activity is requiring a force of 10–25 pounds to move objects most of the time*.

   Can he/she perform heavy work?

   Activity is requiring a force of 25–50 pounds to move objects most of the time*.

   Can he/she perform very heavy work?

   Activity is requiring a force of more than 50 pounds to move objects most of the time*.

   (*Extracted from Dictionary of Occupational Titles provided by the United States Department of Labor, www.occupationalinfo.org)

Answer

Cannot pursue any employment	5
Can perform only sheltered employment	4
Can return to alternate employment with less strenuous work with less salary	3
Can obtain full-time new employment or previous full-time employment and perform the work requiring increased effort	2
or	
Cannot work at height or work involving fire or work involving unguarded machinery because of restriction due to seizures	
Can obtain new employment with less salary or return to original/alternate employment but with reduced working hours	1
Can return to original employment or better full-time employment	0
Not applicable, e.g., after retirement	0
Housewife (refer household activities vide supra)	
(In comparison to pre-morbid level of occupation)	

32 Economic transactions and management

Questions	Reference score	Assigned score
Can he/she transact money from ATM?		
Can he/she perform bank transaction? Can he/she purchase goods using money/credit cards/debit cards?		
Cannot transact money from ATM/Bank, purchase goods using money/credit cards/debit cards	5	
Cannot transact money from ATM/Bank, purchase goods using money/credit cards/debit cards without personal assistance	4	
Cannot transact money from ATM/Bank, but purchase goods using money only and cannot use credit cards/debit cards	3	
Can transact money from ATM/Bank, use money/credit cards/debit cards for purchasing goods with difficulty or increased effort	2	
Can transact money from ATM/Bank, use money/credit cards/debit cards for purchasing goods but take more time than normal duration	1	
Can transact money from ATM/Bank, use money/debit cards/credit cards for purchasing goods	0	
(In comparison to pre-morbid level of functioning)		

Table 20.9 Activity Participation Skill Assessment Scale Community—Social-civic life

33 Community life

Questions	Reference score	Assigned score
Can he/she participate in local social clubs/social groups?		
Can he/she participate in his/her professional academies or exclusive social groups?		
Can he/she participate in marriage functions, initiation functions, funeral functions?		
Answer		
Cannot participate in any community meetings/ functions	5	
Can participate community meetings/functions assisted by caregiver	4	
Can participate community meetings/functions only with mobility aids or assistive devices	3	
Can participate community meetings/functions only with difficulty or increased effort	2	
Can participate community meetings/functions less frequently	1	
Can normally participate in informal and formal community meetings/functions	0	

(In comparison to pre-morbid level of participation in community)

34 Recreation

Questions	Reference score	Assigned score
Can he/she participate in games/sports?		
Can he/she attend fine arts or cultural events such as cinema, museum, and musical shows?		
Can he/she dance?		
Can he/she participate in hobbies?		
Can he/she able to visit friends, relatives or meeting informally in public places?		
Answer		
Cannot participate or attend leisure and recreational activity	5	
Can participate or attend recreational and leisure activity only with the assistance of trainer/caregiver	4	
Can participate or attend recreational and leisure activity only with mobility aids/ assistive devices if facility for wheelchair accessibility exists	3	
Can participate or attend recreational and leisure activity only with increased effort	2	
Can participate or attend recreational and leisure activity at slow pace	1	
Can participate or attend recreational and leisure activity normally	0	

(In comparison to pre-morbid level of functioning)

35 Religious functions and activities

Questions	Reference score	Assigned score
Can he/she participate in religious ceremonies in church/mosque/temple?		
Can he/she participate in religious or spiritual activities in church/mosque/ temple/spiritual contemplation?		
Answer		
Cannot participate in religious ceremonies/activities	5	
Can participate in religious activities/perform ceremonies only with the help of caregiver	4	

(Continued)

Table 20.9 (*Continued*) Activity Participation Skill Assessment Scale Community—Social-civic life

Can participate in religious activities/perform ceremonies with mobility aids or assistive devices	3	
Can participate in religious activities/perform religious ceremonies only in alternate way or personally non-gratifying manner	2	
Can participate religious activities/perform ceremonies at a slow pace (or) infrequently	1	
Can participate normally	0	
(*In comparison to pre-morbid levels*)		

36 Activity in political system and citizenship

Questions	Reference score	Assigned score
Can he/she participate in political and governmental life as a citizen? Can he/she franchise vote?		

Answer

Cannot participate in political/governmental life and franchise vote	5	
Can participate in political/governmental life and franchise vote with the help of a caregiver. Independent decision-making may not be possible	4	
Can participate in political/governmental life and franchise vote with mobility aids and assistive devices	3	
Can participate in political/governmental life with increased effort and franchise vote. Independent and yet indecisive	2	
Can participate partially in political/governmental life and franchise vote in an alternate way but independent, decisive, and yet, clumsy in decision-making	1	
Can normally participate in political/governmental life and franchise vote	0	

REFERENCE

1. *International Classification of Functioning, Disability and Health.* Geneva, Switzerland: World Health Organization; 2001. p. 213.

21

Environmental factors

21.1 ENVIRONMENTAL FACTORS

Environmental factors refer to factors existing in a person's immediate living surroundings. It comprises physical factors, namely built infrastructure (living places and workplaces) and goods for preserving health (water, food, air, etc.). Physical factors also include goods used in personal life (e.g., clothes, furniture, communication devices), transporting system used for commuting, systems required for education, employment, and health services. The social factors (environment) include relationships, such as immediate family, extended family, peers, employers, community participation and social institutions for cultural activities, such as spiritual and religious practices. The attitudinal environment includes the attitude of the individual or society exerting a positive influence and negative influence over his/her functioning, for example, motivation or discrimination (1–3). Thus, an intricate relationship exists between the health condition of the person and the environmental and personal factors, both of which tend to modify the severity of the disability.

Artificial limbs, appliances, crutches, wheelchairs, and walking canes hinder the mobility of a person due to a lack of architectural modifications in the environment. Mobility barriers at home and in the community, assistive technology facilitators for communication, mobility and transportation, and social support influence participation in rehabilitation programs. Social support enhances the reintegration of the person into the home and society (4).

Architectural design for a barrier-free environment alleviates or eliminates limitation of activity and enhances the participation of the person with a disability in his/her social life. The work table, reading table, dining table, sinks in the kitchen and restroom with a space of 700 mm height and width of 850 mm and depth of 600 mm for knee clearance, and a public dealing counter with a 900 mm high with clear space underneath facilitate wheelchair accessibility. Similarly slope of 1:20 in the ramp and 1:12 in the curb, and <1:48 in bus stop boarding and alighting areas and rail platforms facilitate free accessibility and mobility

in a wheelchair. Elevators with a minimum dimension of 1000 × 1300 mm and a minimum door opening of 800 mm and a restroom with a space of 1500 mm diameter facilitate wheelchair access and maneuverability. A provision for seats with detachable or flip-up armrests located on a level floor area at the end of the row in a conference hall, movie theatre, and auditorium accommodate persons in a wheelchair. The design of cantilevered tables or tables without a central pedestal accommodates wheelchair users in restaurants. Tactile guide strips of 600 mm width on the ramp, tactile markings on the handrails, and tactile surfaces with line-type blocks indicating the correct path, and dot-type blocks in the pathway indicating areas of hazards assist people with visual impairment. Similarly tactile or rubber tile of 900 × 900 mm in the pedestrian crossing and textured tactile strips separating a pathway from a vehicular area assist the person with visual impairment. The audio signals in the starting point of a pedestrian crossing, alarm signals in the exit door during an emergency situation, and Braille or elevated, or embossed, text in a bold, contrasting type in the signage and elevator control panel assists the person with visual impairment during their mobility. An assistive listening system with transmitter, receiver, and coupling devices transmit audio signals to a hearing aid by eliminating or decreasing background noise by induction loop, radio frequency, infrared system, or direct-wired equipment. The assistive listening system provides better perception in public telephones and conference halls. Visual signals in a pedestrian crossing, flashlight in the elevator, emergency flashlight in exit door during emergency situations assist the person with hearing impairment (5–7).

Attitude toward disability refers to a cognitive process and behavioral process involving judgment and reactions, either favorable or unfavorable, toward a person with disability (8). The opinion formed by the person may impose inferiority status upon the person with disability. It may be due to ignorance, fear, misunderstanding, and hate. They may not appreciate and experience the true innate potential of the person with a disability.

21.2 "ENVIRONMENTAL FACTORS MEASUREMENT SCALE"

The "Environmental Factors Measurement Scale" comprises hundreds of variables under the domains of assistive technology services, architectural design with facilitators and barriers, social security and health services, and the attitudinal environment (Tables 21.1 through 21.14).

Integrated Evaluation of Disability quantifies the severity of environmental barriers using a severity scale. The severity scale grades the disability into 0 or 0%–4% for no disability, 1 or 5%–24% for mild disability, and 2 or 25%–49% for moderate disability. Furthermore, it grades the disability into 3 or 50%–74% for severe disability, 4 or 75%–94% for profound disability, and 5 or 95%–100% for complete disability.

Table 21.1 Environmental Factors Measurement Scale—Assistive technology

No	Assistive technology services	Lack of assistive technology services	Assigned score
	Vital organ impairment		
1	Does a facility exist to avail Continuous Positive Airway Pressure (CPAP) or Bilevel Positive Airway Pressure (BiPAP) devices or phrenic nerve stimulation device to assist respiration in his/her immediate environment?	1	
2	Does a facility exist to undergo pacing (placement of Cardiac Pacemaker) in his/her immediate environment?	1	
	Impairment of bladder and bowel		
3	Does a facility exist to avail sacral neuromodulation therapy to control bladder and bowel movement in his/her immediate environment?	1	
	Motor impairment		
4	Does a facility exist to avail artificial limb in his/her immediate environment?	1	
5	Does a facility exist to avail appliances in his/her immediate environment?	1	
6	Does a facility exist to avail transfer equipment, a hoist or other such devices, in his/her immediate environment?	1	
7	Does a facility exist to avail assistive devices, namely walking aids, in his/her immediate environment?	1	
8	Does a facility exist to avail mobility aids, namely manual wheelchair/motorized wheelchair, in his/her immediate environment?	1	
9	Does a facility exist to avail special cars/van/scooters or modified vehicles in his/her immediate environment to commute from one place to another?	1	
10	Does a facility exist to avail "Typing System" to enter, retrieve data in the computer, Robotic Arm, Environmental Control System, "Phone System" to communicate over extended distance?	1	
	Visual impairment		
11	Is there a facility to avail assistive technology services namely "type reader" or Text to Speech (TTS) for converting text to speech using synthesized speech in his/her immediate environment?	1	
12	Is there any facility to avail assistive technology services namely orientation system to locate a geographical location in his/her immediate environment?	1	
13	Is there any facility to avail assistive technology services namely recording system for transcribing and retrieving in his/her immediate environment?	1	
14	Is there any facility to avail assistive technology services namely intraocular lens in his/her immediate environment?	1	
	Hearing impairment		
15	Does a facility exist to avail assistive technology services namely cochlear implants, hearing aids, FM auditory trainers in his/her immediate environment?	1	

(Continued)

Table 21.1 (*Continued*) Environmental Factors Measurement Scale—Assistive technology

No	Assistive technology services	Lack of assistive technology services	Assigned score
16	Does a facility exist to avail assistive technology services, namely, "Alert system" using lights or vibration in his/her immediate environment?	1	
17	Does a facility exist to avail assistive technology services namely telecommunication display devices/text telephones exist in his/her immediate environment? Text telephones transfer coded signals through a telephone network for interactive text-based communication.	1	
18	Does a facility exist to avail assistive technology services, namely "Speech recognition system," in his/her immediate environment? Speech recognition system is a device with a software program to convert words or phrases in a speech into a readable format.	1	
	Impairment of language function		
19	Is there any facility to avail augmentative alternative communication technology such as alphabet or picture symbol boards, a computer-based system for synthesis of speech in his/her immediate environment?	1	
	Assistive technology for daily living		
20	Does a facility exist for environmental control systems, such as electronic devices to operate an air conditioner, television, computers, and other appliances, exist in his/her home/workplace?	1	

Table 21.2 Environmental Factors Measurement Scale—Architectural design—Motor impairment: Signage, ramps, and doors

No	Signage, ramps, and doors	Lack of architectural facilitators	Assigned score
21	Is there signage visible, simple without glare even at night in the entrance and inside building?	1	
22	Is an international symbol of accessibility displayed inside and outside the building?	1	
23	Does ramp with sufficient width, the hard and non-slippery surface including tactile marking strips, a slope with a gradient of 1:20, landing at the place of change of direction and the bottom and top of a ramp, and handrails on both sides of the entire length of ramp exist?	1	
24	Does ramp with a maximum width of 1000 mm and slip-resistant surface for wheelchair mobility exist?	1	
25	Do the exterior and interior door have adequate width, and level thresholds in the doorway for wheelchair access exist?	1	
26	Do power assisted doors with increased opening interval or sliding doors or swinging doors with outward opening hinges with a mechanism for effortless opening, and lever style door handle exist?	1	
27	Do low set windows exist to enable a person in a wheelchair to open and close the window without effort?	1	
28	Do low set electrical fixtures exist to enable a person in a wheelchair for operating controls with minimum force exist?	1	

Based on the "Accessibility for the Disabled: A Design Manual for a Barrier-Free Environment, United Nations 2003–2004."

Table 21.3 Environmental Factors Measurement Scale—Architectural design—Motor impairment: Steps, stairs, and corridors

No	Steps, stairs, and corridors	Lack of architectural facilitators	Assigned score
29	Do steps and stairs with adequate width for one-way traffic or two-way traffic exist? Do slip resistant surface, uniform risers and tread without nosing for indoor stairs, intermediate landing for the difference in the level of more than 2.5 m, handrails on both sides of the stairs, landing extending beyond the stairs at bottom and top of the stairs, tactile strip with contrasting color exist?	1	
30	Do round handrails fix firmly to the wall/supporting structure at a suitable height above the floor level of the step and ramp with adequate space between the wall and handrail? A tactile strip of 900 mm with contrasting color incorporated at the bottom and top edge of the handrails?	1	
31	Do public corridors with an unobstructed width allowing two wheelchairs and full maneuvering of a wheelchair, and slip resistant floor with drinking fountains, public telephone housed in a recess outside the pathway exist?	1	

Based on the "Accessibility for the Disabled: A Design Manual for a Barrier-Free Environment, United Nations 2003–2004."

Table 21.4 Environmental Factors Measurement Scale—Architectural design—Motor impairment: Elevators

No	Elevators	Lack of architectural facilitators	Assigned score
32	Do the elevators with adequate dimension, sufficient door opening for wheelchair access and maneuver, hand rails on three sides, slip resistant floor surface, maximum stop precision, control panel at an accessible height with numerals embossed in the control buttons for tactile selection of floors exist?	1	
33	Do the call buttons located at an accessible height from the floor, provision for minimum door opening interval of 5 seconds, and audio signal and visual display to forecast arrival of the elevator for each floor exist?	1	
34	Do the entrance and exit of the escalators have two flat steps and steps of the escalator identifiable by yellow guide strip along the sides and back of the steps?	1	

Based on the "Accessibility for the Disabled: A Design Manual for a Barrier-Free Environment, United Nations 2003–2004."

Table 21.5 Environmental Factors Measurement Scale—Architectural design—Motor impairment: Kitchen

No	Kitchen	Lack of architectural facilitators	Assigned score
35	Do the "U"-shaped kitchen have an adequate work area, wide door with lever type handle for wheelchair access and maneuver?	1	
36	Do the countertop or height adjustable counter, sinks with clear space underneath for knee clearance, single lever faucet, sliding drawers on either side of the sink, detachable cabinetry under the kitchen work surface, kitchen wall cabinet either power adjusted cabinets or pull-down shelves exist? Do insulation of underside of the cooktop to prevent burns, electric burner or oven with controls fixed on the front panel, the minimum operating force of the controls for the appliances, or touchpad or tactile controls with raised buttons and low set electrical fixtures exist?	1	
37	Do dishwasher and bottom-drawer freezer type refrigerator with a clear floor area from the center of the kitchen exist?	1	
	Dining, reading, and working surfaces		
38	Does the reading/work/dining table exist with clear space underneath for knee clearance for wheelchair accessibility?	1	

Based on the "Accessibility for the Disabled: A Design Manual for a Barrier-Free Environment, United Nations 2003–2004."

Table 21.6 Environmental Factors Measurement Scale—Architectural design—Motor impairment: Rest room

No	Rest room	Lack of architectural facilitators	Assigned score
39	Does the restroom have sufficient space for maneuvering wheelchair with slip resistant floor, self-closing pivoted doors open outward? Is the Toilet seat at accessible height from the floor with adequate space from the midline of the toilet seat to the adjacent wall? Do grab bar fixed behind the water closet and adjacent walls of the water closet, flush controls either automatic or hand operating with minimum effort fixed on the open side of the water closet and toilet paper dispenser mounted at an accessible height above the floor?	1	
40	Does the washbasin with its top edge at an accessible height from the floor and lever type handle for faucets exist?	1	
41	Does the bathtub with specified dimension exist with provision for permanent bathtub seat or a detachable in-tub seat at the head end of the tub and with two grab bars on the back wall above the brim of the bathtub and one at the head end and another at the control end of the bathtub? Do shower stalls with adequate dimension with shower seat, shower head with a long hose, and horizontal grab bar in the back and side walls away from the entrance?	1	
42	Does full-length urinal or urinal with the protruding lip at the optimum height from the floor with sufficient space on either side, urine shield, grab bars and automatic or hand-operated flush control exist?	1	
43	Does hot water pipes have insulation?	1	

Based on the "Accessibility for the Disabled: A Design Manual for a Barrier-Free Environment, United Nations 2003–2004."

Table 21.7 Environmental Factors Measurement Scale—Architectural design—Motor impairment: Public utility services

No	Public utility services	Lack of architectural facilitators	Assigned score
44	Does drinking water fountain fixed at the optimum height from the floor and control with effortless operation exist?	1	
45	Does a public dealing counters exist at optimum height with clear underneath space and depth for wheelchair accessibility?	1	
46	Do accessible open book stacks, equipment, and other facilities in the library for wheelchair users, and a separate room for assistance for reading exist?	1	
47	Is there a provision of seats with detachable or flip-up armrests located in a level floor area at the end of the row in a conference hall, movie theatre, sports auditorium?	1	
48	Does thermostat exist to protect persons with impaired thermoregulation?	1	
49	Do minimum slope of the boarding and alighting areas in the bus stop, and rail platform exist for wheelchair access, and maneuver, provision for accessible seating and other facilities exist in the bus, aircraft, and train as well as in bus/train stations and air terminals?	1	
50	Does cantilevered tables or tables without central pedestal exist in restaurants, and a minimum of one room with restroom, etc., designed for wheelchair users exist on the ground floor of the hotel?	1	
51	Does the public telephone booth with folding seats for wheelchair accessibility, low set telephones with elevated touch buttons, coin slot fixed at optimum height exist?	1	
52	Does the letter slot in the mailbox exist at optimum height?	1	
53	Does provision of fire alarm systems in public use areas, employee work areas, lodging and residential facilities with audible alarm signals exist to indicate emergency situations?	1	

Based on the "Accessibility for the Disabled: A Design Manual for a Barrier-Free Environment, United Nations 2003–2004."

Table 21.8 Environmental Factors Measurement Scale—Architectural design—Motor impairment: Foot path

No	Foot path	Lack of architectural facilitators	Assigned score
54	Whether footpath with slip resistant even surface and beveled edges with sufficient width, optimum slope across a path, and curb ramp with adequate width, slip resistant surface and slope to bridge the difference in level between road and pathway at building entrance, pedestrian crossing, parking space and drop-off areas exist?	1	
55	Whether street furniture such as benches, mailboxes, telephone booths, public toilets, newspaper kiosks, shop awnings, advertising signs exist outside the path of travel without any obstruction?		
56	Whether resting areas along the footpath namely bench with the backrest of optimum dimension and sufficient adjoining space to accommodate wheelchair exist?		
57	Whether pedestrian crossing has a slip-resistant surface with provision for traffic control signals, pedestrian push button system, and allowing sufficient time to cross the road?	1	

Based on the "Accessibility for the Disabled: A Design Manual for a Barrier-Free Environment, United Nations 2003–2004."

Table 21.9 Environmental Factors Measurement Scale—Architectural design—Motor impairment: Parking area

No	Parking area	Lack of architectural facilitators	Assigned score
58	Whether parking space of adequate width including an access aisle between two ordinary parking areas, minimum height clearance for indoor parking, near accessible elevator or exit, and near the entrance with guiding signs and international symbol toward parking area exist?	1	
59	Whether textured tactile marking strip exist to separate the pathway from vehicular area to caution transition zone during crossing?	1	
60	Whether drop-off area of sufficient width including aisle at bus stops exists nearby from the entrance to pick up or drop off persons with impairment of function as well as to load and upload luggage?	1	

Based on the "Accessibility for the Disabled: A Design Manual for a Barrier-Free Environment, United Nations 2003–2004."

Table 21.10 Environmental Factors Measurement Scale—Architectural design—Visual impairment: Signage, door, ramp, stairs, elevator

No	Signage, door, ramp, stairs, elevator	Lack of architectural facilitators	Assigned score
61	Whether any signage in Braille or embossed or text with bold color contrasted letter exist in the entrance of the building?	1	
62	Whether there is the provision of international symbols of accessibility in a contrasting color?	1	
63	Whether the entrance door painted with contrasting color to assist persons with low vision?	1	
64	Whether tactile markings on the handrails of exit and around the knob of the exit door exist?	1	
65	Whether ramp exist with slip-resistant surface and tactile marking strips?	1	
66	Whether tactile marking strip of specified width extending over the whole stairs along with tactile strip incorporated at the bottom and top edge of the handrails exist?	1	
67	Whether the lifts/elevator has a control panel with the button of adequate diameter, and numerals embossed in the control buttons for tactile selection of floors?	1	
68	Whether the provision of audio signals namely bell exist to indicate the arrival of the elevator for each floor?	1	
69	Whether door frame of the elevator/lift painted with a contrasting color to assist persons with low vision?	1	

Based on the "Accessibility for the Disabled: A Design Manual for a Barrier-Free Environment, United Nations 2003–2004."

Table 21.11 Environmental Factors Measurement Scale—Architectural design—Visual impairment: Pathway and public utility services

No	Pathway, and public utility services	Lack of architectural facilitators	Assigned score
70	Whether a pathway with guide strip with contrasting color exist?	1	
71	Whether tactile surfaces with line-type blocks indicating the correct path, dot-type blocks exist to indicate hazards or rubber tiles with both tactile and acoustic guidance in the pathway exist?	1	
72	Whether tactile marking strips or signage in bright color or alarm signals exist around obstruction?	1	
73	Whether pedestrian guide strip toward traffic light pole with push button, tactile tile, or rubber tile incorporated in the pedestrian crossing, provision of audio signals at the beginning of the pedestrian crossing, and provision of sufficient time for crossing the road exist?	1	
74	Whether tactile marking strips exist in places of change of route or direction sign in bright and contrasting color letters to orient and reach a place of destination?	1	
75	Whether there is provision for alarm signals to identify facilities?	1	
76	Whether there is the provision of a minimum of one push-button type telephone with raised numbers/letters in public telephone booth?	1	
77	Whether text to speech (TTS) synthesis system or assistance for reading exist in a separate room in a library?	1	

Based on the "Accessibility for the Disabled: A Design Manual for a Barrier-Free Environment, United Nations 2003–2004."

Table 21.12 Environmental Factors Measurement Scale—Architectural design—Hearing impairment

No	Signage, elevator, pathway, and public utility services	Lack of architectural facilitators	Assigned score
78	Whether there is provision for signage with contrasting color and bold letter?		
79	Whether there is provision for indication of the arrival of the elevator by flashlight for each floor?		
80	Whether there is provision for flashing of emergency light in the door or elevator?		
81	Whether visual signals exist in pedestrian pathway/crossing?		
82	Whether assistance for reading exist in a separate room in a library?		
83	Whether the public telephone booths exist with a minimum of one telephone with a hearing aid and amplifiers to improve the perception of hearing? (Assistive listening system with transmitter, receiver and coupling devices for transmitting audio signals to hearing aid by eliminating or decreasing background noise for better perception by induction loop, radio frequency, infrared system, or direct-wired equipment in public telephone)		
84	Whether speech recognition system exist in conference hall?		

Based on the "Accessibility for the Disabled: A Design Manual for a Barrier-Free Environment, United Nations 2003–2004."

Table 21.13 Environmental Factors Measurement Scale—Social security and health services, systems, and polices

No	Social security and health services, systems, and policies	Lack of social security services	Assigned score
85	Does disability related pension subsist for the person with disability?	1	
86	Does subsidy exist for assisted technology related equipment/devices?	1	
87	Does priority for admission in educational courses exist for the person with a disability?	1	
88	Does provision for suitable employment exist for the person with a disability?	1	
89	Does tax exemption available to the person with a disability?	1	
90	Does subsistence for the construction of barrier-free house available to the person with a disability?	1	
91	Do health services provide facilities for medical rehabilitation free of cost or by insurance?	1	

Table 21.14 Environmental Factors Measurement Scale—Attitudinal environment

No	Attitude of immediate and extended family members, friends, employers, and society	Attitudinal barriers exist	Assigned score
92	Does the spouse develop divorce attitude toward his/her wife/husband because of his/her disability	1	
93	Do immediate family members exhibit inhibitory attitude to spend time and money toward rehabilitation management because of loss or limitation of productivity of the person with disability to support his/her family	1	
94	Do parents or primary caretakers place the children with disability in alternative care rather than keeping them with their family	1	
95	Do extended family members and friends ignore the person with disability because of disability	1	
96	Is there inhibition of the employers to recruit eligible persons because of underestimation of the potential of the person with disability	1	
97	Whether there is lack of supportive attitude of the employers to provide reasonable accommodation in the workplace for persons with disability	1	
98	Whether the society has a stereotyped attitude that persons with disability are burden to the society?	1	
99	Whether the society has a prejudice that persons with disability are defective and deviant and cannot participate in and contribute to society? Does the society underestimate that the persons with disability have abilities at a low ebb, and cannot perform the task like a person without a disability?	1	
100	Whether the society has a superstitious belief that persons with disability are associated with evil spirit or suffering from disability due to sin and hence attach stigma?	1	

REFERENCES

1. *International Classification of Functioning, Disability and Health.* Geneva, Switzerland: World Health Organization; 2001. p. 213.

2. *International Classification of Functioning, Disability and Health.* Geneva, Switzerland: World Health Organization; 2001. p. 171.

3. Barnett E, Casper M. A definition of "social environment". *Am J Public Health.* 2001;91(3):465.

4. *Impact Assessment Guidelines.* In: European Commission, editor. European Commission; 2009. p. 35.

5. United Nations. *Accessibility for the Disabled - A Design Manual for Barrier Free Environment.* In: Department of Economic and Social Affairs DfSPaD, editor. 2003–2004.

6. *ADA and ABA Accessibility Guidelines for Buildings and Facilities.* Federal Register; 2004 and 2005.

7. *Guidelines and Space Standard for Barrier Free Built Environment for Disabled and Elderly Persons.* In: Department CPW, editor. Ministry of Urban Affairs & Employment, India; 1998.

8. Zheng Q, Tian Q, Hao C, Gu J, Tao J, Liang Z et al. Comparison of attitudes toward disability and people with disability among caregivers, the public, and people with disability: Findings from a cross-sectional survey. *BMC Public Health.* 2016;16(1):1024.

Personal factors

22.1 PERSONAL FACTORS AND "PERSONAL FACTORS MEASUREMENT SCALE"

Typical personal factors include age, gender, race, education, habits, behavior, and working and earning capacity. *Integrated Evaluation of Disability* focuses mainly on the behavior of the person toward their disability and working and earning capacity. The behavior of the person indicates acceptance of their disability and performance of daily activities, participation in educational/vocational pursuits and social life with residual physical abilities, and mental faculty to attain personal and social self-sufficiency. "Personal Factors" comprise six factors for the evaluation of the behavior of the person with a disability and five variables for evaluating working and earning capacity. *Integrated Evaluation of Disability* developed scales for the evaluation of the behavior of the person toward his/her disability, and a methodology for assessing working and earning capacity based on the pre-morbid working and earning capacity and present working and earning capacity (Tables 22.1 through 22.6).

Table 22.1 Personal Factors Measurement Scale—Behavior toward health

1 Question: Behavior of the person with disability toward health	Reference score	Assigned score
Does the person with disability cooperate for feeding himself/herself to maintain nutrition? Does the person with disability cooperate for initial treatment and further rehabilitation programs?		
Answer:		
The person with disability does not accept his/her disability, develops aggressive behavior and suicidal tendency, and rejects food, initial treatment, and further rehabilitation programs	5	
The person with disability develops depression and does not cooperate for feeding to maintain nutrition and rehabilitation program to regain function	4	
The person with disability does not cooperate in feeding to maintain nutrition and rehabilitation program to regain function	3	
The person with disability cooperates partially for eating and drinking and undergo rehabilitation management irregularly after counseling	2	
The person with disability cooperates fully for eating and drinking and undergoes rehabilitation programs regularly only after counseling	1	
The person with disability cooperates for eating and drinking and undergoes rehabilitation management even without counseling	0	

Table 22.2 Personal Factors Measurement Scale—Behavior toward self-care

2 Question: Behavior of the person toward self-care	Reference score	Assigned score
Does the person with a disability perform or cooperate for washing and drying whole body/caring body parts in the presence of preserved skills for self-care?		
Does the person with disability care for or cooperate for caring skin, face, teeth, scalp, nails, and genitals in the presence of preserved skills for self-care?		
Does the person with a disability perform or cooperate for toileting in the presence of preserved skills for self-care?		
Does the person with a disability perform or cooperate for dressing in the presence of preserved skills for self-care?		
Answer:		
The person with disability does not cooperate for self-care and exhibits aggressive behavior and suicidal tendency	5	
The person with disability does not cooperate for self-care and exhibits depression	4	
The person with disability does not cooperate for self-care	3	
The person with disability cooperates partially for self-care after counseling	2	
The person with disability cooperates fully for self-care after counseling	1	
The person with disability normally cooperates with all activities relating to self-care	0	

Table 22.3 Personal Factors Measurement Scale—Behavior toward communication

3 Question: Behavior of the person—communication	Reference score	Assigned score
Does the perso n with a disability communicate in the presence of preserved communication skills?		
Answer:		
The person with a disability has preserved communication. He/she does not communicate because of elective mutism and exhibits aggressive behavior and suicidal tendency	5	
The person with a disability has preserved communication and exhibits a paucity of communication. He/she answers only in monosyllables or by gestures	4	
The person with a disability has preserved communication but answers only to questions directed at him/her. There is no spontaneity of communication	3	
The person with a disability has preserved communications and exchanges with limited audiences such as family members and friends only after counseling	2	
The person with a disability had preserved communications and communicates with everyone after counseling	1	
The person with disability normally communicates with everyone even without counseling	0	

Table 22.4 Personal Factors Measurement Scale—Behavior toward education

4	Question: Behavior of the person with disability toward learning Whether the person with a disability accepts learning or resumes education in the presence of preserved mental faculty?	Reference score	Assigned score
	Answer:		
	The person with a disability does not cooperate for continuing education and exhibits aggressive behavior and suicidal tendency	5	
	The person with a disability does not refuse but lacks motivation for continuing to learn	4	
	The person with a disability cooperates for continuing education but only sporadically	3	
	The person with a disability has lack of spontaneity but continues to cooperate in learning	2	
	The person with disability resumes learning/education regularly only after counseling	1	
	The person with disability resumes education without counseling	0	

Table 22.5 Personal Factors Measurement Scale—Behavior toward work and employment

5	Question: Behavior of the person—Work and employment Does the person with a disability accept and resume work or training in the presence of preserved occupational or work skills?	Reference score	Assigned score
	Answer:		
	The person with a disability does not cooperate for continuing his/her work or training and exhibits aggressive behavior and suicidal tendency	5	
	The person with a disability does not refuse but has poor executive skills due to lack of motivation in pursuing his/her occupation	4	
	The person with disability continues to cooperate but is unable to sustain his/her motivation and execution	3	
	The person with a disability can sustain his/her motivation and execution only under supervision. Spontaneous plan and execution are lacking	2	
	The person with a disability has adequate motivation, execution, and spontaneity but only after counseling and under supervision	1	
	The person with a disability accepts and resumes employment even without counseling or supervision	0	

Table 22.6 Personal Factors Measurement Scale—Behavior toward social life

6	Question: Behavior of the person—Social life Is the person with a disability able to maintain normal social relationship?	Reference score	Assigned score
	Answer:		
	The person with a disability exhibits physical and verbally aggressive cum disruptive behavior in social life	5	
	The person with a disability remains withdrawn. Though willing he/she is unable to participate in social life	4	
	The person with a disability attempts to sustain a social life but only with the inner circle of family/known members	3	
	The person with a disability can sustain a social interaction but without any spontaneity and on continued efforts by others and counseling	2	
	The person with a disability maintains spontaneous social relationship with everyone only on positive intervention by others and after counseling	1	
	The person with disability maintains normal social relationship with everyone even without counseling	0	

22.2 "WORKING AND EARNING CAPACITY MEASUREMENT SCALE"

The primary fundamental rights of a person are food, shelter, and education. If the person with a disability is responsible and providing food, shelter, and education to the family members during his/her pre-morbid state, loss of his/her earning capacity due to the disability can serve as one of the determinants to claim compensation and disability benefits.

The vocational potential and earning capacity depends on the following variables:

1. Mental faculty
2. Educational qualification, specialization, and specialized training
3. Pre-morbid vocational status namely permanent/temporary/full-time/part-time employment including career development, work attendance, rapport with colleagues, experience, and skills
4. The personality of the person namely resilient/overcontrolled/under controlled
5. Vocational adjustment and occupational interests, career motivation, capacity for retraining, transferable skills, need for retraining/additional training, and vocational accomplishments and failures
6. The propensity for occupational safety

The Americans with Disabilities Act (ADA) emphasizes aptitude and skill rather than impairment as one of the selection criteria for employment of the person with a disability. The ADA defines some modifications as "reasonable accommodations." "Reasonable accommodation" means a modification or alteration of a job or work environment to allow a qualified or eligible employee to participate in the application process, to do the essential functions of the job, and avail of the benefits. It includes modification of the physical environment of the job to make it accessible for wheelchair, restructuring of the job, reallocating to a vacant job, and modifying the work schedule to suit a person with poor endurance or attend to treatment. It further recommends providing equipment (such as a hearing telephone amplifier for a person with hearing impairment), modifying training material, modifying the policy to conduct oral examination for persons with dyslexia, and a provision of qualified readers or interpreters for a person with visual and hearing impairment (1).

Vocational assessment is based "on the job evaluation" or *Functie Identificatie System* (FIS). FIS is a computer system that analyses the person for a job regarding his/her limitations and capabilities against the demands of a job. Both the methods assess the vocational potential of a person and opportunities for a job as well as his/her limitations for a job. Vocation counseling conveys to the person about his vocational potential and limitations. He/she may require vocational training and may undergo vocational adaptation and reintegration program including accommodation for the person in the workplace before vocational placement. The program selects three potential jobs based on the capabilities toward the requirements or demands of a job. Disability due to loss of income refers to the difference between pre-morbid income and income of the best-paid second job among three best-paid jobs identified by the above methods (2).

Clinical tools for the evaluation of impairment of function and structure, "Activity Participation Skill Assessment Scale," "Personal Factors Measuring Scale," and "Environmental Factors Measurement Scale" are necessary to compute a whole person disability.

The severity of disability determines either total inability to pursue the original employment or option for alternate employment. Furthermore, the residual physical ability, psychological reserve, residual vocational skills, and workplace accommodation may determine vocational output and the potential for earning in the original or alternate employment.

Pre-morbid earning capacity may serve as a reference to calculate the loss of earning capacity.

Persons with a work-related injury may seek secondary gain and may malinger for compensation. Hence, it is mandatory that a vocational evaluator assesses and determines the person's vocational potential and earning capacity to resume initial employment or to choose suitable alternate employment as well as loss of earning with above perspectives in mind (3) (Tables 22.7 through 22.10).

Table 22.7   Working and Earning Capacity Measurement Scale—Pre-morbid employment

Status of employment	Working capacity	Earning capacity	Loss of income
Returns to pre-morbid employment	Works full time with 100% work output	Obtains 100% of pre-morbid level of salary/income	Nil
Returns to pre-morbid employment	Works at reduced working hours/reduced work output	Obtains 90% of pre-morbid level of salary/income	10% of pre-morbid salary/income
		Obtains 80% of pre-morbid level of salary/income	20% of pre-morbid salary/income
		Obtains 70% of pre-morbid level of salary/income	30% of pre-morbid salary/income
		Obtains 60% of pre-morbid level of salary/income	40% of pre-morbid salary/income
		Obtains 50% of pre-morbid level of salary/income	50% of pre-morbid salary/income
		Obtains 40% of pre-morbid level of salary/income	60% of pre-morbid salary/income
		Obtains 30% of pre-morbid level of salary/income	70% of pre-morbid salary/income
		Obtains 20% of pre-morbid level of salary/income	80% of pre-morbid salary/income
		Obtains 10% of pre-morbid level of salary/income	90% of pre-morbid salary/income

Table 22.8   Working and Earning Capacity Measurement Scale—Alternate employment

Status of employment	Working capacity	Earning capacity	Loss of income
Returns to alternate employment	Works full time with 100% work output	Obtains 100% of pre-morbid level of salary/income	Nil
Returns to alternate employment	Works at reduced working hours/ reduced work output	Obtains 90% of pre-morbid level of salary/income	10% of pre-morbid salary/income
		Obtains 80% of pre-morbid level of salary/income	20% of pre-morbid salary/income
		Obtains 70% of pre-morbid level of salary/income	30% of pre-morbid salary/income
		Obtains 60% of pre-morbid level of salary/income	40% of pre-morbid salary/income
		Obtains 50% of pre-morbid level of salary/income	50% of pre-morbid salary/income
		Obtains 40% of pre-morbid level of salary/income	60% of pre-morbid salary/income
		Obtains 30% of pre-morbid level of salary/income	70% of pre-morbid salary/income
		Obtains 20% of pre-morbid level of salary/income	80% of pre-morbid salary/income
		Obtains 10% of pre-morbid level of salary/income	90% of pre-morbid salary/income

Table 22.9 Working and Earning Capacity Measurement Scale—Self-employment

Status of employment	Working capacity	Earning capacity	Loss of income
Performs self-employment	Performs full-time work with 100% work output	Obtains 100% of pre-morbid level of salary/income	Nil
	Works at reduced working hours/ reduced work output	Obtains 90% of pre-morbid level of salary/income	10% of pre-morbid salary/income
		Obtains 80% of pre-morbid level of salary/income	20% of pre-morbid salary/income
		Obtains 70% of pre-morbid level of salary/income	30% of pre-morbid salary/income
		Obtains 60% of pre-morbid level of salary/income	40% of pre-morbid salary/income
		Obtains 50% of pre-morbid level of salary/income	50% of pre-morbid salary/income
		Obtains 40% of pre-morbid level of salary/income	60% of pre-morbid salary/income
		Obtains 30% of pre-morbid level of salary/income	70% of pre-morbid salary/income
		Obtains 20% of pre-morbid level of salary/income	80% of pre-morbid salary/income
		Obtains 10% of pre-morbid level of salary/income	90% of pre-morbid salary/income

Table 22.10 Working and Earning Capacity Measurement Scale—Sheltered employment

Status of employment	Working capacity	Earning capacity	Loss of income
Performs sheltered employment	Performs full-time work with 100% output	Obtains 100% of pre-morbid level of salary/income	Nil
	Works at reduced working hours/reduced work output	Obtains 90% of pre-morbid level of salary/income	10% of pre-morbid salary/income
		Obtains 80% of pre-morbid level of salary/income	20% of pre-morbid salary/income
		Obtains 70% of pre-morbid level of salary/income	30% of pre-morbid salary/income
		Obtains 60% of pre-morbid level of salary/income	40% of pre-morbid salary/income
		Obtains 50% of pre-morbid level of salary/income	50% of pre-morbid salary/income
		Obtains 40% of pre-morbid level of salary/income	60% of pre-morbid salary/income
		Obtains 30% of pre-morbid level of salary/income	70% of pre-morbid salary/income
		Obtains 20% of pre-morbid level of salary/income	80% of pre-morbid salary/income
		Obtains 10% of pre-morbid level of salary/income	90% of pre-morbid salary/income
Unemployed	Total inability to perform work	Earning capacity -Nil	100% of pre-morbid salary/income

REFERENCES

1. *The ADA: Your Responsibilities as an Employer.* In: Commission TUSEEO, editor. Washington, DC: Department of Justice, Office on the Americans with Disabilities Act; 2008.

2. Thornton P, Lunt N. *Employment Policies for Disabled People in Eighteen Countries: A Review.* York, UK: Social Policy Research Unit, University of York; 1997.

3. Shahnasarian M. *Assessment of Earning Capacity,* 2nd ed. Tucson, AZ: Lawyers & Judges Publishing Company; 2004.

23

"Ready Reckoner Impairment Table"

Integrated Evaluation of Disability designed the "Ready Reckoner Impairment Table" to easing clinicians practicing disability evaluation save time. Integrated Evaluation of Disability developed the "Ready Reckoner Impairment Table" based on the Pilot Study with the "Clinical Model" about 300 clinical conditions each with different clinical presentations (Tables 23.1 through 23.291).

23.1 READY RECKONER: HIGHER FUNCTIONS AND CRANIAL NERVES

23.1.1 Vegetative state

23.1.2 Seizure disorders

Table 23.1 Seizure disorders—Whole person impairment

Impairment class	Severity profile—Seizure disorders	Maximum impairment 50%
Class 1	Focal/generalized seizures under control with mono or multi-therapy without recurrence (Assigns impairment for burden of treatment compliance, and stigma until the antiepileptic drugs are withdrawn)	5%
Class 2	Focal seizures with preserved consciousness developing recurrence every month with mono/multi-pharmacotherapy	15%
Class 3	Focal seizures with impairment of consciousness,	25%

Impairment class	Severity profile—Seizure disorders	Maximum impairment 50%
	developing recurrence every month with mono/multi-pharmacotherapy	
Class 4	Persistent focal seizure occurring every day/week with impairment of consciousness refractory to pharmacotherapy	37%
Class 4	Generalized seizures, developing recurrence every month with mono/multi-pharmacotherapy	37%
Class 5	Persistent generalized seizures with recurrence every day/week refractory to multi-pharmacotherapy	50%

23.1.3 Mental retardation

Table 23.2 Mental retardation—Whole person impairment

Disability Class	Clinical scales Wechsler's scale/Raven's matrices	Reference impairment median score
Class 1	IQ: 71–84	4%
Class 2	IQ: 50–70	14%
Class 3	IQ: 25–49	39%
Class 4	IQ: <25	63%

23.1.4 Insomnia

Table 23.3 Insomnia: Whole person impairment

Impairment class	Severity profile of chronic insomnia	Maximum impairment 37%
Class 1	1. Difficulty in falling asleep 2. Difficulty in staying asleep 3. Final early awakening 4. Non-restorative sleep with feeling of unrefreshed after early morning 5. Sleep efficiency 75% 6. Day time fatigue, and sleepiness	5%
Class 2	1. Difficulty in falling asleep 2. Difficulty in staying asleep 3. Final early awakening 4. Non-restorative sleep with feeling of unrefreshed after early morning 5. Sleep efficiency 50%–74% 6. Daytime fatigue, sleepiness during driving and increased risk of injury	15%
Class 3	1. Difficulty in falling asleep 2. Difficulty in staying asleep 3. Final early awakening 4. Non-restorative sleep with feeling of unrefreshed after early morning 5. Sleep efficiency 25%–49% 6. Daytime fatigue, increased risk of injury during driving and cognitive deficiencies	25%
Class 4	1. Difficulty in falling asleep 2. Difficulty in staying asleep 3. Final early awakening 4. Non-restorative sleep with feeling of unrefreshed after early morning 5. Sleep efficiency <25% 6. Daytime fatigue, sleepiness during driving with increased risk of injury and cognitive deficiencies 7. Depression 8. Abuse of alcohol and substance	37%

Note: If there is associated cognitive impairment, additional impairment of cognitive function.

23.1.5 Cognitive function

1. Attention function: 1%
2. Memory: 2%
3. Orientation: 3%
4. Auditory perception: 3%
5. Visual perception: 3%
6. Visuospatial: 4%
7. Abstraction: 5%
8. Organization and planning: 5%
9. Judgment: 5%
10. Problem solving: 5%

23.1.6 Language function

1. Global aphasia: 50%
2. Receptive aphasia: 37%
3. Receptive dysphasia: 25%
4. Expressive aphasia: 25%
5. Expressive dysphasia: 15%
6. Speech apraxia: 25%

23.1.7 Articulation function

Table 23.4 Articulation function—Whole person impairment

Class 1 Dysarthria	Speech is understandable but with initialization difficulty, less distinct sounds, and impaired stress or rhythm	5%
Class 2 Dysarthria	Speech is not clear with indistinct sounds and poorly understandable	15%
Class 3 Anarthria	Not able to speak or Speech is unintelligible	25%
Class 1 Stuttering	Stuttering occurring occasionally	0%
Class 2 Stuttering	Stuttering occurring during periods of excitation	5%
Class 3 Stuttering	Stuttering occurring all the time	15%

23.1.8 Voice function

Table 23.5 Voice function—Whole person impairment

Dysphonia—Class 1	Impairment of phonatory quality such as flutter, creak, tremor	5%
Dysphonia—Class 2	Impairment of resonance such as nasal tone, e.g., in cleft palate	10%
Dysphonia—Class 3	Impairment of pitch, loudness, and quality of voice— breathiness or hoarseness strangled or strained voice	15%
Aphonia—Class 4	Not able to produce voice	25%

23.1.9 Swallowing function

Table 23.6 Impairment of oral, pharyngeal, and esophageal swallowing functions

Impairment class	Criteria	Reference impairment score
Class 1	Difficulty in swallowing with drooling of saliva or drooling during drinking liquids or accumulation of solid food in the alveoli of mouth	2.5%
Class 2	Prolonged duration of meal with sensation of holding of food in the throat	5.0%
Class 3	Difficulty in swallowing with nasal regurgitation and/or occasional choking Difficulty in swallowing with nasal regurgitation and on-and-off choking or Limited swallowing ability by modifying food consistency	15%
Class 4	Difficulty in swallowing with frequent nasal regurgitation and choking or Limited swallowing ability by modifying food consistency, and postural techniques and compensatory maneuvers to minimize the risk of aspiration	25%
Class 5	Inability to swallow, develop significant aspiration on attempted swallowing and require feeding by nasogastric tube or PEG (Percutaneous Endoscopic Gastrostomy)	50%

23.1.10 Olfactory function

Table 23.7 Olfactory function—Whole person impairment

Class 1	Hyposmia	2.5%
Class 2	Anosmia	5%

23.1.11 Oculomotor function

Table 23.8 Ptosis—Whole person impairment

Class 1	Ptosis: Distance between the center of the upper lid margin and light reflex in primary gaze (Margin reflex distance—MRD1): 2 mm of droop	1.25%
Class 2	Ptosis: Distance between the center of the upper lid margin and light reflex in primary gaze (Margin reflex distance—MRD1): 3 mm of droop	2.5%
Class 3	Ptosis: Distance between the center of the Upper lid margin and light reflex in primary gaze (Margin reflex distance—MRD1): ≥4 mm of droop	5%

23.1.12 Oculomotor, trochlear, and abducent nerve functions

Table 23.9 Diplopia—Whole person impairment

Class 1	Diplopia score 1–5	5%
Class 2	Diplopia score 6–10	10%
Class 3	Diplopia score 11–15	15%
Class 4	Diplopia score 16–20	20%
Class 5	Diplopia score 21–25	25%

23.1.13 Trigeminal nerve function

1. Complete impairment of sensory and motor functions of the trigeminal nerve: 15%
2. Partial impairment of trigeminal nerve: 5%

23.1.14 Facial nerve function

1. Complete unilateral facial paralysis due to lower motor neuron lesion: 15%
2. Partial unilateral facial paralysis due to lower motor neuron lesion: 7.5%
3. Complete unilateral facial paralysis due to upper motor neuron lesion: 10%
4. Partial unilateral facial paralysis due to upper motor neuron lesion: 5%

23.1.15 Vestibular function

1. Episodic spinning vertigo, nausea, and vomiting
2. Horizontal or rotatory-horizontal nystagmus
3. Positive sharpened Romberg

23.1.16 Hypoglossal nerve function

1. Complete unilateral lesion with dysarthria and dysphagia with drooling: 10%
2. Incomplete unilateral lesion with dysphagia and dysarthria: 7.5%.

23.2 READY RECKONER—CEREBRAL PALSY

Table 23.10 Spastic cerebral palsy MAS 1, 1+, 2

Crural monoplegia MAS 1	3.258%		
Brachial monoplegia MAS 1	3.415%		
Paraplegia MAS 1	8%		
Quadriparesis MAS 1	14%		
Crural monoplegia MAS 1+	5%		
Brachial monoplegia MAS 1+	6%		
Paraplegia MAS 1+	12%		
Quadriparesis MAS 1+	22%		
Crural monoplegia MAS 2	7%		
Brachial monoplegia MAS 2	9%		
Paraplegia MAS 2	17%		
Quadriparesis MAS 2	32%		
Quadriparesis MAS 2	Dysarthria Class 1 (5%)	35%	
Quadriparesis MAS 2	Dysarthria Class 1 (5%)	Bilateral equinus deformity (4%)	38%

Table 23.11 Spastic cerebral palsy MAS 3

Crural monoplegia MAS 3	9%			
Brachial monoplegia MAS 3	12%			
Paraplegia MAS 3	23%			
Quadriparesis MAS 3	40%			
Quadriparesis MAS 3	Dysarthria Class 2 (15%)	49%		
Quadriparesis MAS 3	Dysarthria Class 2 (15%)	Neurogenic bladder (25%)		62%
Quadriparesis MAS 3	Dysarthria Class 2 (15%)	Neurogenic bladder (25%)	Constipation Class 1 (5%)	64%
Quadriparesis MAS 3	Dysarthria Class 2 (15%)	Neurogenic bladder (25%)	Constipation Class 1 (5%), Bilateral equinus deformity (4%)	65%

Table 23.12 Spastic cerebral palsy MAS 4

Crural monoplegia MAS 4	11%			
Brachial monoplegia MAS 4	13%			
Paraplegia MAS 4	26%			
Quadriplegia MAS 4	44%			
Quadriplegia MAS 4	Dysarthria Class 2 (15%)	52%		
Quadriplegia MAS 4	Dysarthria Class 2 (15%)	Neurogenic bladder (25%)	64%	
Quadriplegia MAS 4	Dysarthria Class 2 (15%)	Neurogenic bladder (25%)	Constipation Class 1 (5%)	66%
Quadriplegia MAS 4	Dysarthria Class 2 (15%)	Neurogenic bladder (25%)	Constipation Class 1 (5%), Bilateral equinus deformity (4%)	67%

Table 23.13 Spastic cerebral palsy—Hemiplegia MAS 1, 1+, 2

Hemiplegia MAS 1	9%			
Hemiplegia MAS 1+	13%			
Hemiplegia MAS 2	18%			
Hemiplegia MAS 2	Dysarthria Class 1 (5%)	22%		
Hemiplegia MAS 2	Dysarthria Class 1 (5%)	Neurogenic bladder (25%)	42%	
Hemiplegia MAS 2	Dysarthria Class 1 (5%)	Neurogenic bladder (25%)	Equinus deformity (2%)	43%

Table 23.14 Spastic cerebral palsy—Hemiplegia MAS 3, dysarthria

Hemiplegia MAS 3	24%				
Hemiplegia MAS 3	Dysarthria Class 2 (15%)	35%			
Hemiplegia MAS 3	Dysarthria Class 2 (15%)	Neurogenic bladder (25%)	51%		
Hemiplegia MAS 3	Dysarthria Class 2 (15%)	Neurogenic bladder (25%)	Constipation Class 1 (5%)	54%	
Hemiplegia MAS 3	Dysarthria Class 2 (15%)	Neurogenic bladder (25%)	Constipation Class 1 (5%)	Equinus deformity (2%)	55%

Table 23.15 Spastic cerebral palsy—Hemiplegia MAS 3, expressive aphasia/dysphasia

Hemiplegia MAS 3	24%				
Hemiplegia MAS 3	Expressive dysphasia (15%)	35%			
Hemiplegia MAS 3	Expressive dysphasia (15%)	Neurogenic bladder (25%)	51%		
Hemiplegia MAS 3	Expressive dysphasia (15%)	Neurogenic bladder (25%)	Constipation Class 1 (5%)	54%	
Hemiplegia MAS 3	Expressive dysphasia (15%)	Neurogenic bladder (25%)	Constipation Class 1 (5%)	Equinus deformity (2%)	55%
Hemiplegia MAS 3	24%				
Hemiplegia MAS 3	Expressive aphasia (25%)	43%			
Hemiplegia MAS 3	Expressive aphasia (25%)	Neurogenic bladder (25%)	57%		
Hemiplegia MAS 3	Expressive aphasia (25%)	Neurogenic bladder (25%)	Constipation Class 1 (5%)	59%	
Hemiplegia MAS 3	Expressive aphasia (25%)	Neurogenic bladder (25%)	Constipation Class 1 (5%)	Equinus deformity (2%)	60%

Table 23.16 Spastic cerebral palsy—Hemiplegia MAS 3: Receptive aphasia/dysphasia

Hemiplegia MAS 3	24%				
Hemiplegia MAS 3	Receptive dysphasia (25%)	43%			
Hemiplegia MAS 3	Receptive dysphasia (25%)	Uninhibited neurogenic bladder (25%)	57%		
Hemiplegia MAS 3	Receptive dysphasia (25%)	Uninhibited neurogenic bladder (25%)	Constipation Class 1 (5%)	59%	
Hemiplegia MAS 3	Receptive dysphasia (25%)	Uninhibited neurogenic bladder (25%)	Constipation Class 1 (5%)	Equinus deformity (2%)	60%
Hemiplegia MAS 3	24%				
Hemiplegia MAS 3	Receptive aphasia (37%)	52%			
Hemiplegia MAS 3	Receptive aphasia (37%)	Neurogenic bladder (25%)	64%		
Hemiplegia MAS 3	Receptive aphasia (37%)	Neurogenic bladder (25%)	Constipation Class 1 (5%)	66%	
Hemiplegia MAS 3	Receptive aphasia (37%)	Neurogenic bladder (25%)	Constipation Class 1 (5%)	Equinus deformity (2%)	67%

Table 23.17 Spastic cerebral palsy—Hemiplegia MAS 4, dysarthria

Hemiplegia MAS 4	26%				
Hemiplegia MAS 4	Dysarthria Class 2 (15%)	37%			
Hemiplegia MAS 4	Dysarthria Class 2 (15%)	Neurogenic bladder (25%)	53%		
Hemiplegia MAS 4	Dysarthria Class 2 (15%)	Neurogenic bladder (25%)	Constipation Class 1 (5%)	55%	
Hemiplegia MAS 4	Dysarthria Class 2 (15%)	Uninhibited neurogenic bladder (25%)	Constipation Class 1 (5%)	Equinus deformity (2%)	56%

Table 23.18 Spastic cerebral palsy—Hemiplegia MAS 4, expressive aphasia/dysphasia

Hemiplegia MAS 4	26%			
Hemiplegia MAS 4	Expressive dysphasia (15%)	37%		
Hemiplegia MAS 4	Expressive dysphasia (15%)	Neurogenic bladder (25%)	53%	
Hemiplegia MAS 4	Expressive dysphasia (15%)	Neurogenic bladder (25%)	Constipation Class 1 (5%)	55%
Hemiplegia MAS 4	Expressive dysphasia (15%)	Neurogenic bladder (25%)	Constipation Class 1 (5%)	Equinus deformity (2%)	56%
Hemiplegia MAS 4	26%			
Hemiplegia MAS 4	Expressive aphasia (25%)	45%		
Hemiplegia MAS 4	Expressive aphasia (25%)	Neurogenic bladder (25%)	59%	
Hemiplegia MAS 4	Expressive aphasia (25%)	Neurogenic bladder (25%)	Constipation Class 1 (5%)	61%
Hemiplegia MAS 4	Expressive aphasia (25%)	Neurogenic bladder (25%)	Constipation Class 1 (5%)	Equinus deformity (2%)	61%

Table 23.19 Spastic cerebral palsy—Hemiplegia MAS 4, receptive aphasia/dysphasia

Hemiplegia MAS 4	26%			
Hemiplegia MAS 4	Receptive dysphasia (25%)	45%		
Hemiplegia MAS 4	Receptive dysphasia (25%)	Neurogenic bladder (25%)	59%	
Hemiplegia MAS 4	Receptive dysphasia (25%)	Neurogenic bladder (25%)	Constipation Class 1 (5%)	61%
Hemiplegia MAS 4	Receptive dysphasia (25%)	Neurogenic bladder (25%)	Constipation Class 1 (5%)	Expressive dysphasia (15%)	61%
Hemiplegia MAS 4	26%			
Hemiplegia MAS 4	Receptive aphasia (37%)	54%		
Hemiplegia MAS 4	Receptive aphasia (37%)	Neurogenic bladder (25%)	65%	
Hemiplegia MAS 4	Receptive aphasia (37%)	Neurogenic bladder (25%)	Constipation Class 1 (5%)	67%
Hemiplegia MAS 4	Receptive aphasia (37%)	Neurogenic bladder (25%)	Constipation Class 1 (5%)	Expressive dysphasia (15%)	68%

Table 23.20 Ataxic cerebral palsy—Grades 1, 2, 3, dysarthria, and equinus deformity

Crural monoplegia grade 1	2%	
Brachial monoplegia—ataxia grade 1	3%	
Paraplegia—ataxia grade 1	5%	
Quadriplegia—ataxia grade 1	12%	
Crural monoplegia—ataxia grade 2	4%	
Brachial monoplegia—ataxia grade 2	5%	
Paraplegia—ataxia grade 2	10%	
Quadriplegia—ataxia grade 2	19%	
Crural monoplegia—ataxia grade 3	8%	
Brachial monoplegia—ataxia grade 3	9%	
Paraplegia—ataxia grade 3	18%	
Quadriplegia—ataxia grade 3	32%	
Quadriplegia—ataxia grade 3	Dysarthria Class 2 (15%)	42%

Table 23.21 Cerebral palsy—Ataxic hemiplegia grades 1, 2, 3, dysarthria, deformity

Ataxic hemiplegia grade 1	7%		
Ataxic hemiplegia grade 1	Dysarthria Class 2 (5%)	11%	
Ataxic hemiplegia grade 2	11%		
Ataxic hemiplegia grade 2	Dysarthria Cass 2 (15%)	24%	
Ataxic hemiplegia grade 2	Dysarthria Class 2 (15%)	Equinus deformity (2%)	26%
Ataxic hemiplegia grade 3	19%		
Ataxic hemiplegia grade 3	Dysarthria Class 2 (15%)	31%	
Ataxic hemiplegia grade 3	Dysarthria Class 2 (15%)	Equinus deformity (2%)	32%

Table 23.22 Dyskinetic cerebral palsy—Chorea grades 1, 2, 3

Chorea grade 1 one lower extremity	2%	
Chorea grade 1 both lower extremities	5%	
Chorea grade 1 one upper extremity	3%	
Chorea grade 1 both upper and lower extremities	10%	
Chorea grade 1 both upper and lower extremities	Dysarthria Class 1 (5%)	14%
Chorea grade 2 one lower extremity	3%	
Chorea grade 2 both lower extremities	6%	
Chorea grade 2 one upper extremity	3%	
Chorea grade 2 both upper and lower extremities	11%	
Chorea grade 2 both upper and lower extremities	Dysarthria Class 2 (15%)	24%
Chorea grade 3 one lower extremity	3%	
Chorea grade 3 both lower extremities	7%	
Chorea grade 3 one upper extremity	4%	
Chorea grade 3 both upper and lower extremities	14%	
Chorea grade 2 both upper and lower extremities	Dysarthria Class 2 (15%)	27%

Table 23.23 Dyskinetic cerebral palsy—Athetosis grades 1, 2, 3

Athetosis grade 1 one lower extremity	2%	
Athetosis grade 1 both lower extremities	5%	
Athetosis grade 1 one upper extremity	3%	
Athetosis grade 1 both upper and lower extremities	10%	
Athetosis grade 1 both upper and lower extremities	Dysarthria Class 1 (5%)	14%

(Continued)

Table 23.23 (*Continued*) Dyskinetic cerebral palsy—Athetosis grades 1, 2, 3

Athetosis grade 2 one lower extremity	3%		
Athetosis grade 2 both lower extremities	6%		
Athetosis grade 2 one upper extremity	3%		
Athetosis grade 2 both upper and lower extremities	11%		
Athetosis grade 2 both upper and lower extremities	Dysarthria Class 2 (15%)	24%	
Athetosis grade 2 both upper and lower extremities	Dysarthria Class 2 (15%)	Dysphagia Class (2.5%)	26%
Athetosis grade 3 one lower extremity	3%		
Athetosis grade 3 both lower extremities	7%		
Athetosis grade 3 one upper extremity	4%		
Athetosis grade 3 both upper and lower extremities	14%		
Athetosis grade 3 both upper and lower extremities	Dysarthria Class 2 (15%)	27%	
Athetosis grade 3 both upper and lower extremities	Dysarthria Class 2 (15%)	Dysphagia Class (5%)	30%

Table 23.24 Dyskinetic cerebral palsy—Dystonia grades 1, 2, 3

Dystonia grade 1 one lower extremity	3%		
Dystonia grade 1 one upper extremity	3%		
Dystonia grade 1 both lower extremities and spine	11%		
Dystonia grade 1 both upper, lower extremities and spine	15%		
Dystonia grade 2 one lower extremity	3%		
Dystonia grade 2 one upper extremity	3%		
Dystonia grade 2 both lower extremities and spine	9%		
Dystonia grade 2 both upper, lower extremities and spine	14%		
Dystonia grade 2 both upper, lower extremities and spine	Dysarthria Class 2 (15%)	27%	
Dystonia grade 2 both upper, lower extremities and spine	Dysarthria Class 2 (15%)	Dysphagia Class (2.5%)	28%
Dystonia grade 3 one lower extremity	4%		
Dystonia grade 3 one upper extremity	4%		
Dystonia grade 3 both lower extremities and spine	9%		
Dystonia grade 3 both upper, lower extremities and spine	17%		
Dystonia grade 3 both upper, lower extremities and spine	Dysarthria Class 2 (15%)	29%	
Dystonia grade 3 both upper, lower extremities and spine	Dysarthria Class 2 (15%)	Dysphagia Class (2.5%)	33%

Table 23.25 Hypotonic cerebral palsy—MRC 4, 3, 2, 1

Brachial monoplegia MRC 4	6%	
Crural monoplegia MRC 4	4%	
Paraplegia MRC 4	8%	
Quadriplegia MRC 4	19%	
Quadriplegia MRC 4	Dysphagia Class 1 (2.5%)	21%
Brachial monoplegia MRC 3	8%	
Crural monoplegia MRC 3	8%	
Paraplegia MRC 3	15%	
Quadriplegia MRC 3	30%	
Quadriplegia MRC 3	Dysphagia Class 2 (5%)	34%
Brachial monoplegia MRC 2	15%	
Crural monoplegia MRC 2	11%	
Paraplegia MRC 2	20%	
Quadriplegia MRC 2	47%	
Quadriplegia MRC 2	Dysphagia Class 2 (5%)	49%
Brachial monoplegia MRC 1	19%	
Crural monoplegia MRC 1	15%	
Paraplegia MRC 1	27%	
Quadriplegia MRC 1	56%	
Quadriplegia MRC 1	Dysphagia Class 2 (5%)	58%

23.3 READY RECKONER—STROKE

Table 23.26 Stroke with MAS 1

Hemiparesis MAS 1 (6%)	6%			
Hemiparesis MAS 1 (6%)	Dysarthria Class 1 (5%)	11%		
Hemiparesis MAS 1 (6%)	Dysarthria Class 1 (5%)	Uninhibited neurogenic bladder (25%)	33%	
Hemiparesis MAS 1 (6%)	Dysarthria Class 1 (5%)	Uninhibited neurogenic bladder (25%)	Equinus deformity (2%)	34%

Table 23.27 Stroke with MAS 1+

Hemiparesis MAS 1+ (12%)	12%			
Hemiparesis MAS 1+ (12%)	Dysarthria Class 2 (15%)	26%		
Hemiparesis MAS 1+ (12%)	Dysarthria Class 2 (15%)	Uninhibited neurogenic bladder (25%)	44%	
Hemiparesis MAS 1+ (12%)	Dysarthria Class 2 (15%)	Uninhibited neurogenic bladder (25%)	Equinus deformity (2%)	45%
Hemiparesis MAS 1+ (12%)	Expressive dysphasia (15%)	26%		
Hemiparesis MAS 1+ (12%)	Expressive dysphasia (15%)	Uninhibited neurogenic bladder (25%)	44%	
Hemiparesis MAS 1+ (12%)	Expressive dysphasia (15%)	Uninhibited neurogenic bladder (25%)	Equinus deformity (2%)	45%

Table 23.28 Stroke with MAS 2

Hemiparesis MAS 2 (15%)	15%			
Hemiparesis MAS 2 (15%)	Dysarthria Class 2 (15%)	28%		
Hemiparesis MAS 2 (15%)	Dysarthria Class 2 (15%)	Equinus deformity (2%)	29%	
Hemiparesis MAS 2 (15%)	Dysarthria Class 2 (15%)	Uninhibited neurogenic bladder (25%)	46%	
Hemiparesis MAS 2 (15%)	Dysarthria Class 2 (15%)	Uninhibited neurogenic bladder (25%)	Equinus deformity (2%)	47%
Hemiparesis MAS 2 (15%)	Expressive dysphasia (15%)	28%		
Hemiparesis MAS 2 (15%)	Expressive dysphasia (15%)	Uninhibited neurogenic bladder (25%)	46%	
Hemiparesis MAS 2 (15%)	Expressive dysphasia (15%)	Uninhibited neurogenic bladder (25%)	Equinus deformity (2%)	47%
Hemiparesis MAS 2 (15%)	Expressive aphasia (25%)	36%		

(Continued)

Table 23.28 (Continued) Stroke with MAS 2

Hemiparesis MAS 2 (15%)	Expressive aphasia (25%)	Uninhibited neurogenic bladder (25%)	52%	
Hemiparesis MAS 2 (15%)	Expressive aphasia (25%)	Uninhibited neurogenic bladder (25%)	Equinus deformity (2%)	53%

Table 23.29 Stroke with MAS 2

Hemiparesis MAS 2 (15%)	15%			
Hemiparesis MAS 2 (15%)	Receptive dysphasia (25%)	36%		
Hemiparesis MAS 2 (15%)	Receptive dysphasia (25%)	Uninhibited neurogenic bladder (25%)	52%	
Hemiparesis MAS 2 (15%)	Receptive dysphasia (25%)	Uninhibited neurogenic bladder (25%)	Equinus deformity (2%)	53%
Hemiparesis MAS 2 (15%)	Receptive aphasia (37%)	46%		
Hemiparesis MAS 2 (15%)	Receptive aphasia (37%)	Uninhibited neurogenic bladder (25%)	60%	
Hemiparesis MAS 2 (15%)	Receptive aphasia (37%)	Uninhibited neurogenic bladder (25%)	Equinus deformity	61%
Hemiparesis MAS 2 (15%)	Receptive aphasia (37%)	Uninhibited neurogenic bladder (25%)	Visual neglect	62%
Hemiparesis MAS 2 (15%)	Receptive aphasia (37%)	Uninhibited neurogenic bladder (25%)	Visual neglect, equinus deformity	62%
Hemiparesis MAS 2 (15%)	Global aphasia (50%)	Uninhibited neurogenic bladder (25%)	Finger deformities and equinus deformity (6%)	71%
Hemiparesis MAS 2 (15%)	Global aphasia (50%)	Uninhibited neurogenic bladder (25%)	Visual neglect, homonymous hemianopia, finger and equinus deformities (4.5%)	82%

Table 23.30 Stroke with MAS 3

Hemiparesis MAS 3 (23%)				
Hemiparesis MAS 3 (23%)	Dysarthria Class 2 (15%)	35%		
Hemiparesis MAS 3 (23%)	Dysarthria Class 2 (15%)	Uninhibited neurogenic bladder (25%)	51%	
Hemiparesis MAS 3 (23%)	Dysarthria Class 2 (15%)	Uninhibited neurogenic bladder (25%)	Equinus deformity (2%)	52%
Hemiparesis MAS 3 (23%)	Expressive dysphasia (15%)	35%		
Hemiparesis MAS 3 (23%)	Expressive dysphasia (15%)	Uninhibited neurogenic bladder (25%)	51%	
Hemiparesis MAS 3 (23%)	Expressive dysphasia (15%)	Uninhibited neurogenic bladder (25%)	Equinus deformity (2%)	52%

Table 23.31 Stroke with MAS 3

Hemiparesis MAS 3 (23%)	Expressive aphasia (15%)	42%		
Hemiparesis MAS 3 (23%)	Expressive aphasia (15%)	Uninhibited neurogenic bladder (25%)	57%	
Hemiparesis MAS 3 (23%)	Expressive aphasia (15%)	Uninhibited neurogenic bladder (25%)	Finger and equinus deformities (6%)	59%
Hemiparesis MAS 3 (23%)	Receptive dysphasia (25%)	42%		
Hemiparesis MAS 3 (23%)	Receptive dysphasia (25%)	Uninhibited neurogenic bladder (25%)	57%	
Hemiparesis MAS 3 (23%)	Receptive dysphasia (25%)	Uninhibited neurogenic bladder (25%)	Finger and equinus deformities (6%)	59%

Table 23.32 Stroke with MAS 3

Hemiparesis MAS 3 (23%)	Receptive aphasia (25%)	52%		
Hemiparesis MAS 3 (23%)	Receptive aphasia (25%)	Uninhibited neurogenic bladder (25%)	64%	
Hemiparesis MAS 3 (23%)	Receptive aphasia (25%)	Uninhibited neurogenic bladder (25%)	Finger and equinus deformities (6%)	65%
Hemiparesis MAS 3 (23%)	Global aphasia (50%)	62%		
Hemiparesis MAS 3 (23%)	Global aphasia (50%)	Uninhibited neurogenic bladder (25%)	71%	
Hemiparesis MAS 3 (23%)	Global aphasia (50%)	Uninhibited neurogenic bladder (25%)	Finger and equinus deformity (4.5%)	72%
Hemiparesis MAS 3 (23%)	Global aphasia (50%)	Uninhibited neurogenic bladder (25%)	Visual neglect (4%), finger and equinus deformity (4.5%)	74%
Hemiparesis MAS 3 (23%)	Global aphasia (50%)	Uninhibited neurogenic bladder (25%)	Visual neglect, Hemianesthesia (60%), finger and equinus deformity	89%
Hemiparesis MAS 3 (23%)	Global aphasia (50%)	Uninhibited neurogenic bladder (25%)	Homonymous hemianopia, Hemianesthesia (60%), finger and equinus deformity	94%

Table 23.33 Stroke with MAS 4

Hemiplegia MAS "4" (25%)	25%			
Hemiplegia MAS "4" (25%)	Dysarthria Class "2" (15%)	37%		
Hemiplegia MAS "4" (25%)	Dysarthria Class "2" (15%)	Uninhibited neurogenic bladder (25%)	52%	
Hemiplegia MAS "4" (25%)	Dysarthria Class "2" (15%)	Uninhibited neurogenic bladder (25%)	Finger and equinus deformity (4.5%)	55%
Hemiplegia MAS "4" (25%)	Dysarthria Class "2" (15%)	Uninhibited neurogenic bladder (25%)	Impaired cortical sensation (10%), and finger and equinus deformity (4.5%)	59%
Hemiplegia MAS "4" (25%)	Dysarthria Class "2" (15%)	Uninhibited neurogenic bladder (25%)	Total loss of visual neglect (4%) and cortical sensation (20%)	63%

Table 23.34 Stroke with MAS 4

Hemiplegia MAS 4 (25%)	Expressive dysphasia (15%)	37%		
Hemiplegia MAS 4 (25%)	Expressive dysphasia (15%)	Uninhibited neurogenic bladder (25%)	52%	
Hemiplegia MAS 4 (25%)	Expressive dysphasia (15%)	Uninhibited neurogenic bladder (25%)	Hemianesthesia (60%)	81%
Hemiplegia MAS 4 (25%)	Expressive dysphasia (15%)	Uninhibited neurogenic bladder (25%)	Hemianesthesia (60%) and visual neglect (4%)	82%
Hemiplegia MAS 4 (25%)	Expressive dysphasia (15%)	Uninhibited neurogenic bladder (25%)	Hemianesthesia (60%) and visual neglect (4%) and finger and equinus deformities (4.5%)	83%

Table 23.35 Stroke with MAS 4

Hemiplegia MAS 4 (25%)	Expressive aphasia (25%)	44%		
Hemiplegia MAS 4 (25%)	Expressive aphasia (25%)	Uninhibited neurogenic bladder (25%)	58%	
Hemiplegia MAS 4 (25%)	Expressive aphasia (25%)	Uninhibited neurogenic bladder (25%)	Hemianesthesia (60%)	83%
Hemiplegia MAS 4 (25%)	Expressive aphasia (25%)	Uninhibited neurogenic bladder (25%)	Hemianesthesia and visual neglect (60% + 6%)	84%
Hemiplegia MAS 4 (25%)	Expressive aphasia (25%)	Uninhibited neurogenic bladder (25%)	Hemianesthesia and visual neglect (60% + 6%) and finger and equinus deformity (6%)	85%

Table 23.36 Stroke with MAS 4

Hemiplegia MAS 4 (25%)	Receptive dysphasia (25%)	44%		
Hemiplegia MAS 4 (25%)	Receptive dysphasia (25%)	Uninhibited neurogenic bladder (25%)	58%	
Hemiplegia MAS 4 (25%)	Receptive dysphasia (25%)	Uninhibited neurogenic bladder (25%)	Hemianesthesia (60%)	83%
Hemiplegia MAS 4 (25%)	Receptive dysphasia (25%)	Uninhibited neurogenic bladder (25%)	Hemianesthesia and visual neglect (60% + 6%)	84%
Hemiplegia MAS 4 (25%)	Receptive dysphasia (25%)	Uninhibited neurogenic bladder (25%)	Hemianesthesia and visual neglect (60% + 6%) and finger and equinus deformity (6%)	85%

Table 23.37 Stroke with MAS 4

Hemiplegia MAS 4 (25%)	Receptive aphasia (37%)	53%		
Hemiplegia MAS 4 (25%)	Receptive aphasia (37%)	Uninhibited neurogenic bladder (25%)	65%	
Hemiplegia MAS 4 (25%)	Receptive aphasia (37%)	Uninhibited neurogenic bladder (25%)	Hemianesthesia (60%)	86%
Hemiplegia MAS 4 (25%)	Receptive aphasia (37%)	Uninhibited neurogenic bladder (25%)	Hemianesthesia and visual neglect (60% + 6%)	86%
Hemiplegia MAS 4 (25%)	Receptive aphasia (37%)	Uninhibited neurogenic bladder (25%)	Hemianesthesia and visual neglect (60% + 6%) and finger and equinus deformity (4.5%)	87%

Table 23.38 Stroke with MAS 4

Hemiplegia MAS 4 (25%)	Global aphasia (50%)	63%		
Hemiplegia MAS 4 (25%)	Global aphasia (50%)	Uninhibited neurogenic bladder (25%)	72%	
Hemiplegia MAS 4 (25%)	Global aphasia (50%)	Uninhibited neurogenic bladder (25%)	Hemianesthesia (60%)	89%
Hemiplegia MAS 4 (25%)	Global aphasia (50%)	Uninhibited neurogenic bladder (25%)	Hemianesthesia and visual neglect (60% + 4%)	89%
Hemiplegia MAS 4 (25%)	Global aphasia (50%)	Uninhibited neurogenic bladder (25%)	Hemianesthesia and visual neglect (60% + 4%) and finger and equinus deformity (4.5%)	90%
Hemiplegia MAS 4 (25%)	Global aphasia (50%)	Uninhibited neurogenic bladder (25%)	Hemianesthesia and homonymous, hemianopia visual neglect (60% + 4%) and finger and equinus deformity (4.5%)	94%

23.4 READY RECKONER—PARKINSONISM

Table 23.39 Parkinsonism—MAS 1, 1+: Quadriparesis, tremor, speech—Monotone

Quadriparesis—MAS 1, Bradykinesia Class 1 (16%)	16%			
Quadriparesis—MAS 1, Bradykinesia Class 1 (16%)	Speech—monotone (5%)	20%		
Quadriparesis—MAS 1+, Bradykinesia Class 1 (20%)	20%			
Quadriparesis—MAS 1+, Bradykinesia Class 1 (20%)	Speech—monotone (5%)	24%		
Quadriparesis—MAS 1+, Bradykinesia Class 1 (20%)	Speech—monotone (5%)	Constipation—Class 1 (5%)	28%	
Quadriparesis—MAS 1+, Bradykinesia Class 1 (20%)	Speech—monotone (5%)	Constipation—Class 1 (5%)	Urgency of micturition (5%)	32%

Table 23.40 Parkinsonism—MAS 2: Quadriparesis, tremor, dysarthria, constipation

Quadriparesis—MAS 2, Bradykinesia Class 2 (35%)	35%			
Quadriparesis—MAS 2, Bradykinesia Class 2 (35%)	Speech—monotone (5%)	38%		
Quadriparesis—MAS 2, Bradykinesia Class 2 (35%)	Speech—monotone (5%)	Hypophonia (25%)	47%	
Quadriparesis—MAS 2, Bradykinesia Class 2 (35%)	Speech—monotone (5%)	Hypophonia (25%)	Constipation—Class 1 (5%)	50%

Table 23.41 Parkinsonism—MAS 2: Quadriparesis, tremor, dysarthria, dysphagia

Quadriparesis—MAS 2, Bradykinesia Class 2 (35%)	35%				
Quadriparesis—MAS 2, Bradykinesia Class 2 (35%)	Speech—monotone (5%)	38%			
Quadriparesis—MAS 2, Bradykinesia Class 2 (35%)	Speech—monotone (5%)	Hypophonia (25%)	47%		
Quadriparesis—MAS 2, Bradykinesia Class 2 (35%)	Speech—monotone (5%)	Hypophonia (25%)	Dysphagia Class 3 (15%)	55%	
Quadriparesis—MAS 2, Bradykinesia Class 2 (35%)	Speech—monotone (5%)	Hypophonia (25%)	Dysphagia Class 3 (15%)	Constipation—Class 2 (15%)	62%
Quadriparesis—MAS 2, Bradykinesia Class 2 (35%)	Speech—monotone (5%)	Hypophonia (25%)	Dysphagia Class 3 (15%)	Constipation—Class 2 (15%)	Urgency of micturition (5%) 64%

Table 23.42 Parkinsonism—MAS 3: Quadriparesis, urge incontinence, erectile function

Quadriparesis— MAS 3, Bradykinesia Class 3 (53%)	53%					
Quadriparesis— MAS 3, Bradykinesia Class 3 (53%)	Dysarthria (15%)	60%				
Quadriparesis— MAS 3, Bradykinesia Class 3 (53%)	Dysarthria (15%)	Hypophonia (25%)	66%			
Quadriparesis— MAS 3, Bradykinesia Class 3 (53%)	Dysarthria (15%)	Hypophonia (25%)	Dysphagia Class 3 (15%)	71%		
Quadriparesis— MAS 3, Bradykinesia Class 3 (53%)	Dysarthria (15%)	Hypophonia (25%)	Dysphagia Class 3 (15%)	Constipation Class 3 (25%)	79%	
Quadriparesis— MAS 3, Bradykinesia Class 3 (53%)	Dysarthria (15%)	Hypophonia (25%)	Dysphagia Class 3 (15%)	Constipation Class 3 (25%)	Urgency incontinence (15%)	82%
Quadriparesis— MAS 3, Bradykinesia Class 3 (53%)	Dysarthria (15%)	Hypophonia (25%)	Dysphagia Class 3 (15%)	Constipation Class 3 (25%)	Urgency incontinence (15%) and erectile dysfunction (15%)	85%

Table 23.43 Parkinsonism—MAS 4: Quadriparesis, urge incontinence, erectile function

Quadriplegia—MAS 4, Bradykinesia Class 3 (56%)	56%					
Quadriplegia—MAS 4, Bradykinesia Class 3 (56%)	Speech is unintelligible (25%)	67%				
Quadriplegia—MAS 4, Bradykinesia Class 3 (56%)	Speech is unintelligible (25%)	Hypophonia (15%)	72%			
Quadriplegia—MAS 4, Bradykinesia Class 3 (56%)	Speech is unintelligible (25%)	Hypophonia (15%)	Dysphagia Class 3 (15%)	76%		
Quadriplegia—MAS 4, Bradykinesia Class 3 (56%)	Speech is unintelligible (25%)	Hypophonia (15%)	Dysphagia Class 3 (15%)	Constipation Class 3 (25%)	82%	
Quadriplegia—MAS 4, Bradykinesia Class 3 (56%)	Speech is unintelligible (25%)	Hypophonia (15%)	Dysphagia Class 3 (15%)	Constipation Class 3 (25%)	Urge incontinence (15%)	85%
Quadriplegia—MAS 4, Bradykinesia Class 3 (56%)	Speech is unintelligible (25%)	Hypophonia (15%)	Dysphagia Class 3 (15%)	Constipation Class 3 (25%)	Urge incontinence (15%) and erectile dysfunction (15%)	87%

23.5 READY RECKONER— EXTRAPYRAMIDAL: DYSKINESIA

Table 23.44 Dyskinesia: Chorea, athetosis, dystonia, and ballismus

Hemichorea, involving upper extremity (3%)	3%	
Hemichorea, involving upper and lower extremities (6%)	6%	
Hemichorea, involving upper and lower extremities (10%)	Dysarthria—Class 1 (5%)	10%
Chorea, involving upper and lower extremities (10%)	10%	
Chorea, involving upper and lower extremities (10%)	Dysarthria—Class 1 (5%)	14%
Chorea, motor weakness MRC 4 and grade 1 hypotonia involving upper and lower extremities (19%)	19%	
Chorea, motor weakness MRC 4 and grade 1 hypotonia involving upper and lower extremities (19%)	Dysarthria—Class 2 (15%)	31%
Athetosis involving upper and lower extremities (10%)	10%	
Athetosis involving upper and lower extremities (10%)	Dysarthria—Class 2 (15%)	23%
Dystonia involving upper and lower extremities. And trunk (12%)	12%	
Dystonia involving upper and lower extremities. And trunk (12%)	Dysarthria—Class 2 (15%)	25%
Hemiballismus (6%)	6%	
Ballismus (15%)	15%	

23.6 READY RECKONER—CEREBELLAR AND SPINOCEREBELLAR ATAXIA

Table 23.45 Cerebellar ataxia, tremor, dysarthria

Cerebellar ataxia Class 1 (11%)	11%	
Cerebellar ataxia Class 1 (11%)	Class 1 dysarthria (5%)	16%
Cerebellar ataxia Class 2 (17%)	17%	
Cerebellar ataxia Class 2 (17%)	Class 2 dysarthria (15%)	30%
Cerebellar ataxia Class 3 (28%)	28%	
Cerebellar ataxia Class 3 (28%)	Class 3 dysarthria (25%)	46%

Table 23.46 Spinocerebellar ataxia, Class 1 cerebellar function, MAS 1, Class 1 dysarthria, impairment of vibration and position sense, pes cavus deformity

Spinocerebellar ataxia with Class 1 cerebellar, MAS 1 (11%)	11%		
Spinocerebellar ataxia with Class 1 cerebellar, MAS 1 (11%)	Class 1 dysarthria (5%)	16%	
Spinocerebellar ataxia with Class 1 cerebellar, MAS 1 (11%)	Impairment of vibration and position sense (42%)	Class 1 dysarthria (5%)	55%
Spinocerebellar ataxia with Class 1 cerebellar, MAS 1 (11%)	Impairment of vibration and position sense upper and lower extremities and spine	Class 1 dysarthria (5%)	Pes cavus deformity (2%) 56%

Table 23.47 Spinocerebellar ataxia, Class 2 cerebellar function, MAS 1+, Class 2 dysarthria and impairment of vibration and position sense, and pes cavus deformity

Spinocerebellar ataxia with Class 2 cerebellar, MAS 1+ (21%)	21%		
Spinocerebellar ataxia with Class 2 cerebellar, MAS 1+ (21%)	Impairment of vibration and position sense upper and lower extremities and spine	58%	
Spinocerebellar ataxia with Class 2 cerebellar, MAS 1+ (21%)	Impairment of vibration and position sense upper and lower extremities and spine	Class 2 dysarthria (15%)	65%
Spinocerebellar ataxia with Class 2 cerebellar, MAS 1+ (21%)	Impairment of vibration and position sense upper and lower extremities and spine	Class 2 dysarthria (15%)	Pes cavus deformity (2%) 65%

Table 23.48 Spinocerebellar ataxia, Class 2 cerebellar function, MAS 1+, Class 2 dysarthria, peripheral neuropathy, and pes cavus deformity

Spinocerebellar ataxia with Class 2 cerebellar, MAS 1+ (21%)	21%			
Spinocerebellar ataxia with Class 2 cerebellar, MAS 1+ (21%)	Peripheral neuropathy	47%		
Spinocerebellar ataxia with Class 2 cerebellar, MAS 1+ (21%)	Peripheral neuropathy	Class 2 dysarthria (15%)	55%	
Spinocerebellar ataxia with Class 2 cerebellar, MAS 1+ (21%)	Peripheral neuropathy	Class 2 dysarthria (15%)	Pes cavus deformity (2%)	56%

Table 23.49 Spinocerebellar ataxia, Class 2, cerebellar, MAS 2, impairment of vibration and position sense, tremor, speech dysarthria, dysphagia, and pes cavus deformity

Spinocerebellar ataxia with Class 2 cerebellar, MAS 2 (27%)	27%			
Spinocerebellar ataxia with Class 2 cerebellar, MAS 2 (27%)	Impairment of vibration and position sense upper and lower extremities and spine	61%		
Spinocerebellar ataxia with Class 2 cerebellar, MAS 2 (27%)	Impairment of vibration and position sense upper and lower extremities and spine	Class 2 dysarthria (15%)	67%	
Spinocerebellar ataxia with Class 2 cerebellar, MAS 2 (27%)	Impairment of vibration and position sense upper and lower extremities and spine	Class 2 dysarthria (15%)	Class 2 dysphagia (5%)	69%
Spinocerebellar ataxia with Class 2 cerebellar, MAS 2 (27%)	Impairment of vibration and position sense upper and lower extremities and spine	Class 2 dysarthria (15%)	Class 2 dysphagia (5%) Pes cavus deformity (2%)	69%

23.7 READY RECKONER—FRIEDREICH'S ATAXIA

Table 23.50 Friedrich's ataxia, sensory impairment, dysarthria, pes cavus deformity

Cerebellar Class 1 motor MRC 3	14%			
Cerebellar Class 1 motor MRC 3	Impairment of vibration and position sense upper and lower extremities and spine	43%		
Cerebellar Class 1 motor MRC 3	Impairment of vibration and position sense upper and lower extremities and spine	Class 1 dysarthria (5%)	45%	
Cerebellar Class 1 motor MRC 3	Impairment of vibration and position sense upper and lower extremities and spine	Class 1 dysarthria (5%)	Pes cavus deformity (2%)	48%

Table 23.51 Friedreich's ataxia, sensory impairment, dysarthria, pes cavus deformity

Cerebellar Class 2 motor MRC 2 (25%)	25%			
Cerebellar Class 2 motor MRC 2 (25%)	Impairment of vibration and position sense upper and lower extremities and spine	50%		
Cerebellar Class 2 motor MRC 2 (25%)	Impairment of vibration and position sense upper and lower extremities and spine	Class 2 dysarthria (15%)	58%	
Cerebellar Class 2 motor MRC 2 (25%)	Impairment of vibration and position sense upper and lower extremities and spine	Class 2 dysarthria (15%)	Scoliosis (5%), foot deformities (4%)	61%

Table 23.52 Friedreich's ataxia, sensory impairment, dysarthria, cardiomyopathy

Cerebellar Class 3 motor MRC 1 (38%)	38%			
Cerebellar Class 3 motor MRC 1 (38%)	Impairment of vibration and position sense upper and lower extremities and spine	59%		
Cerebellar Class 3 motor MRC 1 (38%)	Impairment of vibration and position sense upper and lower extremities and spine	Class 3 dysarthria (25%)	69%	
Cerebellar Class 3 motor MRC 1 (38%)	Impairment of vibration and position sense upper and lower extremities and spine	Class 3 dysarthria (25%)	Class 2 dysphagia (5%)	71%
Cerebellar Class 3 motor MRC 1 (38%)	Impairment of vibration and position sense upper and lower extremities and spine	Class 3 dysarthria (25%)	Class 2 dysphagia (5%), Class 2 cardiomyopathy	78%
Cerebellar Class 3 motor MRC 1 (38%)	Impairment of vibration and position sense upper and lower extremities and spine	Class 3 dysarthria (25%)	Class 2 dysphagia (5%), Class 2 cardiomyopathy (25%), scoliosis (5%), foot deformities (4%)	80%

Table 23.53 Friedreich's ataxia, sensory impairment, dysarthria, cardiomyopathy, dysrhythmia

Cerebellar Class 3 motor MRC 1 (38%)	38%			
Cerebellar Class 3 motor MRC 1 (38%)	Impairment of vibration and position sense upper and lower extremities and spine	59%		
Cerebellar Class 3 motor MRC 1 (38%)	Impairment of vibration and position sense upper and lower extremities and spine	Class 3 dysarthria (25%)	69%	
Cerebellar Class 3 motor MRC 1 (38%)	Impairment of vibration and position sense upper and lower extremities and spine	Class 3 dysarthria (25%)	Class 2 dysphagia (5%)	71%
Cerebellar Class 3 motor MRC 1 (38%)	Impairment of vibration and position sense upper and lower extremities and spine	Class 3 dysarthria (25%)	Class 2 dysphagia (25%), Class 2 cardiomyopathy	78%
Cerebellar Class 3 motor MRC 1 (38%)	Impairment of vibration and position sense upper and lower extremities and spine	Class 5 dysarthria (25%)	Class 2 dysphagia (5%), Class 2 cardiomyopathy (25%), Class 4 dysrhythmia (25%)	83%
Cerebellar Class 3 motor MRC 1 (38%)	Impairment of vibration and position sense upper and lower extremities and spine	Class 5 dysarthria (25%)	Class 2 dysphagia (5%), Class 2 cardiomyopathy (25%), Class 4 dysrhythmia (25%), scoliosis (5%), foot deformities (4%)	85%

23.8 READY RECKONER—SCI: CERVICAL CORD

Table 23.54 SCI C3 and/or C4 tetraplegia: MAS 1, 1+ urgency of micturition

Tetraplegia: MAS 1 (18%)	18%			
Tetraplegia: MAS 1 (18%)	Urgency of micturition (5%)	22%		
Tetraplegia: MAS 1+ (25%)	25%			
Tetraplegia: MAS 1+ (25%)	Partial sensory loss	59%		
Tetraplegia: MAS 1+ (25%)	Partial sensory loss	Urgency with incontinence (15%)	66%	
Tetraplegia: MAS 1+ (25%)	Partial sensory loss	Urgency with incontinence (15%)	Constipation Class 1 (5%)	67%

Table 23.55 SCI C3 and/or C4 Tetraplegia: MAS 2, reflex bladder, constipation

Tetraplegia: MAS 2 (34%)	34%				
Tetraplegia: MAS 2 (34%)	Partial sensory loss	64%			
Tetraplegia: MAS 2 (34%)	Partial sensory loss	Reflex bladder (25%)	73%		
Tetraplegia: MAS 2 (34%)	Partial sensory loss	Reflex bladder (25%)	Constipation Class 2 (10%)	76%	
Tetraplegia: MAS 2 (34%)	Partial sensory loss	Reflex bladder (25%)	Constipation Class 2 (10%)	Erectile dysfunction, infertility (15% + 15%)	83%
Tetraplegia: MAS 2 (34%)	Partial sensory loss	Reflex bladder (25%)	Constipation Class 2 (10%)	Erectile dysfunction, infertility (15% + 15%)	Bilateral equinus deformity (2% + 2%)	84%

Table 23.56 SCI C3 and/or C4 Tetraplegia: MAS 3, bladder dyssynergia, constipation

Tetraplegia: MAS 3 (40%)	40%				
Tetraplegia: MAS 3 (40%)	Complete sensory loss	84%			
Tetraplegia: MAS 3 (40%)	Complete sensory loss	Bladder dyssynergia (37%)	90%		
Tetraplegia: MAS 3 (40%)	Complete sensory loss	Bladder dyssynergia (37%)	Constipation Class 3 (15%)	91%	
Tetraplegia: MAS 3 (40%)	Complete sensory loss	Bladder dyssynergia (37%)	Constipation Class 3 (15%)	Erectile dysfunction, infertility (15% + 15%)	94%
Tetraplegia: MAS 3 (40%)	Complete sensory loss	Bladder dyssynergia (37%)	Constipation Class 3 (15%)	Erectile dysfunction, infertility (15% + 15%)	Class 3 respiratory muscle paralysis (50%)	97%
Tetraplegia: MAS 3 (40%)	Complete sensory loss	Bladder dyssynergia (37%)	Constipation Class 3 (15%)	Erectile dysfunction, infertility (15% + 15%)	Class 3 respiratory muscle paralysis (50%), bilateral equinus deformity (2% + 2%)	97%

Table 23.57 SCI C3 and/or C4 Tetraplegia—MAS 4, incontinence of bladder

Tetraplegia: MAS 4 (45%)	45%					
Tetraplegia: MAS 4 (45%)	Complete sensory loss	85%				
Tetraplegia: MAS 4 (45%)	Complete sensory loss	Incontinence of bladder requiring catheterization (50%)	93%			
Tetraplegia: MAS 4 (45%)	Complete sensory loss	Incontinence of bladder requiring catheterization (50%)	Constipation Class 3 (15%)	94%		
Tetraplegia: MAS 4 (45%)	Complete sensory loss	Incontinence of bladder requiring catheterization (50%)	Constipation Class 3 (15%)	Erectile dysfunction, infertility (15% + 15%)	96%	
Tetraplegia: MAS 4 (45%)	Complete sensory loss	Incontinence of bladder requiring catheterization (50%)	Constipation Class 3 (15%)	Erectile dysfunction, infertility (15% + 15%)	Class 3 respiratory muscle paralysis (50%)	98%
Tetraplegia: MAS 4 (45%)	Complete sensory loss	Incontinence of bladder requiring catheterization (50%)	Constipation Class 3 (15%)	Erectile dysfunction, infertility (15% + 15%)	Respiratory muscle paralysis (50%), bilateral equinus deformity (2% + 2%)	98%

Table 23.58 SCI C5: Tetraplegia: MAS 1, 1+, urgency of micturition, constipation

Tetraplegia: MAS 1 (18%)	18%			
Tetraplegia: MAS 1 (18%)	Urgency of micturition (5%)	22%		
Tetraplegia: MAS 1+ (25%)	25%			
Tetraplegia: MAS 1+ (25%)	Partial sensory loss	59%		
Tetraplegia: MAS 1+ (25%)	Partial sensory loss	Urgency with incontinence (15%)	66%	
Tetraplegia: MAS 1+ (25%)	Partial sensory loss	Urgency with incontinence (15%)	Constipation Class 1 (5%)	67%

Table 23.59 SCI C5: Tetraplegia—MAS 2, reflex bladder, constipation

Tetraplegia: MAS 2 (34%)	34%				
Tetraplegia: MAS 2 (34%)	Partial sensory loss	64%			
Tetraplegia: MAS 2 (34%)	Partial sensory loss	Reflex bladder (25%)	73%		
Tetraplegia: MAS 2 (34%)	Partial sensory loss	Reflex bladder (25%)	Constipation Class 2 (10%)	76%	
Tetraplegia: MAS 2 (34%)	Partial sensory loss	Reflex bladder (25%)	Constipation Class 2 (10%)	Erectile dysfunction, infertility (15% + 15%)	83%
Tetraplegia: MAS 2 (34%)	Partial sensory loss	Reflex bladder (25%)	Constipation Class 2 (10%)	Erectile dysfunction, infertility (15% + 15%)	Bilateral equinus deformity (2% + 2%) 84%

Table 23.60 SCI C5: Tetraplegia—MAS 3, bladder dyssynergia, constipation

Tetraplegia: MAS 3 (39%)	39%				
Tetraplegia: MAS 3 (39%)	Complete sensory loss	84%			
Tetraplegia: MAS 3 (39%)	Complete sensory loss	Bladder dyssynergia requiring sphincter management (37%)	90%		
Tetraplegia: MAS 3 (39%)	Complete sensory loss	Bladder dyssynergia requiring sphincter management (37%)	Constipation Class 3 (15%)	91%	
Tetraplegia: MAS 3 (39%)	Complete sensory loss	Bladder dyssynergia requiring sphincter management (37%)	Constipation Class 3 (15%)	Erectile dysfunction, infertility (15% + 15%)	94%
Tetraplegia: MAS 3 (39%)	Complete sensory loss	Bladder dyssynergia requiring sphincter management (37%)	Constipation Class 3 (15%)	Erectile dysfunction, infertility (15% + 15%)	Bilateral equinus deformity (2% + 2%) 94%

Table 23.61 SCI C5: Tetraplegia—MAS 4, incontinence of bladder, constipation

Tetraplegia: MAS 4 (44%)	44%				
Tetraplegia: MAS 4 (44%)	Complete sensory loss	85%			
Tetraplegia: MAS 4 (44%)	Complete sensory loss	Incontinence of bladder requiring catheterization (50%)	93%		
Tetraplegia: MAS 4 (44%)	Complete sensory loss	Incontinence of bladder requiring catheterization (50%)	Constipation Class 3 (15%)	94%	
Tetraplegia: MAS 4 (44%)	Complete sensory loss	Incontinence of bladder requiring catheterization (50%)	Constipation Class 3 (15%)	Erectile dysfunction, infertility (15% + 15%)	96%
Tetraplegia: MAS 4 (44%)	Complete sensory loss	Incontinence of bladder requiring catheterization (50%)	Constipation Class 3 (15%)	Erectile dysfunction, infertility (15% + 15%)	Bilateral equinus deformity (2% + 2%) 96%

Table 23.62 SCI C6: Tetraplegia—MAS 1, 1+ and urgency of micturition, constipation

Tetraplegia: MAS 1 (18%)	18%			
Tetraplegia: MAS 1 (18%)	Urgency of micturition (5%)	22%		
Tetraplegia: MAS 1+ (24%)	24%			
Tetraplegia: MAS 1+ (24%)	Partial sensory loss	54%		
Tetraplegia: MAS 1+ (24%)	Partial sensory loss	Urgency with incontinence of bladder (15%)	61%	
Tetraplegia: MAS 1+ (24%)	Partial sensory loss	Urgency with incontinence of bladder (15%)	Constipation Class 1	63%

Table 23.63 SCI C6: Tetraplegia—MAS 2, reflex bladder, constipation

Tetraplegia: MAS 2 (33%)	33%				
Tetraplegia: MAS 2 (33%)	Partial sensory loss	59%			
Tetraplegia: MAS 2 (33%)	Partial sensory loss	Reflex bladder (25%)	69%		
Tetraplegia: MAS 2 (33%)	Partial sensory loss	Reflex bladder (25%)	Constipation Class 2 (10%)	72%	
Tetraplegia: MAS 2 (33%)	Partial sensory loss	Reflex bladder (25%)	Constipation Class 2 (10%)	Erectile dysfunction, infertility (15% + 15%)	81%
Tetraplegia: MAS 2 (33%)	Partial sensory loss	Reflex bladder (25%)	Constipation Class 2 (10%)	Erectile dysfunction, infertility (15% + 15%)	Bilateral equinus deformity (2% + 2%) 81%

Table 23.64 SCI C6: Tetraplegia—MAS 3, bladder dyssynergia, constipation

Tetraplegia: MAS 3 (38%)	38%				
Tetraplegia: MAS 3 (38%)	Complete sensory loss	78%			
Tetraplegia: MAS 3 (38%)	Complete sensory loss	Bladder dyssynergia requiring sphincter management (37%)	86%		
Tetraplegia: MAS 3 (38%)	Complete sensory loss	Bladder dyssynergia requiring sphincter management (37%)	Constipation Class 2 (10%)	88%	
Tetraplegia: MAS 3 (38%)	Complete sensory loss	Bladder dyssynergia requiring sphincter management (37%)	Constipation Class 2 (10%)	Erectile dysfunction, infertility (15% + 15%)	92%
Tetraplegia: MAS 3 (38%)	Complete sensory loss	Bladder dyssynergia requiring sphincter management (37%)	Constipation Class 2 (10%)	Erectile dysfunction, infertility (15% + 15%)	Bilateral equinus deformity and finger deformities (10%) 92%

Table 23.65 SCI C6—Tetraplegia: MAS 4, urgency of micturition, constipation

Tetraplegia: MAS 4 (43%)	43%					
Tetraplegia: MAS 4 (43%)	Complete sensory loss	80%				
Tetraplegia: MAS 4 (43%)	Complete sensory loss	Incontinence of bladder requiring catheterization (50%)	90%			
Tetraplegia: MAS 4 (43%)	Complete sensory loss	Incontinence of bladder requiring catheterization (50%)	Constipation Class 3 (15%)	91%		
Tetraplegia: MAS 4 (43%)	Complete sensory loss	Incontinence of bladder requiring catheterization (50%)	Constipation Class 3 (15%)	Erectile dysfunction, infertility (15% + 15%)	94%	
Tetraplegia: MAS 4 (43%)	Complete sensory loss	Incontinence of bladder requiring catheterization (50%)	Constipation Class 3 (15%)	Erectile dysfunction, infertility (15% + 15%)	Bilateral Equinus Deformity and Finger Deformities (10%)	94%

Table 23.66 SCI C7: Tetraplegia—MAS 1, 1+, urgency of micturition, constipation

Tetraplegia: MAS 1 (18%)	18%			
Tetraplegia: MAS 1 (18%)	Urgency of micturition (5%)	22%		
Tetraplegia: MAS 1+ (24%)	24%			
Tetraplegia: MAS 1+ (24%)	Partial sensory loss	49%		
Tetraplegia: MAS 1+ (24%)	Partial sensory loss	Urgency with incontinence of bladder (15%)	57%	
Tetraplegia: MAS 1+ (24%)	Partial sensory loss	Urgency with incontinence of bladder (15%)	Constipation Class 1 (5%)	59%

Table 23.67 SCI C7: Tetraplegia—MAS 2, reflex bladder, constipation

Tetraplegia: MAS 2 (32%)	32%				
Tetraplegia: MAS 2 (32%)	Partial sensory loss	55%			
Tetraplegia: MAS 2 (32%)	Partial sensory loss	Reflex bladder (25%)	66%		
Tetraplegia: MAS 2 (32%)	Partial sensory loss	Reflex bladder (25%)	Constipation Class 2 (10%)	69%	
Tetraplegia: MAS 2 (32%)	Partial sensory loss	Reflex bladder (25%)	Constipation Class 2 (10%)	Erectile dysfunction, infertility (15% + 15%)	79%
Tetraplegia: MAS 2 (32%)	Partial sensory loss	Reflex bladder (25%)	Constipation Class 2 (10%)	Erectile dysfunction, infertility (15% + 15%)	Bilateral equinus deformity (2% + 2%)	79%

Table 23.68 SCI C7: Tetraplegia—MAS 3, bladder dyssynergia, constipation

Tetraplegia: MAS 3 (37%)	37%					
Tetraplegia: MAS 3 (37%)	Complete sensory loss	73%				
Tetraplegia: MAS 3 (37%)	Complete sensory loss	DSD requiring sphincter management (37%)	83%			
Tetraplegia: MAS 3 (37%)	Complete sensory loss	DSD requiring sphincter management (37%)	Constipation Class 3 (15%)	85%		
Tetraplegia: MAS 3 (37%)	Complete sensory loss	DSD requiring sphincter management (37%)	Constipation Class 3 (15%)	Erectile dysfunction, infertility (15% + 15%)	90%	
Tetraplegia: MAS 3 (37%)	Complete sensory loss	DSD requiring sphincter management (37%)	Constipation Class 3 (15%)	Erectile dysfunction, infertility (15% + 15%)	Bilateral equinus deformity and finger deformities (10%)	91%

Table 23.69 SCI C7: Tetraplegia—MAS 4, incontinence of bladder, constipation

Tetraplegia: MAS 4 (41%)	41%					
Tetraplegia: MAS 4 (41%)	Complete sensory loss	75%				
Tetraplegia: MAS 4 (41%)	Complete sensory loss	Incontinence of bladder requiring catheter (50%)	87%			
Tetraplegia: MAS 4 (41%)	Complete sensory loss	Incontinence of bladder requiring catheter (50%)	Constipation Class 3 (15%)	89%		
Tetraplegia: MAS 4 (41%)	Complete sensory loss	Incontinence of bladder requiring catheter (50%)	Constipation Class 3 (15%)	Erectile dysfunction, infertility (15% + 15%)	92%	
Tetraplegia: MAS 4 (41%)	Complete sensory loss	Incontinence of bladder requiring catheter (50%)	Constipation Class 3 (15%)	Erectile dysfunction, infertility (15% + 15%)	Bilateral equinus deformity and finger deformities (10%)	93%

Table 23.70 SCI C8: Tetraplegia—MAS 1, 1+, urgency of micturition, constipation

Tetraplegia: MAS 1 (13%)	13%			
Tetraplegia: MAS 1 (13%)	Urgency of micturition (5%)	18%		
Tetraplegia: MAS 1+ (18%)	18%			
Tetraplegia: MAS 1+ (18%)	Partial sensory loss	40%		
Tetraplegia: MAS 1+ (18%)	Partial sensory loss	Urgency with incontinence of micturition	49%	
Tetraplegia: MAS 1+ (18%)	Partial sensory loss	Urgency with incontinence of micturition	Constipation Class 1 (5%)	52%

Table 23.71 SCI C8: Tetraplegia—MAS 2, reflex bladder, constipation

Tetraplegia: MAS 2 (24%)	24%					
Tetraplegia: MAS 2 (24%)	Partial sensory loss	45%				
Tetraplegia: MAS 2 (24%)	Partial sensory loss	Reflex bladder (25%)	59%			
Tetraplegia: MAS 2 (24%)	Partial sensory loss	Reflex bladder (25%)	Constipation Class 2 (10%)	63%		
Tetraplegia: MAS 2 (24%)	Partial sensory loss	Reflex bladder (25%)	Constipation Class 2 (10%)	Erectile dysfunction, infertility (15% + 15%)	74%	
Tetraplegia: MAS 2 (24%)	Partial sensory loss	Reflex bladder (25%)	Constipation Class 2 (10%)	Erectile dysfunction, infertility (15% + 15%)	Bilateral equinus deformity (2% + 2%)	75%

Table 23.72 SCI C8: Tetraplegia—MAS 3, bladder dyssynergia, constipation

Tetraplegia: MAS 3 (29%)	29%					
Tetraplegia: MAS 3 (29%)	Complete sensory loss	64%				
Tetraplegia: MAS 3 (29%)	Complete sensory loss	DSD requiring sphincter management (37%)	77%			
Tetraplegia: MAS 3 (29%)	Complete sensory loss	Bladder dyssynergia requiring sphincter management (37%)	Constipation Class 3 (15%)	80%		
Tetraplegia: MAS 3 (29%)	Complete sensory loss	Bladder dyssynergia requiring sphincter management (37%)	Constipation Class 3 (15%)	Erectile dysfunction, infertility (15% + 15%)	86%	
Tetraplegia: MAS 3 (29%)	Complete sensory loss	Bladder dyssynergia requiring sphincter management (37%)	Constipation Class 3 (15%)	Erectile dysfunction, infertility (15% + 15%)	Bilateral equinus deformity and finger deformities (10%)	87%

Table 23.73 SCI C8: Tetraplegia—MAS 4, incontinence of bladder, constipation

Tetraplegia: MAS 4 (32%)	32%					
Tetraplegia: MAS 4 (32%)	Complete sensory loss	65%				
Tetraplegia: MAS 4 (32%)	Complete sensory loss	Incontinence of bladder requiring catheterization (50%)	83%			
Tetraplegia: MAS 4 (32%)	Complete sensory loss	Incontinence of bladder requiring catheterization (50%)	Constipation Class 3 (15%)	85%		
Tetraplegia: MAS 4 (32%)	Complete sensory loss	Incontinence of bladder requiring catheterization (50%)	Constipation Class 3 (15%)	Erectile dysfunction, infertility (15% + 15%)	90%	
Tetraplegia: MAS 4 (32%)	Complete sensory loss	Incontinence of bladder requiring catheterization (50%)	Constipation Class 3 (15%)	Erectile dysfunction, infertility (15% + 15%)	Bilateral equinus deformity and finger deformities (10%)	90%

Table 23.74 SCI T1: Tetraplegia—MAS 1, 1+ urgency of micturition, constipation

Tetraplegia: MAS 1 (12%)	12%			
Tetraplegia: MAS 1 (12%)	Urgency of micturition (5%)	16%		
Tetraplegia: MAS 1+ (16%)	16%			
Tetraplegia: MAS 1+ (16%)	Partial sensory loss	37%		
Tetraplegia: MAS 1+ (16%)	Partial sensory loss	Urgency incontinence (15%)	47%	
Tetraplegia: MAS 1+ (16%)	Partial sensory loss	Urgency incontinence (15%)	Constipation Class 1 (5%)	49%

Table 23.75 SCI T1: Tetraplegia—MAS 2, reflex bladder, constipation

Tetraplegia: MAS 2 (22%)	22%				
Tetraplegia: MAS 2 (22%)	Partial sensory loss	41%			
Tetraplegia: MAS 2 (22%)	Partial sensory loss	Reflex bladder (25%)	56%		
Tetraplegia: MAS 2 (22%)	Partial sensory loss	Reflex bladder (25%)	Constipation Class 2 (10%)	61%	
Tetraplegia: MAS 2 (22%)	Partial sensory loss	Reflex bladder (25%)	Constipation Class 2 (10%)	Erectile dysfunction, infertility (15% + 15%)	72%
Tetraplegia: MAS 2 (22%)	Partial sensory loss	Reflex bladder (25%)	Constipation Class 2 (10%)	Erectile dysfunction, infertility (15% + 15%)	Bilateral equinus deformity (2% + 2%) 73%

Table 23.76 SCI T1: Tetraplegia—MAS 3, bladder dyssynergia (DSD), constipation

Tetraplegia: MAS 3 (25%)	25%					
Tetraplegia: MAS 3 (25%)	Complete sensory loss	59%				
Tetraplegia: MAS 3 (25%)	Complete sensory loss	Bladder dyssynergia (DSD) (37%)	74%			
Tetraplegia: MAS 3 (25%)	Complete sensory loss	Bladder dyssynergia (DSD) (37%)	Constipation Class 3 (15%)	78%		
Tetraplegia: MAS 3 (25%)	Complete sensory loss	Bladder dyssynergia (DSD) (37%)	Constipation Class 3 (15%)	Erectile dysfunction, infertility (15% + 15%)	85%	
Tetraplegia: MAS 3 (25%)	Complete sensory loss	Bladder dyssynergia (DSD) (37%)	Constipation Class 3 (15%)	Erectile dysfunction, infertility (15% + 15%)	Bilateral equinus deformity and finger deformities (10%)	85%

Table 23.77 SCI T1: Tetraplegia—MAS 4, bladder incontinence, constipation

Tetraplegia: MAS 4 (27%)	27%					
Tetraplegia: MAS 4 (27%)	Complete sensory loss	60%				
Tetraplegia: MAS 4 (27%)	Complete sensory loss	Incontinence of bladder requiring catheterization (50%)	80%			
Tetraplegia: MAS 4 (27%)	Complete sensory loss	Incontinence of bladder requiring catheterization (50%)	Constipation Class 3 (15%)	83%		
Tetraplegia: MAS 4 (27%)	Complete sensory loss	Incontinence of bladder requiring catheterization (50%)	Constipation Class 3 (15%)	Erectile dysfunction, infertility (15% + 15%)	88%	
Tetraplegia: MAS 4 (27%)	Complete sensory loss	Incontinence of bladder requiring catheterization (50%)	Constipation Class 3 (15%)	Erectile dysfunction, infertility (15% + 15%)	Bilateral equinus deformity and finger deformities (10%)	89%

23.9 READY RECKONER—SCI: DORSAL CORD

Table 23.78 SCI D4 Paraplegia: MAS 1, 1+, partial sensory loss, urgency of micturition

Paraplegia MAS 1 (9%)	9%			
Paraplegia MAS 1 (9%)	Urgency of micturition (5%)	14%		
Paraplegia MAS 1+ (14%)	14%			
Paraplegia MAS 1+ (14%)	Partial sensory loss	34%		
Paraplegia MAS 1+ (14%)	Partial sensory loss	Urgency incontinence (15%)	44%	
Paraplegia MAS 1+ (14%)	Partial sensory loss	Urgency incontinence (15%)	Constipation Class 1 (5%)	47%

Table 23.79 SCI D4 Paraplegia: MAS 2, partial sensory loss, reflex bladder

Paraplegia MAS 2 (19%)	19%				
Paraplegia MAS 2 (19%)	Partial sensory loss	38%			
Paraplegia MAS 2 (19%)	Partial sensory loss	Reflex bladder (25%)	53%		
Paraplegia MAS 2 (19%)	Partial sensory loss	Reflex bladder (25%)	Constipation Class 2 (10%)	58%	
Paraplegia MAS 2 (19%)	Partial sensory loss	Reflex bladder (25%)	Constipation Class 2 (10%)	Erectile dysfunction and infertility (15% + 15%)	71%
Paraplegia MAS 2 (19%)	Partial sensory loss	Reflex bladder (25%)	Constipation Class 2 (10%)	Erectile dysfunction and infertility (15% + 15%), bilateral equinus deformity	72%

Table 23.80 SCI D4 Paraplegia: MAS 3, complete sensory loss, bladder dyssynergia

Paraplegia MAS 3 (23%)	23%				
Paraplegia MAS 3 (23%)	Complete sensory loss	56%			
Paraplegia MAS 3 (23%)	Complete sensory loss	Bladder dyssynergia (37%)	72%		
Paraplegia MAS 3 (23%)	Complete sensory loss	Bladder dyssynergia (37%)	Constipation Class 3 (15%)	76%	
Paraplegia MAS 3 (23%)	Complete sensory loss	Bladder dyssynergia (37%)	Constipation Class 3 (15%)	Erectile dysfunction (15%), infertility (15%)	83%
Paraplegia MAS 3 (23%)	Complete sensory loss	Bladder dyssynergia (37%)	Constipation Class 3 (15%)	Erectile dysfunction (15%), infertility (15%), bilateral equinus deformity (4%)	84%

Table 23.81 SCI D4 Paraplegia: MAS 4, complete sensory loss, bladder dyssynergia

Paraplegia MAS 4 (26%)	26%				
Paraplegia MAS 4 (26%)	Complete sensory loss	58%			
Paraplegia MAS 4 (26%)	Complete sensory loss	Incontinence of bladder requiring catheterization (50%)	79%		
Paraplegia MAS 4 (26%)	Complete sensory loss	Incontinence of bladder requiring catheterization (50%)	Constipation Class 3 (15%)	82%	
Paraplegia MAS 4 (26%)	Complete sensory loss	Incontinence of bladder requiring catheterization (50%)	Constipation Class 3 (15%)	Erectile dysfunction (15%), infertility (15%)	87%
Paraplegia MAS 4 (26%)	Complete sensory loss	Incontinence of bladder requiring catheterization (50%)	Constipation Class 3 (15%)	Erectile dysfunction (15%), infertility (15%), bilateral equinus deformity (4%)	88%

Table 23.82 SCI D7 Paraplegia: MAS 1, 1+, urgency of micturition

Paraplegia MAS 1 (9%)	9%			
Paraplegia MAS 1 (9%)	Urgency of micturition (5%)	14%		
Paraplegia MAS 1+ (13%)	13%			
Paraplegia MAS 1+ (13%)	Partial sensory loss	32%		
Paraplegia MAS 1+ (13%)	Partial sensory loss	Urgency incontinence (15%)	42%	
Paraplegia MAS 1+ (13%)	Partial sensory loss	Urgency incontinence (15%)	Constipation Class 1 (5%)	45%

Table 23.83 SCI D7 Paraplegia: MAS 2, partial sensory loss, reflex bladder

Paraplegia MAS 2 (17%)	17%			
Paraplegia MAS 2 (17%)	Partial sensory loss	36%		
Paraplegia MAS 2 (17%)	Partial sensory loss	Reflex bladder (25%)	52%	
Paraplegia MAS 2 (17%)	Partial sensory loss	Reflex bladder (25%)	Constipation Class 2 (10%)	57%
Paraplegia MAS 2 (17%)	Partial sensory loss	Reflex bladder (25%)	Constipation Class 2 (10%)	Erectile dysfunction (15%), infertility (15%)	70%
				Erectile dysfunction (15%), infertility (15%), bilateral equinus deformity (4%)	71%

Table 23.84 SCI D7 Paraplegia: MAS 3, complete sensory loss, bladder dyssynergia

Paraplegia MAS 3 (23%)	23%			
Paraplegia MAS 3 (23%)	Complete sensory loss	54%		
Paraplegia MAS 3 (23%)	Complete sensory loss	Bladder dyssynergia (37%)	71%	
Paraplegia MAS 3 (23%)	Complete sensory loss	Bladder dyssynergia (37%)	Constipation Class 3 (15%)	75%
Paraplegia MAS 3 (23%)	Complete sensory loss	Bladder dyssynergia (37%)	Constipation Class 3 (15%)	Erectile dysfunction (15%), infertility (15%)	83%
Paraplegia MAS 3 (23%)	Complete sensory loss	Bladder dyssynergia (37%)	Constipation Class 3 (15%)	Erectile dysfunction (15%), infertility (15%), bilateral equinus deformity (4%)	83%

Table 23.85 SCI D7 Paraplegia: MAS 4, complete sensory loss, bladder incontinence

Paraplegia MAS 4 (26%)	26%			
Paraplegia MAS 4 (26%)	Complete sensory loss	56%		
Paraplegia MAS 4 (26%)	Complete sensory loss	Incontinence of bladder requiring catheterization (50%)	78%	
Paraplegia MAS 4 (26%)	Complete sensory loss	Incontinence of bladder requiring catheterization (50%)	Constipation Class 3 (15%)	81%
Paraplegia MAS 4 (26%)	Complete sensory loss	Incontinence of bladder requiring catheterization (50%)	Constipation Class 3 (15%)	Erectile dysfunction (15%), infertility (15%)	87%
Paraplegia MAS 4 (26%)	Complete sensory loss	Incontinence of bladder requiring catheterization (50%)	Constipation Class 3 (15%)	Erectile dysfunction (15%), infertility (15%), bilateral equinus deformity (4%)	87%

Table 23.86 SCI D10 Paraplegia: MAS 1, 1+ urgency of micturition

Paraplegia MAS 1 (9%)	9%			
Paraplegia MAS 1 (9%)	Urgency of micturition (5%)	14%		
Paraplegia MAS 1+ (14%)	14%			
Paraplegia MAS 1+ (14%)	Partial sensory loss	32%		
Paraplegia MAS 1+ (14%)	Partial sensory loss	Urgency incontinence (15%)	42%	
Paraplegia MAS 1+ (14%)	Partial sensory loss	Urgency incontinence (15%)	Constipation Class 1 (5%)	45%

Table 23.87 SCI D10 Paraplegia: MAS 2, partial sensory loss, reflex bladder

Paraplegia MAS 2 (19%)	19%			
Paraplegia MAS 2 (19%)	Partial sensory loss	35%		
Paraplegia MAS 2 (19%)	Partial sensory loss	Reflex bladder (25%)	51%	
Paraplegia MAS 2 (19%)	Partial sensory loss	Reflex bladder (25%)	Constipation Class 2 (10%)	56%
Paraplegia MAS 2 (19%)	Partial sensory loss	Reflex bladder (25%)	Constipation Class 2 (10%)	Erectile dysfunction (15%), infertility (15%)	69%
Paraplegia MAS 2 (19%)	Partial sensory loss	Reflex bladder (25%)	Constipation Class 2 (10%)	Erectile dysfunction (15%), infertility (15%), bilateral equinus deformity (4%)	71%

Table 23.88 SCI D10 Paraplegia: MAS 3, complete sensory loss, bladder dyssynergia

Paraplegia MAS 3 (23%)	23%			
Paraplegia MAS 3 (23%)	Complete sensory loss	52%		
Paraplegia MAS 3 (23%)	Complete sensory loss	Bladder dyssynergia (37%)	70%	
Paraplegia MAS 3 (23%)	Complete sensory loss	Bladder dyssynergia (37%)	Constipation Class 3 (15%)	74%
Paraplegia MAS 3 (23%)	Complete sensory loss	Bladder dyssynergia (37%)	Constipation Class 3 (15%)	Erectile dysfunction (15%), infertility (15%)	82%
Paraplegia MAS 3 (23%)	Complete sensory loss	Bladder dyssynergia (37%)	Constipation Class 3 (15%)	Erectile dysfunction (15%), infertility (15%), bilateral equinus deformity (4%)	83%

Table 23.89 SCI D10 Paraplegia: MAS 4, complete sensory loss, bladder incontinence

Paraplegia MAS 4 (26%)	26%			
Paraplegia MAS 4 (26%)	Complete sensory loss	54%		
Paraplegia MAS 4 (26%)	Complete sensory loss	Incontinence of bladder requiring catheterization (50%)	77%	
Paraplegia MAS 4 (26%)	Complete sensory loss	Incontinence of bladder requiring catheterization (50%)	Constipation Class 3 (15%)	80%
Paraplegia MAS 4 (26%)	Complete sensory loss	Incontinence of bladder requiring Catheterization (50%)	Constipation Class 3 (15%)	Erectile dysfunction (15%), Infertility (15%)	86%
Paraplegia MAS 4 (26%)	Complete sensory loss	Incontinence of bladder requiring catheterization (50%)	Constipation Class 3 (15%)	Erectile dysfunction (15%), infertility (15%), bilateral equinus deformity (4%)	87%

Table 23.90 SCI D12 Paraplegia: MAS 1, 1+ urgency of micturition

Paraplegia MAS 1 (9%)	9%		
Paraplegia MAS 1 (9%)	Urgency of micturition (5%)	13%	
Paraplegia MAS 1+ (13%)	13%		
Paraplegia MAS 1+ (13%)	Partial sensory loss	30%	
Paraplegia MAS 1+ (13%)	Partial sensory loss	Urgency with incontinence (15%)	40%
Paraplegia MAS 1+ (13%)	Partial sensory loss	Urgency with incontinence (15%)	Constipation Class 2 (10%)	43%

Table 23.91 SCI D12 Paraplegia: MAS 2, reflex bladder, Class 3 constipation

Paraplegia MAS 2 (17%)	17%				
Paraplegia MAS 2 (17%)	Partial sensory loss	33%			
Paraplegia MAS 2 (17%)	Partial sensory loss	Reflex bladder (25%)	50%		
Paraplegia MAS 2 (17%)	Partial sensory loss	Reflex bladder (25%)	Constipation Class 3 (15%)	55%	
Paraplegia MAS 2 (17%)	Partial sensory loss	Reflex bladder (25%)	Constipation Class 3 (15%)	Erectile dysfunction (15%), infertility (15%)	68%
Paraplegia MAS 2 (17%)	Partial sensory loss	Reflex bladder (25%)	Constipation Class 3 (15%)	Erectile dysfunction (15%), infertility (15%), bilateral equinus deformity (4%)	70%

Table 23.92 SCI D12 Paraplegia: MAS 3, complete sensory loss, bladder dyssynergia

Paraplegia MAS 3 (21%)	21%				
Paraplegia MAS 3 (21%)	Complete sensory loss	49%			
Paraplegia MAS 3 (21%)	Complete sensory loss	Bladder dyssynergia (37%)	68%		
Paraplegia MAS 3 (21%)	Complete sensory loss	Bladder dyssynergia (37%)	Constipation Class 3	73%	
Paraplegia MAS 3 (21%)	Complete sensory loss	Bladder dyssynergia (37%)	Constipation Class 3 (15%)	Erectile dysfunction (15%), infertility (15%)	81%
Paraplegia MAS 3 (21%)	Complete sensory loss	Bladder dyssynergia (37%)	Constipation Class 3 (15%)	Erectile dysfunction (15%), infertility (15%), bilateral equinus deformity (4%)	82%

Table 23.93 SCI D12 Paraplegia: MAS 4, complete sensory loss, bladder incontinence

Paraplegia MAS 4 (24%)	24%				
Paraplegia MAS 4 (24%)	Complete sensory loss	51%			
Paraplegia MAS 4 (24%)	Complete sensory loss	Incontinence of bladder requiring catheterization (50%)	76%		
Paraplegia MAS 4 (24%)	Complete sensory loss	Incontinence of bladder requiring catheterization (50%)	Constipation Class 3 (15%)	79%	
Paraplegia MAS 4 (24%)	Complete sensory loss	Incontinence of bladder requiring catheterization (50%)	Constipation Class 3 (15%)	Erectile dysfunction (15%), infertility (15%)	86%
Paraplegia MAS 4 (24%)	Complete sensory loss	Incontinence of bladder requiring catheterization (50%)	Constipation Class 3 (15%)	Erectile dysfunction (15%), infertility (15%), bilateral equinus deformity (4%)	86%

23.10 READY RECKONER—SCI: CENTRAL CORD SYNDROME

Table 23.94 Central cord syndrome C4: Tetraplegia, sensory impairment-sacral sparing

Upper extremity: MAS 2 Lower extremity: MAS 1 (26%)	26%			
Upper extremity: MAS 2 Lower extremity: MAS 1 (26%)	Sensory impairment with sacral sparing	56%		
Upper extremity: MAS 3 Lower extremity: MAS 1+ (35%)	35%			
Upper extremity: MAS 3 Lower extremity: MAS 1+ (35%)	Sensory impairment with sacral sparing	79%		
Upper extremity: MAS 3 Lower extremity: MAS 1+ (35%)	Sensory impairment with sacral sparing	Retention of urine (50%)	89%	
Upper extremity: MAS 3 Lower extremity: MAS 1+ (35%)	Sensory impairment with sacral sparing	Retention of urine (50%)	Constipation Class 3 (15%)	91%

Table 23.95 Central cord syndrome C5: Tetraplegia, sensory impairment-sacral sparing

Upper extremity: MAS 2 Lower extremity: MAS 1 (25%)	25%			
Upper extremity: MAS 2 Lower extremity: MAS 1 (25%)	Sensory impairment with sacral sparing	56%		
Upper extremity: MAS 3 Lower extremity: MAS 1+ (33%)	33%			
Upper extremity: MAS 3 Lower extremity: MAS 1+ (33%)	Sensory impairment with sacral sparing	75%		
Upper extremity: MAS 3 Lower extremity: MAS 1+ (33%)	Sensory impairment with sacral sparing	Retention of urine (50%)	88%	
Upper extremity: MAS 3 Lower extremity: MAS 1+ (33%)	Sensory impairment with sacral sparing	Retention of urine (50%)	Constipation Class 3 (15%)	89%

Table 23.96 Central cord syndrome C6: Tetraplegia, sensory impairment-sacral sparing

Upper extremity: MAS 2 Lower extremity: MAS 1 (23%)	23%			
Upper extremity: MAS 2 Lower extremity: MAS 1 (23%)	Sensory impairment with sacral sparing	48%		
Upper extremity: MAS 3 Lower extremity: MAS 1+ (33%)	33%			
Upper extremity: MAS 3 Lower extremity: MAS 1+ (33%)	Sensory impairment with sacral sparing	65%		
Upper extremity: MAS 3 Lower extremity: MAS 1+ (33%)	Sensory impairment with sacral sparing	Retention of urine (50%)	83%	
Upper extremity: MAS 3 Lower extremity: MAS 1+ (33%)	Sensory impairment with sacral sparing	Retention of urine (50%)	Constipation Class 3 (15%)	85%

Table 23.97 Central cord syndrome C7: Tetraplegia, sensory impairment-sacral sparing

Upper extremity: MAS 2 Lower extremity: MAS 1 (24%)	24%			
Upper extremity: MAS 2 Lower extremity: MAS 1 (24%)	Sensory impairment with sacral sparing	44%		
Upper extremity: MAS 3 Lower extremity: MAS 1+ (31%)	31%			
Upper extremity: MAS 3 Lower extremity: MAS 1+ (31%)	Sensory impairment with sacral sparing	59%		
Upper extremity: MAS 3 Lower extremity: MAS 1+ (31%)	Sensory impairment with sacral sparing	Retention of urine (50%)	79%	
Upper extremity: MAS 3 Lower extremity: MAS 1+ (31%)	Sensory impairment with sacral sparing	Retention of urine (50%)	Constipation Class 3 (15%)	82%

23.11 READY RECKONER—ANTERIOR CORD SYNDROME

Table 23.98 Anterior cord lesion D4 paraplegia: MAS 1, 1+, 2 sparing of dorsal column, micturition dysfunction

Paraplegia MAS 1	9%			
Paraplegia MAS 1	Urgency of micturition (5%)	14%		
Paraplegia MAS 1+	14%			
Paraplegia MAS 1+	Partial sensory loss with sparing of dorsal column	34%		
Paraplegia MAS 1+	Partial sensory loss with sparing of dorsal column	Urgency incontinence of bladder (15%)	44%	
Paraplegia MAS 1+	Partial sensory loss with sparing of dorsal column	Urgency incontinence of bladder (15%)	Constipation Class 1 (5%)	47%
Paraplegia MAS 2	18%			
Paraplegia MAS 2	Partial sensory loss with sparing of dorsal column	38%		
Paraplegia MAS 2	Partial sensory loss with sparing of dorsal column	Reflex bladder (25%)	53%	
Paraplegia MAS 2	Partial sensory loss with sparing of dorsal column	Reflex bladder (25%)	Constipation Class 2 (10%)	58%

Table 23.99 Anterior cord lesion D4 paraplegia: MAS 3, sparing of dorsal column, micturition dysfunction, erectile dysfunction

Paraplegia MAS 3	22%				
Paraplegia MAS 3	Partial sensory loss with sparing of dorsal column	40%			
Paraplegia MAS 3	Partial sensory loss with sparing of dorsal column	Bladder dyssynergia (37%)	62%		
Paraplegia MAS 3	Partial sensory loss with sparing of dorsal column	Bladder dyssynergia (37%)	Constipation Class 3 (15%)	68%	
Paraplegia MAS 3	Partial sensory loss with sparing of dorsal column	Bladder dyssynergia (37%)	Constipation Class 3 (15%)	Erectile dysfunction and infertility (30%)	78%

Table 23.100 Anterior cord lesion D4 paraplegia: MAS 4, sparing of dorsal column, micturition dysfunction, erectile dysfunction, bilateral equinus deformity

Paraplegia MAS 4	25%				
Paraplegia MAS 4	Partial sensory loss with sparing of dorsal column	43%			
Paraplegia MAS 4	Partial sensory loss with sparing of dorsal column	Incontinence of bladder requiring catheterization (50%)	71%		
Paraplegia MAS 4	Partial sensory loss with sparing of dorsal column	Incontinence of bladder requiring catheterization (50%)	Constipation Class 3 (15%)	76%	
Paraplegia MAS 4	Partial sensory loss with sparing of dorsal column	Incontinence of bladder requiring catheterization (50%)	Constipation Class 3 (15%)	Erectile dysfunction and infertility (30%)	83%
Paraplegia MAS 4	Partial sensory loss with sparing of dorsal column	Incontinence of bladder requiring catheterization (50%)	Constipation Class 3 (15%)	Erectile dysfunction and infertility (30%), bilateral equinus deformity (4%)	84%

Table 23.101 Anterior cord lesion D7 paraplegia: MAS 1, 1+, sparing of dorsal column, micturition dysfunction

Paraplegia MAS 1	9%			
Paraplegia MAS 1	Urgency of micturition (5%)	13%		
Paraplegia MAS 1+	13%			
Paraplegia MAS 1+	Partial sensory loss with sparing of dorsal column	32%		
Paraplegia MAS 1+	Partial sensory loss with sparing of dorsal column	Urgency incontinence of bladder (15%)	42%	
Paraplegia MAS 1+	Partial sensory loss with sparing of dorsal column	Urgency incontinence of bladder (15%)	Constipation Class 1 (5%)	45%

Table 23.102 Anterior cord lesion D7 paraplegia: MAS 2, sparing of dorsal column, micturition dysfunction, erectile dysfunction

Paraplegia MAS 2	17%			
Paraplegia MAS 2	Partial sensory loss with sparing of dorsal column	36%		
Paraplegia MAS 2	Partial sensory loss with sparing of dorsal column	Reflex bladder (25%)	52%	
Paraplegia MAS 2	Partial sensory loss with sparing of dorsal column	Reflex bladder (25%)	Constipation Class 2 (10%)	57%
Paraplegia MAS 2	Partial sensory loss with sparing of dorsal column	Reflex bladder (25%)	Constipation Class 2 (10%)	Erectile dysfunction and infertility (30%)	70%
Paraplegia MAS 2	Partial sensory loss with sparing of dorsal column	Reflex bladder (25%)	Constipation Class 2 (10%)	Erectile dysfunction and infertility (30%), bilateral equinus deformity (4%)	71%

Table 23.103 Anterior cord lesion D7 paraplegia: MAS 3, sparing of dorsal column, micturition dysfunction, erectile dysfunction

Paraplegia MAS 3	22%			
Paraplegia MAS 3	Partial sensory loss with sparing of dorsal column	39%		
Paraplegia MAS 3	Partial sensory loss with sparing of dorsal column	Bladder dyssynergia (37%)	61%	
Paraplegia MAS 3	Partial sensory loss with sparing of dorsal column	Bladder dyssynergia (37%)	Constipation Class 3 (15%)	68%
Paraplegia MAS 3	Partial sensory loss with sparing of dorsal column	Bladder dyssynergia (37%)	Constipation Class 3 (15%)	Erectile dysfunction and infertility (30%)	77%

Table 23.104 Anterior cord lesion D7 paraplegia: MAS 4, sparing of dorsal column, micturition dysfunction, erectile dysfunction

Paraplegia MAS 4	25%			
Paraplegia MAS 4	Partial sensory loss with sparing of dorsal column	41%		
Paraplegia MAS 4	Partial sensory loss with sparing of dorsal column	Incontinence of bladder requiring catheterization (50%)	71%	
Paraplegia MAS 4	Partial sensory loss with sparing of dorsal column	Incontinence of bladder requiring catheterization (50%)	Constipation Class 3 (15%)	75%
Paraplegia MAS 4	Partial sensory loss with sparing of dorsal column	Incontinence of bladder requiring catheterization (50%)	Constipation Class 3 (15%)	Erectile dysfunction and infertility (30%) 83%
Paraplegia MAS 4	Partial sensory loss with sparing of dorsal column	Incontinence of bladder requiring catheterization (50%)	Constipation Class 3 (15%)	Erectile dysfunction and infertility (30%), bilateral equinus deformity (4%) 83%

23.12 READY RECKONER—SCI: BROWN-SÉQUARD SYNDROME: CERVICAL SPINE

Table 23.105 Brown-Séquard C4, MAS 1+, urgency incontinence, and constipation

Ipsilateral motor loss: MAS 1+ (13%)	13%			
Ipsilateral motor loss: MAS 1+ (13%)	Ipsilateral proprioception, contralateral pain and temperature loss	53%		
Ipsilateral motor loss: MAS 1+ (13%)	Ipsilateral proprioception, contralateral pain and temperature loss	Urgency with incontinence of bladder (15%)	60%	
Ipsilateral motor loss: MAS 1+ (13%)	Ipsilateral proprioception, contralateral pain and temperature loss	Urgency with incontinence of bladder (15%)	Class 1 constipation (5%)	62%

Table 23.106 Brown-Séquard C4, MAS 2, reflex bladder and constipation

Ipsilateral motor loss: MAS 2 (17%)	17%			
Ipsilateral motor loss: MAS 2 (17%)	Ipsilateral proprioception, contralateral pain and temperature loss	55%		
Ipsilateral motor loss: MAS 2 (17%)	Ipsilateral proprioception, contralateral pain and temperature loss	Reflex bladder (25%)	66%	
Ipsilateral motor loss: MAS 2 (17%)	Ipsilateral proprioception, contralateral pain and temperature loss	Reflex bladder (25%)	Constipation Class 2 (10%)	70%

Table 23.107 Brown-Séquard C4, MAS 2, bladder dyssynergia, and constipation

Ipsilateral motor loss: MAS 3 (24%)	24%			
Ipsilateral motor loss: MAS 3 (24%)	Ipsilateral proprioception, contralateral pain and temperature loss	59%		
Ipsilateral motor loss: MAS 3 (24%)	Ipsilateral proprioception, contralateral pain and temperature loss	Bladder dyssynergia (37%)	74%	
Ipsilateral motor loss: MAS 3 (24%)	Ipsilateral proprioception, contralateral pain and temperature loss	Bladder dyssynergia (37%)	Constipation Class 3 (15%)	78%

Table 23.108 Brown-Séquard C4, MAS 4, incontinence of bladder, and constipation

Ipsilateral motor loss: MAS 4 (27%)	27%			
Ipsilateral motor loss: MAS 4 (27%)	Ipsilateral proprioception, contralateral pain and temperature loss	61%		
Ipsilateral motor loss: MAS 4 (27%)	Ipsilateral proprioception, contralateral pain and temperature loss	Incontinence of bladder requiring catheterization (50%)	81%	
Ipsilateral motor loss: MAS 4 (27%)	Ipsilateral proprioception, contralateral pain and temperature loss	Incontinence of bladder requiring catheterization (50%)	Constipation Class 3 (15%)	83%

Table 23.109 Brown-Séquard C5, MAS 1+, urgency incontinence, and constipation

Ipsilateral motor loss: MAS 1+ (13%)	13%			
Ipsilateral motor loss: MAS 1+ (13%)	Ipsilateral proprioception, contralateral pain and temperature loss	53%		
Ipsilateral motor loss: MAS 1+ (13%)	Ipsilateral proprioception, contralateral pain and temperature loss	Urgency incontinence of bladder (15%)	60%	
Ipsilateral motor loss: MAS 1+ (13%)	Ipsilateral proprioception, contralateral pain and temperature loss	Urgency incontinence of bladder (15%)	Constipation Class 1 (5%)	62%

Table 23.110 Brown-Séquard C5, MAS 2, reflex bladder, and constipation

Ipsilateral motor loss: MAS 2 (17%)	17%			
Ipsilateral motor loss: MAS 2 (17%)	Ipsilateral proprioception, contralateral pain and temperature loss	57%		
Ipsilateral motor loss: MAS 2 (17%)	Ipsilateral proprioception, contralateral pain and temperature loss	Reflex bladder (25%)	68%	
Ipsilateral motor loss: MAS 2 (17%)	Ipsilateral proprioception, contralateral pain and temperature loss	Reflex bladder (25%)	Constipation Class 2 (10%)	71%

Table 23.111 Brown-Séquard C5, MAS 3, bladder dyssynergia, and constipation

Ipsilateral motor loss: MAS 3 (24%)	24%			
Ipsilateral motor loss: MAS 3 (24%)	Ipsilateral proprioception, contralateral pain and temperature loss	59%		
Ipsilateral motor loss: MAS 3 (24%)	Ipsilateral proprioception, contralateral pain and temperature loss	Bladder dyssynergia (37%)	74%	
Ipsilateral motor loss: MAS 3 (24%)	Ipsilateral proprioception, contralateral pain and temperature loss	Bladder dyssynergia (37%)	Constipation Class 3 (15%)	78%

Table 23.112 Brown-Séquard C5, MAS 4, bladder incontinence and constipation

Ipsilateral motor loss: MAS 4 (27%)	27%			
Ipsilateral motor loss: MAS 4 (27%)	Ipsilateral proprioception, contralateral pain and temperature loss	61%		
Ipsilateral motor loss: MAS 4 (27%)	Ipsilateral proprioception, contralateral pain and temperature loss	Incontinence of bladder requiring catheterization (50%)	80%	
Ipsilateral motor loss: MAS 4 (27%)	Ipsilateral proprioception, contralateral pain and temperature loss	Incontinence of bladder requiring catheterization (50%)	Constipation Class 3 (15%)	83%

Table 23.113 Brown-Séquard C6, MAS 1+, urge incontinence—Bladder and constipation

Ipsilateral motor loss: MAS 1+ (13%)	13%			
Ipsilateral motor loss: MAS 1+ (13%)	Ipsilateral proprioception, contralateral pain and temperature loss	46%		
Ipsilateral motor loss: MAS 1+ (13%)	Ipsilateral proprioception, contralateral pain and temperature loss	Urgency incontinence of bladder (15%)	54%	
Ipsilateral motor loss: MAS 1+ (13%)	Ipsilateral proprioception, contralateral pain and temperature loss	Urgency incontinence of bladder (15%)	Constipation Class 1 (5%)	57%

Table 23.114 Brown-Séquard C6, MAS 2, reflex bladder—Bladder and constipation

Ipsilateral motor loss: MAS 2 (21%)	17%			
Ipsilateral motor loss: MAS 2 (21%)	Ipsilateral proprioception, contralateral pain and temperature loss	49%		
Ipsilateral motor loss: MAS 2 (21%)	Ipsilateral proprioception, contralateral pain and temperature loss	Reflex bladder (25%)	62%	
Ipsilateral motor loss: MAS 2 (21%)	Ipsilateral proprioception, contralateral pain and temperature loss	Reflex bladder (25%)	Constipation Class 2 (10%)	66%

Table 23.115 Brown-Séquard C6, MAS 3, bladder dyssynergia, and constipation

Ipsilateral motor loss: MAS 3 (23%)	23%			
Ipsilateral motor loss: MAS 3 (23%)	Ipsilateral proprioception, contralateral pain and temperature loss	53%		
Ipsilateral motor loss: MAS 3 (23%)	Ipsilateral proprioception, contralateral pain and temperature loss	Bladder dyssynergia (37%)	71%	
Ipsilateral motor loss: MAS 3 (23%)	Ipsilateral proprioception, contralateral pain and temperature loss	Bladder dyssynergia (37%)	Constipation Class 3 (15%)	75%

Table 23.116 Brown-Séquard C6, MAS 4, bladder incontinence and constipation

Ipsilateral motor loss: MAS 4 (26%)	26%			
Ipsilateral motor loss: MAS 4 (26%)	Ipsilateral proprioception, contralateral pain and temperature loss	55%		
Ipsilateral motor loss: MAS 4 (26%)	Ipsilateral proprioception, contralateral pain and temperature loss	Incontinence of bladder requiring catheterization (50%)	77%	
Ipsilateral motor loss: MAS 4 (26%)	Ipsilateral proprioception, contralateral pain and temperature loss	Incontinence of bladder requiring catheterization (50%)	Constipation Class 3 (15%)	81%

Table 23.117 Brown-Séquard C7, MAS 1+, urgency incontinence bladder, constipation

Ipsilateral motor loss: MAS 1+ (12%)	12%			
Ipsilateral motor loss: MAS 1+ (12%)	Ipsilateral proprioception, contralateral pain and temperature loss	41%		
Ipsilateral motor loss: MAS 1+ (12%)	Ipsilateral proprioception, contralateral pain and temperature loss	Urgency incontinence of bladder (15%)	50%	
Ipsilateral motor loss: MAS 1+ (12%)	Ipsilateral proprioception, contralateral pain and temperature loss	Urgency incontinence of bladder (15%)	Constipation Class 1 (5%)	53%

Table 23.118 Brown-Séquard C7, MAS 2, reflex bladder, constipation

Ipsilateral motor loss: MAS 2 (16%)	16%			
Ipsilateral motor loss: MAS 2 (16%)	Ipsilateral proprioception, contralateral pain and temperature loss	44%		
Ipsilateral motor loss: MAS 2 (16%)	Ipsilateral proprioception, contralateral pain and temperature loss	Reflex bladder (25%)	58%	
Ipsilateral motor loss: MAS 2 (16%)	Ipsilateral proprioception, contralateral pain and temperature loss	Reflex bladder (25%)	Constipation Class 2 (10%)	62%

Table 23.119 Brown-Séquard C7, MAS 3, bladder dyssynergia, constipation

Ipsilateral motor loss: MAS 3 (22%)	22%			
Ipsilateral motor loss: MAS 3 (22%)	Ipsilateral proprioception, contralateral pain and temperature loss	48%		
Ipsilateral motor loss: MAS 3 (22%)	Ipsilateral proprioception, contralateral pain and temperature loss	Bladder dyssynergia (37%)	67%	
Ipsilateral motor loss: MAS 3 (22%)	Ipsilateral proprioception, contralateral pain and temperature loss	Bladder dyssynergia (37%)	Constipation Class 3 (15%)	72%

Table 23.120 Brown-Séquard C7, MAS 4, incontinence bladder—Catheterization

Ipsilateral motor loss: MAS 4 (25%)	25%			
Ipsilateral motor loss: MAS 4 (25%)	Ipsilateral proprioception, contralateral pain and temperature loss	50%		
Ipsilateral motor loss: MAS 4 (25%)	Ipsilateral proprioception, contralateral pain and temperature loss	Incontinence of bladder requiring catheterization (50%)	75%	
Ipsilateral motor loss: MAS 4 (25%)	Ipsilateral proprioception, contralateral pain and temperature loss	Incontinence of bladder requiring catheterization (50%)	Constipation Class 3 (15%)	79%

Table 23.121 Brown-Séquard C8, MAS 1+, urgency incontinence of bladder

Ipsilateral motor loss: MAS 1+ (10%)	10%			
Ipsilateral motor loss: MAS 1+ (10%)	Ipsilateral proprioception, contralateral pain and temperature loss	35%		
Ipsilateral motor loss: MAS 1+ (10%)	Ipsilateral proprioception, contralateral pain and temperature loss	Urgency incontinence of bladder (15%)	44%	
Ipsilateral motor loss: MAS 1+ (10%)	Ipsilateral proprioception, contralateral pain and temperature loss	Urgency incontinence of bladder (15%)	Constipation Class 1 (5%)	47%

Table 23.122 Brown-Séquard C8, MAS 2, reflex bladder, constipation

Ipsilateral motor loss: MAS 2 (13%)	13%			
Ipsilateral motor loss: MAS 2 (13%)	Ipsilateral proprioception, contralateral pain and temperature loss	37%		
Ipsilateral motor loss: MAS 2 (13%)	Ipsilateral proprioception, contralateral pain and temperature loss	Reflex bladder (25%)	53%	
Ipsilateral motor loss: MAS 2 (13%)	Ipsilateral proprioception, contralateral pain and temperature loss	Reflex bladder (25%)	Constipation Class 2 (10%)	57%

Table 23.123 Brown-Séquard C8, MAS 3, bladder dyssynergia, constipation

Ipsilateral motor loss: MAS 3 (16%)	16%			
Ipsilateral motor loss: MAS 3 (16%)	Ipsilateral proprioception, contralateral pain and temperature loss	39%		
Ipsilateral motor loss: MAS 3 (16%)	Ipsilateral proprioception, contralateral pain and temperature loss	Bladder dyssynergia (37%)	62%	
Ipsilateral motor loss: MAS 3 (16%)	Ipsilateral proprioception, contralateral pain and temperature loss	Bladder dyssynergia (37%)	Constipation Class 3 (15%)	67%

Table 23.124 Brown-Séquard C8, MAS 4, incontinence of bladder—Catheterization

Ipsilateral motor loss: MAS 4 (19%)	19%			
Ipsilateral motor loss: MAS 4 (19%)	Ipsilateral proprioception, contralateral pain and temperature loss	41%		
Ipsilateral motor loss: MAS 4 (19%)	Ipsilateral proprioception, contralateral pain and temperature loss	Incontinence of bladder requiring catheterization (40%)	70%	
Ipsilateral motor loss: MAS 4 (19%)	Ipsilateral proprioception, contralateral pain and temperature loss	Incontinence of bladder requiring catheterization (40%)	Constipation Class 3 (15%)	75%

Table 23.125 Brown-Séquard T1, MAS 1+, urgency incontinence of bladder

Ipsilateral motor loss: MAS 1+ (9%)	9%			
Ipsilateral motor loss: MAS 1+ (9%)	Ipsilateral proprioception, contralateral pain and temperature loss	32%		
Ipsilateral motor loss: MAS 1+ (9%)	Ipsilateral proprioception, contralateral pain and temperature loss	Urgency incontinence of bladder (15%)	42%	
Ipsilateral motor loss: MAS 1+ (9%)	Ipsilateral proprioception, contralateral pain and temperature loss	Urgency incontinence of bladder (15%)	Constipation Class 1 (5%)	45%

Table 23.126 Brown-Séquard T1, MAS 2, reflex bladder, constipation

Ipsilateral motor loss: MAS 2 (12%)	12%			
Ipsilateral motor loss: MAS 2 (12%)	Ipsilateral proprioception, contralateral pain and temperature loss	34%		
Ipsilateral motor loss: MAS 2 (12%)	Ipsilateral proprioception, contralateral pain and temperature loss	Reflex bladder (25%)	50%	
Ipsilateral motor loss: MAS 2 (12%)	Ipsilateral proprioception, contralateral pain and temperature loss	Reflex bladder (25%)	Constipation Class 2 (10%)	55%

Table 23.127 Brown-Séquard T1, MAS 3, bladder dyssynergia, constipation

Ipsilateral motor loss: MAS 3 (14%)	14%			
Ipsilateral motor loss: MAS 3 (14%)	Ipsilateral proprioception, contralateral pain and temperature loss	36%		
Ipsilateral motor loss: MAS 3 (14%)	Ipsilateral proprioception, contralateral pain and temperature loss	Bladder dyssynergia (37%)	60%	
Ipsilateral motor loss: MAS 3 (14%)	Ipsilateral proprioception, contralateral pain and temperature loss	Bladder dyssynergia (37%)	Constipation Class 3 (15%)	66%

Table 23.128 Brown-Séquard T1, MAS 4, incontinence of bladder catheterization

Ipsilateral motor loss: MAS 4 (15%)	15%			
Ipsilateral motor loss: MAS 4 (15%)	Ipsilateral proprioception, contralateral pain and temperature loss	37%		
Ipsilateral motor loss: MAS 4 (15%)	Ipsilateral proprioception, contralateral pain and temperature loss	Incontinence of bladder requiring catheterization (50%)	68%	
Ipsilateral motor loss: MAS 4 (15%)	Ipsilateral proprioception, contralateral pain and temperature loss	Incontinence of bladder requiring catheterization (50%)	Constipation Class 3 (15%)	73%

23.13 READY RECKONER—SCI: BROWN-SÉQUARD SYNDROME: DORSAL SPINE

Table 23.129 Brown-Séquard T4, MAS 1+, urgency incontinence-bladder, constipation

Ipsilateral motor loss: MAS 1+ (8%)	8%			
Ipsilateral motor loss: MAS 1+ (8%)	Ipsilateral proprioception, contralateral pain and temperature loss	30%		
Ipsilateral motor loss: MAS 1+ (8%)	Ipsilateral proprioception, contralateral pain and temperature loss	Urgency incontinence of bladder (15%)	40%	
Ipsilateral motor loss: MAS 1+ (8%)	Ipsilateral proprioception, contralateral pain and temperature loss	Urgency incontinence of bladder (15%)	Constipation Class 1 (5%)	43%

Table 23.130 Brown-Séquard T4, MAS 2, reflex bladder, constipation

Ipsilateral motor loss: MAS 2 (10%)	10%			
Ipsilateral motor loss: MAS 2 (10%)	Ipsilateral proprioception, contralateral pain and temperature loss	33%		
Ipsilateral motor loss: MAS 2 (10%)	Ipsilateral proprioception, contralateral pain and temperature loss	Reflex bladder (25%)	49%	
Ipsilateral motor loss: MAS 2 (10%)	Ipsilateral proprioception, contralateral pain and temperature loss	Reflex bladder (25%)	Constipation Class 2 (10%)	54%

Table 23.131 Brown-Séquard T4, MAS 3, bladder dyssynergia, constipation

Ipsilateral motor loss: MAS 3 (13%)	13%			
Ipsilateral motor loss: MAS 3 (13%)	Ipsilateral proprioception, contralateral pain and temperature loss	33%		
Ipsilateral motor loss: MAS 3 (13%)	Ipsilateral proprioception, contralateral pain and temperature loss	Bladder dyssynergia (37%)	58%	
Ipsilateral motor loss: MAS 3 (13%)	Ipsilateral proprioception, contralateral pain and temperature loss	Bladder dyssynergia (37%)	Constipation Class 3 (15%)	64%

Table 23.132 Brown-Séquard T4, MAS 4, incontinence of bladder—Catheterization

Ipsilateral motor loss: MAS 4 (14%)	14%			
Ipsilateral motor loss: MAS 4 (14%)	Ipsilateral proprioception, contralateral pain and temperature loss	34%		
Ipsilateral motor loss: MAS 4 (14%)	Ipsilateral proprioception, contralateral pain and temperature loss	Incontinence of bladder requiring catheterization (50%)	67%	
Ipsilateral motor loss: MAS 4 (14%)	Ipsilateral proprioception, contralateral pain and temperature loss	Incontinence of bladder requiring catheterization (50%)	Constipation Class 3 (15%)	72%

Table 23.133 Brown-Séquard T7, MAS 1+, urgency incontinence bladder, constipation

Ipsilateral motor loss: MAS 1+ (7%)	7%			
Ipsilateral motor loss: MAS 1+ (7%)	Ipsilateral proprioception, contralateral pain and temperature loss	28%		
Ipsilateral motor loss: MAS 1+ (7%)	Ipsilateral proprioception, contralateral pain and temperature loss	Urgency incontinence of bladder (15%)	38%	
Ipsilateral motor loss: MAS 1+ (7%)	Ipsilateral proprioception, contralateral pain and temperature loss	Urgency incontinence of bladder (15%)	Constipation Class 1 (5%)	41%

Table 23.134 Brown-Séquard T7, MAS 2, reflex bladder, constipation

Ipsilateral motor loss: MAS 2 (11%)	9%			
Ipsilateral motor loss: MAS 2 (11%)	Ipsilateral proprioception, contralateral pain and temperature loss	29%		
Ipsilateral motor loss: MAS 2 (11%)	Ipsilateral proprioception, contralateral pain and temperature loss	Reflex bladder (25%)	47%	
Ipsilateral motor loss: MAS 2 (11%)	Ipsilateral proprioception, contralateral pain and temperature loss	Reflex bladder (25%)	Constipation Class 2 (10%)	52%

Table 23.135 Brown-Séquard T7, MAS 3, bladder dyssynergia, constipation

Ipsilateral motor loss: MAS 3 (12%)	12%			
Ipsilateral motor loss: MAS 3 (12%)	Ipsilateral proprioception, contralateral pain and temperature loss	31%		
Ipsilateral motor loss: MAS 3 (12%)	Ipsilateral proprioception, contralateral pain and temperature loss	Bladder dyssynergia (37%)	57%	
Ipsilateral motor loss: MAS 3 (12%)	Ipsilateral proprioception, contralateral pain and temperature loss	Bladder dyssynergia (37%)	Constipation Class 3 (15%)	63%

Table 23.136 Brown-Séquard T7, MAS 4, incontinence of bladder catheterization

Ipsilateral motor loss: MAS 4 (14%)	14%			
Ipsilateral motor loss: MAS 4 (14%)	Ipsilateral proprioception, contralateral pain and temperature loss	33%		
Ipsilateral motor loss: MAS 4 (14%)	Ipsilateral proprioception, contralateral pain and temperature loss	Incontinence of bladder requiring catheterization (50%)	66%	
Ipsilateral motor loss: MAS 4 (14%)	Ipsilateral proprioception, contralateral pain and temperature loss	Incontinence of bladder requiring catheterization (50%)	Constipation Class 3 (15%)	71%

Table 23.137 Brown-Séquard T10, MAS 1+, urgency incontinence-bladder, constipation

Ipsilateral motor loss: MAS 1+ (7%)	7%			
Ipsilateral motor loss: MAS 1+ (7%)	Ipsilateral proprioception, contralateral pain and temperature loss	25%		
Ipsilateral motor loss: MAS 1+ (7%)	Ipsilateral proprioception, contralateral pain and temperature loss	Urgency incontinence of bladder (15%)	37%	
Ipsilateral motor loss: MAS 1+ (7%)	Ipsilateral proprioception, contralateral pain and temperature loss	Urgency incontinence of bladder (15%)	Constipation Class 1 (5%)	40%

Table 23.138 Brown-Séquard T10, MAS 2, reflex bladder, constipation

Ipsilateral motor loss: MAS 2 (9%)	9%			
Ipsilateral motor loss: MAS 2 (9%)	Ipsilateral proprioception, contralateral pain and temperature loss	27%		
Ipsilateral motor loss: MAS 2 (9%)	Ipsilateral proprioception, contralateral pain and temperature loss	Reflex bladder (25%)	45%	
Ipsilateral motor loss: MAS 2 (9%)	Ipsilateral proprioception, contralateral pain and temperature loss	Reflex bladder (25%)	Constipation Class 2 (10%)	51%

Table 23.139 Brown-Séquard T10, MAS 3, bladder dyssynergia, constipation

Ipsilateral motor loss: MAS 3 (12%)	12%			
Ipsilateral motor loss: MAS 3 (12%)	Ipsilateral proprioception, contralateral pain and temperature loss	30%		
Ipsilateral motor loss: MAS 3 (12%)	Ipsilateral proprioception, contralateral pain and temperature loss	Bladder dyssynergia (37%)	56%	
Ipsilateral motor loss: MAS 3 (12%)	Ipsilateral proprioception, contralateral pain and temperature loss	Bladder dyssynergia (37%)	Constipation Class 3 (15%)	62%

Table 23.140 Brown-Séquard T10, MAS 4, incontinence of bladder on catheterization

Ipsilateral motor loss: MAS 4 (14%)	14%			
Ipsilateral motor loss: MAS 4 (14%)	Ipsilateral proprioception, contralateral pain and temperature loss	31%		
Ipsilateral motor loss: MAS 4 (14%)	Ipsilateral proprioception, contralateral pain and temperature loss	Incontinence of bladder requiring catheterization (50%)	65%	
Ipsilateral motor loss: MAS 4 (14%)	Ipsilateral proprioception, contralateral pain and temperature loss	Incontinence of bladder requiring catheterization (50%)	Constipation Class 3 (15%)	71%

Table 23.141 Brown-Séquard T12, MAS 1+, urgency incontinence bladder, constipation

Ipsilateral motor loss: MAS 1+ (6%)	6%			
Ipsilateral motor loss: MAS 1+ (6%)	Ipsilateral proprioception, contralateral pain and temperature loss	24%		
Ipsilateral motor loss: MAS 1+ (6%)	Ipsilateral proprioception, contralateral pain and temperature loss	Urgency incontinence of bladder (15%)	36%	
Ipsilateral motor loss: MAS 1+ (6%)	Ipsilateral proprioception, contralateral pain and temperature loss	Urgency incontinence of bladder (15%)	Constipation Class 1 (5%)	39%

Table 23.142 Brown-Séquard T12, MAS 2, reflex bladder, constipation

Ipsilateral motor loss: MAS 2 (10%)	10%			
Ipsilateral motor loss: MAS 2 (10%)	Ipsilateral proprioception, contralateral pain and temperature loss	27%		
Ipsilateral motor loss: MAS 2 (10%)	Ipsilateral proprioception, contralateral pain and temperature loss	Reflex bladder (25%)	45%	
Ipsilateral motor loss: MAS 2 (10%)	Ipsilateral proprioception, contralateral pain and temperature loss	Reflex bladder (25%)	Constipation Class 2 (10%)	51%

Table 23.143 Brown-Séquard T12, MAS 3, bladder dyssynergia, constipation

Ipsilateral motor loss: MAS 3 (12%)	12%			
Ipsilateral motor loss: MAS 3 (12%)	Ipsilateral proprioception, contralateral pain and temperature loss	29%		
Ipsilateral motor loss: MAS 3 (12%)	Ipsilateral proprioception, contralateral pain and temperature loss	Bladder dyssynergia (37%)	55%	
Ipsilateral motor loss: MAS 3 (12%)	Ipsilateral proprioception, contralateral pain and temperature loss	Bladder dyssynergia (37%)	Constipation Class 3 (15%)	62%

Table 23.144 Brown-Séquard T12, MAS 4, incontinence of bladder catheterization

Ipsilateral motor loss: MAS 4 (15%)	15%			
Ipsilateral motor loss: MAS 4 (15%)	Ipsilateral proprioception, contralateral pain and temperature loss	31%		
Ipsilateral motor loss: MAS 4 (15%)	Ipsilateral proprioception, contralateral pain and temperature loss	Incontinence of bladder requiring catheterization (50%)	65%	
Ipsilateral motor loss: MAS 4 (15%)	Ipsilateral proprioception, contralateral pain and temperature loss	Incontinence of bladder requiring catheterization (50%)	Constipation Class 3 (15%)	71%

23.14 READY RECKONER—CONUS LESION

Table 23.145 Conus lesion: MRC 4,3, sensory impairment, neurogenic bladder

Conus MRC 4	9%		
Conus MRC 4	Partial sensory loss	23%	
Conus MRC 4	Partial sensory loss	Voiding by Credé maneuver (15%)	34%
Conus MRC 3	12%		
Conus MRC 3	Partial sensory loss	25%	
Conus MRC 3	Partial sensory loss	Voiding by Credé maneuver (15%)	36%

Table 23.146 Conus lesion: MRC 2,1, sensory impairment, neurogenic bladder

Conus MRC 2	13%			
Conus MRC 2	Partial sensory loss	25%		
Conus MRC 2	Partial sensory loss	Voiding by Credé maneuver with residual urine (25%)	44%	
Conus MRC 2	Partial sensory loss	Voiding by Credé maneuver with residual urine (25%)	Erectile dysfunction and infertility (30%)	61%
Conus MRC 1	14%			
Conus MRC 1	Complete sensory loss	37%		
Conus MRC 1	Complete sensory loss	Incontinence of bladder requiring catheterization (50%)	69%	
Conus MRC 1	Complete sensory loss	Incontinence of bladder requiring catheterization (50%)	Incontinence of bowel (37%)	80%
Conus MRC 1	Complete sensory loss	Incontinence of bladder requiring catheterization (50%)	Incontinence of bowel (37%)	Erectile dysfunction and infertility (30%)	86%

Table 23.147 Conus lesion: MRC 0, sensory impairment, neurogenic bladder

Conus MRC 0	15%			
Conus MRC 0	Complete sensory loss	38%		
Conus MRC 0	Complete sensory loss	Incontinence of bladder requiring catheterization	69%	
Conus MRC 0	Complete sensory loss	Incontinence of bladder requiring catheterization	Incontinence of bowel (37%)	80%
Conus MRC 0	Complete sensory loss	Incontinence of bladder requiring catheterization	Incontinence of bowel (37%)	Erectile dysfunction and infertility (30%)	86%

23.15 READY RECKONER—CAUDA EQUINUS LESION

Table 23.148 Cauda equinus lesion: Symmetrical motor weakness MRC 4,3,2

Symmetrical weakness of BLL MRC 4	8%		
Symmetrical weakness of BLL MRC 3	11%		
Symmetrical weakness of BLL MRC 3	Partial sensory loss	23%	
Symmetrical weakness of BLL MRC 2	13%		
Symmetrical weakness of BLL MRC 2	Partial sensory loss	25%	
Symmetrical weakness of BLL MRC 2	Partial sensory loss	Voiding by Credé maneuver (15%)	36%

Table 23.149 Cauda equinus lesion: Symmetrical motor weakness MRC 1, 0

Symmetrical weakness of BLL MRC 1	14%				
Symmetrical weakness of BLL MRC 1	Complete sensory loss	37%			
Symmetrical weakness of BLL MRC 1	Complete sensory loss	Incontinence of bladder requiring catheterization (50%)	69%		
Symmetrical weakness of BLL MRC 1	Complete sensory loss	Incontinence of bladder requiring catheterization (50%)	Incontinence of bowel (37%)	80%	
Symmetrical weakness of BLL MRC 1	Complete sensory loss	Incontinence of bladder requiring catheterization (50%)	Incontinence of bowel (37%)	Erectile dysfunction and infertility (30%)	86%
Symmetrical weakness of BLL MRC 0	15%				
Symmetrical weakness of BLL MRC 0	Complete sensory loss	38%			
Symmetrical weakness of BLL MRC 0	Complete sensory loss	Incontinence of bladder requiring catheterization (50%)	69%		
Symmetrical weakness of BLL MRC 0	Complete sensory loss	Incontinence of bladder requiring catheterization (50%)	Incontinence of bowel (37%)	80%	
Symmetrical weakness of BLL MRC 0	Complete sensory loss	Incontinence of bladder requiring catheterization (50%)	Incontinence of bowel (37%)	Erectile dysfunction and infertility (30%)	86%

Table 23.150 Cauda equinus lesion: Asymmetrical motor weakness MRC 4/3,3/2,2/1

Asymmetrical weakness of BLL MRC 4/MRC 3	9%		
Asymmetrical weakness of BLL MRC 3/MRC 2	11%		
Asymmetrical weakness of BLL MRC 3/MRC 2	Ipsilateral intact sensation, contralateral partial sensory loss	18%	
Asymmetrical weakness of BLL MRC 2/MRC 1	13%		
Asymmetrical weakness of BLL MRC 2/MRC 1	Ipsilateral impairment of sensation, contralateral complete sensory loss	28%	
Asymmetrical weakness of BLL MRC 2/MRC 1	Ipsilateral impairment of sensation, contralateral complete sensory loss	Voiding by Credé maneuver (15%)	38%

Table 23.151 Cauda equinus lesion: Asymmetrical motor weakness MRC 1/0

Asymmetrical weakness of BLL MRC 1/MRC 0	14%			
Asymmetrical weakness of BLL MRC 1/MRC 0	Ipsilateral partial sensory loss, contralateral complete sensory loss	32%		
Asymmetrical weakness of BLL MRC 1/MRC 0	Ipsilateral partial sensory loss, contralateral complete sensory loss	Incontinence of bladder requiring catheterization (50%)	66%	
Asymmetrical weakness of BLL MRC 1/MRC 0	Ipsilateral partial sensory loss, contralateral complete sensory loss	Incontinence of bladder requiring catheterization (50%)	Incontinence of bowel (37%)	79%
Asymmetrical weakness of BLL MRC 1/MRC 0	Ipsilateral partial sensory loss, contralateral complete sensory loss	Incontinence of bladder requiring catheterization (50%)	Incontinence of bowel (37%)	Erectile dysfunction and infertility (30%)	85%

Table 23.152 Cauda equinus lesion: Unilateral motor weakness MRC 1/0

Unilateral weakness RLL MRC 4	6%	
Unilateral weakness RLL MRC 3	7%	
Unilateral weakness RLL MRC 3	Partial sensory loss RLL	14%
Unilateral weakness RLL MRC 2	8%	
Unilateral weakness RLL MRC 2	Partial sensory loss RLL	15%
Unilateral weakness RLL MRC 1	9%	
Unilateral weakness RLL MRC 1	Partial sensory loss RLL	22%
Unilateral weakness RLL MRC 0	9%	
Unilateral weakness RLL MRC 0	Partial sensory loss RLL	22%

23.16 READY RECKONER—MOTOR NEURON DISEASE

Table 23.153 Primary lateral sclerosis: MAS 1, 1+ facial weakness, dysarthria, drooling whole person impairment

Quadriparesis MAS 1 (18%)	18%			
Quadriparesis MAS 1 (18%)	UMN facial paresis (5%)	22%		
Quadriparesis MAS 1 (18%)	UMN facial paresis (5%)	Dysarthria Class 1 (5%)	26%	
Quadriparesis MAS 1 (18%)	UMN facial paresis (5%)	Dysarthria Class 1 (5%)	Dysphagia Class 1 (2.5%)	28%
Quadriparesis MAS 1+ (22%)	22%			
Quadriparesis MAS 1+ (22%)	UMN facial paresis (5%)	26%		
Quadriparesis MAS 1+ (22%)	UMN facial paresis (5%)	Dysarthria Class 1 (5%)	30%	
Quadriparesis MAS 1+ (22%)	UMN facial paresis (5%)	Dysarthria Class 1 (5%)	Dysphagia Class 1 (2.5 %)	32%

Table 23.154 Primary lateral sclerosis: MAS 2, 3 facial weakness, dysarthria, drooling whole person impairment

Quadriparesis MAS 2 (35%)	35%			
Quadriparesis MAS 2 (35%)	UMN facial paresis (5%)	38%		
Quadriparesis MAS 2 (35%)	UMN facial paresis (5%)	Dysarthria Class 1 (5%)	41%	
Quadriparesis MAS 2 (35%)	UMN facial paresis (5%)	Dysarthria Class 1 (5%)	Dysphagia Class 2 (5%)	42%
Quadriparesis MAS 3 (41%)	41%			
Quadriparesis MAS 3 (41%)	UMN facial palsy (10%)	46%		
Quadriparesis MAS 3 (41%)	UMN facial palsy (10%)	Dysarthria Class 2 (15%)	55%	
Quadriparesis MAS 3 (41%)	UMN facial palsy (10%)	Dysarthria Class 2 (15%)	Dysphagia Class 4 (25%)	61%
Quadriparesis MAS 3 (41%)	UMN facial palsy (10%)	Dysarthria Class 2 (15%)	Dysphagia Class 4 (25%). Urgency incontinence of bladder (15%)	67%
Quadriparesis MAS 3 (41%)	UMN facial palsy (10%)	Dysarthria Class 2 (15%)	Dysphagia Class 4 (25%). Urgency incontinence of bladder (15%), respiratory muscle paralysis Class 2 (25%)	75%

Table 23.155 Primary lateral sclerosis: MAS 4, facial weakness, dysarthria, drooling whole person impairment

Quadriparesis MAS 4 (44%)	44%				
Quadriparesis MAS 4 (44%)	UMN facial palsy (10%)	49%			
Quadriparesis MAS 4 (44%)	UMN facial palsy (10%)	Dysarthria Class 2 (15%)	57%		
Quadriparesis MAS 4 (44%)	UMN facial palsy (10%)	Dysarthria Class 2 (15%)	Dysphagia Class 5 (50%)	79%	
Quadriparesis MAS 4 (44%)	UMN facial palsy (10%)	Dysarthria Class 2 (15%)	Dysphagia Class 5 (50%)	Urgency incontinence of bladder (15%)	82%
Quadriparesis MAS 4 (44%)	UMN facial palsy (10%)	Dysarthria Class 2 (15%)	Dysphagia Class 5 (50%)	Urgency incontinence of bladder (15%), respiratory muscle weakness Class 3 (50%)	91%
Quadriparesis MAS 4 (44%)	UMN facial palsy (10%)	Dysarthria Class 2 (15%)	Dysphagia Class 5 (50%)	Urgency incontinence of bladder (15%), respiratory muscle weakness Class 3 (50%), equinus deformity (4%)	91%

Table 23.156 MND—MND—ALS C5—UE: MRC 4,3,2,1.0 LE: MAS 1,1+,2,3,4 whole person impairment

Quadriparesis MAS 1 (18%)	18%		
Quadriparesis MAS 1+ (27%)	27%		
Quadriparesis MAS 2 (37%)	37%		
Quadriparesis MAS 2 (37%)	Respiratory muscle paralysis Class 1 (15%)	46%	
Quadriparesis MAS 2 (37%)	Respiratory muscle paralysis Class 1 (15%)	Bilateral claw hand deformity (3%)	48%
Quadriparesis MAS 3 (48%)	48%		
Quadriparesis MAS 3 (48%)	Respiratory muscle paralysis Class 1 (15%)	56%	
Quadriparesis MAS 3 (48%)	Respiratory muscle paralysis Class 1 (15%)	Bilateral claw hand deformity (3%)	57%
Quadriparesis MAS 4 (51%)	51%		
Quadriparesis MAS 4 (51%)	Respiratory muscle paralysis Class 2 (25%)	63%	
Quadriparesis MAS 4 (51%)	Respiratory muscle paralysis Class 2 (25%)	Bilateral claw hand and equinus deformities (7%)	66%

Table 23.157 MND—MND—ALS C6—UE: MRC 4,3,2,1.0 LE: MAS 1,1+,2,3,4 whole person impairment

Quadriparesis MAS 1 (17%)	17%		
Quadriparesis MAS 1+ (25%)	25%		
Quadriparesis MAS 2 (35%)	35%		
Quadriparesis MAS 2 (35%)	Respiratory muscle paralysis Class 1 (15%)	45%	
Quadriparesis MAS 2 (35%)	Respiratory muscle paralysis Class 1 (15%)	Bilateral claw hand deformity (3%)	46%
Quadriparesis MAS 3 (46%)	46%		
Quadriparesis MAS 3 (46%)	Respiratory muscle paralysis Class 1 (15%)	54%	
Quadriparesis MAS 3 (46%)	Respiratory muscle paralysis Class 1 (15%)	Bilateral claw hand deformity (3%)	55%
Quadriparesis MAS 4 (49%)	49%		
Quadriparesis MAS 4 (49%)	Respiratory muscle paralysis Class 2 (25%)	61%	
Quadriparesis MAS 4 (49%)	Respiratory muscle paralysis Class 2 (25%)	Bilateral claw hand and equinus deformities (7%)	64%

Table 23.158 MND—ALS C7—UE: MRC 4,3,2,1.0 LE: MAS 1,1+,2,3,4 whole person impairment

Quadriparesis MAS 1 (18%)	18%		
Quadriparesis MAS 1+ (27%)	27%		
Quadriparesis MAS 2 (35%)	35%		
Quadriparesis MAS 2 (35%)	Respiratory muscle paralysis Class 1 (15%)	45%	
Quadriparesis MAS 2 (35%)	Respiratory muscle paralysis Class 1 (15%)	Bilateral claw hand deformity (3%)	46%
Quadriparesis MAS 3 (44%)	44%		
Quadriparesis MAS 3 (44%)	Respiratory muscle paralysis Class 1 (15%)	53%	
Quadriparesis MAS 3 (44%)	Respiratory muscle paralysis Class 1 (15%)	Bilateral claw hand deformity (3%)	54%
Quadriparesis MAS 4 (47%)	47%		
Quadriparesis MAS 4 (47%)	Respiratory muscle paralysis Class 2 (25%)	60%	
Quadriparesis MAS 4 (47%)	Respiratory muscle paralysis Class 2 (25%)	Bilateral claw hand and equinus deformities (7%)	63%

Table 23.159 MND—ALS C8—UE: MRC 4,3,2,1.0 LE: MAS 1,1+,2,3,4 whole person impairment

Quadriparesis MAS 1 (11%)	11%		
Quadriparesis MAS 1+ (22%)	22%		
Quadriparesis MAS 2 (25%)	25%		
Quadriparesis MAS 2 (25%)	Respiratory muscle paralysis Class 1 (15%)	36%	
Quadriparesis MAS 2 (25%)	Respiratory muscle paralysis Class 1 (15%)	Bilateral claw hand deformity (3%)	38%
Quadriparesis MAS 3 (36%)	36%		
Quadriparesis MAS 3 (36%)	Respiratory muscle paralysis Class 1 (15%)	45%	
Quadriparesis MAS 3 (36%)	Respiratory muscle paralysis Class 1 (15%)	Bilateral claw hand deformity (3%)	47%
Quadriparesis MAS 4 (38%)	38%		
Quadriparesis MAS 4 (38%)	Respiratory muscle paralysis Class 2 (25%)	54%	
Quadriparesis MAS 4 (38%)	Respiratory muscle paralysis Class 2 (25%)	Bilateral claw hand and equinus deformity (7%)	57%

Table 23.160 MND—ALS T1—UE: MRC 4,3,2,1.0 LE: MAS 1,1+,2,3,4 whole person impairment

Quadriparesis MAS 1 (10%)	10%		
Quadriparesis MAS 1+ (18%)	18%		
Quadriparesis MAS 2 (22%)	22%		
Quadriparesis MAS 2 (22%)	Respiratory muscle paralysis Class 1 (15%)	34%	
Quadriparesis MAS 2 (25%)	Respiratory muscle paralysis Class 1 (15%)	Bilateral claw hand deformity (3%)	36%
Quadriparesis MAS 3 (29%)	29%		
Quadriparesis MAS 3 (29%)	Respiratory muscle paralysis Class 1 (15%)	39%	
Quadriparesis MAS 3 (29%)	Respiratory muscle paralysis Class 1 (15%)	Bilateral claw hand deformity (3%)	41%
Quadriparesis MAS 4 (32%)	32%		
Quadriparesis MAS 4 (32%)	Respiratory muscle paralysis Class 2 (25%)	49%	
Quadriparesis MAS 4 (32%)	Respiratory muscle paralysis Class 2 (25%)	Bilateral claw hand and equinus deformity (10%)	53%

Table 23.161 MND—Progressive muscular atrophy: MRC 4—Whole person impairment

Quadriparesis MAS 4 (20%)	20%		
Quadriparesis MAS 3 (30%)	30%		
Quadriparesis MAS 2 (42%)	42%		
Quadriparesis MAS 2 (42%)	Respiratory muscle paralysis Class 1 (15%)	51%	
Quadriparesis MAS 2 (42%)	Respiratory muscle paralysis Class 1 (15%)	Bilateral claw hand deformity (3%)	52%
Quadriparesis MAS 1 (54%)	54%		
Quadriparesis MAS 1 (54%)	Respiratory muscle paralysis Class 2 (25%)	66%	
Quadriparesis MAS 1 (54%)	Respiratory muscle paralysis Class 2 (25%)	Bilateral claw hand deformity (3%)	67%

Table 23.162 MND—Bulbar palsy: Dysarthria, facial weakness, dysphagia, respiratory muscle weakness, and central hypoventilation: Whole person impairment

Facial palsy LMN incomplete (10%)	10%			
Facial palsy LMN incomplete (10%)	Dysarthria Class 1 (5%)	14%		
Facial palsy LMN incomplete (10%)	Dysarthria Class 1 (5%)	Dysphagia Class 4 (25%)	36%	
Facial palsy LMN complete (19%)	19%			
Facial palsy LMN complete (19%)	Dysarthria Class 2 (15%)	31%		
Facial palsy LMN complete (19%)	Dysarthria Class 2 (15%)	Dysphagia Class 5 (50%)	66%	
Facial palsy LMN complete (19%)	Dysarthria Class 2 (15%)	Dysphagia Class 5 (50%)	Hypoventilation: Respiratory failure (50%)	83%

Table 23.163 MND—Spino-bulbar-muscular atrophy: MRC 2, dysarthria, facial weakness, dysphagia, respiratory muscle weakness—Whole person impairment

Quadriparesis MAS 2 (44%)	44%				
Quadriparesis MAS 2 (44%)	Dysarthria Class 1 (5%)	47%			
Quadriparesis MAS 2 (44%)	Dysarthria Class 1 (5%)	Dysphagia Class 4 (25%)	60%		
Quadriparesis MAS 2 (44%)	Dysarthria Class 1 (5%)	Dysphagia Class 4 (25%)	Respiratory muscle paralysis Class 2 (25%)	70%	
Quadriparesis MAS 2 (43%)	Dysarthria Class 1 (5%)	Dysphagia Class 4 (25%)	Respiratory muscle paralysis Class 2 (25%)	Bilateral claw hand deformity (3%)	71%

Table 23.164 MND—Spino-bulbar-muscular atrophy: MRC 1, dysarthria, facial weakness, dysphagia, respiratory muscle weakness, hypoventilation, deformities whole person impairment

Quadriparesis MAS 1 (55%)	55%				
Quadriparesis MAS 1 (55%)	Dysarthria Class 2 (15%)	62%			
Quadriparesis MAS 1 (55%)	Dysarthria Class 2 (15%)	Dysphagia Class 5 (50%)	81%		
Quadriparesis MAS 1 (55%)	Dysarthria Class 2 (15%)	Dysphagia Class 5 (50%)	Respiratory muscle paralysis Class 3 (50%)	90%	
Quadriparesis MAS 1 (55%)	Dysarthria Class 2 (15%)	Dysphagia Class 5 (50%)	Respiratory muscle paralysis Class 3 (50%)	Hypoventilation: Respiratory failure (50%)	95%
Quadriparesis MAS 1 (55%)	Dysarthria Class 2 (15%)	Dysphagia Class 5 (50%)	Respiratory muscle paralysis Class 3 (50%)	Hypoventilation: Respiratory failure (50%), bilateral claw hand deformity (5%)	95%

Table 23.165 MND—Spinal muscular atrophy type II/III/IV: Proximal muscles MRC 4,3 whole person impairment

Proximal muscles shoulder and hip, knee: MRC 4	8%				
Proximal muscles shoulder, elbow and hip, knee: MRC 3	12%				
Proximal muscles shoulder, elbow, dorsolumbar spine hip, knee: MRC 2	21%				
Proximal muscles shoulder, elbow, dorsolumbar spine hip, knee: MRC 2	Dysarthria Class 1 (5%)	25%			
Proximal muscles shoulder, elbow, dorsolumbar spine hip, knee: MRC 2	Dysarthria Class 1 (5%)	Dysphagia Class 3 (15%)	36%		
Proximal muscles shoulder, elbow, dorsolumbar spine hip, knee: MRC 2	Dysarthria Class 1 (5%)	Dysphagia Class 3 (15%)	Respiratory muscle paralysis Class 2 (25%)	52%	
Proximal muscles shoulder, elbow, dorsolumbar spine hip, knee: MRC 2	Dysarthria Class 1 (5%)	Dysphagia Class 3 (15%)	Respiratory muscle paralysis Class 2 (25%)	Scoliosis (5%)	55%

Table 23.166 MND—Spinal muscular atrophy type II/III/IV: Proximal muscles MRC 2,1 whole person impairment

Proximal muscles shoulder, elbow, dorsolumbar spine hip, knee: MRC 1	28%				
Proximal muscles shoulder, elbow, dorsolumbar spine hip, knee: MRC 1	Dysarthria Class 2 (15%)	39%			
Proximal muscles shoulder, elbow, dorsolumbar spine hip, knee: MRC 1	Dysarthria Class 2 (15%)	Dysphagia Class 4 (25%)	54%		
Proximal muscles shoulder, elbow, dorsolumbar spine hip, knee: MRC 1	Dysarthria Class 2 (15%)	Dysphagia Class 4 (25%)	Respiratory muscle paralysis Class 2 (25%)	66%	
Proximal muscles shoulder, elbow, dorsolumbar spine hip, knee: MRC 1	Dysarthria Class 2 (15%)	Dysphagia Class 4 (25%)	Respiratory muscle paralysis Class 2 (25%)	Scoliosis (10%)	69%

23.17 READY RECKONER—PERIPHERAL NERVE LESIONS: UPPER EXTREMITY

Table 23.167 Brachial plexus lesion—Total arm: Whole person impairment

Lower motor neuron lesion MRC 4	5%	
Lower motor neuron lesion MRC 3	7%	
Lower motor neuron lesion MRC 3	Partial sensory loss	20%
Lower motor neuron lesion MRC 2	10%	
Lower motor neuron lesion MRC 2	Partial sensory loss	23%
Lower motor neuron lesion MRC 1	15%	
Lower motor neuron lesion MRC 1	Complete sensory loss	41%
Lower motor neuron lesion MRC 0	17%	
Lower motor neuron lesion MRC 0	Complete sensory loss	42%

Table 23.168 C5,6,7 Brachial plexus palsy—Whole person impairment

Lower motor neuron lesion MRC 4	3%	
Lower motor neuron lesion MRC 3	4%	
Lower motor neuron lesion MRC 3	Partial sensory loss	13%
Lower motor neuron lesion MRC 2	7%	
Lower motor neuron lesion MRC 2	Partial sensory loss	16%
Lower motor neuron lesion MRC 1	11%	
Lower motor neuron lesion MRC 1	Complete sensory loss	28%
Lower motor neuron lesion MRC 0	12%	
Lower motor neuron lesion MRC 0	Complete sensory loss	28%

Table 23.169 C5,6 Brachial plexus palsy—Whole person impairment

Lower motor neuron lesion MRC 4	2%	
Lower motor neuron lesion MRC 3	3%	
Lower motor neuron lesion MRC 3	Partial sensory loss	8%
Lower motor neuron lesion MRC 2	4%	
Lower motor neuron lesion MRC 2	Partial sensory loss	10%
Lower motor neuron lesion MRC 1	7%	
Lower motor neuron lesion MRC 1	Complete sensory loss	17%
Lower motor neuron lesion MRC 0	7%	
Lower motor neuron lesion MRC 0	Complete sensory loss	17%

Table 23.170 C7,8,T1 Brachial plexus palsy—Whole person impairment

Lower motor neuron lesion MRC 4	4%	
Lower motor neuron lesion MRC 3	5%	
Lower motor neuron lesion MRC 3	Partial sensory loss	14%
Lower motor neuron lesion MRC 2	8%	
Lower motor neuron lesion MRC 2	Partial sensory loss	17%
Lower motor neuron lesion MRC 1	13%	
Lower motor neuron lesion MRC 1	Complete sensory loss	29%
Lower motor neuron lesion MRC 0	14%	
Lower motor neuron lesion MRC 0	Complete sensory loss	30%

Table 23.171 C8,T1 Brachial plexus palsy—Whole person impairment

Lower motor neuron lesion MRC 4	2%	
Lower motor neuron lesion MRC 3	3%	
Lower motor neuron lesion MRC 3	Partial sensory loss	8%
Lower motor neuron lesion MRC 2	4%	
Lower motor neuron lesion MRC 2	Partial sensory loss	9%
Lower motor neuron lesion MRC 1	7%	
Lower motor neuron lesion MRC 1	Complete sensory loss	17%
Lower motor neuron lesion MRC 0	7%	
Lower motor neuron lesion MRC 0	Complete sensory loss	18%

Table 23.172 Circumflex humeral nerve palsy—Whole person impairment

Lower motor neuron lesion MRC 4	0.12%	
Lower motor neuron lesion MRC 3	1%	
Lower motor neuron lesion MRC 3	Partial sensory loss	1%
Lower motor neuron lesion MRC 2	2%	
Lower motor neuron lesion MRC 2	Partial sensory loss	3%
Lower motor neuron lesion MRC 1	3%	
Lower motor neuron lesion MRC 1	Complete sensory loss	3%
Lower motor neuron lesion MRC 0	3%	
Lower motor neuron lesion MRC 0	Complete sensory loss	3%

Table 23.173 Musculocutaneous nerve palsy—Whole person impairment

Muscle power MRC 4	0.09%	
Muscle power MRC 3	1%	
Muscle power MRC 3	Partial sensory loss	2%
Muscle power MRC 2	2%	
Muscle power MRC 2	Partial sensory loss	3%
Muscle power MRC 1	3%	
Muscle power MRC 1	Complete sensory loss	5%
Muscle power MRC 0	3%	
Muscle power MRC 0	Complete sensory loss	5%

Table 23.174 Radial nerve palsy—Whole person impairment

Muscle power MRC 4	1%	
Muscle power MRC 3	2%	
Muscle power MRC 3	Partial sensory loss	7%
Muscle power MRC 2	5%	
Muscle power MRC 2	Partial sensory loss	9%
Muscle power MRC 1	8%	
Muscle power MRC 1	Complete sensory loss	17%
Muscle power MRC 0	9%	
Muscle power MRC 0	Complete sensory loss	17%

Table 23.175 Posterior interosseous nerve palsy—Whole person impairment

Muscle power MRC 4	1%
Muscle power MRC 3	2%
Muscle power MRC 2	4%
Muscle power MRC 1	5%
Muscle power MRC 0	5%

Table 23.176 Median nerve palsy—Whole person impairment

Muscle power MRC 4	3%		
Muscle power MRC 3	3%		
Muscle power MRC 3	Partial sensory loss	8%	
Muscle power MRC 2	5%		
Muscle power MRC 2	Partial sensory loss	10%	
Muscle power MRC 1	7%		
Muscle power MRC 1	Complete sensory loss	17%	
Muscle power MRC 1	Complete sensory loss	Claw hand	17%
Muscle power MRC 0	7%		
Muscle power MRC 0	Complete sensory loss	17%	
Muscle power MRC 0	Complete sensory loss	Claw hand	18%

Table 23.177 Anterior interosseous nerve palsy—Whole person impairment

Muscle power MRC 3	0.27%
Muscle power MRC 2	1.00%
Muscle power MRC 1	1.00%
Muscle power MRC 0	1.00%

Table 23.178 Median nerve—Carpal tunnel: Whole person impairment

Muscle power MRC 4	1%		
Muscle power MRC 3	2%		
Muscle power MRC 3	Partial sensory loss	6%	
Muscle power MRC 2	2%		
Muscle power MRC 2	Partial sensory loss	6%	
Muscle power MRC 1	4%		
Muscle power MRC 1	Complete sensory loss	12%	
Muscle power MRC 1	Complete sensory loss	Claw hand	12%
Muscle power MRC 0	4%		
Muscle power MRC 0	Complete sensory loss	12%	
Muscle power MRC 0	Complete sensory loss	Claw hand	13%

Table 23.179 Ulnar nerve palsy at the level of elbow—Whole person impairment

Muscle power MRC 4	1%		
Muscle power MRC 3	1%		
Muscle power MRC 3	Partial sensory loss	3%	
Muscle power MRC 2	2%		
Muscle power MRC 2	Partial sensory loss	4%	
Muscle power MRC 1	2%		
Muscle power MRC 1	Complete sensory loss	6%	
Muscle power MRC 1	Complete sensory loss	Claw hand	7%
Muscle power MRC 0	3%		
Muscle power MRC 0	Complete sensory loss	7%	
Muscle power MRC 0	Complete sensory loss	Claw hand	7%

Table 23.180 Ulnar nerve palsy at Guyon's canal—Whole person impairment

Muscle power MRC 4	1%		
Muscle power MRC 3	1%		
Muscle power MRC 3	Partial sensory loss	2%	
Muscle power MRC 2	2%		
Muscle power MRC 2	Partial sensory loss	3%	
Muscle power MRC 1	2%		
Muscle power MRC 1	Complete sensory loss	5%	
Muscle power MRC 1	Complete sensory loss	Claw hand	5%
Muscle power MRC 0	2%		
Muscle power MRC 0	Complete sensory loss	5%	
Muscle power MRC 0	Complete sensory loss	Claw hand	6%

23.18 READY RECKONER—PERIPHERAL NERVE LESION: LOWER EXTREMITY

Table 23.181 Sciatic nerve palsy—Whole person impairment

Muscle power MRC 4	3%	
Muscle power MRC 3	5%	
Muscle power MRC 3	Partial sensory loss	11%
Muscle power MRC 2	7%	
Muscle power MRC 2	Partial sensory loss	13%
Muscle power MRC 1	10%	
Muscle power MRC 1	Complete sensory loss	22%
Muscle power MRC 0	10%	
Muscle power MRC 0	Complete sensory loss	23%

Table 23.182 Tibial nerve palsy—Whole person impairment

Muscle power MRC 4	2%	
Muscle power MRC 3	3%	
Muscle power MRC 3	Partial sensory loss	7%
Muscle power MRC 2	5%	
Muscle power MRC 2	Partial sensory loss	8%
Muscle power MRC 1	7%	
Muscle power MRC 1	Complete sensory loss	14%
Muscle power MRC 0	7%	
Muscle power MRC 0	Complete sensory loss	14%
Tarsal tunnel syndrome	3%	
Tarsal tunnel syndrome	Complete sensory loss	9%

Table 23.183 Medial plantar nerve palsy—Whole person impairment

Muscle power MRC 4	1%	
Muscle power MRC 3	2%	
Muscle power MRC 3	Partial sensory loss	4%
Muscle power MRC 2	2%	
Muscle power MRC 2	Partial sensory loss	4%
Muscle power MRC 1	2%	
Muscle power MRC 1	Complete sensory loss	6%
Muscle power MRC 0	2%	
Muscle power MRC 0	Complete sensory loss	6%

Table 23.184 Lateral plantar nerve palsy—Whole person impairment

Muscle power MRC 4	1%	
Muscle power MRC 3	1%	
Muscle power MRC 3	Partial sensory loss	2%
Muscle power MRC 2	1%	
Muscle power MRC 2	Partial sensory loss	2%
Muscle power MRC 1	2%	
Muscle power MRC 1	Complete sensory loss	3%
Muscle power MRC 0	2%	
Muscle power MRC 0	Complete sensory loss	3%

Table 23.185 Common peroneal nerve palsy—Whole person impairment

Muscle power MRC 4	2%	
Muscle power MRC 3	3%	
Muscle power MRC 3	Partial sensory loss	6%
Muscle power MRC 2	5%	
Muscle power MRC 2	Partial sensory loss	8%
Muscle power MRC 1	7%	
Muscle power MRC 1	Complete sensory loss	13%
Muscle power MRC 0	7%	
Muscle power MRC 0	Complete sensory loss	14%

Table 23.186 Superficial peroneal nerve palsy—Whole person impairment

Muscle power MRC 4	1%	
Muscle power MRC 3	1%	
Muscle power MRC 3	Partial sensory loss	3%
Muscle power MRC 2	1%	
Muscle power MRC 2	Partial sensory loss	3%
Muscle power MRC 1	1%	
Muscle power MRC 1	Complete sensory loss	5%
Muscle power MRC 0	2%	
Muscle power MRC 0	Complete sensory loss	5%

Table 23.187 Deep peroneal nerve palsy—Whole person impairment

Muscle power MRC 4	2%	
Muscle power MRC 3	3%	
Muscle power MRC 3	Partial sensory loss	3%
Muscle power MRC 2	4%	
Muscle power MRC 2	Partial sensory loss	4%
Muscle power MRC 1	6%	
Muscle power MRC 1	Complete sensory loss	6%
Muscle power MRC 0	6%	
Muscle power MRC 0	Complete sensory loss	6%

23.19 READY RECKONER—MYASTHENIA GRAVIS

Table 23.188 Generalized myasthenia gravis—MRC 3, Class 3 dysphagia and Class 2 bilateral ptosis: Whole person impairment

Upper extremities	13%				
Upper extremities	Spine	16%			
Upper extremities	Spine	Lower extremities	24%		
Upper extremities	Spine	Lower extremities	Dysphagia Class 3 (15%)	35%	
Upper extremities	Spine	Lower extremities	Dysphagia Class 2 (15%)	Bilateral ptosis Class 2 (5%)	38%

Table 23.189 Generalized myasthenia gravis—MRC 4, Class 2 dysphagia and Class 1 bilateral ptosis: Whole person impairment

Upper extremities	7%				
Upper extremities	Spine	9%			
Upper extremities	Spine	Lower extremities	14%		
Upper extremities	Spine	Lower extremities	Dysphagia Class 2 (5%)	19%	
Upper extremities	Spine	Lower extremities	Dysphagia Class 2 (5%)	Bilateral ptosis Class 1 (2.5%)	21%

Table 23.190 Focal myasthenia gravis—MRC 3, Class 3 dysphagia and Class 2 bilateral ptosis: Whole person impairment

Upper extremities—proximal muscles: Muscle power MRC 3	3%				
Upper extremities—proximal muscles: Muscle power MRC 3	Spinal muscles: Muscle power MRC 3	4%			
Upper extremities—proximal muscles: Muscle power MRC 3	Spinal muscles: Muscle power MRC 3	Lower extremities—proximal muscles: Muscle power MRC 3	7%		
Upper extremities—proximal muscles: Muscle power MRC 3	Spinal muscles: Muscle power MRC 3	Lower extremities—proximal muscles: Muscle power MRC 3	Dysphagia Class 3 (15%)	21%	
Upper extremities—proximal muscles: Muscle power MRC 3	Spinal muscles: muscle power MRC 3	Lower extremities—proximal muscles: Muscle power MRC 3	Dysphagia Class 3 (15%)	Bilateral ptosis Class 2 (5%)	25%

Table 23.191 Focal myasthenia gravis—MRC 4, Class 2 dysphagia and Class 1 bilateral ptosis: Whole person impairment

Upper extremities—proximal muscles: Muscle power MRC 4	1%				
Upper extremities—proximal muscles: Muscle power MRC 4	Spinal muscles	2%			
Upper extremities—proximal muscles: muscle power MRC 4	Spinal muscles	Lower extremities—proximal muscles: Muscle power MRC 4	4%		
Upper extremities—proximal muscles: muscle power MRC 4	Spinal muscles	Lower extremities—proximal muscles: Muscle power MRC 4	Dysphagia Class 2 (5%)	9%	
Upper extremities—proximal muscles: muscle Power MRC 4	Spinal muscles	Lower extremities—proximal muscles: Muscle power MRC 4	Dysphagia Class 2 (5%)	Bilateral ptosis Class 2 (2.5%)	11%

Table 23.192 Ocular myasthenia gravis with Class 2 bilateral ptosis and diplopia whole person impairment

Bilateral ptosis Class 2 (5%)	5%		
Bilateral ptosis Class 2 (5%)	Diplopia—score 6–10	10%	15%

23.20 READY RECKONER—MUSCULAR DYSTROPHY

Table 23.193 Duchenne/Becker muscular dystrophy—Lower and/or upper extremities early ambulatory stage: Whole person impairment

Lower extremities: Muscle power MRC 3–4	8%	
Upper extremities: Proximal muscle power MRC 4	3%	
Upper extremities: Proximal muscle power MRC 4	Lower extremities: Muscle power MRC 3–4	12%

Table 23.194 Duchenne/Becker muscular dystrophy—Proximal muscles upper extremities, muscles of lower extremities, neck and trunk, respiratory muscle weakness late ambulatory stage: Whole person impairment

Upper extremities: Muscle power MRC 2–3	11%			
Upper extremities: Muscle power MRC 2–3	Cervical and dorsolumbar spine: Muscle power MRC 2–3	13%		
Upper extremities: Muscle power MRC 2–3	Cervical and dorsolumbar spine: Muscle power MRC 2–3	Lower extremities: Muscle power MRC 2–3	26%	
Upper extremities: Muscle power MRC 2–3	Cervical and dorsolumbar spine: Muscle power MRC 2–3	Lower extremities: Muscle power MRC 2–3	Respiratory muscle paralysis Class 1 (15%)	38%
Upper extremities: Muscle power MRC 2–3	Cervical and dorsolumbar spine: Muscle power MRC 2–3	Lower extremities: Muscle power MRC 2–3	Respiratory muscle paralysis Class 1 (15%)	Bilateral equinus deformity (4%) 40%

Table 23.195 Duchenne/Becker muscular dystrophy—Proximal muscles upper extremities, muscles of lower extremities, neck and trunk, respiratory muscle weakness late ambulatory stage: Whole person impairment

Upper extremities: Muscle power MRC 2–3	11%			
Upper extremities: Muscle power MRC 2–3	Cervical and dorsolumbar spine: Muscle power MRC 2–3	13%		
Upper extremities: Muscle power MRC 2–3	Cervical and dorsolumbar spine: Muscle power MRC 2–3	Lower extremities: Muscle power MRC 1–2	32%	
Upper extremities: Muscle power MRC 2–3	Cervical and dorsolumbar spine: Muscle power MRC 2–3	Lower extremities: Muscle power MRC 1–2	Dysphagia Class 1 (5%)	35%
Upper extremities: Muscle power MRC 2–3	Cervical and dorsolumbar spine: Muscle power MRC 2–3	Lower extremities: Muscle power MRC 1–2	Dysphagia Class 1 (5%)	Respiratory muscle paralysis Class 2 (25%) 52%
Upper extremities: Muscle power MRC 2–3	Cervical and dorsolumbar spine: Muscle power MRC 2–3	Lower extremities: Muscle power MRC 1–2	Dysphagia Class 1 (5%)	Respiratory muscle paralysis Class 2 (25%), bilateral equinus deformity (4%) 54%

Table 23.196 Duchenne/Becker muscular dystrophy—Proximal muscles upper extremities, muscles of lower extremities, neck and trunk, respiratory muscle weakness, cardiomyopathy: Non-ambulatory stage: Whole person impairment

Upper extremities: Muscle power MRC 2–3	9%				
Upper extremities: Muscle power MRC 2–3	Cervical and dorsolumbar spine: Muscle power MRC 2–3	13%			
Upper extremities: Muscle power MRC 2–3	Cervical and dorsolumbar spine: Muscle power MRC 2–3	Lower extremities: Muscle power MRC 1–2	31%		
Upper extremities: Muscle power MRC 2–3	Cervical and dorsolumbar spine: Muscle power MRC 2–3	Lower extremities: Muscle power MRC 1–2	Cardiomyopathy Class 3 (15%)	41%	
Upper extremities: Muscle power MRC 2–3	Cervical and dorsolumbar spine: Muscle power MRC 2–3	Lower extremities: Muscle power MRC 1–2	Cardiomyopathy Class 3 (15%)	Respiratory muscle paralysis Class 2 (25%)	56%
Upper extremities: Muscle power MRC 2–3	Cervical and dorsolumbar spine: Muscle power MRC 2–3	Lower extremities: Muscle power MRC 1–2	Cardiomyopathy Class 4 (25%)	Respiratory muscle paralysis Class 2 (25%), scoliosis Class 1 (2.5%), and bilateral equinus deformity (4%)	60%

Table 23.197 Duchenne/Becker muscular dystrophy—Proximal muscles upper extremities, muscles of lower extremities, neck and trunk, respiratory muscle weakness, cardiomyopathy: Non-ambulatory stage: Whole person impairment

Upper extremities: Muscle power MRC 1–3	22%				
Upper extremities: Muscle power MRC 1–3	Cervical and dorsolumbar spine: Muscle power MRC 1–2	28%			
Upper extremities: Muscle power MRC 1–3	Cervical and dorsolumbar spine: Muscle power MRC 1–2	Lower extremities: Muscle power MRC 0–2	46%		
Upper extremities: Muscle power MRC 1–3	Cervical and dorsolumbar spine: Muscle power MRC 1–2	Lower extremities: Muscle power MRC 0–2	Cardiomyopathy Class 4 (25%)	59%	
Upper extremities: Muscle power MRC 1–3	Cervical and dorsolumbar spine: Muscle power MRC 1–2	Lower extremities: Muscle power MRC 0–2	Cardiomyopathy Class 4 (25%)	Respiratory muscle paralysis Class 2 (25%)	70%
Upper extremities: Muscle power MRC 1–3	Cervical and dorsolumbar spine: Muscle power MRC 1–2	Lower extremities: Muscle power MRC 0–2	Cardiomyopathy Class 4 (25%)	Respiratory muscle paralysis Class 2 (25%), scoliosis Class 2 (5%), and bilateral equinus deformity (4%)	72%

Table 23.198 Duchenne/Becker muscular dystrophy—Proximal muscles upper extremities, muscles of lower extremities, neck and trunk, respiratory muscle weakness, cardiomyopathy: Non-ambulatory stage: Whole person impairment

Upper extremities: Muscle power MRC 1–3	22%				
Upper extremities: Muscle power MRC 1–3	Cervical and dorsolumbar spine: Muscle power MRC 1–2	28%			
Upper extremities: Muscle power MRC 1–3	Cervical and dorsolumbar spine: Muscle power MRC 1–2	Lower extremities: Muscle power MRC 0–2	46%		
Upper extremities: Muscle power MRC 1–3	Cervical and dorsolumbar spine: Muscle power MRC 1–2	Lower extremities: Muscle power MRC 0–2	Dysphagia Class 2 (5%)	48%	
Upper extremities: Muscle power MRC 1–3	Cervical and dorsolumbar spine: Muscle power MRC 1–2	Lower extremities: Muscle power MRC 0–2	Dysphagia Class 2 (5%)	Cardiomyopathy Class 4 (25%)	61%
Upper extremities: Muscle power MRC 1–3	Cervical and dorsolumbar spine: Muscle power MRC 1–2	Lower extremities: Muscle power MRC 0–2	Dysphagia Class 2 (5%)	Cardiomyopathy Class 4 (25%), respiratory muscle paralysis Class 3 (50%)	81%
Upper extremities: Muscle power MRC 1–3	Cervical and dorsolumbar spine: Muscle power MRC 1–2	Lower extremities: Muscle power MRC 0–2	Dysphagia Class 2 (5%)	Cardiomyopathy Class 4 (25%), respiratory muscle paralysis Class 3 (50%), scoliosis Class 3 (10%), and bilateral equinus deformity (4%)	83%

Table 23.199 Symmetrical facioscapulohumeral muscular dystrophy—Bilateral—Facial, shoulder and ankle dorsiflexors and peronei: Whole person impairment

Upper extremities: Shoulder girdle and shoulder—muscle power MRC 4	4%		
Upper extremities: Shoulder girdle and shoulder—muscle power MRC 4	Lower extremities: Ankle dorsiflexors and peronei—muscle power MRC 4	8%	
Upper extremities: Shoulder girdle and shoulder—muscle power MRC 4	Lower extremities: Ankle dorsiflexors and peronei—muscle power MRC 4	Bilateral facial muscle weakness (10%), dysarthria Class 1 (5%)	21%
Upper extremities: Shoulder girdle, shoulder and elbow—muscle power—MRC 3	5%		
Upper extremities: Shoulder girdle, shoulder and elbow—muscle power—MRC 3	Lower extremities: Muscle power MRC 3—ankle dorsiflexors and peronei	12%	
Upper extremities: Shoulder girdle, shoulder and elbow—muscle power—MRC 3	Lower extremities: Muscle power MRC 3—ankle dorsiflexors and peronei	Bilateral facial muscle weakness (5%), dysarthria Class 1 (5%), dysphagia Class 1 (2.5%)	27%

Table 23.200 Symmetrical facioscapulohumeral muscular dystrophy—Bilateral—Facial, shoulder, elbow, and hip, knee, ankle, foot: Whole person impairment

Upper extremities: Shoulder and shoulder girdle and elbow—muscle power MRC 2	10%		
Upper extremities: Shoulder and shoulder girdle and elbow—muscle power MRC 2	Lower extremities: Hip, knee—muscle power MRC 3, ankle dorsiflexors and peronei—muscle power MRC 2	20%	
Upper extremities: Shoulder and shoulder girdle and elbow—muscle power MRC 2	Lower extremities: Hip, knee—muscle power MRC 3, ankle dorsiflexors and peronei—muscle power MRC 2	Bilateral facial muscle weakness (10%), dysarthria Class 2 (15%), dysphagia Class 2 (5%)	44%
Upper extremities: Shoulder and shoulder girdle and elbow—muscle power MRC 1	11%		
Upper extremities: Shoulder and shoulder girdle and elbow—muscle power MRC 1	Lower extremities: Hip, knee—muscle power MRC 3, ankle dorsiflexors and peronei—muscle power MRC 2	27%	
Upper extremities: Shoulder and shoulder girdle and elbow—muscle power MRC 1	Lower extremities: Hip, knee—muscle power MRC 3, ankle dorsiflexors and peronei—muscle power MRC 2	Bilateral facial muscle weakness (10%), dysarthria Class 2 (15%), dysphagia Class 2 (5%)	49%

Table 23.201 Unilateral facioscapulohumeral muscular dystrophy—Facial, shoulder and/or, elbow and ankle dorsiflexors and peronei—MRC 4 and MRC 3: Whole person impairment

Upper extremity: Shoulder girdle and shoulder—muscle power MRC 4	2%		
Upper extremity: Shoulder girdle and shoulder—muscle power MRC 4	Lower extremity: Ankle dorsiflexors and peronei—muscle power MRC 4	4%	
Upper extremity: Shoulder girdle and shoulder—muscle power MRC 4	Lower extremity: Ankle dorsiflexors and peronei—muscle power MRC 4	Unilateral facial muscle weakness (5%), dysarthria Class 1 (5%)	14%
Upper extremity: Shoulder girdle, shoulder and elbow—muscle power—MRC 3	3%		
Upper extremity: Shoulder girdle, shoulder and elbow—muscle power—MRC 3	Lower extremity: Ankle dorsiflexors and peronei—muscle power MRC 3	5%	
Upper extremity: Shoulder girdle, shoulder, and elbow—muscle power—MRC 3	Lower extremity: Ankle dorsiflexors and peronei—muscle power MRC 3	Unilateral facial muscle weakness (5%), dysarthria Class 1 (5%), dysphagia Class 1 (2.5%)	18%

Table 23.202 Unilateral facioscapulohumeral muscular dystrophy—Facial, shoulder, elbow, and hip, knee, and ankle and foot: Whole person impairment

Upper extremity: Shoulder girdle, shoulder, and elbow—muscle power MRC 2	5%		
Upper extremity: Shoulder girdle, shoulder, and elbow—muscle power MRC 2	Lower extremity: Hip and knee—muscle power MRC 3, ankle and foot—muscle power MRC 2	11%	
Upper extremity: Shoulder girdle, shoulder, and elbow—muscle power MRC 2	Lower extremity: Hip and knee—muscle power MRC 3, ankle and foot—muscle power MRC 2	Unilateral facial muscle weakness (5%), dysarthria Class 2 (15%), dysphagia Class 2 (5%)	33%
Upper extremity: Shoulder girdle, shoulder, and elbow—muscle power MRC 1	5%		
Upper extremity: Shoulder girdle, shoulder, and elbow—muscle power MRC 1	Lower extremity: Hip and knee—MRC muscle power MRC 2, ankle and foot—muscle power MRC 1	14%	
Upper Extremity: Shoulder girdle, shoulder, and elbow—muscle power MRC 1	Lower extremity: Hip and knee—MRC muscle power MRC 2, ankle and foot—muscle power MRC 1	Unilateral facial muscle weakness (5%), dysarthria Class 2 (15%), dysphagia Class 2 (5%)	36%

Table 23.203 Limb girdle muscular dystrophy involving proximal muscles of upper and lower extremities: MRC 4 and MRC 3—Whole person impairment

Upper extremities: Muscle power MRC 4	4%		
Upper extremities: Muscle power MRC 4	Lower extremities: Muscle power MRC 4	10%	
Upper extremities: Muscle power MRC 3	8%		
Upper extremities: Muscle power MRC 3	Lower extremities: Muscle power MRC 3	14%	
Upper extremities: Muscle power MRC 3	Lower extremities: Muscle power MRC 3	Bilateral equinus deformity (4%)	17%

Table 23.204 Limb girdle muscular dystrophy involving proximal muscles of upper and lower extremities: MRC 2—Whole person impairment

Upper extremities: Muscle power MRC 2	12%				
Upper extremities: Muscle power MRC 2	Abdominal muscles: Muscle power MRC 3	13%			
Upper extremities: Muscle power MRC 2	Abdominal muscles: Muscle power MRC 3	Lower extremities: Muscle power MRC 2	27%		
Upper extremities: Muscle power MRC 2	Abdominal muscles: Muscle power MRC 3	Lower extremities: Muscle power MRC 2	Cardiomyopathy Class 1 (5%)	31%	
Upper extremities: Muscle power MRC 2	Abdominal muscles: Muscle power MRC 3	Lower extremities: Muscle power MRC 2	Cardiomyopathy Class 1 (5%)	Bilateral hearing: 61–80 dB	51%
Upper extremities: Muscle power MRC 2	Abdominal muscles: Muscle power MRC 3	Lower extremities: Muscle power MRC 2	Cardiomyopathy Class 1 (5%)	Bilateral hearing: 61–80 dB, dysphagia Class 2 (5%)	54%
Upper extremities: Muscle power MRC 2	Abdominal muscles: Muscle power MRC 3	Lower extremities: Muscle power MRC 2	Cardiomyopathy Class 1 (5%)	Bilateral hearing: 61–80 dB, dysphagia Class 2 (5%), bilateral equinus deformity (4%)	56%

Table 23.205 Limb girdle muscular dystrophy involving proximal muscles of upper and lower extremities: MRC 1—Whole person impairment

Upper extremities: Muscle power MRC 1	17%				
Upper extremities: Muscle power MRC 1	Abdominal muscles: Muscle power MRC 2–3	20%			
Upper extremities: Muscle power MRC 1	Abdominal muscles: Muscle power MRC 2–3	Lower extremities: Muscle power MRC 1	36%		
Upper extremities: Muscle power MRC 1	Abdominal muscles: Muscle power MRC 2–3	Lower extremities: Muscle power MRC 1	Cardiomyopathy Class 3 (15%)	46%	
Upper extremities: Muscle power MRC 1	Abdominal muscles: Muscle power MRC 2–3	Lower extremities: Muscle power MRC 1	Cardiomyopathy Class 3 (15%)	Respiratory muscle paralysis Class 1 (15%)	54%
Upper extremities: Muscle power MRC 1	Abdominal muscles: Muscle power MRC 2–3	Lower extremities: Muscle power MRC 1	Cardiomyopathy Class 3 (15%)	Respiratory muscle paralysis Class 1 (15%), IQ (18%)	60%
Upper extremities: Muscle power MRC 1	Abdominal muscles: Muscle power MRC 2–3	Lower extremities: Muscle power MRC 1	Cardiomyopathy Class 3 (15%),	Respiratory muscle paralysis Class 1 (15%), IQ (18%), bilateral hearing 61–89 dB (30%)	72%
Upper extremities: Muscle power MRC 1	Abdominal muscles: Muscle power MRC 2–3	Lower extremities: Muscle power MRC 1	Cardiomyopathy Class 3 (15%)	Respiratory muscle paralysis Class 1 (15%), IQ (18%), bilateral hearing 61–89 dB (30%), dysphagia Class 2 (5%)	74%
Upper extremities: Muscle power MRC 1	Abdominal muscles: Muscle power MRC 2–3	Lower extremities: Muscle power MRC 1	Cardiomyopathy Class 3 (15%)	Respiratory muscle paralysis Class 1 (15%), IQ: 50%–70%, bilateral hearing 61–89 dB (30%), dysphagia Class 2 (5%), bilateral equinus deformity (4%)	75%

Table 23.206 Congenital muscular dystrophy involving muscles of upper and lower extremities, and spine, dysphagia, mental retardation—Whole person impairment

Upper extremities: Muscle power MRC 2	23%				
Upper extremities: Muscle power MRC 2	Truncal muscles: Muscle power MRC 2–3	26%			
Upper extremities: Muscle power MRC 2	Truncal muscles: Muscle power MRC 2–3	Lower extremities: Muscle power MRC 2	40%		
Upper extremities: Muscle power MRC 2	Truncal muscles: Muscle power MRC 2–3	Lower Extremities: Muscle power MRC 2	IQ: 50%–70%	48%	
Upper extremities: Muscle power MRC 2	Truncal muscles: Muscle power MRC 2–3	Lower Extremities: Muscle power MRC 2	IQ: 50%–70%	Dysphagia Class 2 (5%)	51%

23.21 READY RECKONER—ANKYLOSIS/LIMITATION OF JOINT MOVEMENT

Table 23.207 Ankylosing spondylitis—Dorsolumbar spine: 25% limitation of movement: Whole person impairment

Dorsolumbar spine—limitation of movement—25%	1%		
Dorsolumbar spine—limitation of movement—25%	VAS 5		6%
Dorsolumbar spine—limitation of movement—25%	Both hips—limitation of movement—25%	6%	
Dorsolumbar spine—limitation of movement—25%	Both hips—limitation of movement—25%	VAS 5	11%

Table 23.208 Ankylosing spondylitis—Dorsolumbar spine and/or hips: 50% limitation of movement: Whole person impairment

Dorsolumbar spine—limitation of movement—50%	2%		
Dorsolumbar spine—limitation of movement—50%	VAS 5	7%	
Dorsolumbar spine—limitation of movement—50%	VAS 5	Restrictive lung disease Class 1 (5%)	11%
Dorsolumbar spine—limitation of movement—50%	2%		
Dorsolumbar spine—limitation of movement—50%	Both hips—limitation of movement—50%	9%	
Dorsolumbar spine—limitation of movement—50%	Both hips—limitation of movement—50%	VAS 5	14%
Dorsolumbar spine—limitation of movement—50%	Both hips—limitation of movement—50%	VAS 5	Restrictive lung disease Class 1 (5%)	18%

Table 23.209 Ankylosing spondylitis—Cervical and dorsolumbar spine: 50% limitation of movement, Class 2 restrictive lung disease: Whole person impairment

Cervical spine and dorsolumbar spine limitation of movement—50%	4%			
Cervical spine and dorsolumbar spine limitation of movement—50%	VAS 5	9%		
Cervical spine and dorsolumbar spine limitation of movement—50%	VAS 5	Restrictive lung disease Class 2 (25%)	31%	
Cervical spine and dorsolumbar spine limitation of movement—50%	VAS 5	Restrictive lung disease Class 2 (25%)	Kyphosis angle: 25°–50° (5%)	35%

Table 23.210 Ankylosing spondylitis—Cervical and dorsolumbar spine and both hips 50% limitation of movement, Class 2 restrictive lung disease: Whole person impairment

Cervical spine and dorsolumbar spine—limitation of movement—50%	4%			
Cervical spine and dorsolumbar spine—limitation of movement—50%	Hips—limitation of movement—50%	11%		
Cervical spine and dorsolumbar spine—limitation of movement—50%	Hips—limitation of movement—50%	VAS 5	16%	
Cervical spine and dorsolumbar spine—limitation of movement—50%	Hips—limitation of movement—50%	VAS 5	Restrictive lung disease Class 2 (25%)	37%
Cervical spine and dorsolumbar spine—limitation of movement—50%	Hips—limitation of movement—50%	VAS 5	Restrictive lung disease Class 2 (25%)	Kyphosis angle: 25°–50° (5%)	40%

Table 23.211 Ankylosing spondylitis—Cervical and dorsolumbar spine—75% limitation of movement, unilateral ankylosis of hip, Class 3 restrictive lung disease: Whole person impairment

Cervical spine and dorsolumbar spine—limitation of movement—75%	5%				
Cervical spine and dorsolumbar spine—limitation of movement—75%	Unilateral ankylosis of hip	6%			
Cervical spine and dorsolumbar spine—limitation of movement—75%	Unilateral ankylosis of hip	VAS 5	11%		
Cervical spine and dorsolumbar spine—limitation of movement—75%	Unilateral ankylosis of hip	VAS 5	Restrictive lung disease Class 3 (37%)	44%	
Cervical spine and dorsolumbar spine—limitation of movement—75%	Unilateral ankylosis of hip	VAS 5	Restrictive lung disease Class 3 (37%)	Kyphosis angle >50° (10%)	49%

Table 23.212 Ankylosing spondylitis—Cervical and dorsolumbar spine—75% limitation of movement, bilateral ankylosis of hip, Class 3 restrictive lung disease: Whole person impairment

Cervical spine and dorsolumbar spine—limitation of movement—75%	5%				
Cervical spine and dorsolumbar spine—limitation of movement—75%	Bilateral ankylosis of hip	15%			
Cervical spine and dorsolumbar spine—limitation of movement—75%	Bilateral ankylosis of hip	VAS 5	19%		
Cervical spine and dorsolumbar spine—limitation of movement—75%	Bilateral ankylosis of hip	VAS 5	Restrictive lung disease Class 3 (37%)	49%	
Cervical spine and dorsolumbar spine—limitation of movement—75%	Bilateral ankylosis of hip	VAS 5	Restrictive lung disease Class 3 (37%)	Kyphosis angle >50° (10%)	54%

Table 23.213 Ankylosing spondylitis—Ankylosis of cervical and dorsolumbar spine with bilateral ankylosis of hip, restrictive lung disease Class 3: Whole person impairment

Ankylosis of cervical spine and dorsolumbar spine	7%				
Ankylosis of cervical spine and dorsolumbar spine	Bilateral ankylosis of hip	17%			
Ankylosis of cervical spine and dorsolumbar spine	Bilateral ankylosis of hip	VAS 5	21%		
Ankylosis of cervical spine and dorsolumbar spine	Bilateral ankylosis of hip	VAS 5	Restrictive lung disease Class 3 (37%)	50%	
Ankylosis of cervical spine and dorsolumbar spine	Bilateral ankylosis of hip	VAS 5	Restrictive lung disease Class 3 (37%)	Kyphosis angle >50° (10%)	55%

Table 23.214 Limitation of movement of shoulder—Whole person impairment

Limitation of movement—25%	1%	
Limitation of movement—25%	VAS 5	6%
Limitation of movement—50%	2%	
Limitation of movement—50%	VAS 5	7%
Limitation of movement—75%	4%	
Limitation of movement—75%	VAS 5	9%
Ankylosis in functional position	6%	
Ankylosis in non-functional position	7%	

Table 23.215 Limitation of movement of elbow—Whole person impairment

Limitation of movement—25%	1%	
Limitation of movement—25%	VAS 5	6%
Limitation of movement—50%	3%	
Limitation of movement—50%	VAS 5	8%
Limitation of movement—75%	4%	
Limitation of movement—75%	VAS 5	9%
Ankylosis in functional position	8%	
Ankylosis in non-functional position	9%	

Table 23.216 Limitation of movement of forearm—Whole person impairment

Limitation of movement—25%	0.33%	
Limitation of movement—25%	VAS 5	5%
Limitation of movement—50%	0.42%	
Limitation of movement—50%	VAS 5	5%
Limitation of movement—75%	1%	
Limitation of movement—75%	VAS 5	6%
Ankylosis in functional position	2%	
Ankylosis in non-functional position	3%	

Table 23.217 Limitation of movement of wrist—Whole person impairment

Limitation of movement—25%	1%	
Limitation of movement—25%	VAS 5	6%
Limitation of movement—50%	2%	
Limitation of movement—50%	VAS 5	7%
Limitation of movement—75%	2%	
Limitation of movement—75%	VAS 5	7%
Ankylosis in functional position	3%	
Ankylosis in non-functional position	4%	

Table 23.218 Ankylosis of hand—Whole person impairment

Ankylosis	MCP + PIP + DIP	MCP	PIP	DIP
Thumb—ankylosis in functional position	7%	3.50%	2.33%	1.16%
Thumb—ankylosis in non-functional position	8%	4.00%	2.66%	1.33%
Index—ankylosis in functional position	4%	2.00%	1.33%	0.66%
Index—ankylosis in non-functional position	5%	2.50%	1.66%	0.83%
Middle finger—ankylosis in functional position	3%	1.5%	1.00%	0.50%
Middle finger—ankylosis in non-functional position	4%	2.00%	1.33%	0.66%
Ring finger—ankylosis in functional position	2%	1.00%	0.66%	0.33%
Ring finger—ankylosis in non-functional position	2%	1.00%	0.66%	0.33%
Little finger—ankylosis in functional position	2%	1.00%	0.66%	0.33%
Little finger—ankylosis in non-functional position	2%	1.00%	0.66%	0.33%

Table 23.219 Limitation of movement of hip—Whole person impairment

Limitation of movement—25%	2%	
Limitation of movement—25%	VAS 3 (3%)	5%
Limitation of movement—50%	3%	
Limitation of movement—50%	VAS 3 (3%)	6%
Limitation of movement—75%	5%	
Limitation of movement—75%	VAS 3 (3%)	8%
Ankylosis of hip joint in functional position	6%	
Ankylosis of hip joint in functional position	VAS 3 (3%)	9%
Ankylosis of hip joint in non-functional position	7%	
Ankylosis of hip joint in non-functional position	VAS 3 (3%)	10%

Table 23.220 Limitation of movement of knee—Whole person impairment

Limitation of movement—25%	2%	
Limitation of movement—25%	VAS 3 (3%)	5%
Limitation of movement—50%	4%	
Limitation of movement—50%	VAS 3 (3%)	6%
Limitation of movement—75%	5%	
Limitation of movement—75%	VAS 3 (3%)	8%
Ankylosis of knee joint in functional position	7%	
Ankylosis of knee joint in functional position	VAS 3 (3%)	10%
Ankylosis of knee joint in non-functional position	8%	
Ankylosis of knee joint in non-functional position	VAS 3 (3%)	11%

Table 23.221 Limitation of movement of ankle—Whole person impairment

Limitation of movement—25%	2%	
Limitation of movement—25%	VAS 3 (3%)	5%
Limitation of movement—50%	3%	
Limitation of movement—50%	VAS 3 (3%)	6%
Limitation of movement—75%	4%	
Limitation of movement—75%	VAS 3 (3%)	7%
Ankylosis of ankle joint in functional position	5%	
Ankylosis of ankle joint in functional position	VAS 3 (3%)	8%
Ankylosis of ankle joint in non-functional position	7%	
Ankylosis of ankle joint in non-functional position	VAS 3 (3%)	10%

Table 23.222 Limitation of movement of foot—Whole person impairment

Limitation of movement—25%	2%	
Limitation of movement—25%	VAS 3 (3%)	5%
Limitation of movement—50%	2%	
Limitation of movement—50%	VAS 3 (3%)	5%
Limitation of movement—75%	3%	
Limitation of movement—75%	VAS 3 (3%)	6%
Ankylosis of subtalar joint in functional position	3%	
Ankylosis of subtalar joint in functional position	VAS 3 (3%)	6%
Ankylosis of subtalar joint in non-functional position	5%	
Ankylosis of subtalar joint in non-functional position	VAS 3 (3%)	7%

Table 23.223 Ankylosis of big toe/2nd/3rd/4th/5th toe—Whole person impairment

Ankylosis of big toe in functional position	1.02%	
Ankylosis of big toe in functional position	VAS 3 (3%)	4%
Ankylosis of big toe in non-functional position	3.99%	
Ankylosis of big toe in non-functional position	VAS 3 (3%)	4.23%
Ankylosis of 2nd or 3rd toe	0.47%	
Ankylosis of 4th or 5th toe	0.40%	

23.22 READY RECKONER— MUSCULOSKELETAL TENDON FUNCTIONS

23.22.1 Tendon functions—Shoulder, elbow, wrist, and hand

1. Full-Thickness Rupture of Rotator Cuff Tendon: 2%
2. Cut Injury/Rupture of Long Head of Biceps Tendon: 1%
3. Cut Injury/Rupture of Triceps tendon at the insertion: 3%
4. Cut Injury/Rupture of Flexor Carpi Radialis: 1%
5. Cut Injury/Rupture of Flexor Carpi Ulnaris: 1%
6. Cut Injury/Rupture of Extensor Carpi Ulnaris: 1%
7. Cut Injury/Rupture of Extensor Carpi Radialis Longus and Brevis: 1%
8. Extensor Digitorum—Dorsum of the Hand: 4%
9. Flexor Digitorum Superficialis & Profundus (Zone 3)— Palm: 7%
10. Flexor Digitorum Superficialis—Zone 3 or 4 in the Wrist/Palm: 5%
11. Flexor Digitorum Profundus—Zone 3 or 4 in the Wrist/Palm: 4%
12. Flexor Digitorum Superficialis—Zone 3 Palm—Index Finger: 3%
13. Flexor Digitorum Profundus—Zone 3 Palm—Index Finger: 2%
14. Flexor Digitorum Superficialis—Zone 3 Palm—Middle Finger: 1%
15. Flexor Digitorum Profundus—Zone 3 Palm—Middle Finger: 1%
16. Flexor Digitorum Superficialis—Zone 3 Palm—Ring Finger: 1%
17. Flexor Digitorum Profundus—Zone 3 Palm—Ring Finger: 1%
18. Flexor Digitorum Superficialis—Zone 3 Palm—Little Finger: 1%
19. Flexor Digitorum Profundus—Zone 3 Palm—Little Finger: 1%
20. Extensor Digitorum—Dorsum of Hand—Index Finger: 1%
21. Extensor Digitorum & Extensor Indicis—Dorsum of Hand—Index Finger: 2%
22. Extensor Digitorum—Dorsum of Hand—Middle Finger: 1%
23. Extensor Digitorum—Dorsum of Hand—Ring Finger: 1%
24. Extensor Digitorum—Dorsum of Hand—Little Finger: 1%
25. Cut Injury of Tendon—Flexor Pollicis Longus of Thumb: 1%
26. Cut Injury of Tendon—Flexor Pollicis Brevis of Thumb: 2%
27. Cut Injury of Tendon—Abductor Pollicis Brevis of Thumb: 2%
28. Cut Injury of Tendon—Abductor Pollicis Longus of Thumb: 1%
29. Cut Injury of Tendon—Extensor Pollicis Longus of Thumb: 1%
30. Cut Injury of Tendon—Extensor Pollicis Brevis of Thumb: 1%

31. Cut Injury of Tendon—Adductor Pollicis of Thumb: 1%
32. Cut Injury of Tendon—Opponens Pollicis of Thumb: 2%
33. Tendon Injury—Flexor Tendons—Zone 2—Index Finger: 2%
34. Tendon Injury—Flexor Tendons—Zone 2—Middle Finger: 1.5%
35. Tendon Injury—Flexor Tendons—Zone 2—Ring Finger: 1%
36. Tendon Injury—Flexor Tendons—Zone 2—Little Finger: 1%
37. Tendon Injury—Flexor Digitorum Profundus—Zone 1—Index Finger: 1.42%
38. Tendon Injury—Flexor Digitorum Profundus—Zone 1—Middle Finger: 0.75%
39. Tendon Injury—Flexor Digitorum Profundus—Zone 1—Ring Finger: 1%
40. Tendon Injury—Flexor Digitorum Profundus—Zone 1—Little Finger: 1%

23.22.2 Tendon functions—Hip, knee, ankle, foot

1. Tendon Injury/Rupture—Adductor Longus and Brevis: 2.5%
2. Tendon Injury/Rupture—Gluteus Medius Tendon: 3%
3. Tendon Injury/Rupture—Hamstring Tendon: 4%
4. Tendon Injury/Rupture—Quadriceps Tendon: 6%
5. Cut Injury/Rupture of Tendo Achilles: 6%
6. Cut Injury/Rupture of Tibialis Anterior, Extensor Digitorum Longus, and Extensor Hallucis Longus: 6%
7. Cut Injury/Rupture of Tibialis Anterior: 4%
8. Cut Injury/Rupture of Extensor Digitorum Longus: 3%
9. Cut Injury/Rupture of Tibialis Posterior: 4%
10. Cut Injury/Rupture of Peronei: 3%
11. Cut Injury/Rupture of—Extensor Hallucis Longus: 1%
12. Cut Injury/Rupture of Tear of Flexor Tendons at the Level of the Sole of the Foot: 3%

23.23 READY RECKONER—UPPER AND LOWER EXTREMITY AMPUTATIONS

23.23.1 Upper extremity amputations

1. Forequarter amputation: 80%
2. Shoulder disarticulation: 79%
3. Transhumeral amputation upper third: 78%
4. Transhumeral amputation middle third: 77%
5. Transhumeral amputation lower third: 76%
6. Elbow disarticulation: 72%
7. Transradial amputation upper third: 70%
8. Transradial amputation middle third: 68%
9. Transradial amputation lower third: 66%
10. Wrist disarticulation: 65%
11. Transmetacarpal amputation all fingers: 55%
12. Carpo-metacarpophalangeal joint amputation four fingers except thumb: 44%

13. Amputation of thumb at carpo-metacarpophalangeal Joint: 31%
14. Transmetacarpal amputation of thumb: 26%
15. Amputation of thumb at metacarpophalangeal Joint: 20%
16. Amputation of thumb at Interphalangeal Joint: 7%
17. Amputation of all fingers including thumb at metacarpophalangeal joint: 45%
18. Amputation of all fingers excepting thumb at metacarpophalangeal joint: 30%
19. Amputation of index finger at carpo-metacarpophalangeal joint: 17%
20. Amputation of index finger at transmetacarpal level: 14%
21. Amputation of index finger at metacarpophalangeal joint: 11%
22. Amputation of index finger at proximal interphalangeal joint: 7%
23. Amputation of index finger at distal interphalangeal joint: 4%
24. Amputation of middle finger at carpo-metacarpophalangeal joint: 17%
25. Amputation of middle finger at transmetacarpal level: 14%
26. Amputation of middle finger at metacarpophalangeal joint: 11%
27. Amputation of middle finger at proximal interphalangeal joint: 7%
28. Amputation of middle finger at distal interphalangeal joint: 4%
29. Amputation of ring finger at carpo-metacarpophalangeal joint: 10%
30. Amputation of ring finger at transmetacarpal level: 8%
31. Amputation of ring finger at metacarpophalangeal joint: 6%
32. Amputation of ring finger at proximal interphalangeal joint: 4%
33. Amputation of ring finger at distal interphalangeal joint: 2%
34. Amputation of little finger at carpo-metacarpophalangeal joint: 10%
35. Amputation of little finger at transmetacarpal level: 8%
36. Amputation of little finger at metacarpophalangeal joint: 6%
37. Amputation of little finger at proximal interphalangeal joint: 4%
38. Amputation of little finger at distal interphalangeal joint: 2%

23.23.2 Amputation of lower extremity

1. Hindquarter amputation: 61%
2. Hip disarticulation: 60%
3. Transfemoral amputation—proximal third: 59%
4. Transfemoral amputation—middle third: 58%
5. Transfemoral amputation—distal third: 55%
6. Knee disarticulation: 54%

7. Trans tibiofibular amputation—proximal third <3″: 53%
8. Trans tibiofibular amputation—proximal third ≥3″: 51%
9. Trans tibiofibular amputation—middle third: 49%
10. Trans tibiofibular amputation—distal third: 47%
11. Ankle disarticulation: 45%
12. Syme's amputation: 38%
13. Chopart-Midtarsal amputation: 27%
14. Lisfranc—Trans metatarsal amputation: 21%
15. Trans metatarsal amputation—all toes: 16%
16. Metatarsophalangeal joint amputation—all toes: 11%
17. Amputation of all toes except big toe: 7%
18. Amputation of big toe at MTP joint: 4%
19. Amputation of big toe at IP joint: 2%
20. Amputation of 2nd toe at MTP joint: 2%
21. Amputation of 2nd toe at PIP joint: 1%
22. Amputation of 2nd toe at DIP joint: 0.5%
23. Amputation of 3rd toe at MTP joint: 2%
24. Amputation of 3rd toe at PIP joint: 1%
25. Amputation of 3rd toe at DIP joint: 0.5%
26. Amputation of 4th toe at MTP joint: 1%
27. Amputation of 4th toe at PIP joint: 0.5%
28. Amputation of 4th toe at DIP joint: 0.25%
29. Amputation of 5th toe at MTP joint: 1%
30. Amputation of 5th toe at PIP joint: 0.5%
31. Amputation of 5th toe at DIP joint: 0.25%

23.24 READY RECKONER—CONGENITAL SKELETAL LIMB DEFICIENCIES

23.24.1 Upper extremity transverse deficiencies

1. Shoulder total transverse deficiency: 80%
2. Upper arm total transverse deficiency: 79%
3. Upper arm upper third transverse deficiency: 78%
4. Upper arm middle third transverse deficiency: 77%
5. Upper arm distal third transverse deficiency: 76%
6. Forearm total transverse deficiency: 72%
7. Forearm upper third transverse deficiency: 70%
8. Forearm middle third transverse deficiency: 68%
9. Forearm distal third transverse deficiency: 66%
10. Carpal total transverse deficiency: 65%
11. Metacarpal total transverse deficiency: 64%
12. Metacarpal partial transverse deficiency: 55%
13. Phalangeal all fingers total transverse deficiency: 45%
14. Phalangeal thumb total transverse deficiency at CMCP: 31%
15. Phalangeal thumb partial transverse deficiency at MCP: 20%
16. Phalangeal thumb partial transverse deficiency at IP: 7%
17. Phalangeal index total transverse deficiency at CMCP: 17%

18. Phalangeal index partial transverse deficiency at MCP: 11%
19. Phalangeal index partial transverse deficiency at PIP: 7%
20. Phalangeal index partial transverse deficiency at DIP: 4%
21. Phalangeal middle finger total transverse deficiency at CMCP: 17%
22. Phalangeal middle finger partial transverse deficiency at MCP: 11%
23. Phalangeal middle finger partial transverse deficiency at PIP: 7%
24. Phalangeal middle finger partial transverse deficiency at DIP: 4%
25. Phalangeal ring finger total transverse deficiency at CMCP: 10%
26. Phalangeal ring finger partial transverse deficiency at MCP: 6%
27. Phalangeal ring finger partial transverse deficiency at PIP: 4%
28. Phalangeal ring finger partial transverse deficiency at DIP: 2%
29. Phalangeal little finger total transverse deficiency at CMCP: 10%
30. Phalangeal little finger partial transverse deficiency at MCP: 6%
31. Phalangeal little finger partial transverse deficiency at PIP: 4%
32. Phalangeal little finger partial transverse deficiency at DIP: 2%

CMCP = Carpo-metacarpophalangeal joint, MCP = Metacarpophalangeal joint, PIP = Proximal interphalangeal joint, DIP = Distal interphalangeal joint.

23.24.2 Lower extremity transverse deficiencies

1. Pelvis total transverse deficiency: 61%
2. Thigh total transverse deficiency: 60%
3. Thigh upper third transverse deficiency: 59%
4. Thigh middle third transverse deficiency: 58%
5. Thigh lower third transverse deficiency: 55%
6. Leg total transverse deficiency: 54%
7. Leg upper third transverse deficiency <3″: 53%
8. Leg upper third transverse deficiency ≥3″: 51%
9. Leg middle third transverse deficiency: 49%
10. Leg lower third transverse deficiency: 47%
11. Tarsal total transverse deficiency: 45%
12. Tarsal partial transverse deficiency: 27%
13. Metatarsal total transverse deficiency: 21%
14. Metatarsal partial transverse deficiency: 16%
15. Phalangeal total transverse deficiency—all toes: 11%

16. Phalangeal total transverse deficiency—Big Toe: 4%
17. Phalangeal partial transverse deficiency—Big Toe: 2%
18. Phalangeal total transverse deficiency 2nd Toe: 2%
19. Phalangeal partial transverse deficiency 2nd Toe: 1%
20. Phalangeal total transverse deficiency 3rd Toe: 2%
21. Phalangeal partial transverse deficiency 3rd Toe: 1%
22. Phalangeal total transverse deficiency 4th Toe: 1%
23. Phalangeal partial transverse deficiency 4th Toe: 0.5%
24. Phalangeal total transverse deficiency 5th Toe: 1%
25. Phalangeal partial transverse deficiency 5th Toe: 0.5%

23.25 READY RECKONER—DWARFISM, DISFIGUREMENT, AND SHORTENING

23.25.1 Dwarfism

"Integrated Evaluation of Disability" assigns an impairment of 1.72% for each inch of shortening from 4'10".

23.25.2 Disfigurement and deformity

Table 23.224 Disfigurement and deformity—Head and neck

Region	Class 1 impairment	Class 2 impairment	Class 3 impairment	Class 4 impairment
Face	Depigmentation, e.g., leukoderma 1%	Hypertrophic scar involving one side of the face 2.5%, both sides of the face 5%	Keloid involving one side of the face 7.5%	Keloid involving both sides 10%
Ear	Depigmentation 0.25%	Hypertrophic scar 0.5%	Keloid 1.0%	Amputation of the pinna of the ear 2.5%
Eye	Scar and loss of hair in the eyebrow, e.g., Burns sequel 0.25%	Entropion/ectropion 0.50%	Corneal opacity 0.75%	Enucleation of one eye 1%
Nose	Saddle nose 1.25%	Saddle nose with keloid 2.5%	Sub-total amputation 3.75%	Total nasal amputation 5%
Mouth	Depigmentation of lip—leukoplakia 0.5%	Microstomia 2.5%	Cleft lip 5%	Cleft lip and palate 10%
Neck	Depigmentation 0.5%	Hypertrophic scar 1.0%	Keloid 2.0%	Torticollis 2.5%

Table 23.225 Disfigurement and deformity—Chest and trunk

Region	Class 1 impairment	Class 2 impairment	Class 3 impairment	Class 4 impairment
Chest	Depigmentation 0.25%	Hypertrophic scar 0.5%	Keloid 1.0%	Band like contracture 2.0%
Breast	Subcutaneous mastectomy 1.0%	Partial mastectomy 2.5%	Total unilateral mastectomy 5.0%	Bilateral total mastectomy 10.0%
Spine—scoliosis/kyphosis cobb/centroid angles		Cobb: 10°–24° 2.5%	Cobb: 25°–49° 5.0%	Cobb: ≥50° 10.0%

Table 23.226 Disfigurement and deformity—Upper extremity

Region	Class 1 impairment	Class 2 impairment	Class 3 impairment	Class 4 impairment
Upper arm	Depigmentation 0.25%	Hypertrophic scar 0.5%	Keloid 0.75%	Contracture 1.0%
Forearm, wrist, and hand	Depigmentation 1.0%	Hypertrophic scar 2.0%	Keloid 3.0%	Contracture, e.g., club hand, claw hand deformity, or Resorption of fingers 4.0%

Table 23.227 Disfigurement and deformity—lower extremity

Region	Class 1 impairment	Class 2 impairment	Class 3 impairment	Class 4 impairment
Hip and thigh			Keloid 0.25%	Deformity 0.5%
Knee and leg			Keloid 0.25%	Deformity 0.5%
Ankle	Depigmentation 0.25%	Hypertrophic scar 0.5%	Keloid 0.75%	Deformity, e.g., equinus deformity, calcaneal deformity 2.0%
Foot including dorsum of foot	Depigmentation 0.25%	Hypertrophic scar 0.5%	Keloid 1.0%	
Foot including sole of the foot	Hypertrophic scar 1.0%	Keloid 2.0%	Pes cavus deformity 2.0%	Club foot 4.0%

23.25.3 Shortening of extremity

"*Integrated Evaluation of Disability*" assigns an impairment of one percent for each inch of shortening of the upper/lower extremity.

23.26 READY RECKONER—BURNS

Table 23.228 Whole body burns—Burns: Head and neck—Class 1 impairment

					Combine impairment by $A + B(100 - A)/100$
Burns face and scalp	Class 1 depigmentation (1%)	Class 1 permanent loss of hair <25% (1.25%)	Class 1—permanent loss of sensation—maxillary or mandibular division (1.25%)	Class 1 loss of sensation C 2 dermatome (0.5%)	3.75%
Eye	Class 1: Scar and loss of hair in the eyebrow both eyes (0.5%)				4.23%
Ear	Class 1 depigmentation (0.25%) Right	Class 1 depigmentation (0.25%) Left	Class 1: Loss of skin over pinna of the ear with intact bare cartilage—right (1.25%)	Class 1: Loss of skin over pinna of the ear with intact bare cartilage—left (1.25%)	7.10%
Nose	Class 1 depigmentation (0.5%)	Class 1: Partial loss of alar lobule of nose (1.25%)			8.73%
Mouth	Class 1 depigmentation (0.5%)				9.19%
Neck	Class 1 depigmentation (0.5%)				9.64%

Table 23.229 Whole body burns—Burns: Chest, trunk, perineum, genitals—Class 1 impairment

			Combine impairment by $A + B(100 - A)/100$
Chest	Class 1 depigmentation (0.25%)	Class 1: Breast—unilateral loss of full thickness skin (1.25%)	11%
Spine—motor function	Limitation of movement—25% (1.71%)		12.52%
Perineum and genitals	Class 1 depigmentation (1.25%)		13.61%

Table 23.230 Whole body burns—Burns: Upper extremities—Class 1 impairment

				Combine impairment by $A + B(100 - A)/100$
Right upper extremity—disfigurement	Class 1 depigmentation—axilla (0.25%)	Class 1 depigmentation—upper arm (0.25%)	Class 1 depigmentation—forearm and hand (1.00%)	14.91%
Right upper extremity—motor function	Limitation of movement—25% (4.17%)			18.45%
Left upper extremity—disfigurement	Class 1 depigmentation—axilla (0.25%)	Class 1 depigmentation—upper arm (0.25%)	Class 1 depigmentation—forearm and hand (1.00%)	19.68%
Left upper extremity—motor function	Limitation of movement—25% (4.17%)			23.02%

Table 23.231 Whole body burns—Burns: Lower extremities—Class 1 impairment

		Combine impairment by $A + B(100 - A)/100$
Right lower extremity—disfigurement	Class 1 depigmentation (0.5%)	23.41%
Left lower extremity—motor function	Limitation of movement—25% (2.59%)	25.39%
Left lower extremity—disfigurement	Class 1 depigmentation (0.5%)	25.76%
Right lower extremity—motor function	Limitation of movement—25% (2.59%)	27.68%
Pain	VAS 3 (3%)	29.85%

Table 23.232 Whole body Burns—Burns: Head and neck—Class 2 impairment

					Combine impairment by A + B(100 − A)/100
Burns face and scalp	Class 2 hypertrophic scar (2.50%)	Class 2 permanent loss of hair 25%–50% (2.50%)	Class 2—permanent loss of sensation—maxillary or mandibular division (1.25%)	Class 2—permanent loss of sensation—maxillary and mandibular division (2.5%) C 2 dermatome (0.5%)	8.00%
Eye	Class 2: entropion/ectropion right eye (0.5%)	Class 2: entropion/ectropion left eye (0.5%)			8.92%
Ear	Class 2 hypertrophic scar (0.50%) right	Class 2 hypertrophic scar (0.50%) left	Class 2: Amputation of the pinna of the ear—right (2.5%)	Class 2: Amputation of the pinna of the ear—left (2.5%)	14.38%
Nose	Class 2 hypertrophic scar (1.0%)	Class 2: Total loss of alar lobule of nose with intact cartilaginous support (2.5%)			17.38%
Mouth	Class 2 hypertrophic scar (1.0%)				18.21%
Neck	Class 2 hypertrophic scar (1.0%)	Partial sensory loss (0.75%)			19.64%

Table 23.233 Whole body burns—Burns: Chest, trunk, perineum, genitals—Class 2 impairment

			Combine impairment by A + B(100 − A)/100
Chest	Class 2 hypertrophic scar (0.50%)	Class 1: Breast—bilateral loss of full thickness skin (2.5%)	22.05%
Spine—motor function	Limitation of movement—50% (3.42%)		24.72%
Perineum and genitals	Class 2 hypertrophic scar (2.5%)		26.60%

Table 23.234 Whole body burns—Burns: Upper extremities—Class 2 impairment

				Combine impairment by A + B(100 − A)/100
Right upper extremity—disfigurement	Class 2 hypertrophic scar—axilla (0.5%)	Class 2 hypertrophic scar—upper arm (0.5%)	Class 2 hypertrophic scar—forearm and hand (2.00%)	28.80%
Right upper extremity—motor function	Limitation of movement—50% (8.36%)			34.76%
Left upper extremity—disfigurement	Class 2 hypertrophic scar—axilla (0.5%)	Class 2 hypertrophic scar—upper arm (0.5%)	Class 2 hypertrophic scar—forearm and hand (2.00%)	36.71%
Left upper extremity—motor function	Limitation of movement—50% (8.36%)			42.01%

Table 23.235 Whole body burns—Burns: Lower extremities—Class 2 impairment

		Combine impairment by A + B(100 − A)/100
Right lower extremity—disfigurement	Class 2 hypertrophic scar (1.0%)	42.59%
Right lower extremity—motor function	Limitation of movement—50% (5.17%)	45.56%
Left lower extremity—disfigurement	Class 2 hypertrophic scar (1.0%)	46.10%
Right lower extremity—motor function	Limitation of movement—50% (5.17%)	48.89%
Pain	VAS 3 (3%)	50.42%

Table 23.236 Whole body burns—Burns: Head and neck—Class 3 impairment

					Combine impairment by A + B(100 − A)/100
Burns face and scalp	Class 3 keloid one side of the face (5.00%)	Class 3 permanent loss of hair 50%–75% (3.75%)	Class 3—permanent loss of sensation—ophthalmic division Class 2—permanent loss of sensation—maxillary or mandibular division (1.25%)	Class 4—permanent loss of sensation—trigeminal nerve (5%) C 2 dermatome (0.75%)	10.00%
Eye	Class 3: Corneal opacity right eye (0.75%)	Class 3: Corneal opacity right eye (0.75%)	Visual impairment of vision (15%)		24.85%
Ear	Class 3 keloid (1.00%) right	Class 3 keloid (1.00%) left	Class 2: Amputation of the pinna of the ear—right (2.5%)	Class 2: Amputation of the pinna of the ear left (2.5%)	30.11%
Nose	Class 2 keloid (2.0%)	Class 3: Sub-total amputation of nose with loss of cartilaginous support (3.75%)	Bilateral anosmia (5.00%)		37.62%
Mouth	Class 3—keloid (2.00%)	Microstomia (1.0%)	Microstomia with inability to smile/drooling (2.5%)		41.05%
Neck	Class 3—keloid (2.00%)	Complete sensory loss (1.5%)			43.12%

Table 23.237 Whole body burns—Burns: Chest, trunk, perineum, genitals—Class 3 impairment

				Combine impairment by A + B(100 − A)/100
Chest	Class 3—keloid (1.00%)	Bilateral total loss of breast (10%)		49.37%
Spine—motor function	Limitation of movement—75% (5.72%)			52.27%
Perineum and genitals	Class 3 keloid (3.75%)	Obliteration of perineum—partial occlusion of anus (2.5%)	Initiation of bowel movement by suppositories (5%)	55.07%

Table 23.238 Whole body burns—Burns: Upper extremities—Class 3 impairment

				Combine impairment by A + B(100 − A)/100
Right upper extremity—disfigurement	Class 3 keloid—axilla (0.75%)	Class 3 keloid—upper arm (0.75%)	Class 3 keloid—forearm and hand (3.00%)	57.09%
Right upper extremity—motor function	Limitation of movement—75% (13.83%)			63.03%
Left upper extremity—disfigurement	Class 3 keloid—axilla (0.75%)	Class 3 keloid—upper arm (0.75%)	Class 3 keloid—forearm and hand (3.00%)	64.69%
Left upper extremity—motor function	Limitation of movement—75% (13.83%)			69.58%

Table 23.239 Whole body burns—Burns: Lower extremities—Class 3 impairment

			Combine impairment by A + B(100 − A)/100
Right lower extremity—disfigurement	Class 3 keloid (2.5%)		70.34%
Right lower extremity—motor function	Limitation of movement—75% (9.84%)		73.26%
Left lower extremity—disfigurement	Class 3 keloid (2.5%)		73.92%
Right lower extremity—motor function	Limitation of movement—75% (9.84%)		76.49%
Pain	VAS 3 (3%)		77.67%
Deformities	Bilateral finger deformities (8%)	Bilateral hip and knee deformities (2%)	79.23%

Table 23.240 Burns: Head and neck—Class 1 impairment

					Combine impairment by $A + B(100 - A)/100$
Burns face and scalp	Class 1 depigmentation (1%)	Class 1 permanent loss of hair <25% (1.25%)	Class 1—permanent loss of sensation—maxillary or mandibular division (1.25%)	Class 1 loss of sensation C 2 dermatome (0.5%)	3.75%
Eye	Class 1: Scar and loss of hair in the eyebrow both eyes (0.5%)				4.23%
Ear	Class 1 depigmentation (0.25%) Right	Class 1 depigmentation (0.25%) Left	Class 1: Loss of skin over pinna of the ear with intact bare cartilage—right (1.25%)	Class 1: Loss of skin over pinna of the ear with intact bare cartilage—left (1.25%)	7.10%
Nose	Class 1 depigmentation (0.5%)	Class 1: Partial loss of alar lobule of nose (1.25%)			8.73%
Mouth	Class 1 depigmentation (0.5%)				9.19%
Neck	Class 1 depigmentation (0.5%)				9.64%
Pain	VAS 3 (3%)				12.35%

Table 23.241 Burns: Head and neck—Class 2 impairment

					Combine impairment by $A + B(100 - A)/100$
Burns face and scalp	Class 2 hypertrophic scar (2.50%)	Class 2 permanent loss of hair 25%–50% (2.50%)	Class 2—permanent loss of sensation—maxillary or mandibular division (1.25%)	Class 2—permanent loss of sensation—maxillary and mandibular division (2.5%) C 2 dermatome (0.5%)	8.00%
Eye	Class 2: entropion/ectropion right eye (0.5%)	Class 2: entropion/ectropion left eye (0.5%)			8.92%
Ear	Class 2 hypertrophic scar (0.50%) right	Class 2 hypertrophic scar (0.50%) left	Class 2: Amputation of the pinna of the ear—right (2.5%)	Class 2: Amputation of the pinna of the ear—left (2.5%)	14.38%

(Continued)

Table 23.241 (*Continued*) Burns: Head and neck—Class 2 impairment

				Combine impairment by $A + B(100 - A)/100$
Nose	Class 2 hypertrophic scar (1.0%)	Class 2: Total loss of alar lobule of nose with intact cartilaginous support (2.5%)		17.38%
Mouth	Class 2 hypertrophic scar (1.0%)			18.21%
Neck	Class 2 hypertrophic scar (1.0%)	Partial sensory loss (0.75%)		19.64%
Pain	VAS 3 (3%)			22.05%

Table 23.242 Burns: Head and neck—Class 3 impairment

					Combine impairment by $A + B(100 - A)/100$
Burns face and scalp	Class 3 keloid one side of the face (5.00%)	Class 3 permanent loss of hair 50%–75% (3.75%)	Class 3—permanent loss of sensation—ophthalmic division Class 2—permanent loss of sensation—maxillary or mandibular division (1.25%)	Class 4—permanent loss of sensation—trigeminal nerve (5%) C 2 dermatome (0.75%)	10.00%
Eye	Class 3: Corneal opacity right eye (0.75%)	Class 3: Corneal opacity right eye (0.75%)	Visual impairment of vision (15%)		24.85%
Ear	Class 3 keloid (1.00%) right	Class 3 keloid (1.00%) left	Class 2: Amputation of the pinna of the ear—right (2.5%)	Class 2: Amputation of the pinna of the ear—left (2.5%)	30.11%
Nose	Class 2 keloid (2.0%)	Class 3: Sub-total amputation of nose with loss of cartilaginous support (3.75%)	Bilateral anosmia (5.00%)		37.62%
Mouth	Class 3—keloid (2.00%)	Microstomia (1.0%)	Microstomia with inability to smile/drooling (2.5%)		41.05%
Neck	Class 3—keloid (2.00%)	Complete sensory loss (1.5%)			43.12%
Pain	VAS 5 (5%)				44.82%

Table 23.243 Burns: Chest, trunk—Class 1 impairment

			Combine impairment by $A + B(100 - A)/100$
Chest	Class 1 depigmentation (0.25%)	Class 1: Breast—unilateral loss of full thickness skin (1.25%)	1.5%
Spine—motor function	Limitation of movement—25% (1.71%)		3.19%
Pain	VAS 3 (3%)		6.09%

Table 23.244 Burns: Chest, trunk—Class 2 impairment

			Combine impairment by A + B(100 − A)/100
Chest	Class 2 hypertrophic scar (0.50%)	Class 1: Breast—bilateral loss of full thickness skin (2.5%)	3.00%
Spine—motor function	Limitation of movement— 50% (3.42%)		6.32%
Pain	VAS 3 (3%)		9.13%

Table 23.245 Burns: Chest, trunk—Class 3 impairment

			Combine impairment by A + B(100 − A)/100
Chest	Class 3—keloid (1.00%)	Bilateral total loss of breast (10%)	11.00%
Spine—motor function	Limitation of movement—75% (5.72%)		16.09%
Pain	VAS 3 (3%)		18.61%

Table 23.246 Burns: Perineum, genitals—Class 1, 2, 3 impairment

		Combine impairment by A + B(100 − A)/100
Perineum and genitals	Class 1 depigmentation (1.25%)	1.25%
Pain	VAS 3 (3%)	4.21%
Perineum and genitals	Class 2 depigmentation (2.5%)	2.5%
Pain	VAS 3 (3%)	5.43%
Perineum and genitals	Class 1 depigmentation (3.75%) Perineal obliteration of anus (2.5%) Initiation of bowel movement by suppositories (5%)	11.25%
Pain	VAS 3 (3%)	13.91%

Table 23.247 Burns: Upper extremities—Class 1 impairment

				Combine impairment by A + B(100 − A)/100
Right upper extremity— disfigurement	Class 1 depigmentation— axilla (0.25%)	Class 1 depigmentation— upper arm (0.25%)	Class 1 depigmentation— forearm and hand (1.00%)	1.50%
Right upper extremity— motor function	Limitation of movement—25% (4.17%)			5.6%
Left upper extremity— disfigurement	Class 1 depigmentation— axilla (0.25%)	Class 1 depigmentation— upper arm (0.25%)	Class 1 depigmentation— forearm and hand (1.00%)	7.02%
Left upper extremity— motor function	Limitation of movement—25% (4.17%)			10.89%
Pain	VAS 3 (3%)			13.57%

Table 23.248 Burns: Upper extremities—Class 2 impairment

				Combine impairment by A + B(100 − A)/100
Right upper extremity—disfigurement	Class 2 hypertrophic scar—axilla (0.5%)	Class 2 hypertrophic scar—upper arm (0.5%)	Class 2 hypertrophic scar—forearm and hand (2.00%)	3.00%
Right upper extremity—motor function	Limitation of movement—50% (8.36%)			11.11%
Left upper extremity—disfigurement	Class 2 hypertrophic scar—axilla (0.5%)	Class 2 Hypertrophic scar—upper arm (0.5%)	Class 2 hypertrophic scar—forearm and hand (2.00%)	13.78%
Left upper extremity—motor function	Limitation of movement—50% (8.36%)			20.99%
Pain	VAS 3 (3%)			23.36%

Table 23.249 Burns: Upper extremities—Class 3 impairment

				Combine impairment by A + B(100 − A)/100
Right upper extremity—disfigurement	Class 3 keloid—axilla (0.75%)	Class 3 keloid—upper arm (0.75%)	Class 3 keloid—forearm and hand (3.00%)	4.50%
Right upper extremity—motor function	Limitation of movement—75% (13.83%)			17.71%
Left upper extremity—disfigurement	Class 3 keloid—axilla (0.75%)	Class 3 keloid—upper arm (0.75%)	Class 3 keloid—forearm and hand (3.00%)	21.41%
Left upper extremity—motor function	Limitation of movement—75% (13.83%)			32.28%
Pain	VAS 3 (3%)			34.32%
Deformities	Bilateral deformity of fingers (8%)			37.60%

Table 23.250 Burns: Lower extremities—Class 1 impairment

		Combine impairment by A + B(100 − A)/100
Right lower extremity—disfigurement	Class 1 depigmentation (0.5%)	0.50%
Left lower extremity—motor function	Limitation of movement—25% (2.59%)	3.07%
Left lower extremity—disfigurement	Class 1 depigmentation (0.5%)	3.56%
Right lower rextremity—motor function	Limitation of movement—25% (2.59%)	6.05%
Pain	VAS 3 (3%)	8.87%

Table 23.251 Burns: Lower extremities—Class 2 impairment

		Combine impairment by A + B(100 − A)/100
Right lower extremity—disfigurement	Class 2 hypertrophic scar (1.0%)	1.00%
Right lower extremity—motor function	Limitation of movement—50% (5.17%)	6.12%
Left lower extremity—disfigurement	Class 2 hypertrophic scar (1.0%)	7.06%
Right lower extremity—motor function	Limitation of movement—50% (5.17%)	11.87%
Pain	VAS 3 (3%)	14.51%

Table 23.252 Whole body burns—Burns: Lower extremities—Class 3 impairment

		Combine impairment by A + B(100 − A)/100
Right lower extremity—disfigurement	Class 3 keloid (2.5%)	2.50%
Right lower extremity—motor function	Limitation of movement—75% (9.84%)	12.09%
Left lower extremity—disfigurement	Class 3 keloid (2.5%)	14.29%
Right lower extremity—motor function	Limitation of movement—75% (9.84%)	22.73%
Pain	VAS 3 (3%)	25.04%
Deformities	Bilateral hip and knee deformities (2%)	26.54%

23.27 READY RECKONER—GENITOURINARY FUNCTION

Table 23.253 Renal function—Chronic renal failure: Whole person impairment

Impairment class	Description of excretory status of kidney function	Reference impairment score
Class 1	When only one kidney is functioning, or one kidney is congenitally absent: Normal safety factor is lost	10%
Class 2	Non-dialysis dependent chronic renal failure with GFR <60 and ≥30 mL/min/1.73 m²	25%
Class 3	Dialysis dependent chronic renal failure with GFR <30 mL/min/1.73 m²	37%
Class 4	End-stage renal failure with GFR <15 mL/min/1.73 m² requiring renal transplantation	50%

Table 23.254 Micturition function—Non-neurogenic lesion: Whole person impairment

Impairment class	Clinical status of micturition function	Impairment	Maximum impairment 15%
Class 1	**Urgency** of micturition without incontinence	5%	
Class 1	**Hesitancy** of micturition	5%	
Class 2	**Urgency** of micturition with incontinence	15%	
Class 2	**Stress incontinence**	15%	

1. Valsalva leak point pressure measures sphincter weakness
2. The urodynamic study assesses sphincter dysfunction
3. Sphincter electromyography ascertains suspected neuropathy

Table 23.255 Micturition function—Neurogenic lesion: Whole person impairment

Impairment class	Clinical status of micturition function	Impairment	Maximum impairment 50%
Class 1	**Urgency** of micturition without incontinence	5%	
Class 1	**Hesitancy** of micturition	5%	
Class 2	**Urgency** of micturition with incontinence	15%	
Class 2	Voiding by abdominal straining (Valsalva Maneuver)/Credé maneuver with no post-void residual urine	15%	
Class 3	Uninhibited neurogenic bladder	25%	
Class 3	(1) Reflex voiding (2) No detrusor sphincter dyssynergia (3) No sensation of desire/fullness/voiding	25%	
Class 4	(1) Reflex voiding (2) Detrusor sphincter dyssynergia (3) No sensation of desire/fullness/voiding associated with detrusor dysfunction (4) Requires alpha blockers or botulinum toxin injection or transurethral sphincterotomy or endo-urethral stents to eliminate post-void residual urine	37%	
Class 5	(1) Inability in initiating micturition resulting in retention/inability to hold urine resulting in incontinence (or) Persistent post-void residual urine even after abdominal straining/Credé maneuver or sphincter management (2) No sensation of desire/fullness/voiding (3) Voiding by catheter/requiring diapers (4) Neurogenic status confirmed by urodynamic study	50%	

Table 23.256 Genital functions—Whole person impairment

Genital functions	Clinical tools	Reference impairment score
Sexual functions	Erectile dysfunction assessed by International Index of Erectile Function questionnaire, nocturnal penile tumescence test, color Doppler ultrasonography; anatomical loss of testes or anatomical loss of penis	15%
Menstrual functions	Primary amenorrhea in reproductive age after maximum medical management	15%
Procreation functions	1. Azoospermia confirmed by hormone or semen analysis and/or vasography before 50 years of age or	15%
	2. Structural and/or functional impairment failing to initiate/continue pregnancy due to cervical/uterine/ovarian/tubal or peritoneal factors before 50 years of age after maximum medical management	15%

23.28 READY RECKONER—SWALLOWING, LIVER, AND DEFECATION FUNCTIONS

Table 23.257 Swallowing functions—Whole person impairment

Impairment class	Criteria	Reference impairment score
Class 1	Difficulty in swallowing with drooling of saliva or drooling during drinking liquids or accumulation of solid food in the alveoli of mouth	2.5%
Class 2	Prolonged duration of meal with sensation of holding of food in the throat Difficulty in swallowing with nasal regurgitation and/or occasional choking	5.0%
Class 3	Difficulty in swallowing with nasal regurgitation and on-and-off choking or Limited swallowing ability by modifying food consistency	15%
Class 4	Difficulty in swallowing with frequent nasal regurgitation and choking or Limited swallowing ability by modifying food consistency, and postural techniques and compensatory maneuvers to minimized the risk of aspiration	25%
Class 5	Inability to swallow, develop significant aspiration on attempted swallowing and require feeding by nasogastric tube or PEG (percutaneous endoscopic gastrostomy)	50%

Table 23.258 Chronic liver failure—Whole person impairment

Impairment class	Encephalopathy	Serum level of bilirubin	INR	Serum level of albumin	Serum level of sodium	Impairment score
Class 1	Anxiety or euphoria	1–2 mg/dL	1.1–2.0	>3.5 gm/dL	136–140 mmol/L	25%
Class 2	1. Lethargy and minor impairment of awareness 2. Impairment of cognition: poor attention span, difficulty in orientation for time and place, difficulty in calculation for addition, subtraction 3. Asterixis (flapping tremor) 4. Inappropriate behavior	2.1–3 mg/dL	2.1–3.0	3.1–3.5 gm/dL	131–135 mmol/L	50%
Class 3	1. Somnolent but arousable 2. Impairment of cognition: lack of orientation for place/time/person 3. Asterixis (flapping tremor), hyperreflexia, and plantar extensor response 4. Bizarre behavior	3.1–4 mg/dL	3.1–4	2.6–3.0 gm/dL	126–130 mmol/L	75%
Class 4	Coma not responding to verbal or painful stimuli	>4 mg/dL	>4	≤2.5 gm/dL	≤125 mmol/L	95%
Class 1	*Integrated Evaluation of Disability* assigns Class 1 impairment to persons who underwent liver transplantation because of burden of treatment compliance					25%

Table 23.259 Bowel movement—Defecation whole person impairment

Impairment class	Nature of impairment	Impairment	Maximum impairment 50%
Class 1	**Constipation** Difficulty in initiating bowel movement and evacuating bowel less than three times per week due to neurological cause and requiring fiber supplements, and suppositories for evacuation of bowel	5%	
Class 2	**Constipation** Difficulty in initiating bowel movement and evacuating bowel less than three times per week due to neurological cause Refractory to fiber supplements and suppositories and Requiring prokinetic agents	10%	
Class 3	**Constipation** Difficulty in initiating bowel movement and evacuating bowel one time per week due to neurological cause and requiring enema for evacuation	15%	
	Constipation Anismus, dyssynergia, descending perineal syndrome	15%	
	Constipation Mechanical obstruction due to partial occlusion of anus, e.g., following burns	15%	
Class 4	**Constipation** Mechanical obstruction due to complete occlusion of anus, e.g., following burns	25%	
Class 5	**Incontinence** Inability in controlling bowel movement resulting in incontinence and Lack of sensation of bowel fullness and movement due to neurological cause and requiring diapers	37%	
Class 6	**Permanent colostomy**	50%	

23.29 READY RECKONER—HEMATOLOGICAL FUNCTIONS

Table 23.260 Chronic anemia—Whole person impairment

Impairment class	Clinical status	Hgb level	Blood transfusion requirement	Reference impairment score
Impairment Class 1	Asymptomatic anemia	110–129 g/L	Not required	0%
Impairment Class 2	Symptomatic anemia without cardiopulmonary limitations	70–109 g/L	Requires occasional transfusion	15%
Impairment Class 3	Symptomatic anemia with cardiopulmonary limitations (palpitations, dyspnea, tachycardia, angina pectoris, dizziness, syncope, de novo ST depression or elevation on the electrocardiogram and new arrhythmia on the ECG)	Less than 70 g/L	Requires monthly transfusion or transfusion dependent for survival	37%

Table 23.261 Chronic lymphoid leukemia—Whole person impairment

Impairment class	Severity of chronic lymphoid leukemia	Reference impairment score
Impairment Class 1	Lymphocytosis only in blood and bone marrow. No symptoms	0%
Impairment Class 2	Lymphocytosis, lymphadenopathy, enlarged spleen or liver	37%
Impairment Class 3	Lymphocytosis, anemia (Hemoglobin ≤100 g/L) and thrombocytopenia (Platelets less than 10,000/μL)	50%

Table 23.262 Thrombocytopenia—Whole person impairment

Severity of thrombocytopenia		Reference impairment score	Maximum impairment 50%
Class 1	Platelet count of 20,000–50,000/μL Bleed only on major trauma or surgery Respond well to prophylactic therapy or blood transfusion	5%	
Class 2	Platelet count of 10,000–20,000/μL Spontaneous bleeding Responding to therapy or blood transfusion	25%	
Class 3	Platelet count of less than 10,000/μL Frequent spontaneous bleeding Refractory to treatment	50%	

Table 23.263 Hemophilia—Whole person impairment

Impairment class	Severity of hemophilia	Reference impairment score	Maximum impairment 50%
Class 1	Persons with more than 5%–40% normal coagulation factor level, i.e., more than 0.05–0.40 IU/mL manifest hemorrhage only during major trauma and surgery.	5%	
Class 2	Persons with 1%–5% normal coagulation factor level, i.e., 0.01–0.05 IU/mL manifest hemorrhage even with mild to moderate trauma for whom factor replacement controls hemorrhage and hemarthrosis	15%	
Class 3	Persons with less than 0.01 IU/mL and less than 1% of normal coagulation factor level manifest spontaneous hemorrhage and hemarthrosis for whom factor replacement controls hemorrhage and hemarthrosis	25%	
Class 4	Replacement of factor could not control spontaneous hemorrhage and hemarthrosis due to FVIII inhibitor Assign additional impairment if there is coexisting hemophilia related chronic arthropathy, nerve lesions, sequel due to intracranial bleeding	50%	

Table 23.264 Impairment class—HIV/AID

Impairment class	Severity	Description of the category	Reference impairment score
Class 1	HIV	Persons with HIV infection under category A on ART: Asymptomatic infection Persistent generalized lymphadenopathy History of acute primary infection	15% (burden of treatment compliance and stigma associated with HIV infection)
Class 2	AIDS	Persons with AIDS disease under category B: Symptomatic infection due to HIV or due to impairment of cell-mediated immunity	25%
Class 3	Advanced AIDS	Persons with AIDS disease under category C with advanced disease with Dementia Cardiac failure Renal failure Hepatic failure Kaposi's sarcoma, lymphoma, etc.	25+%

23.30 READY RECKONER—CARDIOVASCULAR FUNCTION

Table 23.265 CAD, and hypertensive heart disease—Whole person impairment

Impairment class and severity of cardiovascular symptoms	Echocardiographic evidence of systolic and/or diastolic function	METs aerobic capacity	Maximum impairment 75%
Class 1: Person experiences fatigue, angina, and dyspnea during moderate-vigorous-physical exertion	Minimal left ventricular systolic dysfunction or diastolic dysfunction (LVEF $\geq$45% to <55% or E = A)	$\geq$3 METs to $\leq$6 METs	15%
Class 2: Person experiences fatigue, angina, and dyspnea during moderate-vigorous-physical exertion	Minimal left ventricular systolic dysfunction and diastolic dysfunction (LVEF $\geq$45% to <55% and E = A)	$\geq$3 METs to $\leq$6 METs	25%
Class 3: Person experiences fatigue, angina, and dyspnea during moderate physical exertion	Moderate left ventricular systolic dysfunction or diastolic dysfunction (LVEF $\geq$30% to <45% or E = A)	<3 METs to $\geq$1.5 METs	37%
Class 4: Person experiences fatigue, angina, and dyspnea during moderate physical exertion	Moderate systolic and diastolic left ventricular dysfunction (LVEF $\geq$30% to <45% and E = A)	<3 METs to $\geq$1.5 METs	50%
Class 5: Person experiences fatigue, angina, and dyspnea during minimal physical exertion and/or at rest	Severe systolic and diastolic left ventricular dysfunction (LVEF <30% and E < A)	<1.5 METs	75%

Table 23.266 Cardiomyopathy—Whole person impairment—75%

Impairment class and severity of cardiovascular symptoms	Nature of intervention	Echocardiographic evidence of systolic and/or diastolic function	Maximum impairment 75%
Class 1: Asymptomatic	Isolated dysrhythmia controlled under Guideline-Directed Medical Therapy—GDMT	Normal left ventricular function and diastolic function LVEF ≥55% to <70% or E > A	5%
Class 2: Palpitation	Isolated dysrhythmia requiring or underwent implantation of pacemaker and/or AICD	Normal left ventricular function and diastolic function LVEF ≥55% to <70% or E > A	10%
Class 3: Person experiences fatigue, angina, and dyspnea during moderate-vigorous-physical exertion, Palpitation, missing of heartbeat, dizziness, sweating, anxiety	Dysrhythmia requiring or underwent implantation of pacemaker and/or AICD	Minimal left ventricular systolic dysfunction or diastolic dysfunction LVEF ≥45% to <55% or E = A	15%
Class 4: Person experiences fatigue, angina, and dyspnea during moderate-vigorous-physical exertion, Palpitation, missing of heartbeat, dizziness, sweating, anxiety	Dysrhythmia requiring or underwent implantation of pacemaker and/or AICD	Minimal left ventricular systolic dysfunction and diastolic dysfunction LVEF ≥45% to <55% and E = A	25%
Class 5: Person experiences fatigue, angina, and dyspnea during moderate physical exertion, Palpitation, missing of heartbeat, dizziness, sweating, anxiety, dyspnea, chest pain, syncope	Dysrhythmia requiring or underwent implantation of pacemaker and/or AICD	Moderate left ventricular systolic dysfunction or diastolic dysfunction (LVEF ≥30% to <45% or E = A)	37%
Class 6: Person experiences fatigue, angina, and dyspnea during moderate physical exertion, Palpitation, missing of heartbeat, dizziness, sweating, anxiety, dyspnea, chest pain, syncope	Dysrhythmia requiring or underwent implantation of pacemaker and/or AICD	Moderate systolic and diastolic left ventricular dysfunction (LVEF ≥30% to <45% and E = A)	50%
Class 7: Person experiences fatigue, angina, and dyspnea during minimal physical exertion and/or at rest, Palpitation, missing of heartbeat, dizziness, sweating, anxiety, dyspnea, chest pain, syncope	Dysrhythmia requiring or underwent implantation of pacemaker and/or AICD	Severe systolic and diastolic left ventricular dysfunction (LVEF <30% and E < A)	75%

Table 23.267 Dysrhythmias—Whole person impairment 75%

Impairment class and severity of cardiovascular symptoms	Nature of intervention	Echocardiographic evidence of systolic and/or diastolic function	Maximum impairment 75%
Class 1: Asymptomatic	Isolated dysrhythmia controlled under Guideline-Directed Medical Therapy—GDMT	Normal left ventricular function and diastolic function LVEF ≥55% to <70% or E > A	5%
Class 2: Palpitation	Isolated dysrhythmia requiring or underwent implantation of pacemaker and/or AICD	Normal left ventricular function and diastolic function LVEF ≥55% to <70% or E > A	10%
Class 3: Palpitation, missing of heartbeat, dizziness, sweating, anxiety	Dysrhythmia requiring or underwent implantation of pacemaker and/or AICD	Minimal left ventricular systolic dysfunction or diastolic dysfunction LVEF ≥45% to <55% or E = A	15%
Class 4: Palpitation, missing of heartbeat, dizziness, sweating, anxiety	Dysrhythmia requiring or underwent implantation of pacemaker and/or AICD	Minimal left ventricular systolic dysfunction and diastolic dysfunction LVEF ≥45% to <55% and E = A	25%
Class 5: Palpitation, missing of heartbeat, dizziness, sweating, anxiety, dyspnea, chest pain, syncope	Dysrhythmia requiring or underwent implantation of pacemaker and/or AICD	Moderate left ventricular systolic dysfunction or diastolic dysfunction (LVEF ≥30% to <45% or E = A)	37%
Class 6: Palpitation, missing of heartbeat, dizziness, sweating, anxiety, dyspnea, chest pain, syncope	Dysrhythmia requiring or underwent implantation of pacemaker and/or AICD	Moderate systolic and diastolic left ventricular dysfunction (LVEF ≥30% to <45% and E = A)	50%
Class 7: Palpitation, missing of heartbeat, dizziness, sweating, anxiety, dyspnea, chest pain, syncope	Dysrhythmia requiring or underwent implantation of pacemaker and/or AICD	Severe systolic and diastolic left ventricular dysfunction (LVEF <30% and E < A)	75%

Table 23.268 Valvular heart diseases—Whole person impairment—75%

Impairment class symptoms	Size of atrium/ ventricle	Systolic and diastolic ventricular function	Impairment score
Class 1: Asymptomatic valvular heart disease	Normal size of atrium/ ventricle	(1) Left ventricular systolic and diastolic function—Normal: LVEF: 55%–70% and E > A (2) Normal pulmonary artery pressure: 8–20 mm of Hg at rest, and normal right ventricular function	5%
Class 2: Symptomatic valvular heart disease—syncope	Mild enlargement of atrium/ventricle	(1) Minimal left ventricular systolic dysfunction LVEF: ≥45 to <55% or minimal diastolic dysfunction: E = A **and/or** (2) Increased pulmonary artery pressure: >20 to ≤30 mm of Hg with normal right ventricular function	15%
Class 3: Symptomatic valvular heart disease—syncope	Mild enlargement of atrium/ventricle	(1) Minimal left ventricular systolic dysfunction LVEF: ≥45 to <55% and minimal diastolic dysfunction: E = A **and/or** (2) Pulmonary hypertension: >30 to ≤50 mm of Hg with normal right ventricular function	25%

(Continued)

Table 23.268 (*Continued*) Valvular heart diseases—Whole person impairment—75%

Impairment class symptoms	Size of atrium/ventricle	Systolic and diastolic ventricular function	Impairment score
Class 4: Symptomatic valvular heart disease—syncope, angina, dyspnea	Moderate enlargement of atrium/ventricle	(1) Moderate left ventricular systolic dysfunction LVEF: ≥30% to <45% or diastolic dysfunction: E = A **and/or** (2) Pulmonary hypertension: >30 to ≤50 mm of Hg with minimal right ventricular dysfunction	37%
Class 5: Symptomatic valvular heart disease—syncope, angina, dyspnea	Moderate enlargement of atrium/ventricle	(1) Moderate left ventricular systolic dysfunction LVEF: ≥30% to <45% and diastolic dysfunction: E = A **and/or** (2) Pulmonary hypertension: >30 to ≤50 mm of Hg with moderate right ventricular dysfunction	50%
Class 6: Symptomatic valvular heart disease—syncope, angina, dyspnea, decreased exercise tolerance	Severe enlargement of atrium/ventricle	(1) Severe left ventricular systolic dysfunction LVEF: <30% and diastolic dysfunction: E < A **and/or** (2) Pulmonary hypertension: >50 mm of Hg with severe right ventricular dysfunction	75%

Table 23.269 Peripheral arterial disease upper/lower extremities—Whole person impairment 10%

Impairment class	Clinical symptoms and/or signs	Clinical tools	Maximum impairment 10%
Class 1	Asymptomatic	Ankle-Brachial Index: 0.71 to ≤0.90	0%
Class 2	Raynaud's phenomena: Triphasic color changes, triggered by exposure to cold, etc.	—	5%
Class 2	Elicits claudication pain on a 6-minute walk test, and refractory to medical management	Ankle-Brachial Index: 0.71 to ≤0.90	5%
Class 3	Resting pain due to acute limb ischemia Contraindication for endovascular interventions and revascularization surgery due to medical reasons	Ankle-Brachial Index: 0.41 to ≤0.70	10%
Class 4	Gangrene and amputation	Ankle-Brachial Index: ≤0.40	According to level of amputation

Table 23.270 Varicose veins—Upper/lower extremities—Whole person impairment 5%

Impairment class	Clinical symptoms and/or signs	Clinical tools	Maximum impairment 10%
Class 1	Asymptomatic varicose veins	Doppler ultrasound—incompetent superficial veins	0%
Class 2	Varicose veins with pain, heaviness of the leg, muscle cramps, edema	Doppler ultrasound—incompetent superficial and deep veins	1%
Class 3	Varicose veins with pain, heaviness of the leg, muscle cramps, edema, and pigmentation with irritation of the skin	Doppler ultrasound—incompetent superficial, deep and perforator veins	2.5%
Class 4	Varicose veins with chronic venous insufficiency and pain, heaviness of the leg, muscle cramps, edema, pigmentation with irritation of the skin, lipodermatosclerosis, trophic changes, venous ulcer, and venous thrombosis	Doppler ultrasound—incompetent superficial, deep and perforator veins	5%

Table 23.271 Lymphedema—Upper/lower extremities—Whole person impairment 5%

Impairment class	Clinical symptoms and/or signs	Maximum impairment
Class 1	Swelling of arm and/or leg Aching of swollen arm and/or leg	1%
Class 2	Swelling of arm and/or leg with disfigurement Aching of swollen arm and/or leg Fibrosis of skin Limitation of ROM of joint	1% + Impairment score according to limitation of ROM of affected joint
Class 3	Swelling of arm and/or leg with disfigurement Aching of swollen arm and/or leg Fibrosis of skin Limitation of ROM of joint Recurrent cellulitis/lymphangitis	2.5% + Impairment score according to limitation of ROM of affected joint
Class 4	Swelling of arm and/or leg with disfigurement Aching of swollen arm and/or leg Fibrosis of skin Limitation of ROM of joint Recurrent cellulitis/lymphangitis Chronic fissuring and ulceration Amyloidosis Lymphangiosarcoma	5% + Impairment score according to limitation of ROM of affected joint + Impairment score according to level of amputation if deemed necessary

23.31 READY RECKONER—PULMONARY FUNCTIONS

Table 23.272 Chronic obstructive pulmonary disease—COPD—Whole person impairment airflow limitation: $FEV_1/FVC <70\%$

Impairment class clinical profile	Exacerbations per year	Post bronchodilator FEV_1	Impairment score reference value
Class 1: History of exposure to risk factors namely tobacco smoke, occupational dusts/chemicals, indoor/outdoor air pollutants and chronic cough	0	Persistent non-reversible airflow obstruction: $FEV_1 \geq 80\%$, predicted	5%
Class 2: History of exposure to risk factors and chronic cough, sputum production, dyspnoea	1–2	Persistent non-reversible airflow obstruction: FEV_1 61%–79%, predicted	25%
Class 3: History of exposure to risk factors, chronic cough, sputum production, dyspnoea	3–4	Persistent non-reversible airflow obstruction: FEV_1 31%–60% predicted	37%
Class 4: History of exposure to risk factors, chronic cough, sputum production, dyspnoea, respiratory failure, right heart failure	>4	Persistent non-reversible airflow obstruction: $FEV_1 \leq 30\%$ predicted	50%

Table 23.273 Asthma—Whole person impairment

Impairment class clinical profile and control	Nocturnal episode	Post bronchodilator FEV_1	Impairment score reference value
Class 1: Variable symptoms—wheezing, tightness of the chest, dry cough, infrequent day time symptoms. Asthma control: PEF rate: ≥80% predicted	1/Month	Post-bronchodilator: $FEV_1 \geq 80\%$, predicted, Reversible airflow obstruction: Post-Bronchodilator increase in FEV_1 of 12% and >200 mL	5%
Class 2: Variable symptoms—wheezing, tightness of the chest, productive cough. Frequent day time symptoms. Asthma control: PEF rate: 70%–79% predicted	1/Fortnight	Post-bronchodilator: $FEV_1 \geq 70\%$–79%, predicted, Reversible airflow obstruction: Post-Bronchodilator increase in FEV_1 of 12% and >200 mL	25%
Class 3: Symptoms—wheezing, tightness of the chest, productive cough, breathlessness. Frequent day time symptoms. Asthma control: PEF rate: 60%–69% predicted	1/Week	Post-bronchodilator: $FEV_1 \geq 60\%$–69%, predicted, Reversible airflow obstruction: Post-Bronchodilator increase in FEV_1 of 12% and >200 mL	37%
Class 4: Persistent symptoms both day and night Asthma control: PEF rate: <60% predicted		Post-bronchodilator $FEV_1 < 60\%$ predicted, Refractory to treatment	50%

Table 23.274 Restrictive lung diseases—Whole person impairment

Impairment class extrinsic lung diseases	TLC and FEV$_1$% predicted	Reference impairment score
Class 1	Decreased TLC <5th percentile FEV$_1$ ≥ 80% predicted	5%
Class 2	Decreased TLC <5th percentile FEV$_1$ 61%–79% predicted	25%
Class 3	Decreased TLC <5th percentile FEV$_1$ 31%–60% predicted	37%
Class 4	Decreased TLC <5th percentile FEV$_1$ ≥ 30% predicted	50%

Table 23.275 Restrictive lung diseases—Whole person impairment

Impairment class intrinsic lung diseases	D$_L$co % predicted (transfer factor)	Reference impairment score
Class 1	>60% and <LLN	5%
Class 2	51%–60%	25%
Class 3	41%–50%	37%
Class 4	≤40%	50%

Table 23.276 Hypercapnic respiratory failure—Whole person impairment

Clinical profile	Measurements	Reference score
Arterial blood gas—PaCO$_2$	>50 mm of Hg	50%
Arterial blood gas—PaO$_2$	<60 mm of Hg	
Pulmonary hypertension	+	
Right ventricular failure	+	
Cor pulmonale	+	

Table 23.277 Respiratory muscle function—Whole person impairment

Impairment class	Clinical indices	Reference impairment score
Class 1	Intercostal muscle paralysis: Rib paradox Abdominal muscle paralysis: Weak cough reflex Vital capacity >2000 to <3000 cc	15%
Class 2	Intercostal muscle paralysis: Rib paradox Abdominal muscle paralysis: Ineffective cough Vital capacity >1000 to ≤2000 cc	25%
Class 3	Unilateral or bilateral diaphragmatic paralysis: Abdominal and rib paradox, absence of cough reflex Recruitment of accessory muscles of respiration Vital capacity ≤1000 cc requiring assisted ventilation	50%
Class 4	Bilateral diaphragmatic paralysis: Abdominal and rib paradox, absence of cough reflex Recruitment of accessory muscles of respiration Vital capacity ≤500 cc requiring assisted ventilation	75%

Table 23.278 Sleep apneas/hypopneas—Whole person impairment

Impairment class	Obstructive/central/mixed apneas or hypopneas	Reference score
Class 1	1. Disturbed sleep, snoring, daytime sleepiness 2. RDI on OSA: 5–15/hour	15%
Class 2	1. Disturbed sleep, snoring, daytime sleepiness, impaired cognition 2. RDI on OSA: 15–30/hour 3. Asymptomatic cardiac arrhythmias	25%
Class 3	1. Disturbed sleep, snoring, daytime sleepiness, impaired cognition 2. RDI on OSA: >30/hour 3. Symptomatic cardiac arrhythmias: Bradyarrhythmias, PVC, atrial fibrillation, atrial flutter	37%
Class 4	1. Disturbed sleep, snoring, daytime sleepiness, impaired cognition 2. RDI on OSA: >30/hour 3. Cardiac arrhythmias 4. Cardiac failure and/or 5. Cor pulmonale	50%

23.32 READY RECKONER—VISUAL FUNCTION

Table 23.279 Distance acuity of monocular vision—Both eyes: Whole person impairment

Impairment class	ICD–10 version: 2015 categories (8)	Presenting distance visual acuity			Reference impairment score acuity of vision	Select impairment score right eye	Select impairment score left eye	Impairment score of both eyes
		Snellen notation	US notation	Decimal notation				
Class 0	Category 0—mild or no visual impairment	Equal to or better than 6/18	Equal to or better than 20/70	Equal to or better than 3/10 (0.3)	0%			
Class 1	Category 1—moderate impairment	Equal to or better than 6/60 Worse than 6/18	Equal to or better than 20/200 Worse than 20/70	Equal to or better than 1/10 (0.1) Worse than 3/10 (0.3)	5%			
Class 2	Category 2—severe impairment	Equal to or better than 3/60 Worse than 6/60	Equal to or better than 20/400 Worse than 20/200	Equal to or better than 1/20 (0.05) Worse than 1/10 (0.1)	15%			
Class 3	Category 3—blindness	Equal to or better than 1/60 Worse than 3/60	Equal to or better than 20/1200 Worse than 20/400	Equal to or better than 1/50 (0.02) Worse than 1/20 (0.05)	25%			
Class 4	Category 4—blindness	Equal to or better than Light Perception Worse than 1/60	Equal to or better than Light Perception Worse than 20/1200	Equal to or better than Light Perception Worse than 1/50 (0.02)	37%			
Class 5	Category 5—blindness	No light perception			42.5%			

Total impairment of right and left eye

Table 23.280 Distance acuity of monocular vision—Impairment of vision in one eye with preserved normal vision in another eye: Whole person impairment

Impairment class	ICD–10 version: 2015 categories (8)	Presenting distance visual acuity			Reference impairment score acuity of vision	Select impairment score of affected eye
		Snellen notation	US notation	Decimal notation		
Class 0	Category 0—mild or no visual impairment	Equal to or better than 6/18	Equal to or better than 20/70	Equal to or better than 3/10 (0.3)	0%	
Class 1	Category 1—moderate impairment	Equal to or better than 6/60	Equal to or better than 20/200	Equal to or better than 1/10 (0.1)	1%	
		Worse than 6/18	Worse than 20/70	Worse than 3/10 (0.3)		
Class 2	Category 2—severe impairment	Equal to or better than 3/60	Equal to or better than 20/400	Equal to or better than 1/20 (0.05)	2.5%	
		Worse than 6/60	Worse than 20/200	Worse than 1/10 (0.1)		
Class 3	Category 3—blindness	Equal to or better than 1/60	Equal to or better than 20/1200	Equal to or better than 1/50 (0.02)	5%	
		Worse than 3/60	Worse than 20/400	Worse than 1/20 (0.05)		
Class 4	Category 4—blindness	Equal to or better than light perception	Equal to or better than light perception	Equal to or better than Light Perception	10%	
		Worse than 1/60	Worse than 20/1200	Worse than 1/50 (0.02)		
Class 5	Category 5—blindness		No light perception		15%	

Table 23.281 Impairment class—Near acuity of vision: Whole person impairment

Impairment class	Distance for letter recognition of 1M print	Reference impairment score binocular vision	Select the impairment score
Class 0	160 cm	0%	
	125 cm		
	100 cm		
	80 cm		
Class 1	63 cm	5%	
	50 cm		
	40 cm		
	32 cm		
Class 2	25 cm	25%	
	20 cm		
	16 cm		
	12 cm		
Class 3	10 cm	50%	
	8 cm		
	6 cm		
	5 cm		
Class 4	4 cm	75%	
	3 cm		
	2.5 cm		
	2 cm		
Class 5	0 cm	85%	

Table 23.282 Impairment class—Monocular field of vision—Impairment: Both eyes 85%

Impairment class	Reference score monocular vision	Impairment of field of vision right eye	Impairment of field of vision left eye	Select the impairment score
Central				
Superior temporal	6.00%			
Superior nasal	6.00%			
Inferior temporal	6.00%			
Inferior nasal	6.00%			
Peripheral				
Vertical superior temporal	2.00%			
Vertical inferior temporal	3.00%			
Vertical superior nasal	2.00%			
Vertical inferior nasal	3.00%			
Horizontal superior temporal	2.75%			
Horizontal inferior temporal	2.75%			
Horizontal superior nasal	1.50%			
Horizontal inferior nasal	1.50%			
	Sum of the impairment score monocular field of vision right and left eye			

Table 23.283 Binocular field of vision—Whole person impairment 85%

Impairment class	Reference impairment score—Binocular vision	Select the impairment score
Central		
Superior nasal—right	12.0%	
Superior nasal—left	12.0%	
Inferior nasal—right	12.0%	
Inferior nasal—left	12.0%	
Peripheral		
Vertical superior nasal—right	4.0%	
Vertical superior nasal—left	4.0%	
Vertical inferior nasal—right	6.0%	
Vertical inferior nasal—left	6.0%	
Horizontal superior temporal—right	4.25%	
Horizontal inferior temporal—right	4.25%	
Horizontal superior temporal—left	4.25%	
Horizontal inferior temporal—left	4.25%	

Table 23.284 Contrast sensitivity—Whole person impairment

Clinical tool—Pelli Robson contrast sensitivity chart	Reference impairment score	Impairment score
Normal contrast sensitivity: Can read all the eight lines without difficulty	0%	
Low contrast sensitivity: Difficulty in reading last three lines	5%	
Poor contrast sensitivity: Cannot read the last three lines	10%	

Table 23.285 Light sensitivity—Whole person impairment

Light sensitivity	Reference impairment score	Maximum impairment 25%
Persistent photophobia even after maximum medical treatment	10%	
Irreversible night blindness even after maximum medical treatment	25%	

Table 23.286 Color vision—Whole person impairment

Impairment class	Clinical tools	Severity of impairment	Impairment score
Class 1	1. Ishihara test	Anomalous dichromacy with yellow and blue deficiency	5%
Class 2	2. Holmes-Wright lantern test	Anomalous dichromacy with red and green deficiency due to protanomaly and deuteranomaly	10%
	3. FM test (Farnsworth Munsell 100 hue test)	Anomalous trichromacy	15%
Class 3	4. Wire test	Dichromacy	20%
Class 4		Monochromacy	25%

Table 23.287 Diplopia—Whole person impairment

Impairment class	Diplopia score	Reference impairment score	Impairment score
Class 1	Diplopia score 1–5	5%	
Class 2	Diplopia score 6–10	10%	
Class 3	Diplopia score 11–15	15%	
Class 4	Diplopia score 16–25	25%	

23.33 READY RECKONER—HEARING FUNCTIONS

Table 23.288 Monaural hearing impairment with normal hearing function in another ear

Impairment class	WHO's grading of hearing impairment	ISO value—Pure tone average of the threshold at 500, 1000, 2000, and 4000 Hz	*Integrated Evaluation of Disability* reference impairment value	% of impairment
Class 0	No impairment	25 dB or better	0%	
Class 1	Slight impairment	25–40 dB	1%	
Class 2	Moderate impairment	41–60 dB	5%	
Class 3	Severe impairment	61–80 dB	10%	
Class 4	Profound impairment including deafness	>80 dB	15%	

Table 23.289 Monaural/binaural hearing impairment—50%

Impairment class	WHO's grading of hearing impairment	ISO value—Pure tone average of the threshold at 500, 1000, 2000, and 4000 Hz	*Integrated Evaluation of Disability* impairment Reference value	% of impairment right ear	% of impairment left ear
Class 0	No impairment	25 dB or better	0%		
Class 1	Slight impairment	25–40 dB	1%		
Class 2	Moderate impairment	41–60 dB	5%		
Class 3	Severe impairment	61–80 dB	15%		
Class 4	Profound impairment including deafness	>80 dB	25%		
		Total whole person impairment for right and left ear			

23.34 READY RECKONER—INTELLECTUAL DISABILITY OR MENTAL RETARDATION

Table 23.290 Intellectual functions—Whole person impairment

Impairment class	Clinical scales Wechsler's scale/Raven's matrices	Reference impairment median score
Class 1	IQ: 71–84	4%
Class 2	IQ: 50–70	14%
Class 3	IQ: 25–49	39%
Class 4	IQ: <25	63%

Table 23.291 Intellectual disability/mental retardation

Disability class	IQ	Impairment IQ	Activity Participation Skill Assessment score	Disability
Disability Class 1 (1%–4%)	70–84 (Median 60%)	4%	2.78%	3.39%
Disability Class 2 (5%–24%)	50–70 (Median 60%)	14%	17.78%	15.89%
Disability Class 3 (25%–49%)	25–49 (Median 37%)	39%	46.67%	42.83%
Disability Class 4 (≥50%)	<25 (Median 12.5%)	63%	63.89%	63.44%

Index

Note: Page numbers in *italic* and **bold** refer to figures and tables, respectively.